Trends in mRNA Vaccine Research

Trends in Drug Discovery
Edited by János Fischer, Christian Klein, Wayne E. Childers

Trends in mRNA Vaccine Research

Edited by Gabor Tamas Szabo and Norbert Pardi

WILEY-VCH

Editors

Gabor Tamas Szabo
BioNTech SE
An der Goldgrube 12
Mainz 55131
Germany

Norbert Pardi
University of Pennsylvania
Perelman School of Medicine
3400 Civic Center Blvd
Philadelphia
PA 19104
USA

Cover Image: © nobeastsofierce/Shutterstock, © Numstocker/Shutterstock

Library of Congress Card No.: applied for

British Library Cataloguing-in-Publication Data
A catalogue record for this book is available from the British Library.

Bibliographic information published by the Deutsche Nationalbibliothek
The Deutsche Nationalbibliothek lists this publication in the Deutsche Nationalbibliografie; detailed bibliographic data are available on the Internet at <http://dnb.d-nb.de>.

Print ISBN: 978-3-527-35058-2
ePDF ISBN: 978-3-527-83837-0
ePub ISBN: 978-3-527-83838-7
oBook ISBN: 978-3-527-83839-4

Typesetting Straive, Chennai, India

Printed and bound by CPI Group (UK) Ltd, Croydon, CR0 4YY

C9783527350582_271124

Contents

Preface

The **Trends in Drug Discovery** book series focuses on recent drug discoveries, including preclinical studies, successful drug development leading to newly approved drugs in major therapeutic fields. The scope of this series includes both small molecule and large molecule drugs including biologics.

Each volume gives an overview of a specific therapeutic field, discusses concepts and technologies, and describes the discoveries of recently approved drugs.

The **series editors** are introduced as follows:

János Fischer (Emeritus Fellow of IUPAC, research advisor at Richter, Hungary) participated in the editing of two book series of Wiley-VCH: Analogue-based Drug Discovery (Vol. 1–3, 2006–2011) and Successful Drug Discovery (Vol. 1–5, 2015–2021).

Christian Klein (Department Head Cancer Immunotherapy and Site Head at the Roche Innovation Center, Zurich, Switzerland) was a coeditor for Successful Drug Discovery, Vol. 3–5.

Wayne E. Childers (Professor of Pharmaceutical Sciences at Temple University School of Pharmacy, Philadelphia, Pennsylvania, United States) was a coeditor for Successful Drug Discovery, Vol. 2–5.

The goals of this book series are to provide the drug discovery community with reference books and to support teaching in the field of drug discovery.

The first volume has the title: **Trends in mRNA Vaccine Research.** Katalin Karikó and Drew Weissman have been recognized with the 2023 Nobel Prize in Physiology or Medicine for their discoveries leading to the development of mRNA vaccines against COVID-19. The book focuses on the promising trends in the field of mRNA vaccine research.

Preface from the Volume Editors

mRNA vaccines received broad attention during the SARS-CoV-2 pandemic, especially after COVID-19 vaccines developed by Moderna and Pfizer-BioNTech demonstrated high effectivity for decreasing hospital admissions and serious COVID-19. The interest towards the mRNA technology was further intensified in 2023 after Katalin Karikó and Drew Weissman received the Nobel Prize in Physiology or Medicine for their discoveries on nucleoside base modifications that enabled the development of safe and effective mRNA vaccines against SARS-CoV-2. mRNA vaccines represent a revolutionary advancement with enormous potential in medicine to target very different diseases by sending information encoded on mRNA to the cells that take up the nucleic acid. To date, the technology demonstrated its viability for infectious disease vaccine development during the SARS-CoV-2 pandemic, and promising results were obtained in the fight against other pathogens, and other indications including cancer or chronic diseases. Publisher Wiley aimed at summarizing the current knowledge and developments on mRNA vaccines in a book as the first volume in a new series focusing on advanced pharmacology therapy developments.

The editors of this volume are grateful for participating in the collection of the valuable chapters written by outstanding researchers of the mRNA vaccine field. The chapters are divided into two main sections.

The first section contains seven chapters summarizing the general knowledge about mRNA vaccines.

Verbeke and colleagues provide a historical overview about the key discoveries during the course of mRNA vaccine development. The chapter focuses on three main topics: first, the discovery, production, and refinement of mRNA as a therapeutic modality; second, the path to find a suitable vehicle to facilitate the safe and efficient delivery of intact mRNA into the target cells; and finally the clinical advancements of mRNA vaccines.

The immune response induced by an optimal mRNA vaccine provide a balanced activation of the innate and the adaptive immune system. The chapter by Esposito and colleagues gives a detailed summary about the immune response induced by the elements of the mRNA vaccine, including the protein-encoding mRNA, the byproducts generated in the *in vitro* transcription reaction and the components of the formulation, as well.

Morais and Yu focus on the use of modified nucleosides in therapeutic mRNA and summarize their effects on mRNA vaccine immunogenicity and mRNA stability extended with a discussion on the main differences between nucleoside-modified and unmodified mRNA vaccines. Features of self-amplifying mRNA (saRNA) vaccines are presented in the chapter written by Lundstrom, focusing on the history of development, the advantages of the platform, and summarizing the current promising developments with saRNA. Circular RNAs (circRNAs) are a type of RNA with increased stability due to their unique closed structure. Synthetic circRNAs have been developed as a novel RNA platform and have demonstrated their potential as new preclinical vaccine candidates. Current achievements with this new platform are summarized by Liu and Zhu.

Upscaling of mRNA production became a hot topic during the SARS-CoV-2 pandemic, as it was critical to produce large amounts of vaccine in a short timeframe. Manufacturing of large amounts of mRNA had challenges and required investment in the technology as described in the chapter written by Stamoula and colleagues.

mRNA vaccines have the potential to induce immunotolerance, and, thus, opening up new indications such as the treatment of autoimmune diseases, allergies, or transplant rejection. This topic is detailed in the chapter written by Gissler and colleagues.

The landscape of mRNA vaccines is continuously and rapidly evolving: the second section of the volume gives examples about some of the novel developments.

The development and approval of the two mRNA COVID-19 vaccines represented a major breakthrough in the fight against the SARS-CoV-2 pandemic. The section starts with a valuable comparison of the performance of the approved COVID-19 mRNA vaccines written by Istvan Tombacz.

Despite significant progress in the prevention and treatment of HIV-1 infection, the virus continues to pose a significant public health threat. A successful vaccine would be a powerful tool for the reduction of the overall burden of the disease. In this section, the current status of the development of mRNA-based preventive or therapeutic vaccines against HIV is described by Paolo Lusso.

Most mRNA vaccines were developed against viruses but vaccine development against other type of pathogens is also important. While Arora and Fikrig summarized mRNA vaccine studies against tick-borne diseases, Versteeg and Pollet detailed the current status and future outlook of mRNA vaccine development against parasites. Aernout and colleagues gave insights into the challenges of mRNA vaccine generation against bacteria through the example of *Mycobacterium tuberculosis*.

Besides mRNA vaccine development for infectious disease indications, mRNA cancer vaccines represent an exciting area of research with promising results in the fight against cancer. Mey and colleagues summarized the recent achievements in this topic in the last chapter.

The current volume is an ideal source for researchers, medical specialists, healthcare workers, public health officers, students, and anyone interested in understanding the trends in mRNA vaccine research.

April 23, 2024

Gabor Tamas Szabo
BioNTech SE, Mainz
Germany

Norbert Pardi
University of Pennsylvania
Perelman School of Medicine
Department of Microbiology
Philadelphia, PA, USA

Part I

How mRNA Vaccines Work

1

A Historical Overview on mRNA Vaccine Development

Rein Verbeke[1,2], *Miffy H.Y. Cheng*[2], *and Pieter R. Cullis*[2]

[1] *Ghent University, Ghent Research Group on Nanomedicines, Faculty of Pharmaceutical Sciences, Ottergemsesteenweg 460, 9000 Ghent, Belgium*
[2] *University of British Columbia, Department of Biochemistry and Molecular Biology, Health Sciences Mall 2350, BC V6T 1Z4 Vancouver, Canada*

1.1 Introduction

In less than one year after the COVID-19 pandemic outbreak, two mRNA vaccines received the first emergency use authorization from the Food and Drug Administration (FDA) and the European Medicines Agency (EMA), i.e. BNT162b2 (Comirnaty) from Pfizer/BioNTech and mRNA-1273 (Spikevax) from Moderna. In Phase 3 clinical trials, these mRNA vaccines were found to be generally safe and up to 95% efficacious after the second dose of vaccination in preventing symptomatic SARS-CoV-2 infection [1, 2]. The outstanding efficacy and unprecedented speed with which these mRNA vaccines were produced and distributed, strongly helped to curtail the burden of the pandemic and prevented millions of deaths [3, 4].

Now proven against COVID-19, there is explosive growth in research and investments in mRNA technology. Most notably, the platform of nucleoside-modified mRNA encapsulated in lipid nanoparticles (LNPs) that is utilized in today's COVID-19 mRNA vaccines is poised to have a rapid transformative effect on the future of medicine. Vaccines based on this platform are now being tested in Phase 3 clinical trials for several viral diseases other than COVID-19, such as against influenza (BNT161 and mRNA-1010), cytomegalovirus (mRNA-1647), and respiratory syncytial virus (mRNA-1345), while many other mRNA vaccines are being (pre)clinically studied to target diseases, such as bacterial and parasitic infections, cancer, and autoimmune diseases. In addition, the ability of the mRNA–LNP platform to deliver genetic information for the temporal production of proteins inside cells makes it a potential key technology to enable gene editing, protein replacement, and other immunotherapeutic approaches [5].

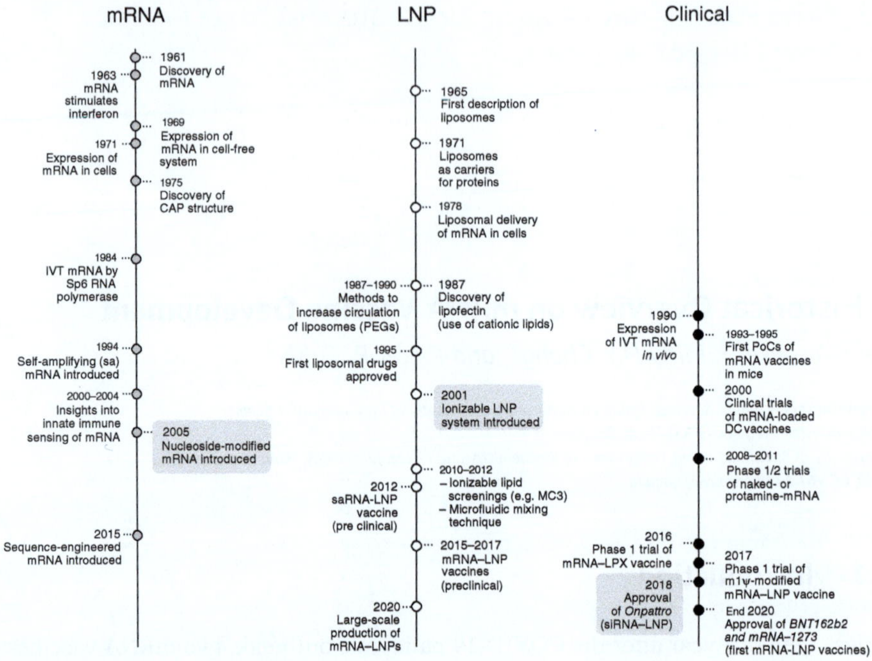

Figure 1.1 Discoveries and milestones in the development of mRNA-based vaccines are subdivided into three parallel timelines of mRNA-, LNP design, and clinical development.

It may seem that the COVID-19 mRNA vaccines came out of the blue, but in fact, decades of research were needed to develop this novel vaccine technology. To understand why it took so long for mRNA vaccines to breakthrough, we need to appreciate the collective efforts made by many scientists and the various problems they have tackled and solved that ultimately led to the development of this first generation of mRNA vaccines. As elucidated by Dowdy, the fundamental problem is that a billion years of evolutionary defenses need to be tackled to successfully deliver RNA. This includes both cellular barriers that have kept foreign RNAs on the outside of cells from invading the inside of cells, as well as the many innate immune defense mechanisms evolved to recognize and destroy foreign RNA [6]. Nonetheless, mRNA represents a most excellent vaccine modality to mimic viral infections, this is to trick the immune system to develop memory against the encoded, pathogen antigen. Indeed, when successfully delivered, mRNA has the potential to process and present encoded antigens through the same cellular machinery as occurring during viral infections, while it may also benefit from the specifically designed immune mechanisms against viruses to prime and promote durable adaptive immune responses, i.e. the immune adjuvant potential of mRNA.

In this first chapter section, a short historical overview is given of the development of mRNA vaccines (Figure 1.1).

1.2 The Path of mRNA as an Unstable and Toxic Product to a New Class of Medicine

1.2.1 The Discovery and *In Vitro* Production of mRNA

In 2015, Cobb wrote an essay that addressed the question of who discovered mRNA. By reconstructing the collective insights and different kinds of evidence gathered during the 1950s through the 1960s, Cobb concluded that mRNA was the product of many years of work by a community of researchers [7]. Ultimately, this research process gained momentum in the summer of 1961, when the nature and properties of mRNA were for the first time described in a theoretical model by Jacob and Monod [8]. In this review article on genetic regulation of protein synthesis, they proposed the existence of an intermediate molecule, or "messenger ribonucleotide" that is produced from DNA and that brings the genetic information to the ribosomes for protein synthesis. At about the same time, experimental support for the existence of mRNA was provided by two different research teams [9, 10]. Both research teams had succeeded in isolating mRNA and demonstrating its association with "pre-existing" ribosomes. This replaced the prevailing theory of the time that new specialized ribosomes are synthesized from the gene, and that these ribosomes are specific for the production of the corresponding protein, i.e. the "one gene – one ribosome – one protein" hypothesis. For detailed information about the remarkable series of events and some of the outstanding experiments that led to the discovery of mRNA, see reference [11].

In 1969, protein synthesis from mRNA inside ribosomes was first demonstrated in cell-free systems. In these experiments, RNA fractions purified from reticulocytes dictated the synthesis of globin when incubated with ribosomes obtained from *Escherichia coli* [12] or a different mammalian species [13]. Later on, the translation of mRNA into hemoglobin was also proven in living cells after the microinjection of 9 s RNA from rabbit reticulocytes into frog oocytes [14, 15]. While these studies might have sparked one's imagination to use mRNA for therapeutic applications, at the time, the focus was solely on understanding its biological function.

In 1984, a simple and efficient method was established for *in vitro* mRNA synthesis using template DNA and a bacteriophage SP6 polymerase that initiates transcription at an SP6 promoter located upstream of the gene of interest [16]. In the following years, T7 and T3 RNA polymerases were also reported for successful *in vitro* transcribed (IVT) RNA synthesis [17–20]. These methods still represent the foundation of how mRNA is manufactured in today's COVID-19 mRNA vaccines. However, a limitation of IVT mRNA production using phage polymerases is that it can give rise to multiple contaminants in the form of short and long double-stranded RNA (dsRNA) strands [21, 22]. These dsRNA byproducts have been shown to be largely responsible for the innate immune response to IVT mRNA, and when not controlled, have the potential to jeopardize the safety and functionality of mRNA vaccines (discussed in more detail below). There is, therefore, continuing interest in optimizing the IVT process of mRNA in order to reduce the formation of dsRNA byproducts, as well as in finding (more) cost-effective purification methods [23–25].

Decades of basic research into the structural characteristics of mRNA and the biological interactions of mRNA with numerous proteins inside the cell not only brought new insights into mRNA metabolism and mRNA translation process but also leveraged IVT mRNA to reach a more optimal design [26]. The genetic information in mRNA is encoded in a codon sequence, where a triplet of adjacent nucleotides specifies an amino acid to be incorporated in a protein, also referred to as the open reading frame (ORF). The ORF is flanked at the 5′ and 3′ positions with start and stop codons. Because most amino acids are encoded by more than one codon, the codon usage in the ORF can be varied, also referred to as synonymous codon usage. Over the years, several strategies have been proposed to optimize codons so as to improve the translation and half-life of the mRNA, including methods of adjusting codons to match host transfer RNA abundances [27] for the enrichment of GC content [28, 29], and to optimize mRNA folds in the construct [30, 31]. It is important, however, to consider that these methods may have unintended effects on the performance of mRNA vaccines, such as altering protein folding and changing the sites of posttranslational modifications that may affect the immunogenicity and function of the encoded antigen, reviewed in [32].

Different nontranslated structural elements are present in eukaryotic mRNA, which were found to have essential roles in different stages of the mRNA life cycle. In 1975, the cap structure was discovered, which is an N7-methylated guanosine linked to the first nucleotide of the RNA via a reverse 5′ to 5′ triphosphate linkage [33–36]. By binding to the eukaryotic initiation factor (eIF) 4E, the cap structure enables the recruitment of translating ribosomes to mRNA. The cap structure and its methylation state are also significant determinants of how the host cell distinguishes itself from nonself RNA, as well as they are important for mRNA stability. At the 3′ end of mRNA, a poly(A) tail made up of a long stretch of repeating adenosine nucleotides was found [37, 38], which functions synergistically with the cap structure to promote translation and regulate mRNA stability [39]. Furthermore, directly upstream and downstream of the ORF, two untranslated regions (UTRs) are positioned, which contain multiple regulatory elements [40]. Since their discovery, continuous efforts and progress have been made in optimizing these structural elements for improved stability and expression of IVT mRNA through empirical screening approaches and computational models [30, 31, 41–43].

Alternative forms of RNA have also been investigated as a therapeutic modality, such as those based on self-amplifying RNA (saRNA) and circular RNA (circRNA). saRNA includes the genetic information for a viral replicase in addition to the vaccine antigen or gene of interest in the ORF sequence and was already introduced in the mid-1990s for vaccine development [44, 45]. This replicase complex typically derived from alphaviruses allows the intracellular amplification of RNA and, in theory, can significantly increase and/or prolong the antigen expression capacity. The replication kinetics of saRNA may provide potential dose-sparing effects, while more prolonged antigen exposure may benefit the quality and duration of vaccine-induced immunity. Another more recent research avenue is the exploration of circRNA. This form of RNA characterized by its closed-ring structure was first reported in 1976 as an independent plant pathogens known as viroids, and later on also found to be prevalent in eukaryotic cells [46, 47]. Due to its unique structure, circRNA is protected from exonuclease-mediated degradation, which may confer improved stability compared to linear mRNA counterparts. Since circRNA lacks a cap and poly(A) tail structure, translation from circRNA into proteins is typically enabled through the insertion of an internal ribosome entry site [48].

1.2.2 The Inflammatory Nature of mRNA

A key bottleneck impeding the therapeutic use of RNA has been its inflammatory capacity. In the early years, it was already demonstrated that mRNA can induce antiviral innate immunity in mammalian cells. In 1957, it was found that adding heat-inactivated influenza virus to cells makes a protein substance that interferes with the replication of viruses, which was called "interferon" [49]. A few years later, it became clear that IFN must act by interfering with the viral RNA metabolism in virus-infected cells [50] and that the viral RNA itself was the component responsible for this antiviral immune reaction [51]. More than 30 years later, the discovery of pathogen recognition receptors by Hoffman and Beutler laid the groundwork for further studies into how mRNA triggers an innate immune response. Several intracellular sensors that are activated by structural features of mRNA were identified. As an example, dsRNA species were shown to be recognized by Toll-like receptor (TLR) 3 in the endosomes [52], and upon arrival in the cytosol by receptors such as Retinoic acid-inducible gene I (RIG-I) [53] and Melanoma differentiation-associated gene 5 (MDA5) [54]. TLR7 and TLR8 were identified as receptors for viral and synthetic single-stranded RNAs and their degradative products [55–58], while the cap1 structure (m7GpppNm) on mRNA was found to be critical to avoid recognition by RIG-I [59, 60]. These discoveries brought explanations of how mammalian cells are capable of distinguishing nonself from self RNA. The reader should refer to the following reviews [61, 62] on this topic for a comprehensive list of RNA sensors, the involved signal transduction pathways, and more details on the molecular basis of mRNA recognition.

The immune recognition of mRNA activates downstream signaling pathways, which leads to the production of inflammatory cytokines, including type I IFNs, inducing in the cells an antiviral state. This has some very important implications for the design of mRNA vaccines and therapeutics. First of all, the immune recognition of mRNA is considered as one of the mechanisms underlying the cause of reactogenicity symptoms, and thus, to a large extent, will determine the safety of mRNA therapeutics. Second, the innate immune response to mRNA can drastically impair the translation of IVT mRNA, thereby reducing the antigen availability for T-cell and B-cell recognition. For example, dsRNA elements in mRNA products are sensed by intracellular enzymes, such as protein kinase R (PKR) and 2′–5′-oligoadenylate synthetase (OAS), which in turn activate other proteins that cause translational shutdown and cell death [63, 64]. Yet, on the upside, the innate immune response to mRNA has the potential to provide an important adjuvant effect on vaccine potency, and it can be argued, maybe even play a crucial role in the success of mRNA vaccines. Indeed, downstream signaling from the RNA sensing receptors also activates the expression of several genes involved in the mobilization and activation of antigen-presenting cells (APCs), while RNA-driven cytokines are capable of exerting direct immune-stimulatory effects on T cells and B cells. Therefore, the most challenging task with mRNA vaccines was to find an optimal mRNA design that could minimize the problems posed by its immune recognition on mRNA translation and vaccine safety while still providing enough adjuvant properties to drive strong vaccine responses against the encoded antigen.

At least part of this problem was overcome by the work of Karikó, Weissman, and colleagues at the University of Pennsylvania (UPenn), who were studying the immune-stimulatory effects of IVT mRNA on dendritic cells (DCs) *in vitro*, i.e. the innate immune cell type specialized in antigen presentation and T-cell activation [65]. By comparing the immune-stimulatory activity of IVT mRNA with RNA types derived from different sources, they found that both bacterial (total) RNA, mammalian mitochondrial RNA, and IVT mRNA primed the DCs to produce high levels of tumor necrosis factor-alpha (TNF-α). In contrast, they found that total-, nuclear-, and cytoplasmic RNAs from mammalian sources were less potent inducers of DC activation, while mammalian transfer RNA was noninflammatory. This finding led the researchers to hypothesize that posttranscriptional modifications commonly present in mammalian RNA, such as pseudouridine and methylated nucleosides, might serve as another molecular signature by which cellular RNA sensors discriminate self-RNA from foreign RNA. When applied to IVT mRNA, modified nucleotides, in particular pseudouridines and their derivatives, indeed protected IVT mRNA from activating the aforementioned RNA sensors; TLR3, TLR7, TLR8, PKR, OAS, RIG-I, and MDA5 [22, 63–66]. Consequently, the use of modified uridines strongly improved the translation and safety profile of IVT mRNA products [67, 68]. It is noteworthy that the following studies also evidenced that the use of modified uridines in the IVT reaction reduces the formation of dsRNA byproducts, which might at least in part explain the reduced immunogenicity of uridine-modified mRNA [22]. In addition, it was shown that pseudouridine not only acts as a major controller of the innate immune activity of IVT mRNA but can also contribute to the intrinsic stability and the dynamics of mRNA molecules with ribosomes, reviewed in [69]. Taken together, the use of modified uridines was a great leap forward for producing more translatable, less immunogenic, and safer IVT mRNA products. Note that for the COVID-19 mRNA vaccines BNT162b2 and mRNA-1273, every uridine residue in the mRNA is replaced with N1-methylpseudouridine (m1ψ).

1.3 How Studying Lipid Bilayer Structures in Cell Membranes Gave Rise to the Eventual Development of Lipid Nanoparticles for RNA Delivery

1.3.1 From Biological Cell Membranes to Liposomal Drugs

RNAs are inherently unstable as they are easily degraded by ribonucleases (RNases), which act as the first line of defense against foreign RNAs as well as allow our cells to regulate RNA metabolism. In addition, the lipid bilayer structure that forms the foundation of cell membranes is uniquely designed to prevent the permeation of such large, negatively charged RNA molecules, protecting the cells from exogenous RNA entering them. Ironically, long-standing efforts to understand the physical properties and functional roles of lipids in cell membranes led scientists to model lipid membrane systems, which have been instrumental in the development of the delivery technology enabling intact nucleic acids to cross these biological barriers; LNPs containing ionizable cationic lipids.

The history of LNPs began in 1964 when Bangham and Horne first described electron microscopy observations of dispersed lecithin (phosphatidylcholine) in water, showing the formation of lamellar "spherulites" structures [70]. In follow-on papers, Bangham and his colleagues described the bimolecular leaflet structure of lecithin vesicles and proved the dispersed phospholipids were spontaneously forming a closed membrane system, i.e. a lipid bilayer completely enclosing an aqueous space [71]. It was Weissmann who named these lipid vesicles "liposomes." Subsequently, the development and characterization of the physical properties of lipids and liposomes quickly followed [72–76]. These studies on the structures that lipids adopt [72] bilayer permeability [77], and membrane fusion [78] helped lay down the cornerstone for the understanding of the biophysical properties of liposomes [79, 80].

In parallel to understanding the membrane biophysics of liposomes, liposome research has extended into areas of therapeutic application. In 1970, Sessa and Weissman first demonstrated that these liposomes have the ability to entrap lysozyme [81], followed by others that started to explore the therapeutic potential of liposomes as drug carriers for enzymes and proteins in rodent models [82–84]. With the experimental methods available at the time, these studies demonstrated that liposomes were removed from the blood within minutes and accumulated in the liver and spleen of the rats, in which liposome-entrapped protein eventually localized in the lysosomes of cells. However, the major initial advances of liposomes as drug delivery systems came with applications for the delivery of anticancer drugs. Two important advances made in the 1980s were the development of the extrusion process for the rapid production of unilamellar vesicles with diameters in the 100 nm size range [85] and the "remote loading" pH gradient technique for efficiently loading liposomal systems with cancer drugs [86, 87].

The third advance involved the development of techniques to increase the circulation lifetime of liposomes following i.v. administration. The incorporation of cholesterol in phosphatidylcholine liposomes reduced bilayer permeability and increased the stability of these systems *in vitro* and *in vivo* [88, 89]. The presence of gangliosides and sphingomyelin reduced liposome clearance rates, which led to the concept of "stealth" liposomes [90]. Incorporation of polyethylene glycol (PEG) lipids further improved the blood circulation half-life of liposomes [91]. PEGylation quickly became popular to improve pharmacokinetics and biodistribution of liposomes, which along with the improvement of liposomal generation (by extrusion) and drug-loading procedures (using pH gradients) have led to the first liposomal drugs for systemic delivery of small molecule drugs to treat fungal infections and a variety of cancers.

With regard to nucleic acid-based drugs, the idea of using liposomes to deliver DNA and RNA into host cells was introduced simultaneously by Dimitriadis and Ostro [92, 93]. Both studies demonstrated the encapsulation and delivery of rabbit globin mRNA and rabbit reticulocyte 9S mRNA into eukaryotic cells by using large unilamellar liposomes. However, these studies were not pursued due to limited transfection potency, lack of scalable methods of manufacture, and poor-encapsulation efficiencies. The introduction of cationic lipids such as 1,2-di-*O*-octadecenyl-3-trimethylammonium propane (DOTMA) rekindled interest in the late 1980s [94, 95]. The electrostatic interaction between the positively charged quaternary ammonium head group of the lipid and the negatively charged phosphate backbone of nucleic acids leads to the formation of "complexes" with high-encapsulation efficiencies. In addition, the cationic lipid has membrane destabilization properties enabling the delivery of nucleic acid payloads across cellular barriers [96, 97]. In 2001, Hafez et al. proposed that the membrane destabilization properties of cationic lipids were related to their ability to form disruptive nonbilayer structures in combination with the negatively charged lipids found in biological membranes ([96]). This research resulted in products such as Lipofectin™, a liposomal composition of the cationic lipid DOTMA and 1,2-dioleoyl-*sn*-glycero-3-phosphatidyl-ethanolamine (DOPE), followed by other polyvalent cationic lipid containing liposomal formulations such as Lipofectamine™ and Transfectam™. These lipofection reagents are commonly used in biochemistry and molecular biology research for the *in vitro* delivery of DNA and RNA in eukaryotic cells.

1.3.2 Ionizable Lipid Nanoparticles for Systemic Delivery of Nucleic Acids

Delivery of nucleic acid-based drugs presents significantly more problems than the delivery of small molecular drugs. In addition to reaching target tissue, the delivery system has to protect the cargo from degradation, facilitate uptake into target cells, and subsequently deliver the cargo into the cytoplasm of target cells. Complexes of DNA or RNA with cationic liposomes result in a heterogeneous mixture of complexes that are relatively unstable and can change properties such as size over time [98]. In addition, cationic lipids can be toxic and cause membrane disruption, hemolysis and induce inflammatory responses limiting therapeutic applications [99, 100].

The major breakthrough for delivering nucleic acid was the introduction of ionizable cationic lipids. In 1994, Bailey and Cullis synthesized 1,2-dioleoyl-3-dimethylammonium propane (DODAP), an ionizable version of a cationic lipid 1,2-dioleoyl-3-trimethylammonium-propane (DOTAP) to study the influence of lipid asymmetry on the fusion of liposomal systems [101]. Subsequently, Cullis and colleagues used lipid-based systems containing ionizable lipids to encapsulate nucleic acids [102]. They showed that DODAP had an apparent pK (pK_a) of approximately 6.5 and that these systems could be used to encapsulate nucleic acids at pH values where the lipids are protonated and positively charged (e.g. pH 4) and that the nucleic acid polymers were retained when the pH was raised to physiological values (pH 7.4). Further investigations showed that these lipid systems had a "solid core" hydrophobic interior surrounded by a lipid monolayer [103]. These systems were called "LNPs" to distinguish them from liposomes, which exhibit bilayer structures. An important benefit of encapsulation using ionizable lipids such as DODAP is that the LNP are effectively neutral at physiological pH, rendering them less toxic than lipid-based systems containing permanently positively charged lipids, allowing systemic administration. In 2001, the first report was published on the therapeutic potential of a lipid formulation composed of DODAP, cholesterol, 1,2-distearoyl-*sn*-glycero-3-phosphocholine, and PEG ceramides for the systemic delivery of antisense oligodeoxynucleotides in mice [104].

Subsequent efforts focused on the delivery of small interfering RNA (siRNA) to the liver following i.v. administration to silence genes in hepatocytes. LNPs containing DODAP were able to induce gene silencing in the liver but only at very high doses (see supplemental information for [105]). This led to the synthesis of 1,2-dilinoleyloxy-3-dimethylaminopropane (DLinDMA), a more stable version of DODAP, which, when formulated in LNP siRNA systems, showed early preclinical promise in nonhuman primates for silencing of apolipoprotein B expression in the liver [106]. Further studies guided by a "rational design" approach to adjust the ionizable lipid pK_a and shape properties to drive the formation of membrane disruptive nonbilayer structures and encourage endosomal escape of siRNA contents resulted in DLin-KC2-DMA. LNP siRNA systems containing DLinKC2DMA exhibited improved gene-silencing properties [105], leading to an intense screening program involving the synthesis of hundreds of ionizable lipids and testing in preclinical animal models to find ionizable lipids with optimal silencing properties when incorporated into LNP siRNA systems. This led to DLin-MC3-DMA [107], which was incorporated into the first RNAi drug to be approved by the FDA [108]. Further iterations focused on the degradability of ionizable lipids led to the inclusion of bio-cleavable ester functions within the lipid acyl chains [109]. Later studies aimed at optimizing the liver transfection properties of LNP systems containing mRNA led to new generations of ionizable lipids incorporating branched structures as illustrated in the SM-102 and ALC-0315 lipid utilized in the mRNA-1273 and BNT162b2 vaccine, respectively [109–111].

A different screening approach was taken by Langer and Anderson from the Massachusetts Institute of Technology, who synthesized a library of ionizable lipid-like polyvalent material called lipidoids; these screens identified potent lipidoids such as C12-200 and generated lipidoid-based LNPs that were used to successfully deliver siRNAs in mice and nonhuman primates [112–114].

The PEG-lipid components also required improvement. A PEG-conjugated lipid is required during formulation to generate small, stable LNP systems [115], however a disadvantage is that the steric barrier created by the PEG coating inhibits the cellular uptake, and thus the transfection potency, of LNP containing nucleic acid-based drugs. Thus, the PEG-lipids employed were designed to diffuse away from the LNP following systemic administration [116]. Previous work has shown that PEG-lipids with short (C_{14}) acyl chains readily exchange out of lipid-based systems if a suitable "sink" is available [117]. In addition to enhanced cellular uptake, another benefit was that the "diffusible" PEG-conjugated lipids mitigate the risk of inducing anti-PEG antibody responses [118, 119]. This unwanted immunogenicity has been associated with accelerated blood clearance and pseudo-allergic reactions upon repeated injections of PEGylated LNPs in preclinical models [120]. Further optimization to balance out the effects of the PEG-conjugated lipid on the efficacy, safety and stability of nucleic-acid loaded LNPs together with the synthesis of the more easily produced PEG-diacylglycerol lipids [121], eventually resulted in the identification of what was to become the gold standard PEG-lipid; 1,2-dimyristoyl-rac-glycero-3-methoxypolyethylene glycol-2000 (DMG-PEG 2000) [122].

A final challenge in the establishment of the LNP technology was to find a reproducible and scalable manufacturing method that could obtain LNPs with high encapsulation efficiencies. Initial work on LNP systems made use of a method based on the ethanol dilution principle first described by Batzri and Korn [123] and followed a three-step procedure: (i) lipid components dissolved in ethanol are diluted in an acidic citrate solution containing nucleic acid to form vesicular structures; (ii) the intermediate mixture is downsized using extrusion; (iii) the mixture is dialyzed to remove ethanol and to raise the pH to 7.4 [104]. This procedure was further optimized by using rapid-mixing devices such as by means of a T-tube junction [124] and microfluidics [125], which allowed for the scalable production of LNP systems with higher encapsulation efficiencies and smaller particle sizes under well defined, reproducible conditions. For more in-depth information on the production of LNPs and how these methods were improved and simplified, the reader is referred to the following reviews [126–128].

Starting from the 2010s, the LNP system became the preferred nonviral delivery system for nucleic acids, which eventually culminated in the clinical approval of the first siRNA-LNP-based product to treat neuropathies associated with hereditary transthyretin amyloidosis, Onpattro® (patisiran) [129]. The clinical approval of Onpattro® was a milestone not only for gene therapies in general but also as a precedent that enabled the clinical progress of mRNA vaccines, as will be discussed in Section 1.4.

1.4 The Journey of Developing Clinical mRNA Vaccines

The exploration of the therapeutic use of IVT mRNA started in the early 1990s with Felgner and coworkers first providing proof-of-concept that naked IVT mRNA or DNA can be translated into protein in living animals [130]. The therapeutic potential of IVT mRNA was first demonstrated in a study where vasopressin-encoding mRNA was injected into the hypothalamus, achieving a temporary reversal of diabetes insipidus in rats [131]. Next, a few pioneering studies reported the usefulness of RNA for immunization in mice; Martinon et al. demonstrated that liposomes containing mRNA encoding the influenza virus nucleoprotein were capable of inducing virus-specific cytotoxic T-cell responses [132]; Conry et al. reported the activation of humoral immune responses by using a naked mRNA vaccine encoding a carcinoembryonic antigen [133]; while Zhou et al. were the first to show the feasibility of a saRNA vaccine [45].

However, before the development of the COVID-19 mRNA vaccines, there was plenty of trial and error, testing many different mRNA designs and delivery approaches. IVT mRNA was first tested in humans using an *ex vivo* approach, where monocyte-derived DCs are transfected with tumor antigen mRNA and reinfused into patients with cancer as a cellular vaccine [134, 135]. Later on, CureVac, a German biotech company founded in 2000, organized the first-in-human clinical trials testing two RNA cancer vaccine approaches for the treatment of melanoma; one based on the direct dermal administration of naked mRNA in combination with granulocyte macrophage colony-stimulating factor as an adjuvant, and the other using mRNA complexed with protamine [136, 137]. Applying the lessons learned from these early clinical trials helped CureVac to systematically develop and test the next generations of mRNA technologies.

These pioneering clinical trials also inspired other researchers/entrepreneurs to come up with novel concepts. Before COVID-19, BioNTech's activities were mainly focused on the field of immuno-oncology, where they have clinically tested various RNA-based technologies for active and passive immunization strategies. In early work, BioNTech evidenced that lymph node-resident DC could be transfected and activated by the direct "intranodal" administration of naked mRNA (using calcium-rich buffers), which resulted in an efficient expansion of T cells against the encoded antigen [138]. The feasibility of this naked mRNA vaccine approach was further demonstrated in patients with melanoma, showing clinical promise in developing T-cell responses against patient-specific neo-epitopes [139]. In 2016, BioNTech introduced another delivery approach for the systemic delivery of unmodified mRNA cancer vaccines using DOTMA/DOPE liposomes [140]. They found that the charge ratio between cationic lipids and mRNA could be used to change the *in vivo* organ transfection of these systems; with lipoplexes exhibiting an excess negative charge specifically targeting DCs in the spleen and lymph nodes. This mRNA vaccine platform is currently being investigated by the company in Phase 1 and Phase 2 clinical trials for various cancer indications, such as monotherapy or in combination with immune checkpoint inhibition [141].

Over the years, the feasibility of the LNP technology has been demonstrated in academic literature for various applications and different nucleic acid cargo. It also became clear that exploiting the interaction of LNPs with immune cells, rather than escaping it, provides opportunities for vaccination and other immunotherapeutic approaches [142, 143]. The first example of combining LNP and RNA as a new vaccine platform was reported by Geall and his colleagues at Novartis in 2012 [144]. An LNP formulation with the ionizable lipid DLinDMA was used to encapsulate a saRNA encoding the fusion glycoprotein of the respiratory syncytial virus. After intramuscular immunization, the saRNA–LNP vaccine demonstrated noninferior immune responses compared to a viral delivery technology in mice with the major advantage of removing the inherent limitations of viral vectors. In the search for a suitable delivery system, the Weissman lab (UPenn) partnered with the LNP-specialized company Acuitas Therapeutics founded by Cullis, Madden, and

Hope in 2009. They first reported on a study that showed the potential of delivering LNPs loaded with m1ψ-modified mRNA via different administration routes in mice [145], followed by several reports on preclinical studies demonstrating the outstanding capacity of this vaccine platform to elicit immune responses against viral pathogens, such as zika, influenza, herpes simplex virus, and human immunodeficiency virus [146–149]. In 2018, this success led to collaborations between BioNTech and Pfizer to co-develop an mRNA influenza vaccine based on these technologies, where it was recently announced by Pfizer that first volunteers have entered a Phase 3 clinical trial [150]. Likewise, CureVac entered an agreement with Acuitas Therapeutics, and before COVID-19, already worked on a prophylactic mRNA–LNP vaccine against rabies by applying their sequence-optimized mRNA platform and Acuitas' LNP technology [151, 152]. In 2017, Moderna was the first company to report interim results from a Phase 1 clinical trial on the immunogenicity and reactogenicity of a m1ψ-modified mRNA–LNP vaccine against H10N8 and H7N9 influenza viruses [153, 154].

So, when the SARS-CoV-2 pandemic hit, several mRNA vaccine platforms had already reached a substantial degree of maturity. This allowed companies such as CureVac, BioNTech/Pfizer, and Moderna to produce clinical-grade mRNA vaccine candidates against SARS-CoV-2 in record times. However, none of these mRNA vaccine platforms had made it to Phase 3 clinical testing before, which made the COVID-19 pandemic the first great opportunity to investigate and compare the potential and safety of these different mRNA vaccine platforms in large-scale clinical trials [155]. The m1ψ-modified mRNA vaccines, BNT162b2 and mRNA-1273, have been the first to get results from Phase 3 clinical trials, and although no direct comparisons were made between the different vaccine candidates, these vaccines have demonstrated a significantly greater efficacy for preventing symptomatic COVID-19 disease (~95%) compared to other mRNA vaccine candidates, e.g. CVnCoV, CureVac's sequence-optimized mRNA vaccine candidate: 47% [156] and ARCT-154, Arcturus's saRNA vaccine candidate: 55% [157]. Note that, all of these mRNA vaccine candidates were using LNPs to enable their delivery following the intramuscular administration route.

1.5 Concluding Remarks

In this chapter section, we focused on some of the fundamental discoveries and technological improvements that contributed to the development of the COVID-19 mRNA vaccines. Here, we highlighted nucleoside modification and ionizable LNPs as two key enabling technologies of this novel vaccine platform, which have drastically increased the therapeutic index and potency of mRNA vaccines.

However, there are many aspects to the success of mRNA vaccines, and we believe that we might soon learn that alternative mRNA vaccine platforms will be clinically useful as well. For SARS-CoV-2 as an example, Providence Therapeutics recently announced positive results from an unmodified uridine mRNA–LNP vaccine (PTX-COVID19-B) that showed noninferior immunogenicity and equal safety compared to BNT162b2 in Phase 2 clinical trial [158]. Also, CureVac has further optimized its COVID-19 mRNA vaccine candidate by adjusting the UTRs and poly(A) tail structure, which achieved greatly improved immunogenicity and protective efficacy compared to their first-generation COVID-19 vaccine in nonhuman primates [41]. For saRNA-based vaccines, it was suggested that modifications or additional measures that could minimize the innate immune response early during saRNA vaccination may prove to be critical to increasing primary expression and the resulting clinical performance [159, 160]. Moreover, there might also be a need to select and/or optimize mRNA vaccine design depending on the disease indication and the types of immune response that correlate with protection. For instance, it was recently demonstrated that LNPs loaded with purified unmodified mRNA elicited a higher $CD8^+$ T-cell response and achieved more effective antitumor immunity in B16-melanoma bearing mice compared to a m1ψ-modified mRNA–LNP counterpart, which highlights the positive effect of unmodified mRNA and the induction of type I IFN responses for cancer vaccination [161]. Interestingly, several studies have also recently demonstrated that the LNP formulation not only enables the delivery of mRNA vaccines but also contributes to their reactogenicity and immunogenicity by providing innate immune stimulation [162–164]. These findings could open up new avenues for the design of more effective and potentially safer mRNA vaccine generations. However, the underlying mechanisms of these LNP adjuvant properties and how these properties can be more fine-tuned remain largely unknown and will require further exploration [165].

Finally, it needs to be mentioned that other factors also helped the rapid development and production of the COVID-19 mRNA vaccines, which were not discussed in this chapter section, such as the prior knowledge that was available on SARS-CoV-1 and other coronaviruses and the huge financial investments and scientific collaborations which allowed some of the steps in the research and development process to be conducted in parallel. Future development of mRNA medicines is poised to benefit from the enormous steps and hurdles taken with respect to various industrial aspects, such as the establishment of supply chain systems for starting materials, the infrastructure that was built for large-scale production of LNP–mRNA products, and the better regulation guidelines that are now set out to bring these products to the market.

Taken together, the development of the COVID-19 mRNA vaccines was a great achievement, which was built on decades of fundamental and translational science. Based on the continuous effort being made by a growing field of multidisciplinary researchers, we believe that multiple therapeutic modalities will become available using (m)RNA technologies for a variety of diseases.

References

1 Baden, L.R., El Sahly, H.M., Essink, B. et al. (2021). Efficacy and safety of the mRNA-1273 SARS-CoV-2 vaccine. *N. Engl. J. Med.* 384 (5): 403–416. https://doi.org/10.1056/NEJMoa2035389.

2 Polack, F.P., Thomas, S.J., Kitchin, N. et al. (2020). Safety and efficacy of the BNT162b2 mRNA Covid-19 vaccine. *N. Engl. J. Med.* 383 (27): 2603–2615. https://doi.org/10.1056/NEJMoa2034577.

3 Di Fusco, M., Marczell, K., Deger, K.A. et al. (2022). Public health impact of the Pfizer-BioNTech COVID-19 vaccine (BNT162b2) in the first year of rollout in the United States. *J. Med. Econ.* 25 (1): 605–617. https://doi.org/10.1080/13696998.2022.2071427.

4 Watson, O.J., Barnsley, G., Toor, J. et al. (2022). Global impact of the first year of COVID-19 vaccination: a mathematical modelling study. *Lancet Infect. Dis.* 22 (9): 1293–1302. https://doi.org/10.1016/S1473-3099(22)00320-6.

5 Rohner, E., Yang, R., Foo, K.S. et al. (2022). Unlocking the promise of mRNA therapeutics. *Nat. Biotechnol.* 40 (11): 1586–1600. https://doi.org/10.1038/s41587-022-01491-z.

6 Dowdy, S.F. (2017). Overcoming cellular barriers for RNA therapeutics. *Nat. Biotechnol.* 35 (3): 222–229. https://doi.org/10.1038/nbt.3802.

7 Cobb, M. (2015). Who discovered messenger RNA? *Curr. Biol.* 25 (13): R526–R532. https://doi.org/10.1016/j.cub.2015.05.032.

8 Jacob, F. and Monod, J. (1961). Genetic regulatory mechanisms in the synthesis of proteins. *J. Mol. Biol.* 3: 318–356. https://doi.org/10.1016/s0022-2836(61)80072-7.

9 Brenner, S., Jacob, F., and Meselson, M. (1961). An unstable intermediate carrying information from genes to ribosomes for protein synthesis. *Nature* 190: 576–581. https://doi.org/10.1038/190576a0.

10 Gros, F., Hiatt, H., Gilbert, W. et al. (1961). Unstable ribonucleic acid revealed by pulse labelling of *Escherichia coli*. *Nature* 190: 581–585. https://doi.org/10.1038/190581a0.

11 Judson, H.F. (1979). *The Eighth Day of Creation*. New York: CSH Press.

12 Laycock, D.G. and Hunt, J.A. (1969). Synthesis of rabbit globin by a bacterial cell free system. *Nature* 221 (5186): 1118–1122. https://doi.org/10.1038/2211118a0.

13 Lockard, R.E. and Lingrel, J.B. (1969). The synthesis of mouse hemoglobin beta-chains in a rabbit reticulocyte cell-free system programmed with mouse reticulocyte 9S RNA. *Biochem. Biophys. Res. Commun.* 37 (2): 204–212. https://doi.org/10.1016/0006-291x(69)90720-7.

14 Gurdon, J.B., Lane, C.D., Woodland, H.R. et al. (1971). Use of frog eggs and oocytes for the study of messenger RNA and its translation in living cells. *Nature* 233 (5316): 177–182. https://doi.org/10.1038/233177a0.

15 Lane, C.D., Marbaix, G., and Gurdon, J.B. (1971). Rabbit haemoglobin synthesis in frog cells: the translation of reticulocyte 9 s RNA in frog oocytes. *J. Mol. Biol.* 61 (1): 73–91. https://doi.org/10.1016/0022-2836(71)90207-5.

16 Melton, D.A., Krieg, P.A., Rebagliati, M.R. et al. (1984). Efficient in vitro synthesis of biologically active RNA and RNA hybridization probes from plasmids containing a bacteriophage SP6 promoter. *Nucleic Acids Res.* 12 (18): 7035–7056. https://doi.org/10.1093/nar/12.18.7035.

17 Milligan, J.F., Groebe, D.R., Witherell, G.W. et al. (1987). Oligoribonucleotide synthesis using T7 RNA polymerase and synthetic DNA templates. *Nucleic Acids Res.* 15 (21): 8783–8798. https://doi.org/10.1093/nar/15.21.8783.

18 Studier, F.W. and Moffatt, B.A. (1986). Use of bacteriophage T7 RNA polymerase to direct selective high-level expression of cloned genes. *J. Mol. Biol.* 189 (1): 113–130. https://doi.org/10.1016/0022-2836(86)90385-2.

19 Tabor, S. and Richardson, C.C. (1985). A bacteriophage T7 RNA polymerase/promoter system for controlled exclusive expression of specific genes. *Proc. Natl. Acad. Sci. U. S. A.* 82 (4): 1074–1078. https://doi.org/10.1073/pnas.82.4.1074.

20 van der Werf, S., Bradley, J., Wimmer, E. et al. (1986). Synthesis of infectious poliovirus RNA by purified T7 RNA polymerase. *Proc. Natl. Acad. Sci. U. S. A.* 83 (8): 2330–2334. https://doi.org/10.1073/pnas.83.8.2330.

21 Baiersdorfer, M., Boros, G., Muramatsu, H. et al. (2019). A facile method for the removal of dsRNA contaminant from in vitro-transcribed mRNA. *Mol. Ther. Nucleic Acids* 15: 26–35. https://doi.org/10.1016/j.omtn.2019.02.018.

22 Mu, X., Greenwald, E., Ahmad, S. et al. (2018). An origin of the immunogenicity of in vitro transcribed RNA. *Nucleic Acids Res.* 46 (10): 5239–5249. https://doi.org/10.1093/nar/gky177.

23 Dousis, A., Ravichandran, K., Hobert, E.M. et al. (2022). An engineered T7 RNA polymerase that produces mRNA free of immunostimulatory byproducts. *Nat. Biotechnol.* 41 (4): 560–568. https://doi.org/10.1038/s41587-022-01525-6.

24 Nelson, J., Sorensen, E.W., Mintri, S. et al. (2020). Impact of mRNA chemistry and manufacturing process on innate immune activation. *Sci. Adv.* 6 (26): eaaz6893. https://doi.org/10.1126/sciadv.aaz6893.

25 Piao, X.J., Yadav, V., Wang, E.D. et al. (2022). Double-stranded RNA reduction by chaotropic agents during in vitro transcription of messenger RNA. *Mol. Ther. Nucleic Acids* 29: 618–624. https://doi.org/10.1016/j.omtn.2022.08.001.

26 Sahin, U., Kariko, K., and Tureci, O. (2014). mRNA-based therapeutics - developing a new class of drugs. *Nat. Rev. Drug Discov.* 13 (10): 759–780. https://doi.org/10.1038/nrd4278.

27 Kane, J.F. (1995). Effects of rare codon clusters on high-level expression of heterologous proteins in *Escherichia coli*. *Curr. Opin. Biotechnol.* 6 (5): 494–500. https://doi.org/10.1016/0958-1669(95)80082-4.

28 Kudla, G., Lipinski, L., Caffin, F. et al. (2006). High guanine and cytosine content increases mRNA levels in mammalian cells. *PLoS Biol.* 4 (6): e180. https://doi.org/10.1371/journal.pbio.0040180.

29 Thess, A., Grund, S., Mui, B.L. et al. (2015). Sequence-engineered mRNA without chemical nucleoside modifications enables an effective protein therapy in large animals. *Mol. Ther.* 23 (9): 1456–1464. https://doi.org/10.1038/mt.2015.103.

30 Leppek, K., Byeon, G.W., Kladwang, W. et al. (2022). Combinatorial optimization of mRNA structure, stability, and translation for RNA-based therapeutics. *Nat. Commun.* 13 (1): 1536. https://doi.org/10.1038/s41467-022-28776-w.

31 Mauger, D.M., Cabral, B.J., Presnyak, V. et al. (2019). mRNA structure regulates protein expression through changes in functional half-life. *Proc. Natl. Acad. Sci. U. S. A.* 116 (48): 24075–24083. https://doi.org/10.1073/pnas.1908052116.

32 Mauro, V.P. and Chappell, S.A. (2014). A critical analysis of codon optimization in human therapeutics. *Trends Mol. Med.* 20 (11): 604–613. https://doi.org/10.1016/j.molmed.2014.09.003.

33 Adams, J.M. and Cory, S. (1975). Modified nucleosides and bizarre 5′-termini in mouse myeloma mRNA. *Nature* 255 (5503): 28–33. https://doi.org/10.1038/255028a0.

34 Furuichi, Y. and Miura, K. (1975). A blocked structure at the 5′ terminus of mRNA from cytoplasmic polyhedrosis virus. *Nature* 253 (5490): 374–375. https://doi.org/10.1038/253374a0.

35 Martin, S.A., Paoletti, E., and Moss, B. (1975). Purification of mRNA guanylyltransferase and mRNA (guanine-7-) methyltransferase from vaccinia virions. *J. Biol. Chem.* 250 (24): 9322–9329. 10.1016/S0021-9258(19)40646-7.

36 Muthukrishnan, S., Both, G.W., Furuichi, Y. et al. (1975). 5′-Terminal 7-methylguanosine in eukaryotic mRNA is required for translation. *Nature* 255 (5503): 33–37. https://doi.org/10.1038/255033a0.

37 Burr, H. and Lingrel, J.B. (1971). Poly A sequences at the 3′ termini of rabbit globin mRNAs. *Nature* 233 (36): 41–43. https://doi.org/10.1038/newbio233041a0.

38 Lim, L. and Canellakis, E.S. (1970). Adenine-rich polymer associated with rabbit reticulocyte messenger RNA. *Nature* 227 (5259): 710–712. https://doi.org/10.1038/227710a0.

39 Passmore, L.A. and Coller, J. (2022). Roles of mRNA poly(A) tails in regulation of eukaryotic gene expression. *Nat. Rev. Mol. Cell Biol.* 23 (2): 93–106. https://doi.org/10.1038/s41580-021-00417-y.

40 Kozak, M. (1984). Compilation and analysis of sequences upstream from the translational start site in eukaryotic mRNAs. *Nucleic Acids Res.* 12 (2): 857–872. https://doi.org/10.1093/nar/12.2.857.

41 Gebre, M.S., Rauch, S., Roth, N. et al. (2022). Optimization of non-coding regions for a non-modified mRNA COVID-19 vaccine. *Nature* 601 (7893): 410–414. https://doi.org/10.1038/s41586-021-04231-6.

42 Holtkamp, S., Kreiter, S., Selmi, A. et al. (2006). Modification of antigen-encoding RNA increases stability, translational efficacy, and T-cell stimulatory capacity of dendritic cells. *Blood* 108 (13): 4009–4017. https://doi.org/10.1182/blood-2006-04-015024.

43 Orlandini von Niessen, A.G., Poleganov, M.A., Rechner, C. et al. (2019). Improving mRNA-based therapeutic gene delivery by expression-augmenting 3′ UTRs identified by cellular library screening. *Mol. Ther.* 27 (4): 824–836. https://doi.org/10.1016/j.ymthe.2018.12.011.

44 Johanning, F.W., Conry, R.M., LoBuglio, A.F. et al. (1995). A Sindbis virus mRNA polynucleotide vector achieves prolonged and high level heterologous gene expression in vivo. *Nucleic Acids Res.* 23 (9): 1495–1501. https://doi.org/10.1093/nar/23.9.1495.

45 Zhou, X., Berglund, P., Rhodes, G. et al. (1994). Self-replicating semliki forest virus RNA as recombinant vaccine. *Vaccine* 12 (16): 1510–1514. https://doi.org/10.1016/0264-410x(94)90074-4.

46 Hsu, M.T. and Coca-Prados, M. (1979). Electron microscopic evidence for the circular form of RNA in the cytoplasm of eukaryotic cells. *Nature* 280 (5720): 339–340. https://doi.org/10.1038/280339a0.

47 Sanger, H.L., Klotz, G., Riesner, D. et al. (1976). Viroids are single-stranded covalently closed circular RNA molecules existing as highly base-paired rod-like structures. *Proc. Natl. Acad. Sci. U. S. A.* 73 (11): 3852–3856. https://doi.org/10.1073/pnas.73.11.3852.

48 Wesselhoeft, R.A., Kowalski, P.S., and Anderson, D.G. (2018). Engineering circular RNA for potent and stable translation in eukaryotic cells. *Nat. Commun.* 9 (1): 2629. https://doi.org/10.1038/s41467-018-05096-6.

49 Isaacs, A. and Lindenmann, J. (1957). Virus interference. I. The interferon. *Proc. R. Soc. Lond. Ser. B Biol. Sci.* 147 (927): 258–267. https://doi.org/10.1098/rspb.1957.0048.

50 De Somer, P., Prinzie, A., Denys, P. Jr., et al. (1962). Mechanism of action of interferon. I. Relationship with viral ribonucleic acid. *Virology* 16: 63–70. https://doi.org/10.1016/0042-6822(62)90202-7.

51 Isaacs, A., Cox, R.A., and Rotem, Z. (1963). Foreign nucleic acids as the stimulus to make interferon. *Lancet* 2 (7299): 113–116. https://doi.org/10.1016/s0140-6736(63)92585-6.

52 Alexopoulou, L., Holt, A.C., Medzhitov, R. et al. (2001). Recognition of double-stranded RNA and activation of NF-kappaB by Toll-like receptor 3. *Nature* 413 (6857): 732–738. https://doi.org/10.1038/35099560.

53 Yoneyama, M., Kikuchi, M., Natsukawa, T. et al. (2004). The RNA helicase RIG-I has an essential function in double-stranded RNA-induced innate antiviral responses. *Nat. Immunol.* 5 (7): 730–737. https://doi.org/10.1038/ni1087.

54 Pichlmair, A., Schulz, O., Tan, C.P. et al. (2009). Activation of MDA5 requires higher-order RNA structures generated during virus infection. *J. Virol.* 83 (20): 10761–10769. https://doi.org/10.1128/JVI.00770-09.

55 Diebold, S.S., Kaisho, T., Hemmi, H. et al. (2004). Innate antiviral responses by means of TLR7-mediated recognition of single-stranded RNA. *Science (New York, N.Y.)* 303 (5663): 1529–1531. https://doi.org/10.1126/science.1093616.

56 Heil, F., Hemmi, H., Hochrein, H. et al. (2004). Species-specific recognition of single-stranded RNA via toll-like receptor 7 and 8. *Science (New York, N.Y.)* 303 (5663): 1526–1529. https://doi.org/10.1126/science.1093620.

57 Tanji, H., Ohto, U., Shibata, T. et al. (2015). Toll-like receptor 8 senses degradation products of single-stranded RNA. *Nat. Struct. Mol. Biol.* 22 (2): 109–115. https://doi.org/10.1038/nsmb.2943.

58 Zhang, Z., Ohto, U., Shibata, T. et al. (2016). Structural analysis reveals that toll-like receptor 7 is a dual receptor for guanosine and single-stranded RNA. *Immunity* 45 (4): 737–748. https://doi.org/10.1016/j.immuni.2016.09.011.

59 Devarkar, S.C., Wang, C., Miller, M.T. et al. (2016). Structural basis for m7G recognition and 2′-O-methyl discrimination in capped RNAs by the innate

immune receptor RIG-I. *Proc. Natl. Acad. Sci. U. S. A.* 113 (3): 596–601. https://doi.org/10.1073/pnas.1515152113.
60 Schuberth-Wagner, C., Ludwig, J., Bruder, A.K. et al. (2015). A conserved histidine in the RNA sensor RIG-I controls immune tolerance to N1-2′O-methylated self RNA. *Immunity* 43 (1): 41–51. https://doi.org/10.1016/j.immuni.2015.06.015.
61 Alameh, M.-G. and Weissman, D. (2022). Chapter 7 - Nucleoside modifications of in vitro transcribed mRNA to reduce immunogenicity and improve translation of prophylactic and therapeutic antigens. In: *RNA Therapeutics* (ed. P.H. Giangrande, V. de Franciscis, and J.J. Rossi), 141–169. Academic Press.
62 Mu, X. and Hur, S. (2021). Immunogenicity of in vitro-transcribed RNA. *Acc. Chem. Res.* 54 (21): 4012–4023. https://doi.org/10.1021/acs.accounts.1c00521.
63 Anderson, B.R., Muramatsu, H., Jha, B.K. et al. (2011). Nucleoside modifications in RNA limit activation of 2′-5′-oligoadenylate synthetase and increase resistance to cleavage by RNase L. *Nucleic Acids Res.* 39 (21): 9329–9338. https://doi.org/10.1093/nar/gkr586.
64 Anderson, B.R., Muramatsu, H., Nallagatla, S.R. et al. (2010). Incorporation of pseudouridine into mRNA enhances translation by diminishing PKR activation. *Nucleic Acids Res.* 38 (17): 5884–5892. https://doi.org/10.1093/nar/gkq347.
65 Karikó, K., Buckstein, M., Ni, H. et al. (2005). Suppression of RNA recognition by Toll-like receptors: the impact of nucleoside modification and the evolutionary origin of RNA. *Immunity* 23 (2): 165–175. https://doi.org/10.1016/j.immuni.2005.06.008.
66 Durbin, A.F., Wang, C., Marcotrigiano, J. et al. (2016). RNAs containing modified nucleotides fail to trigger RIG-I conformational changes for innate immune signaling. *mBio* 7 (5): e00833-16. https://doi.org/10.1128/mBio.00833-16.
67 Andries, O., Mc Cafferty, S., De Smedt, S.C. et al. (2015). N(1)-methylpseudouridine-incorporated mRNA outperforms pseudouridine-incorporated mRNA by providing enhanced protein expression and reduced immunogenicity in mammalian cell lines and mice. *J. Control. Release* 217: 337–344. https://doi.org/10.1016/j.jconrel.2015.08.051.
68 Karikó, K., Muramatsu, H., Welsh, F.A. et al. (2008). Incorporation of pseudouridine into mRNA yields superior nonimmunogenic vector with increased translational capacity and biological stability. *Mol. Ther.* 16 (11): 1833–1840. https://doi.org/10.1038/mt.2008.200.
69 Morais, P., Adachi, H., and Yu, Y.T. (2021). The critical contribution of pseudouridine to mRNA COVID-19 vaccines. *Front. Cell Dev. Biol.* 9: 789427. https://doi.org/10.3389/fcell.2021.789427.
70 Bangham, A.D. and Horne, R.W. (1964). Negative staining of phospholipids and their structural modification by surface-active agents as observed in the electron microscope. *J. Mol. Biol.* 8 (5): 660–668. https://doi.org/10.1016/S0022-2836(64)80115-7.
71 Bangham, A.D., Standish, M.M., Watkins, J.C. et al. (1967). The diffusion of ions from a phospholipid model membrane system. *Protoplasma* 63 (1): 183–187. 10.1007/BF01248030 .

72 Cullis, P.R. and de Kruijff, B. (1979). Lipid polymorphism and the functional roles of lipids in biological membranes. *Biochim. Biophys. Acta* 559 (4): 399–420. https://doi.org/10.1016/0304-4157(79)90012-1.

73 Papahadjopoulos, D., Mayhew, E., Poste, G. et al. (1974). Incorporation of lipid vesicles by mammalian cells provides a potential method for modifying cell behaviour. *Nature* 252 (5479): 163–166. https://doi.org/10.1038/252163a0.

74 Papahadjopoulos, D., Poste, G., and Schaeffer, B.E. (1973). Fusion of mammalian cells by unilamellar lipid vesicles: influence of lipid surface charge, fluidity and cholesterol. *Biochim. Biophys. Acta Biomembr.* 323 (1): 23–42. https://doi.org/10.1016/0005-2736(73)90429-X.

75 Papahadjopoulos, D., Poste, G., Schaeffer, B.E. et al. (1974). Membrane fusion and molecular segregation in phospholipid vesicles. *Biochim. Biophys. Acta Biomembr.* 352 (1): 10–28. https://doi.org/10.1016/0005-2736(74)90175-8.

76 Papahadjopoulos, D., Vail, W.J., Jacobson, K. et al. (1975). Cochleate lipid cylinders: formation by fusion of unilamellar lipid vesicles. *Biochim. Biophys. Acta* 394 (3): 483–491. https://doi.org/10.1016/0005-2736(75)90299-0.

77 Deamer, D.W. and Bramhall, J. (1986). Permeability of lipid bilayers to water and ionic solutes. *Chem. Phys. Lipids* 40 (2–4): 167–188. https://doi.org/10.1016/0009-3084(86)90069-1.

78 Cullis, P.R. and Hope, M.J. (1978). Effects of fusogenic agent on membrane structure of erythrocyte ghosts and the mechanism of membrane fusion. *Nature* 271 (5646): 672–674. https://doi.org/10.1038/271672a0.

79 Cullis, P.R., Hope, M.J., Bally, M.B. et al. (1997). Influence of pH gradients on the transbilayer transport of drugs, lipids, peptides and metal ions into large unilamellar vesicles. *Biochim. Biophys. Acta* 1331 (2): 187–211.

80 Nicolau, C. and Gregoriadis, G. (1998). Demetrios Papahadjopoulos (1934-98). *Nature* 396 (6707): 118. https://doi.org/10.1038/24052.

81 Sessa, G. and Weissmann, G. (1970). Incorporation of lysozyme into liposomes: a model for structure-linked latency. *J. Biol. Chem.* 245 (13): 3295–3301. https://doi.org/10.1016/S0021-9258(18)62994-1.

82 Gregoriadis, G., Leathwood, P.D., and Ryman, B.E. (1971). Enzyme entrapment in liposomes. *FEBS Lett.* 14 (2): 95–99. https://doi.org/10.1016/0014-5793(71)80109-6.

83 Gregoriadis, G. and Ryman, B.E. (1972). Fate of protein-containing liposomes injected into rats. *Eur. J. Biochem.* 24 (3): 485–491. https://doi.org/10.1111/j.1432-1033.1972.tb19710.x.

84 Gregoriadis, G. and Ryman, B.E. (1972). Lysosomal localization of β-fructofuranosidase-containing liposomes injected into rats. Some implications in the treatment of genetic disorders. *Biochem. J.* 129 (1): 123–133. https://doi.org/10.1042/bj1290123.

85 Hope, M.J., Bally, M.B., Webb, G. et al. (1985). Production of large unilamellar vesicles by a rapid extrusion procedure: characterization of size distribution, trapped volume and ability to maintain a membrane potential. *Biochim. Biophys. Acta* 812 (1): 55–65. https://doi.org/10.1016/0005-2736(85)90521-8.

86 Madden, T.D., Harrigan, P.R., Tai, L.C. et al. (1990). The accumulation of drugs within large unilamellar vesicles exhibiting a proton gradient: a survey. *Chem. Phys. Lipids* 53 (1): 37–46. https://doi.org/10.1016/0009-3084(90)90131-a.

87 Mayer, L., Bally, M., and Cullis, P. (1986). Uptake of adriamycin into large unilamellar vesicles in response to a pH gradient. *Biochim. Biophys. Acta* 857 (1): 123–126.

88 Gregoriadis, G. and Davis, C. (1979). Stability of liposomes in vivo and in vitro is promoted by their cholesterol content and the presence of blood cells. *Biochem. Biophys. Res. Commun.* 89 (4): 1287–1293. https://doi.org/10.1016/0006-291x(79)92148-x.

89 Papahadjopoulos, D., Jacobson, K., Nir, S. et al. (1973). Phase transitions in phospholipid vesicles. Fluorescence polarization and permeability measurements concerning the effect of temperature and cholesterol. *Biochim. Biophys. Acta* 311 (3): 330–348. https://doi.org/10.1016/0005-2736(73)90314-3.

90 Allen, T.M. and Chonn, A. (1987). Large unilamellar liposomes with low uptake into the reticuloendothelial system. *FEBS Lett.* 223 (1): 42–46. https://doi.org/10.1016/0014-5793(87)80506-9.

91 Klibanov, A.L., Maruyama, K., Torchilin, V.P. et al. (1990). Amphipathic polyethyleneglycols effectively prolong the circulation time of liposomes. *FEBS Lett.* 268 (1): 235–237. https://doi.org/10.1016/0014-5793(90)81016-H.

92 Dimitriadis, G.J. (1978). Translation of rabbit globin mRNA introduced by liposomes into mouse lymphocytes. *Nature* 274 (5674): 923–924. https://doi.org/10.1038/274923a0.

93 Ostro, M.J., Giacomoni, D., Lavelle, D.O.N. et al. (1978). Evidence for translation of rabbit globin mRNA after liposomemediated insertion into a human cell line. *Nature* 274 (5674): 921–923. https://doi.org/10.1038/274921a0.

94 Felgner, P.L., Gadek, T.R., Holm, M. et al. (1987). Lipofection: a highly efficient, lipid-mediated DNA-transfection procedure. *Proc. Natl. Acad. Sci. U. S. A.* 84 (21): 7413–7417. https://doi.org/10.1073/pnas.84.21.7413.

95 Malone, R.W., Felgner, P.L., and Verma, I.M. (1989). Cationic liposome-mediated RNA transfection. *Proc. Natl. Acad. Sci. U. S. A.* 86 (16): 6077–6081. https://doi.org/10.1073/pnas.86.16.6077.

96 Hafez, I.M., Maurer, N., and Cullis, P.R. (2001). On the mechanism whereby cationic lipids promote intracellular delivery of polynucleic acids. *Gene Ther.* 8 (15): 1188–1196. https://doi.org/10.1038/sj.gt.3301506.

97 Zelphati, O. and Szoka, F.C. Jr., (1996). Mechanism of oligonucleotide release from cationic liposomes. *Proc. Natl. Acad. Sci. U. S. A.* 93 (21): 11493–11498. https://doi.org/10.1073/pnas.93.21.11493.

98 Chonn, A. and Cullis, P.R. (1998). Recent advances in liposome technologies and their applications for systemic gene delivery. *Adv. Drug Deliv. Rev.* 30 (1): 73–83. https://doi.org/10.1016/S0169-409X(97)00108-7.

99 Campbell, P.I. (1983). Toxicity of some charged lipids used in liposome preparations. *Cytobios* 37 (145): 21–26.

100 Filion, M.C. and Phillips, N.C. (1997). Toxicity and immunomodulatory activity of liposomal vectors formulated with cationic lipids toward immune effector cells. *Biochim. Biophys. Acta* 1329 (2): 345–356. https://doi.org/10.1016/S0005-2736(97)00126-0.

101 Bailey, A.L. and Cullis, P.R. (1994). Modulation of membrane fusion by asymmetric transbilayer distributions of amino lipids. *Biochemistry* 33 (42): 12573–12580. https://doi.org/10.1021/bi00208a007.

102 Semple, S.C., Klimuk, S.K., Harasym, T. et al. (1998). High efficiency encapsulation of charged therapeutic agents in lipid vesicles. WO/1998/051278, filed 14 May 1998.

103 Leung, A.K.K., Hafez, I.M., Baoukina, S. et al. (2012). Lipid nanoparticles containing siRNA synthesized by microfluidic mixing exhibit an electron-dense nanostructured core. *J. Phys. Chem. C* 116 (34): 18440–18450. https://doi.org/10.1021/jp303267y.

104 Semple, S.C., Klimuk, S.K., Harasym, T.O. et al. (2001). Efficient encapsulation of antisense oligonucleotides in lipid vesicles using ionizable aminolipids: formation of novel small multilamellar vesicle structures. *Biochim. Biophys. Acta* 1510 (1–2): 152–166. https://doi.org/10.1016/s0005-2736(00)00343-6.

105 Semple, S.C., Akinc, A., Chen, J. et al. (2010). Rational design of cationic lipids for siRNA delivery. *Nat. Biotechnol.* 28 (2): 172–176. https://doi.org/10.1038/nbt.1602.

106 Zimmermann, T.S., Lee, A.C., Akinc, A. et al. (2006). RNAi-mediated gene silencing in non-human primates. *Nature* 441 (7089): 111–114. https://doi.org/10.1038/nature04688.

107 Jayaraman, M., Ansell, S.M., Mui, B.L. et al. (2012). Maximizing the potency of siRNA lipid nanoparticles for hepatic gene silencing in vivo. *Angew. Chem. Int. Ed. Eng.* 51 (34): 8529–8533. https://doi.org/10.1002/anie.201203263.

108 Adams, D., Gonzalez-Duarte, A., O'Riordan, W.D. et al. (2018). Patisiran, an RNAi therapeutic, for hereditary transthyretin amyloidosis. *N. Engl. J. Med.* 379 (1): 11–21. https://doi.org/10.1056/NEJMoa1716153.

109 Maier, M.A., Jayaraman, M., Matsuda, S. et al. (2013). Biodegradable lipids enabling rapidly eliminated lipid nanoparticles for systemic delivery of RNAi therapeutics. *Mol. Ther.* 21 (8): 1570–1578.

110 Ansell, S.M. and Du, X. (2016). Lipid and lipid nanoparticle formulation for delivery of nucleic acids. US Patent 10,166,298 B2, filed 28 October 2016.

111 Hassett, K.J., Benenato, K.E., Jacquinet, E. et al. (2019). Optimization of lipid nanoparticles for intramuscular administration of mRNA vaccines. *Mol. Ther. Nucleic Acids* 15: 1–11. https://doi.org/10.1016/j.omtn.2019.01.013.

112 Akinc, A., Goldberg, M., Qin, J. et al. (2009). Development of lipidoid-siRNA formulations for systemic delivery to the liver. *Mol. Ther.* 17 (5): 872–879. https://doi.org/10.1038/mt.2009.36.

113 Akinc, A., Zumbuehl, A., Goldberg, M. et al. (2008). A combinatorial library of lipid-like materials for delivery of RNAi therapeutics. *Nat. Biotechnol.* 26 (5): 561–569. https://doi.org/10.1038/nbt1402.

114 Love, K.T., Mahon, K.P., Levins, C.G. et al. (2010). Lipid-like materials for low-dose, in vivo gene silencing. *Proc. Natl. Acad. Sci. U. S. A.* 107 (5): 1864–1869. https://doi.org/10.1073/pnas.0910603106.

115 Maurer, N., Wong, K.F., Stark, H. et al. (2001). Spontaneous entrapment of polynucleotides upon electrostatic interaction with ethanol-destabilized cationic liposomes. *Biophys. J.* 80 (5): 2310–2326. https://doi.org/10.1016/S0006-3495(01)76202-9.

116 Mui, B.L., Tam, Y.K., Jayaraman, M. et al. (2013). Influence of polyethylene glycol lipid desorption rates on pharmacokinetics and pharmacodynamics of siRNA lipid nanoparticles. *Mol. Ther. Nucleic Acids* 2 (12): e139. https://doi.org/10.1038/mtna.2013.66.

117 Holland, J.W., Hui, C., Cullis, P.R. et al. (1996). Poly(ethylene glycol)–lipid conjugates regulate the calcium-induced fusion of liposomes composed of phosphatidylethanolamine and phosphatidylserine. *Biochemistry* 35 (8): 2618–2624. https://doi.org/10.1021/bi952000v.

118 Judge, A., McClintock, K., Phelps, J.R. et al. (2006). Hypersensitivity and loss of disease site targeting caused by antibody responses to PEGylated liposomes. *Mol. Ther.* 13 (2): 328–337. https://doi.org/10.1016/j.ymthe.2005.09.014.

119 Semple, S.C., Harasym, T.O., Clow, K.A. et al. (2005). Immunogenicity and rapid blood clearance of liposomes containing polyethylene glycol-lipid conjugates and nucleic acid. *J. Pharmacol. Exp. Ther.* 312 (3): 1020–1026. https://doi.org/10.1124/jpet.104.078113.

120 Dams, E.T., Laverman, P., Oyen, W.J. et al. (2000). Accelerated blood clearance and altered biodistribution of repeated injections of sterically stabilized liposomes. *J. Pharmacol. Exp. Ther.* 292 (3): 1071–1079. https://www.ncbi.nlm.nih.gov/pubmed/10688625.

121 Ambegia, E., Ansell, S., Cullis, P. et al. (2005). Stabilized plasmid–lipid particles containing PEG-diacylglycerols exhibit extended circulation lifetimes and tumor selective gene expression. *Biochim. Biophys. Acta Biomembr.* 1669 (2): 155–163. https://doi.org/10.1016/j.bbamem.2005.02.001.

122 Heyes, J., Hall, K., Tailor, V. et al. (2006). Synthesis and characterization of novel poly (ethylene glycol)-lipid conjugates suitable for use in drug delivery. *J. Control. Release* 112 (2): 280–290. https://doi.org/10.1016/j.jconrel.2006.02.012.

123 Batzri, S. and Korn, E.D. (1973). Single bilayer liposomes prepared without sonication. *Biochim. Biophys. Acta* 298 (4): 1015–1019. https://doi.org/10.1016/0005-2736(73)90408-2.

124 Jeffs, L.B., Palmer, L.R., Ambegia, E.G. et al. (2005). A scalable, extrusion-free method for efficient liposomal encapsulation of plasmid DNA. *Pharm. Res.* 22 (3): 362–372. https://doi.org/10.1007/s11095-004-1873-z.

125 Belliveau, N.M., Huft, J., Lin, P.J. et al. (2012). Microfluidic synthesis of highly potent limit-size lipid nanoparticles for in vivo delivery of siRNA. *Mol. Ther. Nucleic Acids* 1: e37. https://doi.org/10.1038/mtna.2012.28.

126 Evers, M.J.W., Kulkarni, J.A., van der Meel, R. et al. (2018). State-of-the-art design and rapid-mixing production techniques of lipid nanoparticles for nucleic acid delivery. *Small Methods* 2 (9): 1700375. https://doi.org/10.1002/smtd.201700375.

127 Kulkarni, J.A., Cullis, P.R., and van der Meel, R. (2018). Lipid nanoparticles enabling gene therapies: from concepts to clinical utility. *Nucleic Acid Ther.* 28 (3): 146–157. https://doi.org/10.1089/nat.2018.0721.

128 Semple, S.C., Leone, R., Barbosa, C.J. et al. (2022). Lipid nanoparticle delivery systems to enable mRNA-based therapeutics. *Pharmaceutics* 14 (2): 398. https://doi.org/10.3390/pharmaceutics14020398.

129 Akinc, A., Maier, M.A., Manoharan, M. et al. (2019). The Onpattro story and the clinical translation of nanomedicines containing nucleic acid-based drugs. *Nat. Nanotechnol.* 14 (12): 1084–1087. https://doi.org/10.1038/s41565-019-0591-y.

130 Wolff, J.A., Malone, R.W., Williams, P. et al. (1990). Direct gene transfer into mouse muscle in vivo. *Science (New York, N.Y.)* 247 (4949 Pt 1): 1465–1468. https://doi.org/10.1126/science.1690918.

131 Jirikowski, G.F., Sanna, P.P., Maciejewski-Lenoir, D. et al. (1992). Reversal of diabetes insipidus in Brattleboro rats: intrahypothalamic injection of vasopressin mRNA. *Science (New York, N.Y.)* 255 (5047): 996–998. https://doi.org/10.1126/science.1546298.

132 Martinon, F., Krishnan, S., Lenzen, G. et al. (1993). Induction of virus-specific cytotoxic T lymphocytes in vivo by liposome-entrapped mRNA. *Eur. J. Immunol.* 23 (7): 1719–1722. https://doi.org/10.1002/eji.1830230749.

133 Conry, R.M., LoBuglio, A.F., Wright, M. et al. (1995). Characterization of a messenger RNA polynucleotide vaccine vector. *Cancer Res.* 55 (7): 1397–1400. https://www.ncbi.nlm.nih.gov/pubmed/7882341.

134 Heiser, A., Coleman, D., Dannull, J. et al. (2002). Autologous dendritic cells transfected with prostate-specific antigen RNA stimulate CTL responses against metastatic prostate tumors. *J. Clin. Invest.* 109 (3): 409–417. https://doi.org/10.1172/JCI14364.

135 Su, Z., Dannull, J., Heiser, A. et al. (2003). Immunological and clinical responses in metastatic renal cancer patients vaccinated with tumor RNA-transfected dendritic cells. *Cancer Res.* 63 (9): 2127–2133. https://www.ncbi.nlm.nih.gov/pubmed/12727829.

136 Weide, B., Carralot, J.P., Reese, A. et al. (2008). Results of the first phase I/II clinical vaccination trial with direct injection of mRNA. *J. Immunother.* 31 (2): 180–188. https://doi.org/10.1097/CJI.0b013e31815ce501.

137 Weide, B., Pascolo, S., Scheel, B. et al. (2009). Direct injection of protamine-protected mRNA: results of a phase 1/2 vaccination trial in metastatic melanoma patients. *J. Immunother.* 32 (5): 498–507. https://doi.org/10.1097/CJI.0b013e3181a00068.

138 Kreiter, S., Selmi, A., Diken, M. et al. (2010). Intranodal vaccination with naked antigen-encoding RNA elicits potent prophylactic and therapeutic antitumoral immunity. *Cancer Res.* 70 (22): 9031–9040. https://doi.org/10.1158/0008-5472.Can-10-0699.

139 Sahin, U., Derhovanessian, E., Miller, M. et al. (2017). Personalized RNA mutanome vaccines mobilize poly-specific therapeutic immunity against cancer. *Nature* 547 (7662): 222. https://doi.org/10.1038/nature23003.

140 Kranz, L.M., Diken, M., Haas, H. et al. (2016). Systemic RNA delivery to dendritic cells exploits antiviral defence for cancer immunotherapy. *Nature* 534 (7607): 396–401. https://doi.org/10.1038/nature18300.

141 Sahin, U., Oehm, P., Derhovanessian, E. et al. (2020). An RNA vaccine drives immunity in checkpoint-inhibitor-treated melanoma. *Nature* 585 (7823): 107–112. https://doi.org/10.1038/s41586-020-2537-9.

142 Basha, G., Novobrantseva, T.I., Rosin, N. et al. (2011). Influence of cationic lipid composition on gene silencing properties of lipid nanoparticle formulations of siRNA in antigen-presenting cells. *Mol. Ther.* 19 (12): 2186–2200. https://doi.org/10.1038/mt.2011.190.

143 Leuschner, F., Dutta, P., Gorbatov, R. et al. (2011). Therapeutic siRNA silencing in inflammatory monocytes in mice. *Nat. Biotechnol.* 29 (11): 1005–1010. https://doi.org/10.1038/nbt.1989.

144 Geall, A.J., Verma, A., Otten, G.R. et al. (2012). Nonviral delivery of self-amplifying RNA vaccines. *Proc. Natl. Acad. Sci. U. S. A.* 109 (36): 14604–14609. https://doi.org/10.1073/pnas.1209367109.

145 Pardi, N., Tuyishime, S., Muramatsu, H. et al. (2015). Expression kinetics of nucleoside-modified mRNA delivered in lipid nanoparticles to mice by various routes. *J. Control. Release* 217: 345–351. https://doi.org/10.1016/j.jconrel.2015.08.007.

146 Awasthi, S., Hook, L.M., Pardi, N. et al. (2019). Nucleoside-modified mRNA encoding HSV-2 glycoproteins C, D, and E prevents clinical and subclinical genital herpes. *Sci. Immunol.* 4 (39): https://doi.org/10.1126/sciimmunol.aaw7083.

147 Pardi, N., Hogan, M.J., Naradikian, M.S. et al. (2018). Nucleoside-modified mRNA vaccines induce potent T follicular helper and germinal center B cell responses. *J. Exp. Med.* 215 (6): 1571–1588. https://doi.org/10.1084/jem.20171450.

148 Pardi, N., Hogan, M.J., Pelc, R.S. et al. (2017). Zika virus protection by a single low-dose nucleoside-modified mRNA vaccination. *Nature* 543 (7644): 248–251. https://doi.org/10.1038/nature21428.

149 Pardi, N., LaBranche, C.C., Ferrari, G. et al. (2019). Characterization of HIV-1 nucleoside-modified mRNA vaccines in rabbits and rhesus macaques. *Mol. Ther. Nucleic Acids* 15: 36–47. https://doi.org/10.1016/j.omtn.2019.03.003.

150 Pfizer. (2022). Pfizer initiates phase 3 study of mRNA-based influenza vaccine. https://www.pfizer.com/news/press-release/press-release-detail/pfizer-initiates-phase-3-study-mrna-based-influenza-vaccine (accessed 9 November 2022).

151 Aldrich, C., Leroux-Roels, I., Huang, K.B. et al. (2021). Proof-of-concept of a low-dose unmodified mRNA-based rabies vaccine formulated with lipid nanoparticles in human volunteers: a phase 1 trial. *Vaccine* 39 (8): 1310–1318. https://doi.org/10.1016/j.vaccine.2020.12.070.

152 Lutz, J., Lazzaro, S., Habbeddine, M. et al. (2017). Unmodified mRNA in LNPs constitutes a competitive technology for prophylactic vaccines. *NPJ Vaccines* 2: 29. https://doi.org/10.1038/s41541-017-0032-6.

153 Bahl, K., Senn, J.J., Yuzhakov, O. et al. (2017). Preclinical and clinical demonstration of immunogenicity by mRNA vaccines against H10N8 and H7N9 influenza viruses. *Mol. Ther.* 25 (6): 1316–1327. https://doi.org/10.1016/j.ymthe.2017.03.035.

154 Feldman, R.A., Fuhr, R., Smolenov, I. et al. (2019). mRNA vaccines against H10N8 and H7N9 influenza viruses of pandemic potential are immunogenic and well tolerated in healthy adults in phase 1 randomized clinical trials. *Vaccine* 37 (25): 3326–3334. https://doi.org/10.1016/j.vaccine.2019.04.074.

155 Verbeke, R., Lentacker, I., De Smedt, S.C. et al. (2021). The dawn of mRNA vaccines: the COVID-19 case. *J. Control. Release* 333: 511–520. https://doi.org/10.1016/j.jconrel.2021.03.043.

156 CureVac. (2021). CureVac provides update on phase 2b/3 trial of first-generation COVID-19 vaccine candidate, CVnCoV. https://www.curevac.com/en/curevac-provides-update-on-phase-2b-3-trial-of-first-generation-covid-19-vaccine-candidate-cvncov/ (accessed 9 November 2022).

157 Arcturus. (2022). Arcturus announces self-amplifying COVID-19 mRNA vaccine candidate ARCT-154 meets primary efficacy endpoint in phase 3 study. https://ir.arcturusrx.com/news-releases/news-release-details/arcturus-announces-self-amplifying-covid-19-mrna-vaccine (accessed 9 November 2022).

158 Providence. (2022). Providence announces positive top-line data from phase 2 primary immunization trial of its mRNA vaccine candidate PTX-COVID19-B in adults. https://providencetherapeutics.com/press-details/providence-announces-positive-top-line-data-from-phase-2-primary-immunization-trial-of-its-mrna-vaccine-candidate-ptx-covid19-b-in-adults.html (accessed 9 November 2022).

159 Low, J. G., de Alwis, R., Chen, S., et al. (2021). A phase 1/2 randomized, double-blinded, placebo controlled ascending dose trial to assess the safety, tolerability and immunogenicity of ARCT-021 in healthy adults. *medRxiv*: 2021.2007.2001.21259831. https://doi.org/10.1101/2021.07.01.21259831

160 Pollock, K.M., Cheeseman, H.M., Szubert, A.J. et al. (2022). Safety and immunogenicity of a self-amplifying RNA vaccine against COVID-19: COVAC1, a phase I, dose-ranging trial. *EClinicalMedicine* 44: 101262. https://doi.org/10.1016/j.eclinm.2021.101262.

161 Sittplangkoon, C., Alameh, M.G., Weissman, D. et al. (2022). mRNA vaccine with unmodified uridine induces robust type I interferon-dependent anti-tumor immunity in a melanoma model. *Front. Immunol.* 13: 983000. https://doi.org/10.3389/fimmu.2022.983000.

162 Alameh, M.G., Tombacz, I., Bettini, E. et al. (2021). Lipid nanoparticles enhance the efficacy of mRNA and protein subunit vaccines by inducing robust T follicular helper cell and humoral responses. *Immunity* 54 (12): 2877–2892 e2877. https://doi.org/10.1016/j.immuni.2021.11.001.

163 Ndeupen, S., Qin, Z., Jacobsen, S. et al. (2021). The mRNA-LNP platform's lipid nanoparticle component used in preclinical vaccine studies is highly inflammatory. *iScience* 24 (12): 103479. https://doi.org/10.1016/j.isci.2021.103479.

164 Tahtinen, S., Tong, A.J., Himmels, P. et al. (2022). IL-1 and IL-1ra are key regulators of the inflammatory response to RNA vaccines. *Nat. Immunol.* 23 (4): 532–542. https://doi.org/10.1038/s41590-022-01160-y.

165 Verbeke, R., Hogan, M.J., Loré, K. et al. (2022). Innate immune mechanisms of mRNA vaccines. *Immunity* 55 (11): 1993–2005. https://doi.org/10.1016/j.immuni.2022.10.014.

2

Immune Responses to mRNA Vaccine

Jean-Yves Exposito†, *Claire Monge*†, *Danielle C. Arruda*†, *and Bernard Verrier*

Laboratoire de Biologie Tissulaire et d'Ingénierie Thérapeutique (LBTI), UMR CNRS 5305, Universite Lyon 1, Institut de Biologie et Chimie des Protéines, 7 passage du Vercors, 69367 Lyon Cedex 07, France

2.1 Introduction

A robust and durable adaptive immune response to a vaccine highly depends on an efficient innate response involving immune signaling and proinflammatory signals. In most of the vaccines, the stimulation of the adaptive immunity is induced by a pathogen-specific antigen and further signals for T-cell activation are triggered by an adjuvant or the vaccine components. The balance between activation and overactivation of the innate immune system has to be carefully thought to control immunogenicity and reactogenicity. The SARS-CoV-2 pandemic urged the development of mRNA-based vaccines, notably the BNT162b2 (Pfizer–BioNTech) and the mRNA-1273 (Moderna). These vaccines are both based on a lipid nanoparticle (LNP) carrying mRNA molecules coding for a stabilized SARS-CoV-2 spike protein (S protein).

The reactogenicity reported for these vaccines is characterized by local and systemic inflammation expressed by symptoms such as pain, swelling, and redness at the injection site as well as transient fever or chills and fatigue after both prime and boost vaccinations [1, 2].

The immunogenicity relies mainly on the production of the S protein and the subsequent humoral and cellular adaptive responses against it. Indeed, after intramuscular (IM) administration, LNPs can either be internalized by muscle cells or by antigen-presenting cells (like dendritic cells [DCs]) near the injection sites or directly within the draining lymph nodes (LNs, lateral axillary lymph node if injection into the deltoid muscle) for LNPs traveling as free particles. After production by the translational machinery, the S protein could either be presented through MHC class I (cross-presentation) or be presented through MHC class II molecules according to their posttranslational modifications [3]. When transported through the proteasome, the S proteins are degraded, and the produced antigenic peptides are transported to the endoplasmic reticulum where they will be loaded into MHC class I receptor for

† These authors contributed equally to this work.

Trends in mRNA Vaccine Research, First Edition. Edited by Gabor Tamas Szabo and Norbert Pardi.

presentation to $CD8^+$ T cells. Alternatively, the binding of viral peptides to MHC class II molecules will allow a presentation to $CD4^+$ T cells.

For instance, BNT162b2 mRNA vaccine injection has been shown to induce robust germinal center reactions in humans, triggering robust humoral immunity [4]. Besides, in the context of COVID-19, numerous clinical studies reported the induction of potent binding and neutralizing anti-spike antibodies together with polyspecific cellular immune response [5]. However, several key observations have been made during the last two years concerning the importance of adjuvant effects induced by each vaccine component, such as mRNA itself and ingredients of the LNP. Indeed, the activation of immune pathways by lipid components of LNP is of interest as it could depend on lipid origins or structure when coupled to polyethylene glycol (PEG) [see part 2.6]. The self-adjuvanticity of mRNA vaccine will rely on different immune mechanisms, from the binding of vaccine components to immune receptors to the activation of immune defenses by specific cell death pathways [6].

2.2 Innate Sensing of RNA Molecules

The innate immunity acts as a first line of defense against pathogens, its activation being dependent on the binding of pathogen-associated molecular patterns (PAMPs) through pattern recognition receptors (PRRs) as already reviewed [7, 8]. The mRNAs used in vaccines are produced *in vitro* (*in vitro* transcribed mRNAs, IVT–mRNAs), and we will first summarize the different innate immunity pathways activated by nonself RNAs (single-stranded RNA [ssRNA] and double-stranded RNA [dsRNA]). An illustration of the major RNA sensing by PRRs and the subsequent pathways is shown in Figure 2.1.

After internalization, a ssRNA is recognized as a PAMP and can be sensed by multiple innate sensors from the PRR family located in the endosome membrane or in the cytosolic compartment. Endosomal sensors of nonself ssRNA are toll-like receptors (TLRs)7 and 13 in mice and TLR7 and TLR8 in humans. In humans, TLR7/TLR8 binds short ssRNAs and nucleosides after RNA degradation by RNase T2 and RNase 2 into the endolysosome [9]. However, due to the existence of a secondary structure in the mRNA molecules or the presence of dsRNA contaminants, other sensors could be activated such as the dsRNA sensor TLR3 [10], also located in the endosome and sensing dsRNAs longer than 40–50 bp [11]. TLRs are expressed in all subtypes of innate immune cells including DCs, macrophages, monocytes, and natural killer cells. Based on the interaction between TLRs and adapter molecules, different signaling pathways can be activated. The stimulation of TLR7/8 activates the myeloid differentiation marker 88 (MyD88)-dependent signaling pathway and results in the expression of proinflammatory cytokines through nuclear factor κB (NF-κB) and activator protein 1 (AP-1) transcription factors and expression of type I interferon (IFN) through IFN regulatory factor 7 (IRF7). The stimulation of TLR3 activates the toll-interleukin-1 receptor domain-containing protein-inducing type I IFN (TRIF)-dependent pathways leading to IRF3 activation, but it is also involved in IRF7 and NF-κB pathways.

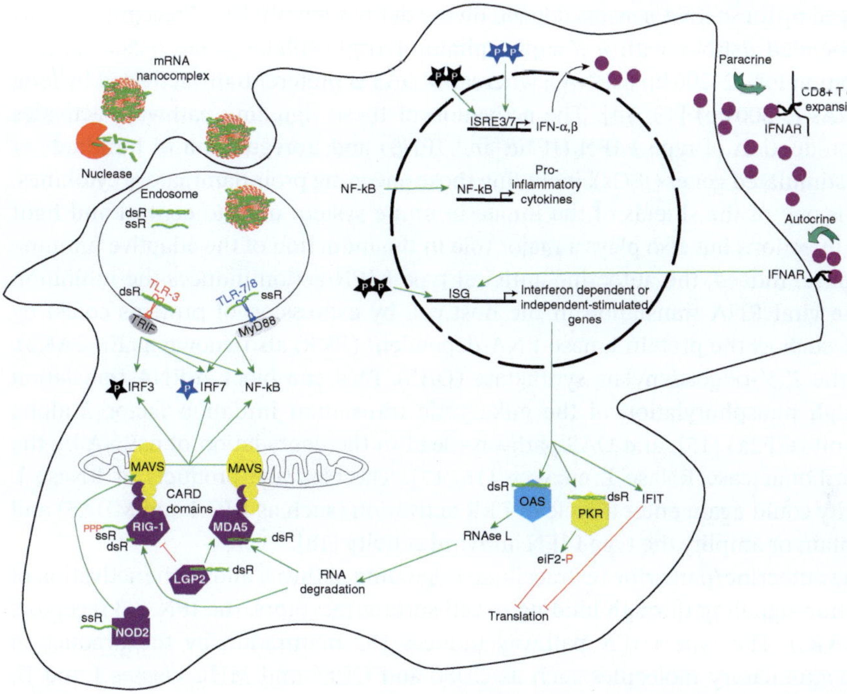

Figure 2.1 From RNA sensing to innate immunity activation. After injection, some mRNA-complexes are uptaken by cells, and will engage different pathways of sensing into the endosome, and in the cytosol after endosomal escape. For more simplicity, only ssRNA and dsRNA sensing are represented in this illustration. Into the endosomal compartment dsRNA and ssRNA are sensed by TLR3 and TLR-7/8 leading to the activation of IFN-α and β genes and pro-inflammatory cytokines genes. Inside the cytosol, other PRR members (RIG-1, MDA5, and NOD2) of the innate immunity pathway are activated by different patterns of ssRNA and dsRNA and after association with MAVS by CARD domain interactions (RIG-I and MDA5) will also activate ISRE3/7 and NF-κB responsive genes. IFN production will be involved in paracrine (CD8$^+$ T cell expansion) and autocrine (activation of ISGs) pathways upon activation of IFNAR receptors. The autocrine pathways will activate some PRR-sensing RNA motifs that might contribute to RNA degradation (OAS) or inhibition of the translation machinery (PKR and IFIT). The production of cytokines and chemokines will lead to antigen-presenting cell (APC) activation.

Cytosolic nonself RNA sensors could be components of the inflammasome from the family of the nucleotide oligomerization domain-like receptors (NLRs) and the retinoic acid-inducible gene-I (RIG-I)-like receptors (RLRs). The nucleotide-binding oligomerization domain 2 (NOD2), also called caspase recruitment domain-containing protein 15 (CARD15), recognize ssRNA and leads to the mitochondrial antiviral signaling protein (MAVS) mediated activation of IRF3. Both the melanoma differentiation-associated (MDA) 5 and RIG-I bind to dsRNA [12]. Both activations of the helicases RIG-I and MDA5 induce interaction of the caspase activation and recruitment domain (CARD) with the MAVS, triggering the expression of proinflammatory cytokines. However, the IFN responses induced by these RNA sensors depend on the dsRNA length. RIG-I recognizes short blunt-ended dsRNA with a 5′-diphosphate or triphosphate group (<500 bp, best activation for 22–200 bp dsRNA), whereas MDA5 is preferentially activated by long dsRNAs (>500 bp) [13, 14]. The activation of these signaling pathways activates the production of type I IFN (IFNα and IFNβ) and upregulation of hundreds of IFN-stimulated genes (ISGs), including those encoding proinflammatory cytokines. IFN is one of the shields of the innate immune system used to control and fight viral infections but also plays a major role in the induction of the adaptive immune response. Indeed, the autocrine antiviral type I IFN action induces the inhibition of the viral RNA translation in the host cell by expression of proteins coded by ISGs, such as the protein kinase RNA-dependent (PKR; also known as EIF2AK2), and the 2′,5′-oligoadenylate synthetase (OAS). PKR can block mRNA translation through phosphorylation of the eukaryotic translation initiation factor 2 alpha subunit (eIF2a) [15], and OAS pathways lead to the degradation of dsRNA by the endoribonuclease RNase L enzyme [16, 17]. The cleavage products of RNase L activity could again enter a cycle of PRR activation (such as RIG-I and MDA5) and maintain or amplify the type I IFN antiviral activity [18].

The autocrine/paracrine (extracellular) signaling pathway allows the activation of immune signaling through binding to cell surface receptors, the IFN α/β receptors (IFNARs). The type I IFN pathway induces DC maturation by the production of co-stimulatory molecules such as CD80 and CD86 and MHC classes I and II. Therefore, the balance between activation of type I IFN and translation inhibition is critical for the efficacy and safety of mRNA vaccines. Decreased mRNA sensing by TLRs or RIG-I could be achieved by nucleoside modification and leads to a reduced or abolished recognition of mRNA by the innate immune system [19]. This is the reason why the currently approved mRNA vaccines contain modified nucleosides to limit type I IFN production and subsequent inhibition of translation by avoiding the recognition of mRNA to immune receptors and limiting PKR and OAS activation [20, 21].

2.3 Innate Immune Response to mRNA Vaccines

The entire immune mechanisms behind the innate immune activation are not yet fully and precisely elucidated. Several studies highlighted cellular pathways involved in the initiation of the immune response in humans, mice, and nonhuman primates [22–26]. However, beyond the direct activation of PRRs of innate immune cells by antigens or adjuvants, some clues are emerging, such as the role of cellular mechanisms at the injection site, relying on the activation of several other pathways caused by stress signals, damaged tissues, or cell death [6, 27] and have been understudied. During pyroptosis (a caspase-dependent form of necrosis) and necroptosis (a form of necrosis that is dependent on receptor-interacting protein kinase 3 signaling), the dying cells release damage-associated molecular patterns (DAMPs) that trigger immature DC activation [28].

2.3.1 Innate Immune Response in Humans

The signature of innate immunity response after BNT162b2 vaccine injection has been studied to decipher markers associated with the quality of antibody production. The IFN cascade is an important parameter to monitor in order to characterize the response to mRNA vaccination [23, 29]. No significant increase of type I IFN plasma level was detected in individuals a few days after immunization with the BNT162b2 vaccine, but a significant increase in IFNγ (type II IFN), CXCL10, and IL-5 expression was measured, as well as an upregulation of mature IL-1β in macrophages, especially after the boost. In their study, Bergamaschi et al. showed that the IL-15/IFN-γ signature could be used as an early immune biomarker for the effective development of vaccine-induced humoral responses [29].

By quantifying the frequency of different subsets of immune cells in peripheral blood before and after BNT162b2 mRNA vaccine injection, several correlations were identified between some immune cell dynamics and vaccine response or adverse effects (reactogenicity). For example, natural killer T-like (NKT) cell dynamics were recognized to correlate with high antibody titers and the severity of systemic symptoms [30]. It was also hypothesized that NK cell subsets participate in the production of IFNγ. In addition, an enhanced innate immune response was highlighted after the second immunization (boost) compared to the first immunization (prime) that only induced a modest innate response [23]. In particular, increased levels of circulating IFNγ and enhanced transcriptional signatures of innate immunity and antiviral immunity were described in myeloid cells after the second immunization. Besides, a strong cytokine signature was also found in individuals who recovered from a previous infection, highlighting the involvement of cytokines in the reactivation of immune responses [29]. Interestingly, gene set enrichment analysis also highlighted that the first boost vaccination induced upregulation of TLR signaling, which was not observed after a single injection [23].

These findings show that a robust adaptive response to SARS-CoV-2 mRNA vaccine is built on a sequence of orchestrated innate mechanisms which differ from the dysregulated innate immune responses to SARS-CoV-2 infection [31]. Severe COVID-19 correlates with alterations in the myeloid cell compartment and weak and delayed IFN response, characterizing SARS-CoV-2 by its capacity to circumvent the innate immune response [32, 33]. However, studies have shown that infected cells, and in particular macrophages, use a "suicide technique" (pyroptosis) to stop the viral cycle by inflammasome activation leading to the production of inflammatory cytokines and cell death by pyroptosis [34]. In parallel, it was evidenced in patients with COVID-19 that the S protein itself is recognized as a PAMP and triggers inflammatory signaling [35]. Based on the fact that mRNA vaccines also induce the production of S protein, studies confirmed that commercially available mRNA vaccines induced NLRP3 inflammasome activation and pyroptosis in macrophages of vaccinated individuals (no discrimination between the two brands used) [36]. This NLRP3 activation (inducing the secretion of IL-1 β) was shown to be S-protein dependent and mediated by C-type lectin receptor (CLR), triggering phosphorylation of the spleen tyrosine kinase (SYK) and NF-κB in circulating macrophages.

Even though the innate immunity pathways activated by the majority of vaccines and adjuvants are dependent on TLR activation, some mRNA vaccines ostensibly also use alternative pathways due to the presence of modified nucleotides, although a TLR might sense LNP components, as suggested by Hogan and Pardi [37]. However, these immune pathways and associated cellular mechanisms are difficult to study in humans. Indeed, most of our knowledge on mRNA innate immunity in humans is only performed by analyzing peripheral blood responses (mainly cytokine expression and circulating cell responses), whereas the use of animal models can provide access to more detailed descriptions of immune responses in tissue, in particular lymphoid organs and cells at the injection site. Indeed, after injection, most LNP from the vaccines are expected to migrate through the lymphatic circulation until reaching lymph nodes to initiate the adaptive immune response. Biodistribution studies in mice after IM injection of LNP–mRNA vaccine against influenza virus have shown that there is an mRNA accumulation in other secondary lymphoid organs, such as the spleen, and in the muscle at the injection site [38].

Although the benefit for basic science is tremendous, the prediction or explanation of human immune responses from animal models are still mitigated and have to be taken with caution because innate immune mechanisms in mice, and in particular the type I IFN and IL-1 response, differ from humans [39–41]. Moreover, due to their pathogen-free housing, laboratory mice have a relatively naive immune system thus complicating the prediction and transposition into clinics [42].

2.3.2 Tissue Innate Immune Response in Mice

As an animal model, mice have been extensively used to unravel immune mechanisms induced by mRNA vaccines. Taking advantage of that nucleoside-modified mRNA can drastically reduce unwanted innate immunity activation, improve mRNA stability [43], and allow increased expression of the antigen *in vivo* [44], different studies have shown that a single dose injection of N1-methylpseudouridine-mRNA vaccine protected mice and nonhuman primates against Zika virus infection [45, 46]. Thus, mRNA from BNT162b2 or mRNA-1273 vaccines relies on cytosolic nonself RNA sensors as both contain N1-methylpseudouridine nucleosides. A study about the impact of BNT162b2 vaccine has been performed in mice and identified that immune signaling is mainly initiated by cytosolic components of the inflammasome [25]. In this study, the authors showed that a high dose of BNT162b2 vaccine in mice did not activate TLR2, 3, 4, 5, 7, nor the NLRP3 inflammasome pathway, nor pyroptosis or necroptosis cell death pathways [25]. They describe the implication of the MDA5-IFNAR1 signaling pathway in the recognition of double-stranded secondary structures of mRNA. Likewise, in human studies, the second immunization in mice led to an enhanced innate immune response. Concomitant with the increased IFNγ levels (and other cytokines including IL-2, CCL2/MCF-1, CCL4/MIP1β, CCL5) compared to the first immunization, enhanced activation of innate cells in the lymph nodes (monocytes, macrophages, and DCs) was also highlighted by the increased levels of CD86 expression. Natural killer and CD8+T cells in the draining lymph nodes were identified as the main producers of circulating IFNγ, confirming the possible contribution of NK subsets in IFNγ production in humans after vaccination. Of note, the study was based on the injection of 5 μg of BNT162b2 vaccine (high dose) in C57BL/6 mice because a dose of 0.2 μg (low dose, corresponding to human dose) induced a 10-fold lower antibody kinetics and a fivefold lower magnitude of T-cell responses.

2.4 mRNA Design and Innate Immunity

As shown in Figure 2.2, all regions and parts of mRNAs have been optimized during the last decades in order to improve the stability and translation efficiency of the mRNAs but also to avoid a strong innate immune response. Before further discussions of these different regions, it is important to note that, in cells, mRNAs are always complex to RNA-binding proteins (RBPs) from their initial transcription into pre-mRNA up to their final degradation. These complexes, called ribonucleoproteins (RNPs), play important functions in mRNA export, stability, and subsequently from translation initiation/elongation to cellular localization/compartmentalization [47, 48]. This is not the case for naked IVT–mRNA present in the different types of nucleic acid platforms, increasing the challenge to use the most optimized mRNAs and protect them from degradation. As we will further discuss below, advances in RNA technology have revealed new paradigms about the regulation of mRNAs, for example, capping homeostasis or non-A nucleosides present in poly(A)-tails.

2.4.1 Cap

In eukaryotic cells, mRNAs are usually capped, harboring at their 5′-end N7-methylated guanosine (^{m7}GpppN or ^{m7}GN) linked to their first nucleotide through a triphosphate linkage. This 5′ modification occurred just after the transcription initiation process of pre-mRNA (20–30 nucleotide long) by RNA polymerase II [49, 50]. mRNA capping and complexing RNPs are involved in different posttranscriptional and regulation steps like pre-mRNA splicing, polyadenylation, and mRNA nuclear export. Other important functions are translational initiation and the 5′ to 3′ looping of mRNA (closed-loop model) facilitating ribosome reentry and translation efficiency, but also mRNA protection from degradation. Further modifications of the sequence surrounding the 5′ m^{7}GN Cap (or Cap 0) are observed in higher eukaryotes, allowing nonself-discrimination during infection. The m^{7}GN mRNA is usually post-modified by 2′-*O*-ribose methyltransferase with the addition of a methyl group in the first transcribed nucleotide (termed cap 1; ^{m7}GNm) or the two first nucleotides (cap 2; ^{m7}GNmNm). Another modification often occurs in ^{m7}G-Am (2′-*O*-methyladenosine)-capped mRNA and consists of the addition of a methyl group to Am nucleoside in position N6. The m6Am mRNA is more stable than other types of capped RNA, this particularity arising from their

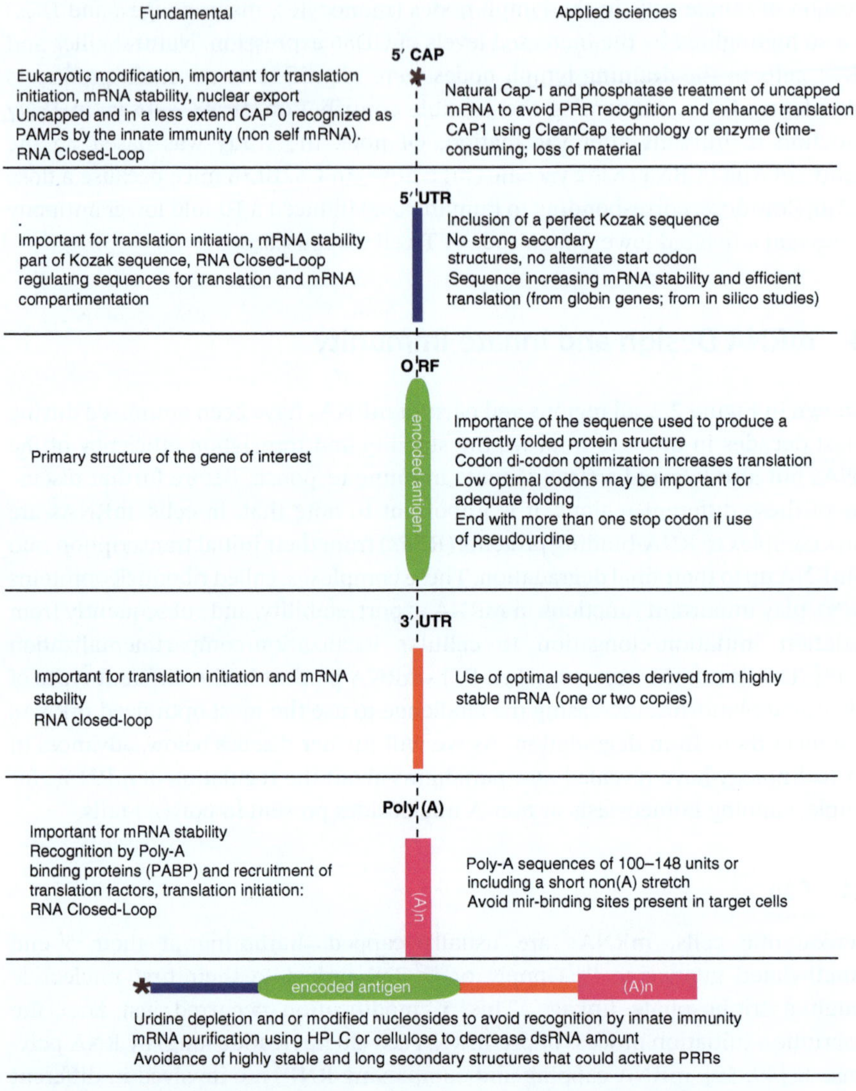

Figure 2.2 mRNA architecture, from the function of the different regions to their optimization in regard to mRNA vaccine use. For each region, the main functions and the optimization approaches used during mRNA design and production are indicated.

lower susceptibility to mRNA-decapping enzyme 2 DCP2 [51]. However, in a more recent study, the depletion of the cap-specific adenosine methyltransferase (PCIF1) involved in this chemical modification did not drastically affect mRNA translation in human cervical carcinoma HeLa or HEK293T (human embryonic kidney cell 293T) cells, but generate a reduced stability in a subset of m6Am-annotated mRNAs that do not represent unusually stable and highly abundant transcripts [52]. Hence, the high stability of abundant mRNAs is not due to the presence of m6Am, but to other intrinsic characteristics.

Uncapped mRNA (5′PPP and 5′PP) and in a less extent $5'^{m7}G$ cap or cap0 mRNA can be recognized and bound by PRRs like RIG-I, triggering the type I IFN activation leading to mRNA translation inhibition. The type I IFN can, in an autocrine manner, induce genes like IFIT (IFN-induced protein with tetratricopeptide repeats), which upon binding to uncapped single-stranded mRNA, outcompetes to eiF4F (Eukaryotic initiation factor 4F), a cap-binding translation initiation factor, and blocks the translation. Some IFIT can also bind to eiF3 and impede the translation [53]. Furthermore, mRNA transport, translation, or stability can be regulated by decapping and recapping mechanisms. This model is called cap homeostasis [54]. In agreement with this concept, uncapped mRNA seems to be more stable than previously defined. Thus, eukaryotic capping and PRRs seem to have evolved to fight against pathogens. The techniques used to obtain the more efficient capping and how this cap addition could lead to innate activation are detailed later.

2.4.2 Untranslated Regions

Sequences flanking the coding sequences are the 5′ and 3′ untranslated regions (UTRs). In coordination with RNA-binding proteins, UTRs play important roles in mRNA location and decay, and in translation efficiency. Some of the first mRNAs characterized by cDNA cloning have been the ones encoding globin. These mRNAs are very stable, with half-lives ranging between 16 and 48 hours instead of a few minutes to several hours, as it is for most of the other mRNAs. Indeed, this high stability allows an accumulation of globin mRNAs in terminally differentiated erythrocyte precursors, where they represent almost 95% of total mRNAs [55]. The stability of globin mRNAs is due in part to their untranslated sequences [56] and explains why UTRs from α- and ß-globins have historically been used to increase mRNA stability.

For therapeutical mRNAs, UTR regions need to be improved, keeping in mind that the impact of these noncoding sequences on the stability and translatability of the mRNA is dependent on multiple factors including species, cell type, cell state, and the coding sequence. Several approaches have been used to develop and improve UTRs in the context of mRNA vaccines to improve mRNA stability and expression in target cells/tissue.

In synergy with the 5′ cap, 5′ UTR is involved in the initiation of translation. The 43S eukaryotic preinitiation complex (40S ribosomal subunit + eukaryotic initiation factors [eIF] + Met initiator tRNA) attaches to the 5′ end of capped mRNA and scans the 5′UTR sequence to find the AUG initiation start codon (AUGi), forms the elongation 80S complex, and initiates the production of the protein. The bases flanking the AUGi codon are important for its efficient recognition and consist of the Kozak sequence, the consensus form being GCC**R**CCAUG**G** (in bold, important bases). However, not all AUGi codons in mRNAs have a strong Kozak sequence, and part of mRNA has some canonical start codon (AUG) and noncanonical start codons (CUG being the most efficient of them) that can be used to generate short peptides, alternate protein, or a longer antigen sequence if this alternate initiation translation is in frame with the AUGi. Hence, in the building of therapeutic mRNA, canonical and noncanonical start codons should be avoided in the 5' UTR to not compete with the right initiation codon.

Strong secondary structures have to be avoided, these sequences can impede ribosome recruitment, scanning, and start codon recognition [57]. However, the secondary structure in the 5′UTR can act at different levels (stability, location of mRNA, translation efficiency) in association with RNA binding proteins [58, 59]. Thus, an important balance between the secondary structure of UTRs and the potential activation of PRRs needs to be carefully addressed during the selection process of new sequences.

A good example of secondary structure concerns the 5′ UTR loop of mRNA encoding proα1(I) and proα2(I) collagen chains. At the protein level, these two chains associate to form a procollagen type I molecule made of 2 α1 and one α2 chains. The type I extracellular matrix collagen is the most abundant protein in vertebrates and is involved in the formation of collagen fibrils. Although knock-in mice lacking a 5′ loop in the proα1(I) mRNA developed normally, the steady-state level of proα1(I) mRNA decreased, and they were more resistant to induced liver fibrosis than wild-type mice [60]. The 5′ loop seems to play an important function during wound healing and pathological fibrosis [61]. Hence, LARP6 (La Ribonucleoprotein 6) is the specific binding protein of the 5′ loop of type I collagen mRNAs. The coordinate binding of LARP6 with vimentin induced a better stability of the mRNAs in a nontranslatable configuration and allowed cells to have a pool of available type I transcripts [62]. After binding to the 5′ loop, LARP6 can subsequently bind to the protein translocation channel SEC61. In addition to other protein interactions, this double interaction allowed an efficient, coordinated production and association of both type I chains into specific SEC61 translocon. LARP6 mutant that did not interact with SEC61 prevented collagen synthesis in a dominant negative manner [63]. This example shows that deciphering the impact of a 5′ UTR (but also 3′UTR) on the stability and the translation efficiency of mRNA is a huge question, and these parameters depend on the RBPs present in targeted cells, the different bindings between the mRNAs and cellular molecules, and the mode of structural assembly of the antigen.

Machine learning is probably a great methodology to optimize 5′UTR [64]. The Optimus 5-prime tool has been developed to build a predictive model of the ribosome loading of 5′UTR sequences [65]. For that, a random library of 5′UTR sequences sharing the same ORF (eGFP) and 3′UTR sequences has been transfected into HEK293 cells, and the mean ribosomal load was measured for each 5′UTR. These data were used to train a convolutional neural network and develop Optimus-5-prime. Using this bioinformatic tool, the relationships between predictive mean ribosome load for a 5′UTR sequence and eGFP expression were tested and were highly correlated. More recently, some high ribosomal loading 5′UTR from this study have been tested and compared to the broadly used 5′UTR of the human ß-globin in different cell lines and primary human–monocyte-derived DCs and confirmed the plus-value of this methodology [66].

As for 5′UTRs, 3′UTRs from highly stable mRNAs have been used to design a mRNA template. Moreover, it has been shown that the use in tandem of the 3′UTR of the ß-globin can improve the mRNA stability compared to one copy of this 3′UTR [67, 68]. An alternative has recently been used, with the presence of the 3′UTR histone stem-loop into a nucleoside unmodified SARS-COV-2-mRNA [24]. In nonpolyadenylated mature replication-dependent histone mRNA, the stem-loop is located at the 3′ end of the transcript and is bounded by the stem-loop binding protein (SLBP). This protein/RNA interaction is important for the nuclear export, the stability/degradation of the mRNA, and its efficient translation. Moreover, the ability of the SLBP/3′histone stem-loop to increase the translation is dependent on the 5′cap [69], similar to the closed-loop model where the poly(A)-5′cap association enhanced the translation [70, 71].

However, at the G2 phase of the cell cycle, the histone mRNAs are quickly degraded [72]. The addition of a poly(A) sequence to the histone 3′stem-loop enhanced the stability and translation efficiency of the mRNA [24]. The identification of 3′UTR sequences allowing high-translation efficiency has also been realized after screening by several rounds of RT-PCR of a pool of derived mRNA fragments included as cDNA into the 3′ end of a reporter gene and electroporated into human DCs [68]. Moreover, this study showed that the more stable mRNA contained fewer miRNA-binding sites in their 3′UTRs. Since miRNAs promote mRNA degradation, their related binding sites should be avoided into 3′ UTR sequences, except if they might impede the translation of the injected mRNA into nontargeted tissues. In addition, some destabilizing sequences can induce a rapid deadenylation and turnover of mRNA after binding to specific RBPs, like AU-rich (ARE) and GU-rich (GRE) elements [73, 74]. Finally, Leppek et al. indicated that the best UTR combinations leading to an efficient translation may be different depending on the mRNA coding sequence and targeted cell types. All these data strongly suggest that modifying UTR sequences should be carefully addressed, both in terms of RBP recruitment and half-life improvement versus PRR activation through deleterious secondary structures [75].

2.4.3 Poly(A)

Addition of adenosines at the 3′ end of the mRNA occurred posttranscriptionally in the nucleus by poly(A) polymerases, although some re-adenylation can occur in the cytoplasm by noncanonical poly(A) polymerases like TENT5C (Terminal Nucleotidyltransferase 5C) [76]. Poly(A)-tail plays important functions in the nuclear export, stability, and translation of the mRNA. Usually, the length of a poly(A) sequence is estimated to be around 200 adenosines, but recent technical advances have shown that the length of this tail is more versatile and is regulated by various enzymes and regulatory mechanisms (for a recent review of these mechanisms and methodologies used to measure the poly(A)-tail length, see Brouze et al. [77]). Hence, Lima et al. [78] have shown in *Caenorhabditis elegans* that highly expressed and translated mRNA rich in optimal codons have a short poly(A)-tail of approximately 30 A, fitting with the binding of a proximal poly-A-binding protein (PABP). In their model, only the proximal poly(A)-PABP is associated with the 5′Cap-translational initiation factors eiF4G and eiF4E, this molecular complex leads to the closed-loop model favoring ribosome reentry, this mRNA–protein interacting complex (cap-eIF4E-eiF4G-PABP-poly(A)-tail) impeding further deadenylation of the poly(A)-tail, mRNA decapping, and subsequent 5′ to 3′ exonucleolytic degradation. Further analysis by this group in other animals (mouse) confirmed that highly translated mRNAs are stable, rich in optimal codons, and possess a short poly(A)-tail. PABP plays an important function in mRNA stability and translatability, this RBP interacts with both translation and deadenylation pathways. By rapidly depleting PABP in human HEK293T and HeLa cells, Kajjo et al. have shown a general decrease in mRNA abundance and stability [79]. However, a deeper analysis indicated that depletion of PABP impacted, more specifically the population of stable mRNA, while more unstable mRNA decay at the same level as in PABP un-depleted cells. These stable mRNAs usually present short 5′ and 3′ UTRs and short poly(A)-tail. In these PABP-depleted cells, the decay of stable mRNA seems to be promoted by the LSM1-7 complex, promoting the decapping of the mRNA by DCP2 and its degradation through the 5′ to 3′ end. This result suggested that PABP-poly(A) interaction is important to protect the mRNA integrity from the LSM1-7 pathway.

The closed-loop model is well accepted in the scientific community, but as indicated by Vicens et al., it will be important to decipher the conformational and temporal dynamics of this 5′–3′ interactive network in the cells [80]. Even if highly stable mRNA seems to have a short poly(A)-tail in their steady-state, several studies have shown that longer poly(A) sequences improve their stability and translation efficiency in different cell lines or in human monocyte-derived DCs (MoDCs) or human primary T cells [66, 67, 81]. All these experiments have been performed with nude *in vitro* transcribed (IVT) mRNAs, the longer poly(A) stretch may allow the recruitment of RBPs before a complete deadenylation process.

Most mRNAs are polyadenylated in the nucleus and, during their lifespan, can undergo different modifications [77]. Into the cytosol, deadenylated and nondeadenylated mRNAs can be polyadenylated by noncanonical poly(A) polymerase [76]. With the use of Tail-seq, mRNAs have been shown to commonly carry non-A stretches at the 3′end of their poly(A)-tail in human cervical cancer HeLa and mouse fibroblast NIH 4T3 cell lines [82]. A large part (80%) of mRNA species has uridine residues at their end at a frequency higher than 2%. These uridylated mRNA harbor short poly(A)-tail (≤25). Guanylation is also observed among 60% of mRNA species at a frequency higher than 2% and is found at the 3′ end of longer poly(A)-tail (>40 units). Finally, cytidine residues can be rarely found at the 3′ terminus of poly(A)-tail. All these modifications are orchestrated by noncanonical poly(A) polymerase and terminal uridylyltransferase. Add of uridine residues by terminal uridylyl transferase TUT4 and TUT7 (also known as Terminal Nucleotidyltransferase TENT3A and TENT3B) in deadenylated mRNA has been shown to play a function in their degradation [83]. By contrast, guanylation of mRNA by TENT4A and TEN4B had a protective effect against rapid deadenylation [84]. Recently, it has also been shown in the parasite Trypanosoma brucei that some poly(A)-tails contained m6A, allowing better stability of the mRNA molecules [85]. In addition, recent works highlighted that nonadenine residues can be found inside the poly(A)-tail [86, 87]. The use of non-A linker into the poly(A)-tail has been shown to not decrease mRNA stability and protein expression [88, 89], and has been used in the Pfizer/BioNTech's BNT-162b2 mRNA.

2.4.4 Coding Sequence

As emphasized in case of the successful COVID-19 mRNA vaccines, the knowledge and the design of the coding sequence is an important step to deliver the correct protein antigen and ensure vaccine effectiveness [90, 91]. In addition to the choice of the antigen, it is important to have a good knowledge of its structure and conformation to allow the induction of neutralizing antibodies. In this case, authors have taken advantage of previous studies showing that the mutation of two proline residues in the MERS (Middle East Respiratory Syndrome) coronavirus spike sequence permitted its production in the prefusion conformation [92, 93]. Spike protein binds to ACE2 (angiotensin converting enzyme-2) receptors, which are the entry door for the virus into the cells. The selection of an optimal antigen structural conformation can be supported by the tools and 3D-protein data available in the RCSB protein data bank [94]. Besides, other changes have been realized in these vaccine mRNAs and concern the codon usage and the preferential use of GC-rich codons leading to uridine depletion. These modifications have been made to enhance translation efficiency and to avoid an over-reaction of innate immunity due to PRR sensing.

The open reading frame (ORF) encoding the antigen can be modified at the codon level to improve the translation efficiency. The different amino acid residues can be encoded by one codon (methionine, tryptophan) or two to six synonymous codons. Moreover, the frequency of synonymous codons is more or less variable between species and genes and is known as the codon bias. Another important point is the amount and frequency of the different tRNA present in the cytoplasm of different cell types. These two features have led to the notion of codon optimality representing the balance between the available pool of the different active tRNAs in the cytoplasm and the needs of the translational machinery for each of them [95]. As indicated by Presnyak et al. [95], common codons are not always optimal, and vice versa for rare codons. Hence, optimal codons are decoded faster than nonoptimal codons, and their distribution and frequency in the ORF impact the translation efficiency and their stability via the decay machinery. The presence of nonoptimal codons decreases the elongation rate, this pausing favorizing the recruitment of the RBP decapping activator and DEAD-Box (Glu-Asp-Ala-Glu box) RNA helicase Dhh1/DDX6 (DDX6, human ortholog of yeast Dhh1) that might trigger mRNA decay [96–98]. According to that, the presence of optimal codons near the AUGi codon increases elongation rates and translation efficiency [99]. Finally, another level of consideration when synonymous changes are realized is that not all the codons are decoded by their cognate tRNA in a standard (Watson–Crick) base pairing interaction [100]. As not all the 61 types of tRNA are present in organisms, some codon-tRNA recognitions involve a wobble interaction (standard base pairing of the two first bases). These wobble interactions have been involved in slow decoding and poor translation. Different strategies have been developed to optimize protein production. For example, the coding sequences can be modified according to codon usage bias, codon-pair bias optimal codons instead of rare codons or tRNA abundance [101–104].

Another alternative to enhance translation can be uridine (U) depletion [105], which minimizes U-rich regions that are recognized by RIG-I and allows an enhancement of protein production. Moreover, this U replacement in the ORF leads to an increase in the GC content, the third base of the codons (GC3). It has been shown that the third base of codons is exceptionally important, GC3 and AT3 codons are associated with stability and instability, respectively, and influence protein expression accordingly [106]. If high GC content can be beneficial for antigen production, it has been assumed that highly stable secondary structures and hairpin loops should be avoided. These structures can disturb some steps of the translation process and be sensed by the innate immune system. However, several studies indicated that highly structured mRNA has a longer half-life, and more interestingly, an improvement of protein expression [75, 107].

As mentioned in several reviews [100, 108], silent substitutions aim to improve mRNA stability and translation efficiency can be detrimental. Hence, the replacement of nonoptimal codons by optimal ones can increase the elongation speed and impede the correct folding of the protein, as exemplified by the loss of activity of the protein encoded by a codon-optimized firefly luciferase (Fluc) mRNA [109]. Another point is that silent substitutions can create cryptic translation initiation sites, allowing the production of undesirable proteins.

2.5 Optimization and Production of mRNA for an Adequate Innate Immune Response

2.5.1 IVT Production

For therapeutical purposes, mRNA is produced *in vitro* (IVT–mRNA) using either a linearized plasmid or an amplified PCR product containing a promoter for a bacteriophage RNA polymerase. The different steps of production and purification are presented in Figure 2.3. For the linearization, if the master vector codes for the mRNA in the poly(A) tail, type II restriction enzyme sites located downstream of the A-tail allow a cutting of the plasmid at the end of the poly(A) stretch. In the absence of an encoded poly(A) tail, the linearization is made at the corresponding 3′-end on the cDNA template, and a subsequent polyadenylation step is required after the IVT. For the PCR amplification, the forward and reverse primers contain a phage RNA polymerase promoter and a poly(T) stretch, respectively, permitting the production of a DNA template ready for the IVT [110]. In the IVT reaction, a phage RNA polymerase (T7, T3, or SP6) is used, with or without the presence of a cap analog and modified nucleosides. In the absence of cap analog, the capping is made by enzymatic reaction after the IVT–mRNA production. During the IVT reaction, several components play an important function in improving the quality and yield of mRNA [111]. Hence, pyrophosphatase can be added to degrade pyrophosphate, a byproduct of the IVT inhibiting the transcription. The IVT reaction also includes Mg^{2+},

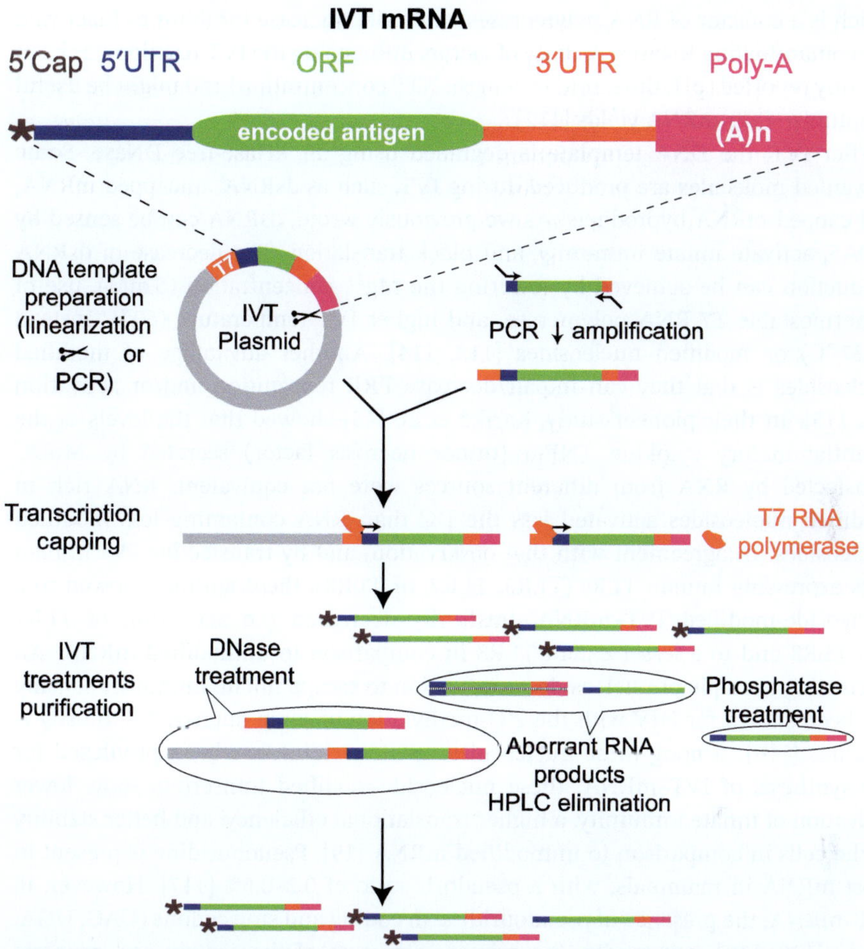

Figure 2.3 *In vitro* transcribed (IVT) mRNA synthesis and purification. The DNA sequence including the different regions of the mRNA sequence is included either in an *in vitro* transcription plasmid or in a PCR DNA fragment. For the vector method, the plasmid is usually linearized by a type II restriction endonuclease in order to finish the transcription at the end of the poly(A) sequence. The poly(A) sequence is usually made of 100–148 units, and in some cases, can be interrupted by a short non-A stretch as shown in previous studies [88, 89] or for the Pfizer-BioNTech BNT162b2 mRNA vaccine. The linearized plasmid or the PCR insert are used for the mRNA production using the T7 RNA polymerase, and with or without modified nucleosides. During this step, the capping can be realized using ARCA or CleanCap technologies. For an enzymatic capping approach, the IVT transcripts are subsequently capped using vaccinia enzyme or an alternative capping enzyme. Unwanted products like DNA, dsRNA, or uncapped mRNA are treated/purified by DNase–RNase-free enzyme, HPLC, or cellulose purification and phosphatase treatment, respectively.

which is a cofactor of RNA polymerases and a ribonuclease inhibitor to inactivate any contaminating RNases. A study of factors influencing the IVT reaction has been recently reported (pH, time, mRNA length, NTP concentration) and might be useful to optimize IVT–mRNA yields [112].

After IVT, the DNA template is degraded using an RNase-free DNase. Some unwanted molecules are produced during IVT, such as dsRNA, uncapped mRNA, and capped mRNA byproducts. As we previously wrote, dsRNA can be sensed by MDA5, activate innate immunity, and block translation. The decrease of dsRNA production can be achieved by lowering the Mg^{2+} concentration (5 mM), use of a thermostable T7 RNA polymerase, and higher IVT temperature (50 °C instead of 37 °C) or modified nucleosides [113, 114]. Another advantage of modified nucleosides is that they can impair/decrease PRR recognition and/or activation [43, 115]. In their pioneer study, Karikó et al. [43] showed that the levels of the proinflammatory cytokine TNF-α (tumor necrosis factor) secreted by MoDC transfected by RNA from different sources were not equivalent. RNA rich in modified nucleosides activated less the DC than RNA containing less modified nucleosides. In agreement with that observation, and by transfecting 293 human cells expressing human TLRs (TLR3, TLR7, or TLR8), these authors showed that nucleoside-modified IVT–mRNA drastically decreased the activation of TLR7 and TLR8 and to a lesser extent TLR3 in comparison to unmodified mRNA. An interesting example of nucleoside modification to escape innate immunity sensing has been shown for HIV with the 2′O-methylation of some nucleosides, mostly A residues [116]. Among these nucleosides, pseudouridine has been privileged for the synthesis of IVT–mRNA, these nucleoside-modified transcripts show lower activation of innate immunity, a higher translational efficiency, and better stability in the cells in comparison to unmodified mRNA [19]. Pseudouridine is present in most mRNA in mammals, with a pseudo/U ratio of 0.2–0.6% [117]. However, in IVT–mRNA, the presence of pseudouridine in coding and stop codons (UAG, UGA, UAA) [118, 119], can modify the primary structure of the protein and generate longer proteins, due to their altered capacity in their base-pairing abilities [120]. Later, the N1-methylpseudouridine has been shown to improve mRNA stability and translation efficiency, decreasing innate immunity activation [45, 121]. Moreover, this modified nucleoside seems to follow better the Watson–Creek base-pairing suggesting a better choice of the tRNA and a more accurate protein synthesis [120]. Altogether, these works suggest that the limitation of dsRNA and the use of modified nucleosides decrease the innate immune activation properties of IVT–mRNA so that antigen production and adaptive immune response would be improved after vaccine injections.

2.5.2 Posttranscriptional Modification

Capping is an important step in the production of IVT–mRNA. The capping can be performed together with mRNA transcription using cap analogs, such as ARCA (anti-reverse Cap analog) or in a later step in an enzymatic reaction (with the vaccinia virus capping enzyme, for example). The ARCA capping leads to moderate capping efficiency (60–80%) and allows the formation of Cap-0 mRNA. To achieve this capping efficiency, a fourfold molar excess of cap analog over GTP is used to minimize the incorporation of a GTP at the +1 transcript position. However, by lowering the GTP concentration, the mRNA yield is decreased during the IVT reaction. The vaccinia capping performed in the presence of the mRNA Cap 2′-*O*-Methyltransferase can be very efficient (close to 100% of Cap-1 structure), but it is time-consuming, and this extra step results in a waste of mRNA during the purification steps. Clean-cap capping system (Trilink product) can be used in the IVT reaction, the Clean-cap capping has been proven to be very efficient with approximately 90–99% of Cap-1 capped mRNA. More recently, some studies have emphasized the promising use of Cap-2 capped mRNA in vaccines. Hence, Cap-2 is enriched on long-lived mRNAs and is a weaker activator of RIG-I than Cap-1 mRNAs [122]. Moreover, by developing a new capping technology (the Purecap method), it has been shown that Cap-2 mRNAs are more efficiently translated (up to fourfolds) than Cap-1 mRNAs in *in vitro* and *in vivo* experiments [123]. The phosphatase treatment of uncapped mRNA can prevent the activation of RIG-I by 5′-triphosphate mRNAs and subsequent activation of the type I IFN pathway and inhibition of mRNA translation [124]. In the case of efficient capping or highly purified capped mRNA, as in the PureCap method, this final step can be avoided.

2.5.3 Purification

The purification of IVT mRNA batches is a central step in mRNA vaccine production to avoid the unwanted activation of innate immunity through nucleic acid contaminants. In this purification procedure, dsRNA and unwanted contaminants (proteins, DNA, nucleosides, ssRNA, and dsRNA byproducts) have to be eliminated. This can be achieved by different types of chromatography, such as high-pressure liquid chromatography (HPLC) or tangential flow filtration techniques [125, 126]. A faster and cheaper purification allowing an efficient dsRNA purification has also been developed [113]. In this latter report, dsRNA is selectively bound to a cellulose-based support. mRNAs purified by cellulose chromatography gave comparable results to those obtained by HPLC-purified mRNA in terms of protein translation efficiency and IFNα induction after their intravenous (IV) injection in mice. This cellulose purification method has also been used in a preclinical study of the SARS-CoV-2 mRNA vaccine [127].

2.6 mRNA Delivery Systems and Immune Response: The Role of Formulation Composition

Naked mRNAs are susceptible to enzymatic degradation in the extracellular environment, and due to their high molecular weight and negative charge, they cannot easily diffuse through the cellular membrane due to electrostatic repulsion. Therefore, the performance of mRNA vaccines is highly dependent on delivery systems that protect mRNA from nucleases and improve their uptake by APCs, such as macrophages and

DCs [128–130]. Moreover, inside the cell, mRNA should escape the endosome and reach the cytoplasm to be translated before its degradation in late endosomes.

Among different formulations for mRNA, LNPs have been the most studied as a vaccine platform [38, 46, 131, 132]. The first LNP for clinical use was approved in 2018 with Onpattro® (patisiran) as siRNA therapeutics for the treatment of polyneuropathy caused by hereditary transthyretin-mediated amyloidosis in adults [133, 134]. More recently, the employment of LNP platform for the delivery of mRNA coding for the spike protein of SARS-CoV-2 by Pfizer–BioNTech (BNT162b2) and Moderna (mRNA-1273) showed outstanding performance that allowed their approbation for emergency clinical use by health regulatory agencies [135–138]. Typically, LNP formulation is composed of four lipids at variable molar ratios: (I) a cationic ionizable lipid, (II) cholesterol, (III) a phospholipid, and (IV) a lipid conjugated to polyethylene glycol (PEG-lipid). The auto-assembly of lipids and nucleoside modified mRNA forming LNPs ensures highly efficient and prolonged protein expression *in vivo* with potent immune responses in different species [38, 121, 139].

The innovation of LNP technology is mostly based on the use of ionizable lipids containing amino groups with $pK_a < 7$. Due to this pH-sensitive property, ionizable lipids are positively charged at acidic pH ($pH < 6.0$) and neutral or slightly charged at $pH = 7.4$ [140]. LNP preparation is performed at pH $\approx$5.0–5.5, a condition in which ionizable lipids are positively charged, allowing prompt self-assembly with mRNA molecules and high-encapsulation efficiency. At physiological conditions, the LNP surface charge becomes close to neutral, which improves biocompatibility and safety profile following injection. In addition, inside endosomes, the ionizable lipids of LNPs become protonated again, which plays an important role in the destabilization of the endosomal membrane and improves mRNA release into the cytosol [129]. However, by using six different types of ionizable cationic lipids to build mRNA–LNP, an alternative to the proton sponge and endosomal bursting has been proposed [141]. In this model, mRNA escape arose from the endosomes with recycling tubules, the membrane linkage could result from interference between the cationic lipids and the lipid structure in the membrane bilayer.

Many studies have explored the effect of modifications on the chemical structure of ionizable lipids and their impact on RNA delivery [140, 142, 143]. The ionizable lipid D-Lin-MC3-DMA (MC3) is one of the optimized lipids containing two unsaturated linoleoyl tails, which was used in the formulation of patisiran. The previous knowledge of ionizable lipids for siRNA delivery contributed to the foundation of LNP development and application for efficient mRNA delivery [144]. Likewise, MC3 has been employed as a benchmark for the comparison and screening of new synthesized ionizable lipids used in mRNA-based LNP design [139, 145, 146]. Among lipid tail structural modifications of MC3, the inclusion of biodegradable properties by the replacement of double bonds by hydrolyzable ester groups increased endosomal escape and mRNA expression with minimal elevation in markers of immune activation (complement components and cytokines), compared to MC3-based LNP, following IV injection in nonhuman primates [147]. Another study showed that the replacement of MC3 by biodegradable ionizable lipids containing ester lipid tails in LNP composition improved tolerability, protein expression, and immunogenicity upon IM administration [139]. Fenton et al. [128, 148] synthesized a series of ionizable lipids including degradable ester linkages, which enable the delivery of nontranslating Cy5 mRNA–LNP predominantly to the liver after IV injection and to a lesser extent (100-fold) to other organs like the spleen. However, they observed that after IV injection of Fluc mRNA–LNP, 85% of the luciferase was produced in the spleen. They hypothesized that electrophilic ester bonds of ionizable lipid mRNA–LNP are sensitive to enzymatic degradation in the liver, although they retain the ability to induce functional protein expression in the spleen. To go further, they injected intravenously a single dose of Cy5 mRNA–LNP and identified that B lymphocytes and monocyte/macrophage population were the main cells labeled with the Cy5 mRNA in the spleen. These results showed that LNP biodistribution must be associated with the characterization of functional delivery of mRNA *in vivo*. Hajj et al. [149] synthesized a library of branched-tail lipids to formulate mRNA-based LNP, and they have found that this sort of ionizable lipid can generate more potent hepatic mRNA expression when compared to their straight-tail counterpart following IV injection. The difference was probably due to the more effective surface ionization of LNP-containing branched-tail lipids at an endosomal pH of 5.0, which could improve endosomal escape. The ionizable lipids used by Moderna and Pfizer–BioNTech, SM-102 and ALC-0315, respectively, have some common features: head group with a tertiary amine, multibranched tails, and ester linkers. This suggests that ionizable lipids with branched tails and degradable structures are probably essential to the clinical application of LNP-formulated mRNA [143].

Meanwhile, the development of mRNA–LNPs as vaccine formulations should consider the envisioned biological application, e.g. cancer immunotherapy or prophylactic vaccines, in order to trigger specific immune response following parenteral administration.

Clinical trials of mRNA-based LNP used in disorders characterized by genetic deficiency of key enzymes and cancer immunotherapy have been tested with IV or intratumorally administration, which leads to a particular environment and interactions with cells or biomolecules, including physical barriers depending on target organ or tissue [129]. Cheng et al. [150] found that direct tissue-tropism of LNP and mRNA delivery beyond liver hepatocytes following IV administration can be achieved using a Selective Organ Targeting (SORT) strategy. This strategy consists of an extra lipid (SORT molecule) in LNP composition at an increased molar percentage that modifies their internal charge. The addition of cationic lipid as a SORT molecule moved the protein expression from the liver (0%) to the spleen (10–15%) and then the lungs (50%). In addition, they showed that the change of a negatively charged lipid (10–40%) to a cationic one led to mRNA translation exclusively in the spleen. Finally, they identified which cell types are transfected in different organs after one single administration of mRNA–LNPs. Studies showed that the hepatic mRNA delivery by LNP depends on the interaction with the serum protein Apo-E, and this interaction could trigger a rearrangement of the LNP structure [151, 152]. Recently, another study demonstrated that LNP–RNA tropism is affected by non-ApoE interactions *in vivo* [153]. Bevers et al. [154] evaluated the correlation between LNP composition and their ability to induce strong CD8+ T-cell response involved in antitumor immunity. Using a design of experiments (DOEs) approach, optimal LNPs composition was identified by a combination of low percentage of PEG-lipid (<0.6%), a high percentage of ionizable lipid (>50%), and a low percentage of the neutral lipid DOPE (<10%). Further, they found a significant correlation between LNP size, which strongly depends on lipid composition, and the relative mRNA expression in the spleen following IV injection in mice and nonhuman primates. Optimal LNPs increased mRNA expression in splenic macrophages and DCs, as well as the functional maturation of splenic DCs and the production of T-cell stimulatory cytokines and chemokines. The antigen-specific $CD8^+$ T cells were essentially activated by type I IFNs, phagocytes, and B cells. In addition, they showed that repeated IV injections of LNPs increased anti-PEG IgM and IgG levels in mouse serum, which did not impair the T-cell response after the vaccine boost.

The report of hypersensitivity reactions following vaccination with Pfizer/BioNTech and Moderna vaccines triggered some suspicion about their safety, mostly related to the presence of PEG-lipid in LNP composition [155, 156]. A possible mechanism that could explain the off-target effects of LNPs is related to hypersensitivity mediated by complement activation, also known as complement activation-related pseudoallergy (CARPA), which has been associated with the administration of PEGylated liposomes such as Doxil [157–159]. One factor that influences the C activation by PEGylated liposomes is their binding to anti-PEG IgG and IgM antibodies [160, 161]. However, the CARPA phenomenon has been observed with IV injection of PEGylated liposomes, whereas COVID mRNA vaccines and a majority of mRNA–LNPs evaluated in preclinical studies or clinical trials against infectious diseases are administered by IM injection [129, 138, 162]. Thus, different protein and cellular interactions and reduced interaction with plasma IgG and IgM could be expected. An *in vitro* study showed a correlation between the preexistence of anti-PEG IgM antibodies and the lysis of LNPs, which trigger the premature release and exposure of encapsulated mRNA to plasma proteins [163]. The mechanism of mRNA release occurs via complement activation and could potentially reduce mRNA–LNP efficacy and off-target effects and toxicity. Recently, the *ex vivo* analysis of plasma samples of individuals vaccinated with two doses of SARS-CoV-2 LNP mRNA vaccines showed that anti-PEG IgG and IgM were significantly boosted by mRNA-1273 and modestly boosted by BNT162b2 [164]. The authors suggested that the difference in PEG immunogenicity between the two vaccines might be due to a higher content of lipid-PEG in mRNA-1273 than the BNT162b2 vaccine. In addition, their results suggested that anti-PEG IgG specifically recognized PEG-lipid in both mRNA vaccines but no other lipids of LNP formulation. However, the neutralizing immune responses of two doses of vaccines were not impacted by the presence of specific anti-PEG antibodies prior to or following BNT162b2 or mRNA-1273 vaccination, and the increase in anti-PEG antibodies was correlated with higher systemic reactogenicity after repeated injection of SARS-CoV-2 LNP mRNA vaccines. Altogether, these results suggest that more extensive *in vivo* studies should be performed to have extended clinical conclusions about the risks of using PEG-lipid in LNP composition.

mRNA–LNP vaccines were tested in different administration routes. It has been shown that administration of a single dose of modified mRNA–LNPs by various parental routes (intraperitoneal, IV, intradermal, subcutaneous, IM, and intratracheal) is able to deliver mRNA with specific expression kinetics depending on the dose and site of injections in mice [121]. The administration of mRNA–LNP led to high levels of neutralizing antibodies (nAbs) against influenza virus, zika virus, and HIV-1 [46, 165–167]. Liang et al. [168] showed that hemagglutinin (HA) modified mRNA–LNPs induced high antibody titers in 25 weeks, without the addition of an adjuvant with ID and IM administration in the rhesus macaque model. Despite the promotion of immune cell infiltration to the injection sites, LNP alone was not able to induce CD80 upregulation which was necessary to induce APCs activation. They identified that mRNA-mediated type I IFN response was responsible for the activation of innate immune cells. The analysis of cell populations showed that monocytes and DCs efficiently promoted LNP uptake and mRNA expression at draining LNs and injection sites. Compared to IM administration, ID injection showed the most durable expression of mRNA-encoded protein. Depending on the site of injection, the antigen production and presentation to $CD4^+$ T cells were likely performed by different APCs subsets and vaccine-specific $CD4^+$ T cells were generated only in draining LNs. Hassett et al. [169] demonstrated that the size of the LNP in the cytomegalovirus mRNA vaccine can strongly affect antibody titers in mice after IM injection, where approximately 100 nm size generates the highest IgG titers. However, in nonhuman primates, no difference in the titers was observed in the tested LNP size range (60–150 nm). They hypothesized that mice are more sensitive to particle size due to the smaller scale of murine lymphatics compared to larger primate lymphatics. Then, differences in the immune responses of mRNA–LNP vaccines could be dependent on anatomical features of animal species used in preclinical studies consequently the translation of the results should be considered cautiously for upcoming clinical studies.

The design of LNPs for mRNA delivery for nonparenteral administration has been studied considering the biological features of target tissues or epithelium, as well as the pharmaceutical formulation that will be administered. Actually, the intranasal (IN) and intratracheal administrations have been explored in order to develop mRNA vaccines against respiratory diseases that are able to induce long-lasting and tissue-specific memory immune responses at the entry site of pathogens [170]. Lokugamage et al. [171] have demonstrated that LNP formulation should be optimized for pulmonary administration by nebulization. In accordance with previous work [150], the inclusion of cationic lipids in LNP formulation is required for efficient lung delivery. They also identified that PEG molarity and PEG-lipid density are critical in LNP design. Even if they could not prove a precise correlation between components and mRNA delivery, they hypothesized that nebulization and lung biology can modify the distribution depending on LNP composition. Recently, Anderluzzi et al. [172] demonstrated that the IN administration of LNP formulations encapsulating the rabies virus glycoprotein (RVG) encoding saRNA induced a low immune response compared to IM and ID administrations, even with the 10-fold higher dose. This low-vaccine efficacy is probably related to the limitation of the IN administration in small animal models. The biodistribution study showed lower retention of LNPs in mice after IN administration compared to IM and ID administration, with most of the LNPs being detected in the throat and stomach. Other types of nanoparticles, all containing cationic lipids in their composition, evaluated in the same study exhibited a similar biodistribution profile but lower total anti-RVG IgG titers than saRNA–LNPs. Importantly, all nanoparticle formulations were administered in liquid form, suggesting that the physicochemical properties of nanoparticles were not able to promote mucoadhesion and/or penetration in the mucosal tissue. Taken together, these results highlight the importance of nanoparticle composition, formulation, and route administration in order to ensure an optimal antigen expression and required immune response.

An important aspect related to mRNA–LNP vaccines is its adjuvant effect, but the mechanism involved is still not completely clear [173]. The immunomodulatory properties of ionizable cationic LNP were described following their coadministration with dengue virus envelope protein [174]. The authors of the study suggested that dengue protein-specific B-cell and $CD4^+/CD8^+$ response decreased when the content of ionizable cationic lipids was reduced in LNP composition. The coadministration of high doses of LNP with tetravalent dengue antigen formulations boosted nAbs against four serotypes of dengue virus following IM vaccination without an increase of biomarkers associated with systemic inflammation or complement activation. It has been shown that uridine- or N1-methylpseudouridine-nucleoside modified mRNA–LNP can exert an adjuvant effect specifically on GC B cells [165, 166]. In this study, IM administration of firefly luciferase combined with influenza PR8 HA protein subunit vaccine strongly increased the number of B cells in the splenic germinal center (GC) when compared to the administration of protein alone. Another study observed that the coadministration of nonionizable cationic LNP without mRNA encapsulated and with split vaccines (SVs) for influenza significantly increased SV-specific total IgG antibodies compared to the administration of SV vaccine alone [175]. Likewise, LNP enhanced the SV-induced neutralization of SV-specific IgG1 and IgG2 in mice after two SC immunizations. *In vitro* stimulation of splenocytes with SV showed that LNP can improve the Th1 response induced by SV. The immune response induced by LNPs strongly protects mice against the H1N1 influenza A virus in a challenge study. Administration of LNPs did not induce local inflammation since the number of inflammatory immune cells did not change when compared to mice that received SV alone. However, the coadministration of LNP with recombinant hemagglutinin (rHA) protein did not improve the rHA-specific antibody response and T-cell response suggesting that the adjuvant effect of nonionizable cationic LNP is dependent of the selected antigen. *In vitro* stimulation of DCs by LNP did not induce cytokine production or enhanced expression of costimulatory molecules on DCs, suggesting that innate immune response is not activated. As proposed by authors, some studies observed that the presence of cationic lipids could be responsible for TLR activation and the adjuvant effect of lipid nanovectors [176–178]. More recently, Alameh et al. [22]

showed that empty LNPs (eLNP, LNP without mRNA) were able to induce robust Tfh cell response and durable protective antibodies when coadministered IM with influenza virus rHA protein in mice. Their results confirmed that eLNP formulation can induce Tfh and GC B cells response after a single IM or ID immunization in mice. The induction of Tfh cells was related to the secretion of IL-6 stimulated by eLNP formulation. The administration of rHA protein and eLNP induced stronger HA-specific long-lived plasma cells (LLPC) and high-affinity memory B cells (MBCs) compared to the coadministration of rHA with the benchmark adjuvant AddaVax™ (MF-59). In addition, the authors showed that vaccination with rHA + eLNP with the ionizable lipid-induced high hemagglutination-inhibition titers following IM administration while rHA adjuvanted with eLNP in the absence of ionizable lipid did not present HAI activity and, thus, lost adjuvant activity. These results highlight the crucial role of ionizable lipids in the adjuvant effect of LNP formulation. However, a complementary effect of mRNA sensing via the MyD88 pathway in the adjuvanticity of N1-methylpseudouridine-modified mRNA–LNP vaccines was also demonstrated in this study. Tahtinen et al. [40] performed a complete study to examine which mechanisms are involved in the reactogenicity of mRNA vaccines. They demonstrated that IL-1 is directly involved in the systemic inflammatory response induced by mRNA vaccines and that innate immune stimulation could be modulated by the antagonism of endogenous IL-1ra. In accordance with previous studies, they showed that the immunostimulatory activity of modified mRNA vaccines is highly dependent on the formulations. Their results showed that mRNA formulated with liposomes (RNA–LPX) confers a robust upregulation of IL-1ra in mice being nonimmunostimulatory and resistant to adverse events. However, mRNA formulated in LNPs exhibited strong innate immune response on human peripheral blood mononuclear cells as observed in individuals vaccinated with mRNA-1273. They observed that empty LNPs without mRNA were able to release IL-1β *in vitro* suggesting that lipids alone could act as inflammatory signals.

The results presented here started to elucidate which parameters are involved in immunogenic and inflammatory responses to mRNA vaccines, and taken together, they could help to overcome the challenge to find the fine adjustment of immune responses to design new generations of more efficient and safe mRNA vaccines. Among the next perspectives, the development of mRNA vaccine formulations able to induce high levels of persistent IgA antibodies and antigen-specific resident memory T cells at the mucosal level is essential to prevent transmission of respiratory pathogens such as influenza virus and SARS-CoV-2.

2.7 Concluding Remarks and Perspectives

Several regions of IVT–mRNA might be recognized as nonself by the PRRs and activate innate immunity, and have to be taken into account during the design of the primary structure, the posttranscriptional modifications and purification procedure. Although an activation of innate immunity is mandatory to stimulate a strong immune response when using mRNA vaccine, an overactivation could lead to an inhibition of the translational machinery of the mRNA as exemplified by the role of type I IFN, and consequently to a lower production and presentation of the selected antigen. However, all mRNA vaccine components can play different functions in innate immune activation [6, 22, 175], and the impact of these interplay has to be evaluated in order to allow a long-lasting antibody and potent cellular immune responses. There is still room for improvement to guide future developments of mRNA vaccines for infectious diseases in order to reduce their reactogenicity while increasing their immunogenicity.

For the mRNA molecule itself, the design of more stable and efficiently translated mRNA will allow to decrease mRNA vaccine doses and their inherent toxicity. The analysis of designed mRNA libraries and the development of *in silico* programs will be useful in achieving this goal [65, 75]. As indicated before, the development of more stable mRNA has to be realized while preserving the structure of the encoded antigen is preserved. In the case of a new antigen, the use of 3D protein data present in the RCSB protein data bank could be helpful [94]. Once mRNA is produced by IVT, formulated into LNP, and stored, the integrity of the mRNA and its functionality have to be checked. Although 70–75% of mRNA integrity was considered to be acceptable in the pandemic context by the European Medicines Agency [179, 180], and even if strong quality control has been implemented, new automated processes are currently being developed to ensure more than 90% intact mRNA in the vaccine. Moreover, due to interactions between mRNA molecules and other components, some chemical modifications of mRNAs can make them unable to produce the full protein, as recently shown [181]. In this study, aldehyde addition to nucleosides was identified, and this adduct would come from some impurities of the ionizable lipid. These data also highlight the need for strong quality control of vaccine batches, implying a fine analysis of new mRNA–LNPs or any other types of mRNA complex.

Although the BNT162b2 and mRNA-1273 vaccines were powerful during the COVID-19 pandemic, several ways of improvement can be done. Hence, the patient's reactogenicity has to be further lowered, the uploading of the mRNA into the cytosol can be increased, and the possible impact of PEG in anaphylactic reactions and the production of anti-PEG antibodies in vaccinated patients should be extensively studied. About the reactogenicity of the COVID-19 mRNA vaccines, the inflammation observed in patients seems to be related to the ionizable lipids of the LNPs, the symptoms being similar to those associated with inflammation triggered by cytokines such as IL-1β and IL-6. Indeed, in mice, LNPs with or without encapsulated mRNA induced a strong inflammation in the site of injection, and activated multiple inflammatory pathways and induced IL-1β and IL-6 [6, 40]. Although the LNP has an important adjuvant function in the efficiency of the mRNA vaccines and acts as a mRNA carrier, novel LNPs, and especially ionizable cationic lipids could reduce the inflammation around the site of administration while allowing a strong immune response. A recent study available as a preprint to date describes a novel multiprotic ionizable lipid allowing the production of mRNA–LNPs with higher potency than MC3 and a lower inflammation around the injection site [182]. An improved loading of mRNA into the cytosol could lead to the reduction of vaccine doses. As indicated by Paramasivam et al. [141], only a small part of the mRNAs is released from endosomes that are rich in recycling tubules. To build the next generation of LNPs, a structure/function analysis between the different components, maybe with a molecular modeling approach, might be a way to increase their potency. This goal could also be achieved by using libraries of ionizable lipids or cholesterol or even other materials to develop non-LNP mRNA carriers. The presence of PEG has been rapidly identified as a potential source of anaphylactic reactions, although this assumption is highly debated. An additional consequence is the induction of antibodies directed against PEG, which could become an issue if the mRNA vaccine becomes the new gold standard in vaccination. We could anticipate that an immune reaction against the vaccine vehicle will appear, thus diminishing the efficacy of the subsequent booster shots, but also a cross-protection against new mRNA vaccines [37]. It should be noted that mRNA-1272, but not BTN162b2 induces antibodies against PEG, one of the suggested reasons being the higher LNP dose used with mRNA-1272 [183]. However, the limited number of subjects studied (especially BTNT162b2 recipients) and future studies including 2/3 booster shots should be realized.

As a preclinical model of vaccination, mice are widely used to evaluate new mRNA formulations. However, as indicated by Tahtinen et al. [40], mice (C57BL/6 and Balb/c) are highly tolerant to mRNA vaccines compared to humans, even at high mRNA doses. In this study, the authors showed that in contrast to humans, mRNA vaccines upregulated IL-1 receptor antagonist (IL-1ra) in mice, an anti-inflammatory cytokine which, upon binding into IL-1 receptor, avoids IL-1 binding and the subsequent inflammatory pathway. The use of IL-1ra$^-$/IL-1ra$^-$ mouse would thus allow a better prediction of what could happen in human assays. Another study realized with C57BL/6 and BNT162b2 vaccine indicated that the innate immunity was not activated via TLR or inflammasome, but the IFNAR-MDA5 pathway. Hence, CD8$^+$ T-cell activation was dependent on type I IFN-dependent MDA5 signaling, with binding of dsRNA to MDA5 [25]. From this study, the short-lasting of antibodies in mRNA-vaccinated patients are questioned, as well as the lack of TLR/RIG-I activation due to the low binding of the modified mRNA to these PRRs. One of the possible alternatives to activate appropriately TLR and RIG-I pathways, and subsequently, the humoral response will be to test unmodified transcripts. In this option, the development of more stable and highly translatable mRNA coupled with a better loading into the targeted cells will be useful to decrease the amount of mRNA injected.

Other alternatives to improve the adaptative immune response could be the addition of adjuvants into the mRNA vaccines, either as PRR agonists or by adding mRNA-encoding chemokines. The persistence of the antigen is also of importance and can be increased by the design of more stable mRNA and structurally well-folded antigens or with the use of self-amplifying RNA or circular RNA. Recent works have described the use of mRNA encoding a multimeric protein (multimerization sequence linked to the antigen one) to better improve the adaptative immune response ([184]), a strategy already used in protein vaccines.

Finally, one of the major concerns of mRNA vaccines is that after injection, the mRNA complexes and encoded antigens are detectable not only at the site of injection but are also widely distributed into the whole-body host. Development of mRNA carriers allowing better retention of the formulated vaccine in lymphoid organs and testing other routes of administration are under progress and will allow a better induction of adaptative immunity and a decrease of vaccine reactogenicity by favoring cross-talk of immune cells in secondary lymphoid organs such as draining lymph nodes. Another challenge will be to develop efficient adjuvants to overcome mucosal tolerance when testing noninvasive mucosal administration route against respiratory pathogens as optimization of mucosal delivery systems remains an unsolved issue.

To conclude, if the mRNA vaccine field is blooming, it appears that having a naked mRNA as the main component of this new vaccine brings a lot of complexities due to its high versatility.

Acknowledgments

This research was funded by BQR Accueil EC 2020 to D.C.A., ANR 616-CE20-002-01554 (Fish RNAVax) to B.V., ANRS ECTZ 119388 to B.V., ANR-21-CE35 60019 (LipoFishVac) to B.V., Eranet ICRAD-Nuc NanoFish/ANR-21-ICRD-0009 to B.V., and ANR-22-CE18-0038 (MucRNAvax) to B.V.

References

1 Baden, L.R., el Sahly, H.M., Essink, B. et al. (2021). Efficacy and Safety of the mRNA-1273 SARS-CoV-2 Vaccine. *N. Engl. J. Med.* 384 (5): 403–416. https://doi.org/10.1056/nejmoa2035389.

2 Polack, F.P., Thomas, S.J., Kitchin, N. et al. (2020). Safety and efficacy of the BNT162b2 mRNA COVID-19 vaccine. *N. Engl. J. Med.* 383 (27): 2603–2615. https://doi.org/10.1056/nejmoa2034577.

3 Rijkers, G.T., Weterings, N., Obregon-Henao, A. et al. (2021). Antigen presentation of mRNA-based and virus-vectored SARS-CoV-2 vaccines. *Vaccine* 9 (8): https://doi.org/10.3390/vaccines9080848.

4 Turner, J.S., O'Halloran, J.A., Kalaidina, E. et al. (2021). SARS-CoV-2 mRNA vaccines induce persistent human germinal centre responses. *Nature* 596 (7870): 109–113. https://doi.org/10.1038/s41586-021-03738-2.

5 Sahin, U., Muik, A., Vogler, I. et al. (2021). BNT162b2 vaccine induces neutralizing antibodies and poly-specific T cells in humans. *Nature* 595 (7868): 572–577. https://doi.org/10.1038/s41586-021-03653-6.

6 Ndeupen, S., Qin, Z., Jacobsen, S. et al. (2021). The mRNA-LNP platform's lipid nanoparticle component used in preclinical vaccine studies is highly inflammatory. *iScience* 24 (12): https://doi.org/10.1016/j.isci.2021.103479.

7 Dolasia, K., Bisht, M.K., Pradhan, G. et al. (2018). TLRs/NLRs: shaping the landscape of host immunity. *Int. Rev. Immunol.* 37 (1): 3–19. https://doi.org/10.1080/08830185.2017.1397656.

8 Guy, C. and Bowie, A.G. (2022). Recent insights into innate immune nucleic acid sensing during viral infection. *Curr. Opin. Immunol.* 78: https://doi.org/10.1016/j.coi.2022.102250.

9 Ostendorf, T., Zillinger, T., Andryka, K. et al. (2020). Immune sensing of synthetic, bacterial, and protozoan RNA by toll-like receptor 8 requires coordinated processing by RNase T2 and RNase 2. *Immunity* 52 (4): 591–605.e6. https://doi.org/10.1016/j.immuni.2020.03.009.

10 Karikó, K., Ni, H., Capodici, J. et al. (2004). mRNA is an endogenous ligand for toll-like receptor 3. *J. Biol. Chem.* 279 (13): 12542–12550. https://doi.org/10.1074/jbc.M310175200.

11 Miyake, K., Saitoh, S.I., Fukui, R. et al. (2021). Dynamic control of nucleic-acid-sensing Toll-like receptors by the endosomal compartment. *Int. Immunol.* 33 (12): 835–840. https://doi.org/10.1093/intimm/dxab037.

12 Barral, P.M., Sarkar, D., Su, Z.-Z. et al. (2009). Functions of the cytoplasmic RNA sensors RIG-I and MDA-5: Key regulators of innate immunity. *Pharmacol. Ther.* 124 (2): 219–234. https://doi.org/10.1016/j.pharmthera.2009.06.012.

13 Chen, Y.G. and Hur, S. (2022). Cellular origins of dsRNA, their recognition and consequences. *Nat. Rev. Mol. Cell Biol.* 23 (4): 286–301. https://doi.org/10.1038/s41580-021-00430-1.

14 Im, J.H., Duic, I., Yoshimura, S.H. et al. (2023). Mechanisms of length-dependent recognition of viral double-stranded RNA by RIG-I. *Sci. Rep.* 13 (1): https://doi.org/10.1038/s41598-023-33208-w.

15 García, M.A., Meurs, E.F., and Esteban, M. (2007). The dsRNA protein kinase PKR: Virus and cell control. *Biochimie* 89 (6–7): 799–811. https://doi.org/10.1016/j.biochi.2007.03.001.

16 Floyd-Smith, G., Slattery, E., and Lengyel, P. (1981). Interferon action: RNA cleavage pattern of a (2′-5′) oligoadenylate-dependent endonuclease. *Science* 212 (4498): 1030–1032. https://doi.org/10.1126/science.6165080.

17 Silverman, R.H. (2007). Viral encounters with 2′,5′-oligoadenylate synthetase and RNase L during the interferon antiviral response. *J. Virol.* 81 (23): 12720–12729. https://doi.org/10.1128/jvi.01471-07.

18 Sadler, A. and Williams, B. (2008). Interferon-inducible antiviral effectors. *Nat. Rev. Immunol.* 8: 559–568. https://doi.org/10.1038/nri2314.

19 Karikó, K., Muramatsu, H., Welsh, F.A. et al. (2008). Incorporation of pseudouridine into mRNA yields superior nonimmunogenic vector with increased translational capacity and biological stability. *Mol. Ther.* 16 (11): 1833–1840. https://doi.org/10.1038/mt.2008.200.

20 Anderson, B.R., Muramatsu, H., Jha, B.K. et al. (2011). Nucleoside modifications in RNA limit activation of 2′-5′- oligoadenylate synthetase and increase resistance to cleavage by RNase L. *Nucleic Acids Res.* 39 (21): 9329–9338. https://doi.org/10.1093/nar/gkr586.

21 Anderson, B.R., Muramatsu, H., Nallagatla, S.R. et al. (2010). Incorporation of pseudouridine into mRNA enhances translation by diminishing PKR activation. *Nucleic Acids Res.* 38 (17): 5884–5892. https://doi.org/10.1093/nar/gkq347.

22 Alameh, M.G., Tombácz, I., Bettini, E. et al. (2021). Lipid nanoparticles enhance the efficacy of mRNA and protein subunit vaccines by inducing robust T follicular helper cell and humoral responses. *Immunity* 54 (12): 2877–2892.e7. https://doi.org/10.1016/j.immuni.2021.11.001.

23 Arunachalam, P.S., Scott, M.K.D., Hagan, T. et al. (2021). Systems vaccinology of the BNT162b2 mRNA vaccine in humans. *Nature* 596 (7872): 410–416. https://doi.org/10.1038/s41586-021-03791-x.

24 Gebre, M.S., Rauch, S., Roth, N. et al. (2022). Optimization of non-coding regions for a non-modified mRNA COVID-19 vaccine. *Nature* 601 (7893): 410–414. https://doi.org/10.1038/s41586-021-04231-6.

25 Li, C., Lee, A., Grigoryan, L. et al. (2022). Mechanisms of innate and adaptive immunity to the Pfizer-BioNTech BNT162b2 vaccine. *Nat. Immunol.* 23 (4): 543–555. https://doi.org/10.1038/s41590-022-01163-9.

26 Valentin, A., Bergamaschi, C., Rosati, M. et al. (2022). Comparative immunogenicity of an mRNA/LNP and a DNA vaccine targeting HIV gag conserved elements in macaques. *Front. Immunol.* 13: https://doi.org/10.3389/fimmu.2022.945706.

27 Pulendran, B., Arunachalam, P.S., and O'Hagan, D.T. (2021). Emerging concepts in the science of vaccine adjuvants. *Nat. Rev. Drug Discov.* 20 (6): 454–475. https://doi.org/10.1038/s41573-021-00163-y.

28 Yatim, N., Cullen, S., and Albert, M.L. (2017). Dying cells actively regulate adaptive immune responses. *Nat. Rev. Immunol.* 17 (4): 262–275. https://doi.org/10.1038/nri.2017.9.

29 Bergamaschi, C., Terpos, E., Rosati, M. et al. (2021). Systemic IL-15, IFN-γ, and IP-10/CXCL10 signature associated with effective immune response to SARS-CoV-2 in BNT162b2 mRNA vaccine recipients. *Cell Rep.* 36 (6): https://doi.org/10.1016/j.celrep.2021.109504.

30 Takano, T., Morikawa, M., Adachi, Y. et al. (2022). Distinct immune cell dynamics correlate with the immunogenicity and reactogenicity of SARS-CoV-2 mRNA vaccine. *Cell Rep. Med.* 3 (5): https://doi.org/10.1016/j.xcrm.2022.100631.

31 Al-Attiyah, R., Safar, H.A., Botras, L. et al. (2022). Immune cells profiles in the peripheral blood of patients with moderate to severe COVID-19 and healthy subjects with and without vaccination with the Pfizer-BioNTech mRNA vaccine. *Front. Immunol.* 13: 851765. https://doi.org/10.3389/fimmu.2022.851765.

32 Hadjadj, J., Yatim, N., Barnabei, L. et al. (2020). Impaired type I interferon activity and inflammatory responses in severe COVID-19 patients. *Science* 369 (6504): 718–724. https://doi.org/10.1126/science.abc6027ï.

33 Schulte-Schrepping, J., Reusch, N., Paclik, D. et al. (2020). Severe COVID-19 is marked by a dysregulated myeloid cell compartment. *Cell* 182 (6): 1419–1440.e23. https://doi.org/10.1016/j.cell.2020.08.001.

34 Sefik, E., Qu, R., Junqueira, C. et al. (2022). Inflammasome activation in infected macrophages drives COVID-19 pathology. *Nature* 606 (7914): 585–593. https://doi.org/10.1038/s41586-022-04802-1.

35 Theobald, S.J., Simonis, A., Georgomanolis, T. et al. (2021). Long-lived macrophage reprogramming drives spike protein-mediated inflammasome activation in COVID-19. *EMBO Mol. Med.* 13 (8): https://doi.org/10.15252/emmm.202114150.

36 Theobald, S.J., Simonis, A., Mudler, J.M. et al. (2022). Spleen tyrosine kinase mediates innate and adaptive immune crosstalk in SARS-CoV-2 mRNA vaccination. *EMBO Mol. Med.* 14 (8): https://doi.org/10.15252/emmm.202215888.

37 Hogan, M.J. and Pardi, N. (2022). mRNA Vaccines in the COVID-19 pandemic and beyond. *Annu. Rev. Med.* 73: 17–39. https://doi.org/10.1146/annurev-med-042420.

38 Bahl, K., Senn, J.J., Yuzhakov, O. et al. (2017). Preclinical and Clinical Demonstration of Immunogenicity by mRNA Vaccines against H10N8 and H7N9 Influenza Viruses. *Mol. Ther.* 25 (6): 1316–1327. https://doi.org/10.1016/j.ymthe.2017.03.035.

39 Harari, D., Abramovich, R., Zozulya, A. et al. (2014). Bridging the species divide: transgenic mice humanized for type-I interferon response. *PLoS One* 9 (1): https://doi.org/10.1371/journal.pone.0084259.

40 Tahtinen, S., Tong, A.J., Himmels, P. et al. (2022). IL-1 and IL-1ra are key regulators of the inflammatory response to RNA vaccines. *Nat. Immunol.* 23 (4): 532–542. https://doi.org/10.1038/s41590-022 01160-y.

41 Zschaler, J., Schlorke, D., and Arnhold, J. (2014). Differences in innate immune response between man and mouse. *Crit. Rev. Immunol.* 34 (5): 433–454. https://doi.org/10.1615/critrevimmunol.2014011600.

42 Tao, L. and Reese, T.A. (2017). Making mouse models that reflect human immune responses. *Trends Immunol.* 38 (3): 181–193. https://doi.org/10.1016/j.it.2016.12.007.

43 Karikó, K., Buckstein, M., Ni, H., and Weissman, D. (2005). Suppression of RNA recognition by Toll-like receptors: the impact of nucleoside modification and the evolutionary origin of RNA. *Immunity* 23 (2): 165–175. https://doi.org/10.1016/j.immuni.2005.06.008.

44 Karikó, K., Muramatsu, H., Keller, J.M., and Weissman, D. (2012). Increased erythropoiesis in mice injected with submicrogram quantities of pseudouridine-containing mRNA encoding erythropoietin. *Mol. Ther.* 20 (5): 948–953. https://doi.org/10.1038/mt.2012.7.

45 Andries, O., Mc Cafferty, S., de Smedt, S.C. et al. (2015). N1-methylpseudouridine-incorporated mRNA outperforms pseudouridine-incorporated mRNA by providing enhanced protein expression and reduced immunogenicity in mammalian cell lines and mice. *J. Control. Release* 217: 337–344. https://doi.org/10.1016/j.jconrel.2015.08.051.

46 Pardi, N., Hogan, M.J., Pelc, R.S. et al. (2017). Zika virus protection by a single low-dose nucleoside-modified mRNA vaccination. *Nature* 543 (7644): 248–251. https://doi.org/10.1038/nature21428.

47 Chouaib, R., Safieddine, A., Pichon, X. et al. (2020). A dual protein-mRNA localization screen reveals compartmentalized translation and widespread co-translational RNA targeting. *Dev. Cell* 54 (6): 773–791.e5. https://doi.org/10.1016/j.devcel.2020.07.010.

48 Lashkevich, K.A. and Dmitriev, S.E. (2021). mRNA Targeting, transport and local translation in eukaryotic cells: from the classical view to a diversity of new concepts. *Mol. Biol.* 55 (4): 507–537. https://doi.org/10.1134/S0026893321030080.

49 Rasmussen, E.B. and Lis, J.T. (1993). In vivo transcriptional pausing and cap formation on three Drosophila heat shock genes (RNA polymerase lI/elongation arrest/RNA capping). *Proc. Natl. Acad. Sci. USA* 90: 7923–7927. https://www.pnas.org.

50 Singh, G., Pratt, G., Yeo, G.W., and Moore, M.J. (2015). The clothes make the mRNA: past and present trends in mRNP fashion. *Annu. Rev. Biochem.* 84: 325–354. https://doi.org/10.1146/annurev-biochem-080111-092106.

51 Mauer, J., Luo, X., Blanjoie, A. et al. (2017). Reversible methylation of m6 Am in the 5′ cap controls mRNA stability. *Nature* 541 (7637): 371–375. https://doi.org/10.1038/nature21022.

52 Boulias, K., Toczydłowska-Socha, D., Hawley, B.R. et al. (2019). Identification of the m6Am methyltransferase PCIF1 reveals the location and functions of m6Am in the transcriptome. *Mol. Cell* 75 (3): 631–643.e8. https://doi.org/10.1016/j.molcel.2019.06.006.

53 Diamond, M.S. (2014). IFIT1: a dual sensor and effector molecule that detects non-2’-O methylated viral RNA and inhibits its translation. *Cytokine Growth Factor Rev.* 25 (5): 543–550. https://doi.org/10.1016/j.cytogfr.2014.05.002.

54 Borden, K.L.B., Culjkovic-Kraljacic, B., and Cowling, V.H. (2021). To cap it all off, again: dynamic capping and recapping of coding and non-coding RNAs to control transcript fate and biological activity. *Cell Cycle* 20 (14): 1347–1360. https://doi.org/10.1080/15384101.2021.1930929.

55 Bastos, R.N. and Volloch, Z. (1977). Messenger RNA population analysis during erythroid differentiation: a kinetical approach. *J. Mol. Biol.* 110: 191–203.

56 Russell, J.E. and Liebhaber, S.A. (1996). The stability of human ß-globin mRNA is dependent on structural determinants positioned within its 3’ untranslated region. *Blood* 87 (12): 5314–5323.

57 Kozak, M. (1986). Influences of mRNA secondary structure on initiation by eukaryotic ribosomes (translational control/insertion mutagenesl/scanning model/RNA stem-and-loop structures/preproinsulin). *Proc. Natl. Acad. Sci. USA* 83: 2850–2854.

58 Jia, L., Mao, Y., Ji, Q. et al. (2020). Decoding mRNA translatability and stability from the 5′ UTR. *Nat. Struct. Mol. Biol.* 27 (9): 814–821. https://doi.org/10.1038/s41594-020-0465-x.

59 Lee, A.S.Y., Kranzusch, P.J., and Cate, J.H.D. (2015). EIF3 targets cell-proliferation messenger RNAs for translational activation or repression. *Nature* 522 (7554): 111–114. https://doi.org/10.1038/nature14267.

60 Parsons, C.J., Stefanovic, B., Seki, E. et al. (2011). Mutation of the 5′-untranslated region stem-loop structure inhibits α1(I) collagen expression in vivo. *J. Biol. Chem.* 286 (10): 8609–8619. https://doi.org/10.1074/jbc.M110.189118.

61 Zhang, Y. and Stefanovic, B. (2016). LARP6 meets collagen mRNA: specific regulation of type I collagen expression. *Int. J. Mol. Sci.* 17 (3): https://doi.org/10.3390/ijms17030419.

62 Challa, A.A. and Stefanovic, B. (2011). A novel role of vimentin filaments: binding and stabilization of collagen mRNAs. *Mol. Cell. Biol.* 31 (18): 3773–3789. https://doi.org/10.1128/mcb.05263-11.

63 Stefanovic, L., Longo, L., Zhang, Y., and Stefanovic, B. (2014). Characterization of binding of LARP6 to the 5' stem-loop of collagen mRNAs: implications for synthesis of type I collagen. *RNA Biol.* 11 (11): 1386–1401. https://doi.org/10.1080/15476286.2014.996467.

64 Castillo-Hair, S.M. and Seelig, G. (2022). Machine learning for designing next-generation mRNA therapeutics. *Acc. Chem. Res.* 55 (1): 24–34. https://doi.org/10.1021/acs.accounts.1c00621.

65 Sample, P.J., Wang, B., Reid, D.W. et al. (2019). Human 5′ UTR design and variant effect prediction from a massively parallel translation assay. *Nat. Biotechnol.* 37 (7): 803–809. https://doi.org/10.1038/s41587-019-0164-5.

66 Linares-Fernández, S., Moreno, J., Lambert, E. et al. (2021). Combining an optimized mRNA template with a double purification process allows strong expression of in vitro transcribed mRNA. *Mol. Ther. Nucleic Acids* 26: 945–956. https://doi.org/10.1016/j.omtn.2021.10.007.

67 Holtkamp, S., Kreiter, S., Selmi, A. et al. (2006). Modification of antigen-encoding RNA increases stability, translational efficacy, and T-cell stimulatory capacity of dendritic cells. *Blood* 108 (13): 4009–4017. https://doi.org/10.1182/blood-2006-04-015024.

68 Orlandini von Niessen, A.G., Poleganov, M.A., Rechner, C. et al. (2019). Improving mRNA-based therapeutic gene delivery by expression-augmenting 3′ UTRs identified by cellular library screening. *Mol. Ther.* 27 (4): 824–836. https://doi.org/10.1016/j.ymthe.2018.12.011.

69 Gallie, D.R., Lewis, N.J., and Marzluff, W.F. (1996). The histone 3′-terminal stem-loop is necessary for translation in Chinese hamster ovary cells. *Nucleic Acids Res.* 24 (10): 1954–1962.

70 Jang, S.K. and Paek, K.Y. (2016). Cap-dependent translation is mediated by 'RNA looping' rather than 'ribosome scanning'. *RNA Biol.* 13 (1): 1–5. https://doi.org/10.1080/15476286.2015.1107700.

71 Michel, Y.M., Poncet, D., Piron, M. et al. (2000). Cap-poly(A) synergy in mammalian cell-free extracts. Investigation of the requirements for poly(A)-mediated stimulation of translation initiation. *J. Biol. Chem.* 275 (41): 32268–32276. https://doi.org/10.1074/jbc.M004304200.

72 Dominski, Z., Yang, X.-C., Kaygun, H. et al. (2003). A 3' exonuclease that specifically interacts with the 3 end of histone mRNA. *Mol. Cell* 12: 295–305.

73 Rattenbacher, B., Beisang, D., Wiesner, D.L. et al. (2010). Analysis of CUGBP1 targets identifies GU-repeat sequences that mediate rapid mRNA decay. *Mol. Cell. Biol.* 30 (16): 3970–3980. https://doi.org/10.1128/mcb.00624-10.

74 Stoecklin, G., Colombi, M., Raineri, I. et al. (2002). Functional cloning of BRF1, a regulator of ARE-dependent mRNA turnover. *EMBO J.* 21 (17): 4709–4718.

75 Leppek, K., Byeon, G.W., Kladwang, W. et al. (2022). Combinatorial optimization of mRNA structure, stability, and translation for RNA-based therapeutics. *Nat. Commun.* 13 (1): https://doi.org/10.1038/s41467-022-28776-w.

76 Bilska, A., Kusio-Kobiałka, M., Krawczyk, P.S. et al. (2020). Immunoglobulin expression and the humoral immune response is regulated by the non-canonical poly(A) polymerase TENT5C. *Nat. Commun.* 11 (1): https://doi.org/10.1038/s41467-020-15835-3.

77 Brouze, A., Krawczyk, P.S., Dziembowski, A., and Mroczek, S. (2023). Measuring the tail: methods for poly(A) tail profiling. *Wiley Interdis. Rev. RNA* 14 (1): e1737. https://doi.org/10.1002/wrna.1737.

78 Lima, S.A., Chipman, L.B., Nicholson, A.L. et al. (2017). Short poly(A) tails are a conserved feature of highly expressed genes. *Nat. Struct. Mol. Biol.* 24 (12): 1057–1063. https://doi.org/10.1038/nsmb.3499.

79 Kajjo, S., Sharma, S., Chen, S. et al. (2022). PABP prevents the untimely decay of select mRNA populations in human cells. *EMBO J.* 41 (6): https://doi.org/10.15252/embj.2021108650.

80 Vicens, Q., Kieft, J.S., and Rissland, O.S. (2018). Revisiting the closed-loop model and the nature of mRNA 5′–3′ communication. *Mol. Cell* 72 (5): 805–812. https://doi.org/10.1016/j.molcel.2018.10.047.

81 Grier, A.E., Burleigh, S., Sahni, J. et al. (2016). pEVL: a linear plasmid for generating mRNA IVT templates with extended encoded poly(A) sequences. *Mol. Ther. Nucleic Acids* 5: e306. https://doi.org/10.1038/mtna.2016.21.

82 Chang, H., Lim, J., Ha, M., and Kim, V.N. (2014). TAIL-seq: genome-wide determination of poly(A) tail length and 3' end modifications. *Mol. Cell* 53 (6): 1044–1052. https://doi.org/10.1016/j.molcel.2014.02.007.

83 Lim, J., Ha, M., Chang, H. et al. (2014). Uridylation by TUT4 and TUT7 marks mRNA for degradation. *Cell* 159 (6): 1365–1376. https://doi.org/10.1016/j.cell.2014.10.055.

84 Lim, J., Kim, D., Lee, Y.-S. et al. (2018). Mixed tailing by TENT4A and TENT4B shields mRNA from rapid deadenylation. *Science* 361 (6403): 701–704. https://doi.org/10.1126/science.aam5794.

85 Viegas, I.J., de Macedo, J.P., Serra, L. et al. (2022). N 6-methyladenosine in poly(A) tails stabilize VSG transcripts. *Nature* 604 (7905): 362–370. https://doi.org/10.1038/s41586-022-04544-0.

86 Legnini, I., Alles, J., Karaiskos, N. et al. (2019). FLAM-seq: full-length mRNA sequencing reveals principles of poly(A) tail length control. *Nat. Methods* 16 (9): 879–886. https://doi.org/10.1038/s41592-019-0503-y.

87 Liu, Y., Nie, H., Liu, H., and Lu, F. (2019). Poly(A) inclusive RNA isoform sequencing (PAIso–seq) reveals wide-spread non-adenosine residues within

RNA poly(A) tails. *Nat. Commun.* 10 (1): https://doi.org/10.1038/s41467-019-13228-9.

88 Stadler, C.R., Bähr-Mahmud, H., Celik, L. et al. (2017). Elimination of large tumors in mice by mRNA-encoded bispecific antibodies. *Nat. Med.* 23 (7): 815–817. https://doi.org/10.1038/nm.4356.

89 Trepotec, Z., Geiger, J., Plank, C. et al. (2019). Segmented poly(A) tails significantly reduce recombination of plasmid DNA without affecting mRNA translation efficiency or half-life. *RNA* 25 (4): 507–518. https://doi.org/10.1261/rna.

90 Jackson, L.A., Anderson, E.J., Rouphael, N.G. et al. (2020). An mRNA vaccine against SARS-CoV-2—preliminary report. *N. Engl. J. Med.* 383 (20): 1920–1931. https://doi.org/10.1056/nejmoa2022483.

91 Mulligan, M.J., Lyke, K.E., Kitchin, N. et al. (2020). Phase I/II study of COVID-19 RNA vaccine BNT162b1 in adults. *Nature* 586 (7830): 589–593. https://doi.org/10.1038/s41586-020-2639-4.

92 Kirchdoerfer, R.N., Wang, N., Pallesen, J. et al. (2018). Stabilized coronavirus spikes are resistant to conformational changes induced by receptor recognition or proteolysis. *Sci. Rep.* 8 (1): 15701. https://doi.org/10.1038/s41598-018-34171-7.

93 Pallesen, J., Wang, N., Corbett, K.S. et al. (2017). Immunogenicity and structures of a rationally designed prefusion MERS-CoV spike antigen. *Proc. Natl. Acad. Sci. USA* 114 (35): E7348–E7357. https://doi.org/10.1073/pnas.1707304114.

94 Goodsell, D.S. and Burley, S.K. (2022). RCSB Protein Data Bank resources for structure-facilitated design of mRNA vaccines for existing and emerging viral pathogens. *Structure* 30 (1): 55–68.e2. https://doi.org/10.1016/j.str.2021.10.008.

95 Presnyak, V., Alhusaini, N., Chen, Y.H. et al. (2015). Codon optimality is a major determinant of mRNA stability. *Cell* 160 (6): 1111–1124. https://doi.org/10.1016/j.cell.2015.02.029.

96 Narula, A., Ellis, J., Taliaferro, J.M., and Rissland, O.S. (2019). Coding regions affect mRNA stability in human cells. *RNA* 25: 1751–1764. https://doi.org/10.1261/rna.

97 Radhakrishnan, A., Chen, Y.H., Martin, S. et al. (2016). The DEAD-Box protein Dhh1p couples mRNA decay and translation by monitoring codon optimality. *Cell* 167 (1): 122–132.e9. https://doi.org/10.1016/j.cell.2016.08.053.

98 Sweet, T., Kovalak, C., and Coller, J. (2012). The dead-box protein dhh1 promotes decapping by slowing ribosome movement. *PLoS Biol.* 10 (6): https://doi.org/10.1371/journal.pbio.1001342.

99 Chu, D., Kazana, E., Bellanger, N. et al. (2014). Translation elongation can control translation initiation on eukaryotic mRNAs. *EMBO J.* 33 (1): 21–34. https://doi.org/10.1002/embj.201385651.

100 Mauro, V.P. (2018). Codon optimization in the production of recombinant biotherapeutics: potential risks and considerations. *BioDrugs* 32 (1): 69–81. https://doi.org/10.1007/s40259-018-0261-x.

101 Alexaki, A., Kames, J., Holcomb, D.D. et al. (2019). Codon and codon-pair usage tables (CoCoPUTs): facilitating genetic variation analyses and recombinant gene design. *J. Mol. Biol.* 431 (13): 2434–2441. https://doi.org/10.1016/j.jmb.2019.04.021.

102 Fuglsang, A. (2003). Codon optimizer: a freeware tool for codon optimization. *Protein Expr. Purif.* 31 (2): 247–249. https://doi.org/10.1016/S1046-5928(03)00213-4.

103 Hanson, G. and Coller, J. (2018). Translation and protein quality control: codon optimality, bias and usage in translation and mRNA decay. *Nat. Rev. Mol. Cell Biol.* 19 (1): 20–30. https://doi.org/10.1038/nrm.2017.91.

104 Yoon, J., Chung, Y.-J., and Lee, M. (2018). STADIUM: species-specific tRNA adaptive index compendium. *Genom. Inform.* 16 (4): e28. https://doi.org/10.5808/gi.2018.16.4.e28.

105 Vaidyanathan, S., Azizian, K.T., Haque, A.K.M.A. et al. (2018). Uridine depletion and chemical modification increase Cas9 mRNA activity and reduce immunogenicity without HPLC purification. *Mol. Ther. Nucleic Acids* 12: 530–542. https://doi.org/10.1016/j.omtn.2018.06.010.

106 Hia, F., Yang, S.F., Shichino, Y. et al. (2019). Codon bias confers stability to human mRNAs. *EMBO Rep.* 20 (11): https://doi.org/10.15252/embr.201948220.

107 Mauger, D.M., Joseph Cabral, B., Presnyak, V. et al. (2019). mRNA structure regulates protein expression through changes in functional half-life. *Proc. Natl. Acad. Sci. USA* 116 (48): 24075–24083. https://doi.org/10.1073/pnas.1908052116.

108 Hia, F. and Takeuchi, O. (2021). The effects of codon bias and optimality on mRNA and protein regulation. *Cell. Mol. Life Sci.* 78 (5): 1909–1928. https://doi.org/10.1007/s00018-020-03685-7.

109 Spencer, P.S., Siller, E., Anderson, J.F., and Barral, J.M. (2012). Silent substitutions predictably alter translation elongation rates and protein folding efficiencies. *J. Mol. Biol.* 422 (3): 328–335. https://doi.org/10.1016/j.jmb.2012.06.010.

110 Oh, S. and Kessler, J.A. (2018). Design, assembly, production, and transfection of synthetic modified mRNA. *Methods* 133: 29–43. https://doi.org/10.1016/j.ymeth.2017.10.008.

111 Geall, A.J., Mandl, C.W., and Ulmer, J.B. (2013). RNA: the new revolution in nucleic acid vaccines. *Semin. Immunol.* 25 (2): 152–159. https://doi.org/10.1016/j.smim.2013.05.001.

112 Rosa, S.S., Nunes, D., Antunes, L. et al. (2022). Maximizing mRNA vaccine production with Bayesian optimization. *Biotechnol. Bioeng.* 119 (11): 3127–3139. https://doi.org/10.1002/bit.28216.

113 Baiersdörfer, M., Boros, G., Muramatsu, H. et al. (2019). A facile method for the removal of dsRNA contaminant from in vitro-transcribed mRNA. *Mol. Ther. Nucleic Acids* 15: 26–35. https://doi.org/10.1016/j.omtn.2019.02.018.

114 Mu, X., Greenwald, E., Ahmad, S., and Hur, S. (2018). An origin of the immunogenicity of in vitro transcribed RNA. *Nucleic Acids Res.* 46 (10): 5239–5249. https://doi.org/10.1093/nar/gky177.

115 Durbin, A.F., Wang, C., Marcotrigiano, J., and Gehrke, L. (2016). RNAs containing modified nucleotides fail to trigger RIG-I conformational changes for innate immune signaling. *MBio* 7 (5): https://doi.org/10.1128/mBio.00833-16.

116 Ringeard, M., Marchand, V., Decroly, E. et al. (2019). FTSJ3 is an RNA 2′-O-methyltransferase recruited by HIV to avoid innate immune sensing. *Nature* 565 (7740): 500–504. https://doi.org/10.1038/s41586-018-0841-4.

117 Li, X., Zhu, P., Ma, S. et al. (2015). Chemical pulldown reveals dynamic pseudouridylation of the mammalian transcriptome. *Nat. Chem. Biol.* 11 (8): 592–597. https://doi.org/10.1038/nchembio.1836.

118 Eyler, D.E., Franco, M.K., Batool, Z. et al. (2019). Pseudouridinylation of mRNA coding sequences alters translation. *Proc. Natl. Acad. Sci. USA* 116 (46): 23068–23074. https://doi.org/10.1073/pnas.1821754116.

119 Karijolich, J. and Yu, Y.T. (2011). Converting nonsense codons into sense codons by targeted pseudouridylation. *Nature* 474 (7351): 395–399. https://doi.org/10.1038/nature10165.

120 Morais, P., Adachi, H., and Yu, Y.T. (2021). The critical contribution of pseudouridine to mRNA COVID-19 vaccines. *Front. Cell Dev. Biol.* 9: https://doi.org/10.3389/fcell.2021.789427.

121 Pardi, N., Tuyishime, S., Muramatsu, H. et al. (2015). Expression kinetics of nucleoside-modified mRNA delivered in lipid nanoparticles to mice by various routes. *J. Control. Release* 217: 345–351. https://doi.org/10.1016/j.jconrel.2015.08.007.

122 Despic, V. and Jaffrey, S.R. (2023). mRNA ageing shapes the Cap2 methylome in mammalian mRNA. *Nature* 614 (7947): 358–366. https://doi.org/10.1038/s41586-022-05668-z.

123 Inagaki, M., Abe, N., Li, Z. et al. (2023). Cap analogs with a hydrophobic photocleavable tag enable facile purification of fully capped mRNA with various cap structures. *Nat. Commun.* 14 (1): https://doi.org/10.1038/s41467-023-38244-8.

124 Hornung, V., Ellegast, J., Kim, S. et al. (2006). 5'-Triphosphate RNA is the ligand for RIG-I. *Science* 314 (5801): 994–997. https://www.science.org.

125 Karikó, K., Muramatsu, H., Ludwig, J., and Weissman, D. (2011). Generating the optimal mRNA for therapy: HPLC purification eliminates immune activation and improves translation of nucleoside-modified, protein-encoding mRNA. *Nucleic Acids Res.* 39 (21): https://doi.org/10.1093/nar/gkr695.

126 Szabó, G.T., Mahiny, A.J., and Vlatkovic, I. (2022). COVID-19 mRNA vaccines: platforms and current developments. *Mol. Ther.* 30 (5): 1850–1868. https://doi.org/10.1016/j.ymthe.2022.02.016.

127 Laczkó, D., Hogan, M.J., Toulmin, S.A. et al. (2020). A single immunization with nucleoside-modified mRNA vaccines elicits strong cellular and humoral immune responses against SARS-CoV-2 in mice. *Immunity* 53 (4): 724–732.e7. https://doi.org/10.1016/j.immuni.2020.07.019.

128 Fenton, O.S., Kauffman, K.J., Kaczmarek, J.C. et al. (2017). Synthesis and biological evaluation of ionizable lipid materials for the in vivo delivery of messenger RNA to B lymphocytes. *Adv. Mater.* 29 (33): https://doi.org/10.1002/adma.201606944.

129 Hou, X., Zaks, T., Langer, R., and Dong, Y. (2021). Lipid nanoparticles for mRNA delivery. *Nat. Rev. Mater.* 6 (12): 1078–1094. https://doi.org/10.1038/s41578-021-00358-0.

130 Lederer, K., Castaño, D., Gómez Atria, D. et al. (2020). SARS-CoV-2 mRNA vaccines foster potent antigen-specific germinal center responses associated with neutralizing antibody generation. *Immunity* 53 (6): 1281–1295.e5. https://doi.org/10.1016/j.immuni.2020.11.009.

131 Alberer, M., Gnad-Vogt, U., Hong, H.S. et al. (2017). Safety and immunogenicity of a mRNA rabies vaccine in healthy adults: an open-label, non-randomised, prospective, first-in-human phase 1 clinical trial. *Lancet* 390 (10101): 1511–1520. https://doi.org/10.1016/S0140-6736(17)31665-3.

132 Feldman, R.A., Fuhr, R., Smolenov, I. et al. (2019). mRNA vaccines against H10N8 and H7N9 influenza viruses of pandemic potential are immunogenic and well tolerated in healthy adults in phase 1 randomized clinical trials. *Vaccine* 37 (25): 3326–3334. https://doi.org/10.1016/j.vaccine.2019.04.074.

133 Adams, D., Gonzalez-Duarte, A., O'Riordan, W.D. et al. (2018). Patisiran, an RNAi therapeutic, for hereditary transthyretin amyloidosis. *N. Engl. J. Med.* 379 (1): 11–21. https://doi.org/10.1056/nejmoa1716153.

134 Weng, Y., Xiao, H., Zhang, J. et al. (2019). RNAi therapeutic and its innovative biotechnological evolution. *Biotechnol. Adv.* 37 (5): 801–825. https://doi.org/10.1016/j.biotechadv.2019.04.012.

135 Dolgin, E. (2021). How COVID unlocked the power of RNA vaccines. *Nature* 589 (7841): 189–191. https://doi.org/10.1038/d41586-021-00019-w.

136 Dolgin, E. (2021). The tangled history of mRNA vaccines. *Nature* 597 (7876): 318–324. https://doi.org/10.1038/d41586-021-02483-w.

137 Kon, E., Elia, U., and Peer, D. (2022). Principles for designing an optimal mRNA lipid nanoparticle vaccine. *Curr. Opin. Biotechnol.* 73: 329–336. https://doi.org/10.1016/j.copbio.2021.09.016.

138 Lee, J., Kim, D., Byun, J. et al. (2022). In vivo fate and intracellular trafficking of vaccine delivery systems. *Adv. Drug Deliv. Rev.* 186: 114325. https://doi.org/10.1016/j.addr.2022.114325.

139 Hassett, K.J., Benenato, K.E., Jacquinet, E. et al. (2019). Optimization of lipid nanoparticles for intramuscular administration of mRNA vaccines. *Mol. Ther. Nucleic Acids* 15: 1–11. https://doi.org/10.1016/j.omtn.2019.01.013.

140 Zhang, Y., Sun, C., Wang, C. et al. (2021). Lipids and lipid derivatives for RNA delivery. *Chem. Rev.* 121 (20): 12181–12277. https://doi.org/10.1021/acs.chemrev.1c00244.

141 Paramasivam, P., Franke, C., Stöter, M. et al. (2022). Endosomal escape of delivered mRNA from endosomal recycling tubules visualized at the nanoscale. *J. Cell Biol.* 221 (2): https://doi.org/10.1083/jcb.202110137.

142 Dolgin, E. (2022). Better lipids to power next generation of mRNA vaccines. *Science* 376 (6594): 680–681. https://doi.org/10.1126/science.adc9449.

143 Han, X., Zhang, H., Butowska, K. et al. (2021). An ionizable lipid toolbox for RNA delivery. *Nat. Commun.* 12 (1): 7233. https://doi.org/10.1038/s41467-021-27493-0.

144 Arteta, M.Y., Kjellman, T., Bartesaghi, S. et al. (2018). Successful reprogramming of cellular protein production through mRNA delivered by functionalized lipid nanoparticles. *Proc. Natl. Acad. Sci. USA* 115 (15): E3351–E3360. https://doi.org/10.1073/pnas.1720542115.

145 Cui, L., Hunter, M.R., Sonzini, S. et al. (2022). Mechanistic studies of an automated lipid nanoparticle reveal critical pharmaceutical properties associated with enhanced mRNA functional delivery in vitro and in vivo. *Small* 18 (9): e2105832. https://doi.org/10.1002/smll.202105832.

146 Patel, S., Ashwanikumar, N., Robinson, E. et al. (2020). Naturally-occurring cholesterol analogues in lipid nanoparticles induce polymorphic shape and enhance intracellular delivery of mRNA. *Nat. Commun.* 11 (1): https://doi.org/10.1038/s41467-020-14527-2.

147 Sabnis, S., Kumarasinghe, E.S., Salerno, T. et al. (2018). A novel amino lipid series for mRNA delivery: improved endosomal escape and sustained pharmacology and safety in non-human primates. *Mol. Ther.* 26 (6): 1509–1519. https://doi.org/10.1016/j.ymthe.2018.03.010.

148 Fenton, O.S., Kauffman, K.J., McClellan, R.L. et al. (2018). Customizable lipid nanoparticle materials for the delivery of siRNAs and mRNAs. *Angew. Chem. Int. Ed.* 57 (41): 13582–13586. https://doi.org/10.1002/anie.201809056.

149 Hajj, K.A., Ball, R.L., Deluty, S.B. et al. (2019). Branched-tail lipid nanoparticles potently deliver mRNA in vivo due to enhanced ionization at endosomal pH. *Small* 15 (6): https://doi.org/10.1002/smll.201805097.

150 Cheng, Q., Wei, T., Farbiak, L. et al. (2020). Selective organ targeting (SORT) nanoparticles for tissue-specific mRNA delivery and CRISPR–Cas gene editing. *Nat. Nanotechnol.* 15 (4): 313–320. https://doi.org/10.1038/s41565-020-0669-6.

151 Dilliard, S.A., Cheng, Q., Siegwart, D.J., and Desimone, J. (2021). On the mechanism of tissue-specific mRNA delivery by selective organ targeting nanoparticles. *Proc. Natl. Acad. Sci. USA* 118 (52): e2109256118. https://doi.org/10.1073/pnas.2109256118/-/DCSupplemental.

152 Sebastiani, F., Yanez Arteta, M., Lerche, M. et al. (2021). Apolipoprotein E binding drives structural and compositional rearrangement of mRNA-containing lipid nanoparticles. *ACS Nano* 15 (4): 6709–6722. https://doi.org/10.1021/acsnano.0c10064.

153 da Silva Sanchez, A.J., Dobrowolski, C., Cristian, A. et al. (2022). Universal barcoding predicts in vivo ApoE-independent lipid nanoparticle delivery. *Nano Lett.* 22 (12): 4822–4830. https://doi.org/10.1021/acs.nanolett.2c01133.

154 Bevers, S., Kooijmans, S.A.A., van de Velde, E. et al. (2022). mRNA-LNP vaccines tuned for systemic immunization induce strong antitumor immunity by engaging splenic immune cells. *Mol. Ther.* 30 (9): 3078–3094. https://doi.org/10.1016/j.ymthe.2022.07.007.

155 Bigini, P., Gobbi, M., Bonati, M. et al. (2021). The role and impact of polyethylene glycol on anaphylactic reactions to COVID-19 nanovaccines. *Nat. Nanotechnol.* 16 (11): 1169–1171. https://doi.org/10.1038/s41565-021-01001-3.

156 de Vrieze, J. (2021). Pfizer's vaccine raises allergy concerns. *Science* 371 (6524): 10–11. https://doi.org/10.1126/science.371.6524.10.

157 Chanan-Khan, A., Szebeni, J., Savay, S. et al. (2003). Complement activation following first exposure to pegylated liposomal doxorubicin (Doxil®): possible role in hypersensitivity reactions. *Ann. Oncol.* 14 (9): 1430–1437. https://doi.org/10.1093/annonc/mdg374.

158 Kong, Y.W. and Dreaden, E.C. (2022). PEG: Will it come back to you? Polyethelyne glycol immunogenicity, COVID vaccines, and the case for new PEG derivatives and alternatives. *Front. Bioeng. Biotechnol.* 10: https://doi.org/10.3389/fbioe.2022.879988.

159 Szebeni, J., Muggia, F., Gabizon, A., and Barenholz, Y. (2011). Activation of complement by therapeutic liposomes and other lipid excipient-based therapeutic products: prediction and prevention. *Adv. Drug Deliv. Rev.* 63 (12): 1020–1030. https://doi.org/10.1016/j.addr.2011.06.017.

160 Kozma, G.T., Shimizu, T., Ishida, T., and Szebeni, J. (2020). Anti-PEG antibodies: properties, formation, testing and role in adverse immune reactions to PEGylated nano-biopharmaceuticals. *Adv. Drug Deliv. Rev.* 154–155: 163–175. https://doi.org/10.1016/j.addr.2020.07.024.

161 Shi, D., Beasock, D., Fessler, A. et al. (2022). To PEGylate or not to PEGylate: immunological properties of nanomedicine's most popular component, polyethylene glycol and its alternatives. *Adv. Drug Deliv. Rev.* 180: https://doi.org/10.1016/j.addr.2021.114079.

162 Maruggi, G., Zhang, C., Li, J. et al. (2019). mRNA as a transformative technology for vaccine development to control infectious diseases. *Mol. Ther.* 27 (4): 757–772. https://doi.org/10.1016/j.ymthe.2019.01.020.

163 Estapé Senti, M., de Jongh, C.A., Dijkxhoorn, K. et al. (2022). Anti-PEG antibodies compromise the integrity of PEGylated lipid-based nanoparticles via complement. *J. Control. Release* 341: 475–486. https://doi.org/10.1016/j.jconrel.2021.11.042.

164 Ju, Y., Lee, W.S., Pilkington, E.H. et al. (2022). Anti-PEG antibodies boosted in humans by SARS-CoV-2 lipid nanoparticle mRNA vaccine. *ACS Nano* 16 (8): 11769–11780. https://doi.org/10.1021/acsnano.2c04543.

165 Pardi, N., Hogan, M.J., Naradikian, M.S. et al. (2018). Nucleoside-modified mRNA vaccines induce potent T follicular helper and germinal center B cell responses. *J. Exp. Med.* 215 (6): 1571–1588. https://doi.org/10.1084/jem.20171450.

166 Pardi, N., Hogan, M.J., Porter, F.W., and Weissman, D. (2018). mRNA vaccines-a new era in vaccinology. *Nat. Rev. Drug Discov.* 17 (4): 261–279. https://doi.org/10.1038/nrd.2017.243.

167 Saunders, K.O., Pardi, N., Parks, R. et al. (2021). Lipid nanoparticle encapsulated nucleoside-modified mRNA vaccines elicit polyfunctional HIV-1 antibodies comparable to proteins in nonhuman primates. *NPJ Vac.* 6 (1): https://doi.org/10.1038/s41541-021-00307-6.

168 Liang, F., Lindgren, G., Lin, A. et al. (2017). Efficient targeting and activation of antigen-presenting cells in vivo after modified mRNA vaccine administration in *Rhesus macaques*. *Mol. Ther.* 25 (12): 2635–2647. https://doi.org/10.1016/j.ymthe.2017.08.006.

169 Hassett, K.J., Higgins, J., Woods, A. et al. (2021). Impact of lipid nanoparticle size on mRNA vaccine immunogenicity. *J. Control. Release* 335: 237–246. https://doi.org/10.1016/j.jconrel.2021.05.021.

170 Roh, E.H., Fromen, C.A., and Sullivan, M.O. (2022). Inhalable mRNA vaccines for respiratory diseases: a roadmap. *Curr. Opin. Biotechnol.* 74: 104–109. https://doi.org/10.1016/j.copbio.2021.10.017.

171 Lokugamage, M.P., Vanover, D., Beyersdorf, J. et al. (2021). Optimization of lipid nanoparticles for the delivery of nebulized therapeutic mRNA to the lungs. *Nat. Biomed. Eng.* 5 (9): 1059–1068. https://doi.org/10.1038/s41551-021-00786-x.

172 Anderluzzi, G., Lou, G., Woods, S. et al. (2022). The role of nanoparticle format and route of administration on self-amplifying mRNA vaccine potency. *J. Control. Release* 342: 388–399. https://doi.org/10.1016/j.jconrel.2021.12.008.

173 Kobiyama, K. and Ishii, K.J. (2022). Making innate sense of mRNA vaccine adjuvanticity. *Nat. Immunol.* 23 (4): 474–476. https://doi.org/10.1038/s41590-022-01168-4.

174 Swaminathan, G., Thoryk, E.A., Cox, K.S. et al. (2016). A tetravalent sub-unit dengue vaccine formulated with ionizable cationic lipid nanoparticle induces significant immune responses in rodents and non-human primates. *Sci. Rep.* 6: https://doi.org/10.1038/srep34215.

175 Shirai, S., Kawai, A., Shibuya, M. et al. (2020). Lipid nanoparticle acts as a potential adjuvant for influenza split vaccine without inducing inflammatory responses. *Vaccine* 8 (3): 1–18. https://doi.org/10.3390/vaccines8030433.

176 Christensen, D., Korsholm, K.S., Andersen, P., and Agger, E.M. (2011). Cationic liposomes as vaccine adjuvants. *Expert Rev. Vaccines* 10 (4): 513–521. https://doi.org/10.1586/erv.11.17.

177 Lonez, C., Bessodes, M., Scherman, D. et al. (2014). Cationic lipid nanocarriers activate toll-like receptor 2 and NLRP3 inflammasome pathways. *Nanomedicine* 10 (4): 775–782. https://doi.org/10.1016/j.nano.2013.12.003.

178 Pizzuto, M., Bigey, P., Lachagès, A.M. et al. (2018). Cationic lipids as one-component vaccine adjuvants: a promising alternative to alum. *J. Control. Release* 287: 67–77. https://doi.org/10.1016/j.jconrel.2018.08.020.

179 Schoenmaker, L., Witzigmann, D., Kulkarni, J.A. et al. (2021). mRNA-lipid nanoparticle COVID-19 vaccines: structure and stability. *Int. J. Pharm.* 601: https://doi.org/10.1016/j.ijpharm.2021.120586.

180 Tinari, S. (2021). The EMA COVID-19 data leak, and what it tells us about mRNA instability. *BMJ* 372: https://doi.org/10.1136/bmj.n627.

181 Packer, M., Gyawali, D., Yerabolu, R. et al. (2021). A novel mechanism for the loss of mRNA activity in lipid nanoparticle delivery systems. *Nat. Commun.* 12 (1): https://doi.org/10.1038/s41467-021-26926-0.

182 Alishetty, S., Carrasco, M., Alameh, M.-G. et al. (2021). Novel lipid nanoparticle provides potent SARS-CoV-2 mRNA vaccine at low dose with low local reactogenicity, high thermostability and limited systemic biodistribution. *Preprint* https://doi.org/10.21203/rs.3.rs-798453/v1.

183 Carreño, J.M., Singh, G., Tcheou, J. et al. (2022). mRNA-1273 but not BNT162b2 induces antibodies against polyethylene glycol (PEG) contained in mRNA-based vaccine formulations. *Vaccine* 40: 6114–6124. https://doi.org/10.1016/j.vaccine.2022.08.024.

184 Mu, Z., Wiehe, K., Saunders, K.O. et al. (2022). mRNA-encoded HIV-1 Env trimer ferritin nanoparticles induce monoclonal antibodies that neutralize heterologous HIV-1 isolates in mice. *Cell Rep.* 38 (11): https://doi.org/10.1016/j.celrep.2022.110514.

3

Modified or Unmodified mRNA Vaccines? – The Biochemistry of Pseudouridine and mRNA Pseudouridylation

Pedro Morais[1,*] *and Yi-Tao Yu*[2]

[1] *ProQR Therapeutics, Innovation Unit, Zernikedreef 9, 2333 CK Leiden, The Netherlands*
[2] *University of Rochester Medical Center, Department of Biochemistry and Biophysics, Center for RNA Biology, 601 Elmwood Avenue, Rochester, NY 14642, USA*

3.1 Pseudouridine (Ψ): The Fifth Nucleoside

RNA encodes genetic information via different nucleobases, but unlike DNA, which has a few modifications beyond the standard nucleobases (mostly methylations), RNA has a much wider chemical diversity. Indeed, more than 150 different RNA nucleoside modifications have been described so far [1, 2]. Today, the exact role of all these RNA modifications is still poorly understood, although it is known that they contribute significantly to gene expression. One of the most abundant RNA modifications is an isomer of uridine, known as pseudouridine (Ψ). Ψ is widespread in nature [3], and it can even be found in the RNA of viruses [4, 5], including the COVID-19 virus [6].

The Ψ nucleoside was first discovered in RNA digests from calf liver and yeast decades ago by thin-layer chromatography (TLC) [7, 8]. Several other RNA modifications were discovered simultaneously, but the unusual properties of Ψ immediately attracted the attention of many research groups. Its importance in the human organism was evident since it could be easily detected in the urine, more substantially in individuals suffering from certain diseases, such as gout [9] or leukemia [10].

Ψ is derived from the U-to-Ψ isomerization (Figure 3.1), a reaction catalyzed by the pseudouridylation machinery present in the cells. Two critical molecular consequences from the isomerization of uridine confer biophysical properties specific to Ψ. First, there are two NH groups in Ψ instead of one in U; second, the bond between the ribose sugar and the Ψ base is the rotatable C—C bond, unlike the case of uridine (constrained N—C glycosidic bond). Specifically, during the U-to-Ψ isomerization, the molecular link between the base and the sugar, the N—C glycosidic bond of U, is broken. The uracil base is then lifted and rotated 180° along the N3–C6 axis, allowing the formation of a new glycosidic C—C covalent bond [11].

* Current Affiliation: BAYER Pharmaceuticals, Research & Development, Drug Metabolism and Pharmacokinetics/Pharmaceutical Sciences, Aprather Weg 18a, 42113 Wuppertal, Germany.

Trends in mRNA Vaccine Research, First Edition. Edited by Gabor Tamas Szabo and Norbert Pardi.

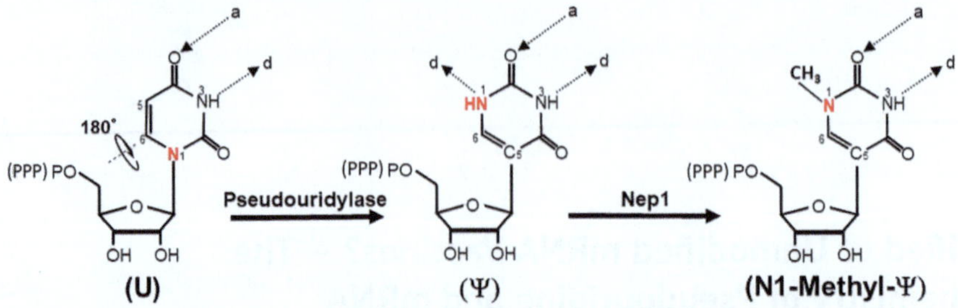

Figure 3.1 Schematic representation of U-to-Ψ isomerization and Ψ-to-N1-methyl-Ψ methylation reactions. Ψ has an extra hydrogen bond donor (-N1H) and a glycosidic rotatable C–C bond. Pseudouridylases catalyze this reaction. The N1-methyl-Ψ is generated by methylation of Ψ at the N1 position by Nep1 (N1-specific Ψ methyltransferase). d, hydrogen bond donor; a, hydrogen bond acceptor; P, 5′ monophosphate; PPP, 5′ triphosphate; O, oxygen; N, nitrogen; C, carbon; H, hydrogen.

The new C—C bond can rotate more freely, thus providing structural flexibility to Ψ. Further, due to the isomerization, Ψ has an extra hydrogen bond donor (N1H) on the major groove side while keeping the two hydrogen bonds in the Watson–Crick face (one acceptor and one donor H-bond). This new molecular configuration of Ψ promotes a C3′-endo conformation of the sugar moiety, leading to improved base stacking properties [12] and additional stability [13]. Nevertheless, despite these changes, Ψ can still base pair with adenosine residues, either via its standard *anti* or even a *syn* conformation [14]. Further, the Ψ–A pair has higher thermodynamic stability than the U–A pair [15].

It has been known for decades that this RNA modification somehow protects RNA against nucleases [16]. In general, pseudouridylation increases RNA stability in solution [17]. Specifically, when uridine is substituted by Ψ (or N1-methyl-Ψ, a Ψ derivative), the resulting RNA is more resistant to in-line hydrolysis (base-catalyzed cleavage of the phosphodiester bond by the 2′-OH sugar group) at the Ψ sites [17]. Interestingly, despite this, the Ψ (or N1-methyl-Ψ) incorporation in the RNA does not seem to change the global RNA structure significantly [17], even though it can alter the RNA local structure [18–20].

3.2 RNA Pseudouridylation Mechanism

The discovery of Ψ prompted scientists to uncover the mechanistic pathway for RNA pseudouridylation in cells. Because of the unusual C—C bond connecting the sugar and the base, two initial hypotheses were proposed. The first was built around the "*rearrangement*" idea, i.e. the enzyme-catalyzed 180° rotation of the base along the N3–C6 axis occurring in a substrate RNA where the target uridine would be already incorporated. The second was known as the "*incorporation*" hypothesis, under which the presynthesized Ψ mononucleotide would be incorporated as ΨTP during transcription [21]. After several years of investigation, the *rearrangement* hypothesis was proven to be the correct one. Specifically, in the experiments performed by Johnson and Söll, ^{14}C–Ψ was formed when ^{14}C(U)-containing RNA was incubated with *Escherichia coli* extracts [22], suggesting that an enzymatic activity would be involved in the pseudouridylation of uridine residues already incorporated in the RNA.

RNA pseudouridylation can be catalyzed in cells by either of the two independent naturally occurring mechanisms, an RNA-independent mechanism (by simple stand-alone protein enzymes), or an RNA-dependent mechanism (by complex box H/ACA RNP enzymes consisting of both RNA and proteins). In addition, pseudouridylation can be achieved by way of artificial guide RNA-targeted pseudouridylation (using artificial box H/ACA guide RNAs). Finally, Ψ can also be incorporated into RNA via *in vitro* transcription reaction. The different processes will be discussed below.

3.2.1 Naturally Occurring RNA Pseudouridylation

The U-to-Ψ isomerization reaction, naturally occurring in cells, is either catalyzed by stand-alone protein enzymes known as Ψ synthases (PUS proteins, and thus an RNA-independent process) or by box H/ACA snoRNPs (small nucleolar ribonucleoproteins), where the RNA component (or a specific box H/ACA RNA) guides site-specific pseudouridylation (and thus an RNA-dependent process) [23]. Either way, natural pseudouridylation in cells is targeted to specific locations in the RNA, and thus, most pseudouridylation sites are highly conserved [24].

3.2.1.1 RNA-independent Pseudouridylation Catalyzed by PUS Enzymes

In eukaryotes, stand-alone Ψ synthase enzymes (PUS) can recognize the target U in the substrate RNA (via sequence or secondary structure recognition) and catalyze the isomerization to Ψ without the intervention of a guide RNA [25].

There are 6 families of PUS proteins (TruA, TruB, RsuA, RluA, TruD, and Pus10) and 10 different PUS enzymes (PUS1 through PUS10) [23, 26]. PUS enzymes can be found in the nucleus, mitochondria, and cytoplasm. Different PUS enzymes can act on mRNA and noncoding RNAs such as tRNA, rRNA, and snRNA [26]. The PUS enzymes have a common active site in which an aspartate residue (located in a conserved catalytic core domain) attacks the target uridine to form an aspartate intermediate, thus breaking the bond between the sugar and the base [27]. Subsequently, the uracil base is rotated 180° along the N3–C6 axis, reestablishing the new C—C bond between the sugar and the base. This mechanism occurs via a glycal intermediate, in which the sugar is deprotonated at the C2′ position by the aspartate in the active site of PUS [11]. The catalytic core domain is flanked by N- and C-terminal extensions and consists of antiparallel β-sheets flanked by α-helices and loops [26]. Recently, with a series of *in silico* molecular modeling simulation studies, Kiss et al. suggested the importance of having an unstable target uridine positioned in the active site of the pseudouridine synthase for pseudouridylation to occur [28].

3.2.1.2 RNA-dependent Pseudouridylation Catalyzed by Box H/ACA snoRNP

RNA pseudouridylation can also be achieved via an RNA-guided mechanism, where the enzymes are RNA–protein complexes (ribonucleoproteins or RNPs),

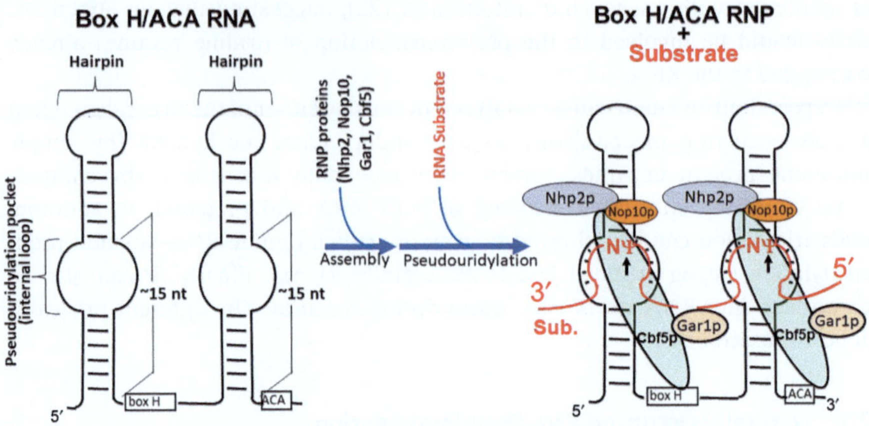

Figure 3.2 Box H/ACA guide RNAs fold into a characteristic hairpin-hinge (box H)-hairpin-tail (box ACA) secondary structure. Each hairpin has a pseudouridylation pocket, i.e. a single-stranded internal loop that base-pairs with the substrate RNA, positioning the target U at the base of the upper stem for isomerization by Cbf5. Usually, the target U is located 15 nt from the H or ACA box (downstream of the 5′ or 3′ hairpin, respectively). RNA-protein complexes (ribonucleoproteins or RNPs), each consisting of one unique box H/ACA RNA (guide RNA) and four common core proteins (Nhp2, Nop10, Gar1, and Cbf5/Dyskerin/NAP57), are responsible for the RNA guided pseudouridylation.

each consisting of one unique box H/ACA RNA (guide RNA) and four common core proteins (Nhp2, Nop10, Gar1, and Cbf5/Dyskerin/NAP57) (Figure 3.2). During pseudouridylation, the guide RNA component base pairs with the substrate RNA, specifying the target uridine to be isomerized by the catalytic component Cbf5 (one of the four core proteins). It is now known that many different types of RNA, including mRNA, rRNA, and snRNA, can be pseudouridylated by this mechanism [29].

Cbf5/Dyskerin/NAP57 (in yeast, humans, and rats, respectively) is characterized as a Ψ synthase [30]. However, Cbf5 has no substrate specificity; instead, it associates with the box H/ACA RNP and relies on the guide RNA (box H/ACA RNA) to specify the target uridine for pseudouridylation. Despite sequence differences, the eukaryotic box H/ACA guide RNAs all fold into a characteristic hairpin-hinge (box H)–hairpin-tail (box ACA) secondary structure. In each hairpin, a single-stranded internal loop sequence recognizes and pairs with the substrate sequences, flanking the target U, specifying the uridine by positioning it at the base of the upper stem for pseudouridylation by Cbf5. The target U is located approximately 15nt from either the H or ACA box (downstream of the 5′ or 3′ hairpin, respectively, see Figure 3.2) [31]. Box H/ACA guide RNAs typically have ~130 nts in length. Given that there are two hairpins in each mammalian box H/ACA RNA, a single box H/ACA RNA can often target two different U residues in one or two separate RNAs. At least eight base pairs between the internal loop of the guide RNA and its substrate sequence are required for pseudouridylation to occur in a specific manner [32, 33].

In recent years, several structural studies have provided much-needed insight into the mechanism of box H/ACA RNA-mediated pseudouridylation, both in archaea and in yeast. The crystal structure of the *Pyrococcus furiosus* box H/ACA RNP (including the four common core proteins and a unique single hairpin box H/ACA RNA), complexed with a substrate RNA, shows an arrangement whereby Cbf5 (the catalytic component), Nop10, and L7Ae (the archaeal homologous of Nhp2) all bind to the upper stem of the hairpin providing alignment of the guide RNA and binding to the substrate RNA [34–36]. The PUA (*P*seudo*U*ridine synthase and *A*rchaeosine transglycosylase) domain of Cbf5 also binds to the lower stem portion and the ACA (or presumably the H) box motif. On the other hand, Gar1 does not interact with the RNA. Instead, it interacts with the thumb loop of Cbf5 and has a role in substrate loading and release from the RNP complex [37]. Another structural study with H/ACA RNP from yeast showed a similar structural arrangement [38], although Nhp2 does not seem to be required for the activity of the box H/ACA RNP.

3.2.2 Artificially Introduced RNA Pseudouridylation

Since Goldberg and Rabinowitz found that Ψ-5′-monophosphate could be converted into its triphosphate version in mammalian cell extracts, suggesting that the Ψ could be somehow incorporated into cellular mRNA via transcription [39], the artificial pseudouridylation of (endogenous or synthetic) RNA has attracted much attention [40]. Because Ψ has unusual properties [41] and confers RNA with stability against nucleases [16] while improving its base-pairing properties [13], it is not surprising that several potential therapeutic applications have been described for this RNA modification, in particular, the ones implementing artificial RNA pseudouridylation [31].

There are two ways to artificially pseudouridylate the RNA. The first is based on the targeted pseudouridylation using artificial guide RNAs (box H/ACA snoRNA), which will be assembled into box H/ACA RNPs in the cell to direct pseudouridylation of a specific uridine within an RNA substrate [42]. The other methodology relies on the addition of Ψ (through ΨTP) to RNA via the standard *in vitro* transcription reaction (Ψ is read as a U by polymerases) [43]. By changing the ratio of ΨTP versus UTP, RNA can be partially or entirely pseudouridylated [44]. Here, we describe both methods.

3.2.2.1 Targeted Pseudouridylation of RNA Using Artificial Guide RNAs

It has been reported that pseudouridylation can be artificially introduced to virtually any uridine sites in any RNA substrates by designer box H/ACA RNAs (guide RNAs) [42, 45, 46]. These designer guide RNAs, consisting of two hairpins, can be based on naturally occurring box H/ACA snoRNAs, in which the pseudouridylation pocket (the internal loop sequences) can be altered to base-pair virtually with any RNA substrate (Figures 3.2 and 3.3). Once the designer box H/ACA RNAs are introduced into cells, they will be complexed with the endogenous four core proteins (Nhp2, Nop10, Gar1, and Cbf5/Dyskerin/NAP57) to form functional box H/ACA RNPs, allowing pseudouridylation at the target site of a substrate RNA, which is either endogenously expressed or exogenously transfected.

RNA-guided pseudouridylation can also be carried out *in vitro*. To develop the *in vitro* system, a yeast strain, where one of the core proteins is tandem affinity

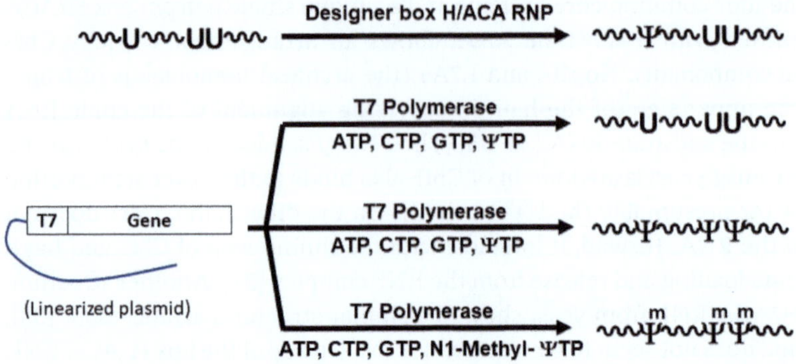

Figure 3.3 Pseudouridylation can be site-specifically performed into virtually any uridine site in any RNA substrate via designer box H/ACA RNAs (guide RNAs). The designer guide RNA is based on naturally occurring box H/ACA guide RNAs, in which the pseudouridylation pocket sequence is changed to base-pair with the new target RNA. Alternatively, pseudouridylation can be achieved via the incorporation of Ψ during the *in vitro* transcription reaction. Usually, in the *in vitro* transcription reaction, mRNA is generated from a linearized plasmid (with a T7 promoter) that is incubated with rNTPs and T7 RNA polymerase. Taking advantage of the base-pairing properties of Ψ, which can base pair with adenosines, it is possible to incorporate Ψ (or N1-methyl-Ψ) in the *in vitro* transcription reaction by replacing UTP with ΨTP (or N1-methyl-ΨTP, or Ψ^{m}TP).

purification (TAP)-tagged, can be used for TAP purification of the total box H/ACA RNP particles. Micrococcal nuclease can then degrade box H/ACA RNAs, thus releasing the four common core proteins from the RNP complexes. Upon inactivating the micrococcal nuclease, a designer box H/ACA RNA (guide RNA) can then be added to the mixture, allowing the reassembly of a new box H/ACA RNP centered on the designer box H/ACA RNA. When the substrate is supplied, the designer box H/ACA RNA can target it for pseudouridylation [45]. In the case of mammalian cells, where the four common core proteins are synthesized in significant excess, there is no need to purify total box H/ACA RNPs. Instead, whole-cell extracts can be prepared. Upon supplement with a designer box H/ACA RNA, a new functional box H/ACA RNP forms in the cell extracts. This newly formed RNP can target its substrate RNA, catalyzing the U-to-Ψ conversion [42].

Various designer box H/ACA RNAs (with different lengths) have been tested in the yeast and mammalian *in vitro* systems. Interestingly, it has been demonstrated that an engineered half-length box H/ACA guide RNA (consisting of only one hairpin) is fully capable of directing site-specific pseudouridylation [47].

3.2.2.2 Incorporation of Ψ During *In Vitro* Transcription of RNA

Using the *in vitro* transcription reaction [48, 49], Ψ can also be incorporated into RNA. Here, the RNA is transcribed from a DNA template, and the transcription is usually under the control of a short promoter recognized by a bacteriophage RNA polymerase [50]. One of the most used polymerases is T7 RNA polymerase, derived from *E. coli* T7 bacteriophage [51], although other similar systems are available (SP6 and T3). Typically, during an *in vitro* transcription reaction, the plasmid is first linearized at the end of the coding sequence with a restriction enzyme. Upon addition of rNTPs and T7 RNA polymerase, transcription occurs, generating an RNA [52]. By replacing the UTP with ΨTP (different ratio) in the rNTP mix, Ψ is incorporated into the transcribed RNA (Figure 3.3). The synthesis of Ψ-modified mRNA via *in vitro* transcription was described in several studies [53–55]. It was initially hypothesized that a mutant T7 RNA polymerase would be required to incorporate modified nucleotides such as ΨTP into the RNA chain during *in vitro* transcription. Padilla and Sousa developed a double-mutant T7 RNA polymerase by introducing two mutations (Y639F/H784A) that made the enzyme more amenable to incorporating modified/noncanonical NTPs such as deoxy, 2′-NH_2, and 2′-F, as well as Ψ [56]. However, it turned out that the standard T7 RNA polymerase was just as effective in incorporating ΨTP [54, 57]. Some important Ψ derivatives, such as N1-methyl-Ψ (discussed later in this chapter), can also be incorporated into transcribing RNA during the standard *in vitro* transcription [58, 59].

Because the *in vitro* transcription of pseudouridylated mRNA can generate several contaminants, such as double-stranded RNA, removing them via HPLC purification was deemed necessary to increase mRNA druggability [60]. These contaminants, which can induce cytokine production, are not a consequence of the use of ΨTP but rather the *in vitro* transcription reaction itself, namely, RNA-dependent RNA polymerase activity self-complementary 3′ extension of the RNA and RNA-primed transcription from RNA templates [60]. Recently, the Karikó lab proposed a novel method to remove such dsRNA contaminants from the *in vitro* transcription reaction using a conventional lab method based on cellulose-based chromatography [61]. This new method can provide high-quality mRNA without the need for HPLC purification.

In the last few years, massive efforts have been undertaken to upscale the *in vitro* transcription reaction of Ψ-modified mRNA to produce billions of mRNA COVID-19 vaccine doses [62]. This was an outstanding achievement, only possible due to the scalability of this enzymatic reaction, which enabled the production of hundreds of kilograms of N1-methyl-Ψ-modified mRNA while following strict regulatory guidelines and complying with current good manufacturing practices (cGMPs).

3.3 Ψ detection in RNA

Since Ψ is so widespread in various RNA species, understanding its cellular function and biological role becomes increasingly important. For this purpose, several techniques were first developed to precisely quantify and map, at the single-nucleoside resolution, this modification in all types of RNA. Fortunately, its physicochemical properties, which are distinct from the physicochemical properties of its uridine isomer, made this task feasible.

Ψ can be detected and quantified in RNA via several chromatographic, electrophoretic, or spectrometric methods, performed once the analyzed RNA is degraded into single nucleosides via nuclease digestion [63]. However, to map the position of Ψ in the RNA, sequencing methods with resolution at the single-nucleoside level become necessary. Nevertheless, Ψ is read as uridine in standard

PCR and RT–PCR reactions [44]. Therefore, novel techniques have been developed to map reliably and sometimes even quantify (or semiquantify) Ψ in transcriptomes [31, 64]. These techniques rely primarily on two methodologies: (i) the indirect identification of Ψ via modification (consisting of a labeling step of Ψ beforehand) and (ii) direct mapping methods (i.e. methods that do not require reverse transcription, PCR, or Ψ derivatization). Here, we will briefly discuss both methodologies.

3.3.1 Indirect Ψ Sequencing Methods

In most cases, indirect sequencing methods rely on the derivatization of Ψ with an electrophilic compound, such as CMCT [*N*-cyclohexyl-*N*′-β-(4-methylmorpholinum ethyl) carbodiimide *p*-tosylate]. While this reagent can also derivatize other nucleobases in the RNA (uridine and guanosine), once the total CMCT-labeled RNA is treated in alkaline conditions, only the Ψ-CMCT subsists. The position of this bulky modified nucleobase can then be mapped via primer extension (cDNA synthesis with a reverse transcriptase), a reaction that will stop one nucleotide before the CMCT-modified Ψ [65, 66]. When coupled with next-generation sequencing technologies, this indirect sequencing method has been applied to transcriptome-wide detection of Ψ in mammalian mRNA [67–70]. Despite the usefulness of this methodology, it still has room for improvement. For example, incomplete alkaline hydrolysis can fail to remove all U- and G-derivatized nucleosides, introducing unwanted false positives. To address this and other limitations, significant developments have been made in direct sequencing methods that do not rely on any derivatization or labeling scheme for the reliable mapping of Ψ.

3.3.2 Direct Ψ Sequencing Methods

Direct sequencing methods promise to detect Ψ (and other modified nucleosides) within any RNA sequence without prior amplification (RT–PCR) or chemical derivatization step (such as CMCT addition reaction for Ψ mapping). However, there are still some challenges with this emerging technology [71], namely the high error rate [72] and the need for a high amount of input material (RNA). Nevertheless, with further exploration, direct sequencing methods will enable long-read nucleic acid sequencing without the bias of the amplification or chemical derivatization step, which is otherwise needed in indirect sequencing methods. Direct sequencing also simultaneously identifies multiple RNA modifications (including Ψ) [73].

One of the direct sequencing techniques that stands out is Nanopore RNA technology [74], which uses a protein pore incorporated in a membrane. When electricity is applied, it creates an electrophoretic field, allowing a DNA or RNA strand to pass through the protein nanopore. A slight but distinct current variation is expected in the electrical field as each nucleoside in the RNA chain crosses the nanopore. The distinct current perturbation results from the nucleoside physicochemical properties, and therefore it is not surprising that Ψ [75] and other RNA modifications, such as N6-methyladenosine [76] can be detected via base-calling algorithms [77, 78]. In fact, this method was used to map RNA modifications, including Ψ sites, in the COVID-19 transcriptome, specifically at positions U27164, U28039, U28759, U28927, and U29418 [6]. It has also been recently used to detect a modified version of Ψ (N1-methyl-Ψ) [59]. These direct sequencing techniques will significantly accelerate the development of epitranscriptomics and its therapeutic applications.

3.4 Impact of Ψ in Pre-mRNA Splicing and Protein Translation

It is well-documented that distinct nucleotides in RNA play an essential role in gene expression and regulation. Therefore, it is not surprising that Ψ, which has a peculiar structure (flexible C—C glycosidic bond and the additional hydrogen bond donor N1H group) and is highly abundant and widespread in a variety of RNAs such as rRNA, tRNA, snRNA, and even mRNA, can have a functional role in processes such as splicing and translation. Below, we will briefly discuss the contribution of Ψ to pre-mRNA splicing and mRNA translation.

3.4.1 Effect of Ψ in snRNA and Pre-mRNA on Pre-mRNA Splicing

During pre-mRNA splicing, five snRNA molecules (U1, U2, U4, U5, and U6 snRNAs) within a large RNA-protein complex known as the spliceosome, interact with each other and with the pre-mRNA to guide the spliceosome assembly and the transesterification reactions [79]. It has been suggested that nucleoside modifications, including Ψ (present in all human snRNAs, particularly in the regions that are known to be functionally important), play critical roles in the recognition and selection of the 5' and 3′ splice sites and the branch site [80–83].

When artificially incorporated into the polypyrimidine tract of pre-mRNA introns, Ψ can also have a negative effect on pre-mRNA splicing [53]. Recently, Martinez et al. used a global sequencing method to map naturally occurring Ψ in pre-mRNAs [84]. Remarkably, several hundreds of Ψ residues are modified co-transcriptionally by Ψ synthases (PUS1, PU7, and RPUSD4) and are often present in the critical intronic motifs (near the splice sites and in the binding sites for RNA-binding proteins). Indeed, at least some of these Ψs can impact splicing efficiency and alternative splicing [84].

3.4.2 Effect of Ψ in rRNA and tRNA on Protein Translation

It has been known for decades that Ψ is present in ribosomal RNA [85]. There are several highly conserved Ψs in rRNAs across species [86], particularly in critical domains, such as the decoding center of ribosomal RNA [87, 88]. It is known that mutations in the enzymes responsible for pseudouridylation of rRNA can lead to disease and that reduced Ψ levels have been observed in patients with dyskeratosis congenita, a severe disease characterized by a failure in the bone marrow and a deficiency in the production of enough blood cells [31].

Furthermore, it has been reported that a lack of Ψ in rRNAs can cause defects in the translation process, suggesting that Ψs in rRNA have a functional role in translation (although the mechanism is still poorly understood). Recently, Zhao et al. compared the CryoEM structural conformation of Ψ-free ribosomes with that of naturally modified ribosomes. They hypothesized that Ψ could contribute to an essential conformation in the rRNA, which plays an important role in protein translation and is absent in Ψ-free ribosomal rRNA [89]. At the molecular level, it is suggested that the N1 atom in the Ψ contributes to stabilizing critical motifs by interacting with the phosphate backbone via water molecules [89].

Since the translational machinery reads the genetic code (nucleoside triplets known as codons) of the mRNA via the anticodon triplets present in the tRNA, it was hypothesized many years ago that RNA modifications such as Ψ in the anticodon could perhaps have an impact on translation. In fact, Tomita identified an unusual decoding phenomenon due to a pseudouridylated mitochondrial tRNA anticodon (GΨU). They found that the presence of a Ψ in the anticodon made it possible to read alternative codons [90]. This alternative decoding would not be possible without Ψ. It should be pointed out that even before this study, there was already a hint that the Ψ in anticodons is crucial for specific natural suppressor tRNAs in plants, such as cytoplasmic $tRNA^{Tyr}$ (GΨA). The Ψ in the middle position of the anticodon could help suppress UAG stop codons in the RNA of tobacco mosaic virus (TMV) [91–93].

3.4.3 Effect of mRNA Pseudouridylation on Nonsense Suppression

More than a decade ago, the Yu Lab showed that pseudouridylation of stop codons could also have a functional role [94]. Karijolich and Yu demonstrated that, in the yeast organism, nonsense codons could be converted into sense codons via site-specific pseudouridylation targeting the first U in a nonsense codon using artificial guide RNAs derived from naturally occurring box H/ACA RNA [94]. The authors identified the amino acids that resulted from the nonsense to sense codon conversion: phenylalanine/tyrosine was incorporated predominantly at the ΨGA codons and threonine/serine largely at the ΨAA and ΨAG codons. The nonsense suppression mechanism via targeted pseudouridylation of nonsense codons was also shown using the bacterial system [95]. In normal translation, release factors bind to stop codons leading to translation termination. It appears that the release factors are outcompeted by some near-cognate tRNAs in binding to pseudouridylated nonsense codons (ΨGA, ΨAG, and ΨAA), even if such interaction is not optimal between codon and anticodon. Fernández et al. studied this interaction by crystalizing the 30S ribosomal unit and the whole 70S ribosome. Their work has demonstrated codon–anticodon (ΨAG–$tRNA^{Ser}$) interactions in the ribosome's catalytic center. The authors observed important characteristics of the binding between pseudouridylated stop codons and the near cognate anticodon of tRNA when comparing with the corresponding ribosomal structures containing unmodified stop codons: On the one hand, Ψ appears to promote an unusual purine–purine base-pairing scheme, involving both Watson–Crick and Hoogsteen hydrogen bonding. On the other hand, the presence of Ψ does not seem to alter the overall duplex structure/geometry; however, it helps increase the base-pairing (Ψ–A) stability and allows the neighboring purine to take a different configuration (*syn* rather than the anti-configuration). The extra hydrogen bond of Ψ (N1H) does not interact with the anticodon or the ribosome structure, but its presence appears to provide an alternate base-pairing scheme allowing a near-cognate codon to be paired. This scheme would explain the novel decoding mechanism [95].

Recently, the Yu Lab presented this targeted pseudouridylation approach to suppress nonsense mutations – mutations that create premature termination codons (PTCs) within disease genes, such as CFTR or IDUA [96], in human cells. The suppression occurs at two different levels. First, targeted pseudouridylation at the PTC results in the suppression of nonsense-mediated mRNA decay (NMD), thus increasing PTC–transcript levels. Second, pseudouridylation at PTC promotes translational readthrough in a target-specific manner. Since this mechanism suppresses the nonsense mRNA-mediated decay pathway and translational termination simultaneously, it could potentially be developed into a new PTC suppression therapy [97]. In this regard, it is also worth mentioning that some short designer box H/ACA guide RNAs (much smaller than the original ones) can be used to pseudouridylate the target RNA (see Section 3.2.2.1). Given that short (and potentially chemically modified) designer guide RNAs are much easier to deliver to cells, it broadens the therapeutic potential of this approach. This study from the Yu Lab was the only one so far where the targeted pseudouridylation of PTCs successfully restored not only the full-length protein but also its function [96].

There are two additional successful examples where targeted pseudouridylation was performed to suppress nonsense mutations. Song et al. recently confirmed that engineered guide RNAs targeting PTCs can promote readthrough in mammalian cells [98]. In addition, the authors identified an isoform of dyskerin (lacking a C-terminal nuclear localization signal) that can significantly enhance the nonsense suppression effect. Another example was provided by Dai et al., where pseudouridine synthase (PUS1) was fused to a dCas13d (catalytically inactive Cas13) to suppress nonsense mutations with a guide RNA designed to target the PTCs [99].

Interestingly, this study from Dai et al. also showed that pseudouridylated stop codons (i.e. ΨGA, ΨAA, and ΨAG) were endogenously detected in mRNAs of human cell lines (HeLa and A549) and mouse tissues [99]. Particularly striking is the fact that in all pseudouridylated stop codons found in mice (a total of 106), there was always a normal stop codon located downstream. The authors were able to confirm, in the case of several protein targets, the expected Western Blot band shift (due to the addition of a small peptide sequence between the pseudouridylated stop codon, which is read-through, and the downstream normal stop codon) [99].

Despite the growing evidence of the effect of mRNA pseudouridylation on nonsense suppression, a recent report suggested that pseudouridylation of a PTC would not lead to translational readthrough [100]. These results from Nir et al. could result from different systems used, namely an artificial system where a PTC-containing, intron-lacking reporter was transiently expressed in human cells, and an endogenous box H/ACA RNA (not abundantly expressed) was utilized to target the PTC [100].

The study of the suppression of nonsense mutations via targeted pseudouridylation, as a potential therapeutic RNA editing modality, is expected to continue to attract attention in the coming years. Nonsense mutations account for approximately 10–20% of all point mutations leading to genetic diseases [101, 102].

Nonsense mutations impact patients at two different molecular levels. First, the presence of a PTC in the middle of a disease gene often activates the surveillance pathway (known as the NMD pathway) that degrades most PTC-containing mRNA. Thus, only a very low amount of transcript is present in the cell. Second, translation terminates prematurely at the PTC. Compared to other RNA-targeting technologies, targeted pseudouridylation can simultaneously suppress both NMD and premature translation termination at the PTC [96, 97].

3.4.4 Effect of mRNA Pseudouridylation on the Coding Specificity of Sense Codons

Beyond nonsense decoding, the Ψ modification can also modulate sense codon decoding. Eyler et al. showed that Ψ could modulate translatability, i.e. how codons are recognized by the translational machinery and anticodons of near-cognate tRNAs [103]. The authors investigated the interactions between the ribosome, $tRNA^{Phe}$, and pseudouridylated mRNA (ΨUU in the A-site) during translation elongation. They found that the 3′ CCA site in the $tRNA^{Phe}$ has more flexibility than the situation where unmodified UUU is complexed in the A-site. Specifically, when a pseudouridylated codon is present in the A-site, the CCA-end of the $tRNA^{Phe}$ cannot form canonical interactions in the A site of the peptidyl transferase center.

Recently, Fujita et al. showed that pseudouridylation of near-cognate non-AUG start codons, such as NUG, enhances translational initiation, regardless of the surrounding sequence context. This appears to be achieved through increased base pairing to the mismatched start codon [104].

Pseudouridylation of mRNA also impacts translation efficiency. Karikó et al. found that incorporating Ψ into *in vitro* transcribed mRNA would produce ten times more protein in human cells [55]. This increase in efficiency was believed to be because pseudouridylated mRNA was less prone to activation of an RNA-dependent kinase (PKR), which ultimately reduces translation efficiency via phosphorylation of eIF-2α, a translation initiation factor 2-alpha [105]. In a series of pull-down experiments, the authors found that pseudouridylated mRNA would bind less efficiently to PKR. Subsequently, Karikó et al. found that the translation efficiency of pseudouridylated mRNA could be further improved by HPLC purification and elimination of contaminants resulting from the *in vitro* transcription reaction [60]. Purified pseudouridylated mRNA was shown to be more efficiently translated *in vivo* than unmodified mRNA [106]. Recently, Leppek et al. also demonstrated that Ψ incorporation in the mRNA could increase the protein output by increasing the in-solution stability of mRNA while not affecting the global RNA structure [17].

3.5 Ψ and the Immune System

Our immune system has evolved to detect nucleic acids from pathogens and certain DNA or RNA modifications in our genome and transcriptome [107, 108]. For example, unmethylated CpG dinucleotides in bacterial DNA have an immunostimulatory effect on our immune cells [109], and overall, DNA methylation plays an essential role in the correct functioning of our cells [110]. On the other hand, our immune system can also recognize structural patterns in the nucleic acids of pathogens, such as double-stranded RNA in viruses [111]. Therefore, before effective mRNA technologies were successfully validated in vaccine applications, a breakthrough was needed to understand better how our immune system differentiates self-RNA from pathogen-derived RNA. Katalin Karikó and Drew Weissman's research groups made significant contributions in this field during the last two decades and will be discussed here.

More than 20 years ago, Weissman et al. realized that, while delivering *in vitro* transcribed mRNA coding for HIV gag protein to dendritic cells, the mRNA was efficiently transfected, and the gag protein was produced, but additionally, the cells built an inflammatory response [112]. At that time, it was known that double-stranded RNA induced interferon production [113], but the exact mechanisms were poorly understood. Ultimately, it was found that double-stranded viral RNA was recognized via toll-like receptors (TLRs) activation, particularly TLR3 [114]. Still, the question following Weissman's 2000 work was how an exogenous RNA built an inflammatory response and how it differed from endogenous RNA in the cell. To answer this question, Karikó et al. compared the immunogenicity of isolated mammalian RNA with *in vitro* transcribed mammalian RNA following the transfection of monocyte-derived dendritic cells [54]. The authors realized that the isolated RNA from mammalian cells produced a lower amount of TNF-α than the *in vitro* transcribed RNA did, thus producing a lower inflammatory response and lower activation of dendritic cells. However, when comparing the effects of *E. coli*-derived RNA (total and tRNA), Karikó et al. found that although *E. coli* total RNA was inflammatory in dendritic cells, the bacterial tRNA had lower immunogenicity in those cells, just as that of isolated mammalian RNA. Given that tRNA (including bacterial tRNA) is heavily modified by pseudouridylation, 2′-O-methylation, and other modifications [115], Karikó et al. decided to assess the effect of a few RNA modifications on mRNA immunogenicity by using *in vitro* transcribed RNA containing RNA modifications such as Ψ (replacing all uridines with Ψs in the *in vitro* transcription reaction). These modified mRNA, especially the Ψ-modified mRNA, when transfected in isolated primary human dendritic cells, produced a less inflammatory response. The lower immunogenicity provided by RNA modifications was corroborated with Ψ-modified (at a single position) synthetic oligoribonucleotides transfected in monocyte-derived dendritic cells [54]. Further, the Weissman/Karikó group confirmed the lower immunogenicity of Ψ-modified mRNA *in vivo* [55] and suggested that Ψ present in the *in vitro* transcribed mRNA could render it more resistant to RNase L-mediated degradation [116]. RNase L is a component of the innate immune response following a viral infection. Ψ could thus act by suppressing the immune recognition of RNA.

Despite all the breakthroughs in this field, the exact mechanism by which uridine replacement by Ψ decreases mRNA immunogenicity might not yet be wholly grasped. Around the time of Karikó and Weissman's groundbreaking studies [54], two independent studies shed some light on the role of uridine in mRNA's immunogenicity. First, Heil et al. implied that an immune response could also be induced by single-stranded RNA and that uridine-rich single-stranded RNA could, in fact, immunostimulate dendritic cells through recognition by two different TLRs, TLR7 and TLR8 [117]. Second, Diebold et al. suggested that TLR7 could recognize repeats of uracil residues in the RNA [118]. The use of Ψ in the mRNA could potentially prevent this interferon-inducing activity of uridines.

Recently, Huang et al. found that cells can increase the pseudouridylation of some endogenous transcripts, particularly the transcripts of interferon-stimulated genes (ISGs), as a response to treatment with interferon [119]. ISGs can play a role in the immune system's ability to resist pathogenic infections.

3.6 Pseudouridylated Versus Unmodified mRNA Vaccines

Following the work from the Weissman/Karikó labs, in which they used the *in vitro* transcription reaction to incorporate Ψ into mRNA for therapeutic or vaccine applications, subsequent studies further consolidated the role of the RNA pseudouridylation as a critical enabling technology for the development of the mRNA technology platform. One of those studies, which caught immense attention, was published by Warren et al. who used synthetic Ψ-modified mRNA for reprogramming human cells and creating induced pluripotent stem cells [120]. The *in vitro* transcribed Ψ-modified mRNA enabled the expression of the four required genes (LF4, c-MYC, OCT4, and SOX2), known as the Yamanaka reprogramming factors, in human fibroblasts, thus avoiding the use of potentially oncogenic viral vectors to transduce the same genes, therefore paving the way for safer cell therapies [121]. Another study emphasizing the promising nature of Ψ-modified mRNA was published in 2013 by Zangi et al. By delivering Ψ-modified mRNA via intramyocardial injection, the authors were able to express human vascular endothelial growth factor-A (VEGF-A) to improve the heart function in a mouse myocardial infarction model [122]. Below, we will discuss the evolution of the Ψ-modified mRNA technology platform, focusing on successful applications of an improved version of Ψ, N1-methyl-Ψ, for mRNA therapeutics/vaccines.

3.6.1 Ψ Successor: N1-methyl-Ψ

The identification of Ψ as a nucleoside substitute for the *in vitro* transcription reaction paved the way to enhance the therapeutic properties of mRNA, and its potential as a vaccine molecule, by either increasing its biological stability and translational efficiency or modulating its intrinsic immunogenicity. Following the initial work by the Weissman/Karikó labs, there was a need to screen new RNA modifications in *in vitro* transcribed mRNA, but there were very few available as ribonucleoside trisphosphates. Fortunately, several ribonucleoside triphosphates derived from synthetic and naturally occurring RNA modifications were made commercially available in the subsequent years. Thus, scientists could assess these modified nucleosides' effect on therapeutic mRNA. It was hoped that novel RNA modifications would boost mRNA's therapeutic and vaccine properties. However, cellular toxicity was observed when some non-natural nucleobases were incorporated into the mRNA. In addition, in a clinical study, the use of a nucleoside analog (Fialuridine, or 1-(2-deoxy-2-fluoro-β-d-arabinofuranosyl)-5-iodouracil) resulted in several deaths due to liver failure [123]. These incidents led scientists in this field to focus on screening naturally occurring RNA modifications [54, 55]. Naturally occurring modified nucleosides incorporated in the mRNA would be well tolerated by our cells and, crucially, have a natural metabolic (i.e. noncytochrome P450-dependent) and excretion pathway in humans, an essential success factor for pharmacokinetics and ADME properties that enable the suitability of mRNA as a drug [124]. In this regard, Ψ is not catabolized in humans and is, thus, directly eliminated in the urine [21].

In recent years, one of the naturally occurring RNA modifications identified with innovation potential for the development of the Ψ-modified mRNA platform technology (and available as a ribonucleoside triphosphate) was N1-methyl-ΨTP (Figure 3.1). Research data generated from this modified nucleotide attracted great attention [58]. In nature, N1-methyl-Ψ is formed following the N1-methylation reaction of Ψ residues by N1-specific Ψ methyltransferase (Nep1), an enzyme known to be present in archaeal and eukaryotic organisms [125]. This RNA modification was first found in 18S rRNA in HeLa cells (the most common human cell line used in research) [126] and later in the tRNA content of several organisms [127]. However, because the current gold-standard identification method for Ψ might not be able to distinguish it from N1-methyl-Ψ, it could very well be that N1-methyl-Ψ is more prevalent in our transcriptome than previously believed [70, 128, 129]. This hypothesis warrants further study, potentially through the novel direct sequencing methods.

From the molecular standpoint, N1-methyl-Ψ differs from Ψ because it does not have the extra hydrogen bond donor group (N1H) (Figure 3.1). Therefore, unlike Ψ, N1-methyl-Ψ can presumably only interact with its nucleoside partner via its canonical Watson–Crick face (hydrogen bonding). Further, N1-methyl-Ψ perhaps cannot wobble base pair with other nucleotides (while Ψ can), although the flexible C5—C1′ bond is common both for Ψ and N1-methyl-Ψ. It is worth noting that the flexibility feature of the C5—C1′ bond (in Ψ and N1-methyl-Ψ) is believed to contribute to better base-stacking and higher hybridization affinity than uridine [13, 130].

Andries et al. observed that, when incorporating N1-methyl-Ψ as a total replacement of uridine during *in vitro* transcription, the resulting mRNA had an even better immunogenicity profile than Ψ-modified mRNA in both mammalian cells and mice [58]. On the other hand, this RNA modification provided mRNA with an improved protein expression and reduced cytotoxicity to the cell [58]. Along this line, Svitkin et al. showed that N1-methyl-Ψ improves mRNA translational capacity by increasing ribosome loading [129]. Other labs later corroborated the improved properties of N1-methyl-Ψ as a technological innovation compared to Ψ in the modified mRNA platform [130, 131].

The discovery of the N1-methyl-Ψ modification was thus a significant milestone, and this RNA modification became another enabling technology for developing mRNA therapeutics and vaccines. N1-methyl-Ψ, like Ψ, would have all its advantages, including the immunosuppressor effect, stability, and translational effect. During the last years, it was hypothesized that, when compared to Ψ, N1-methyl-Ψ could also have the additional benefit of enhanced mRNA coding fidelity due to the lack of the extra hydrogen bond donor group (N1H, present in Ψ but absent in N1-methyl-Ψ – Figure 3.1) [128]. A recently published study by Kim et al. confirmed that N1-methyl-Ψ does not interfere with coding accuracy compared to uridines [14]. In addition, the authors suggested that N1-methyl-Ψ is less prone to errors by reverse transcriptase (i.e. misincorporation events) than Ψ is during primer extension reactions. Further, Chen et al. compared the fidelity of N1-methyl-Ψ and Ψ incorporation and showed that the former is incorporated during the *in vitro* transcription reaction with a higher fidelity [132].

Pardi et al. showed that an LNP formulation could be successfully used to deliver N1-methyl-Ψ-modified mRNA *in vivo* (mice) via different systemic or local routes (subcutaneous, intramuscular, intradermal, intratracheal, intravenous, and intraperitoneal) and express the protein in sustained fashion [133]. A similar platform technology (LNP-formulated N1-methyl-Ψ-modified mRNA) was used to protect nonhuman primates [134] and mice [135] successfully against Zika virus infection. Several studies followed, confirming the advantages of using N1-methyl-Ψ as a replacement for uridine and as an improvement over Ψ in *in vitro* transcribed therapeutic mRNA [136–140].

3.6.2 Nucleoside-modified COVID-19 mRNA Vaccines

The lack of effective antiviral drugs against COVID-19 and the limited efficacy of all the preventive measures at the beginning of the pandemic made it clear that only effective vaccines could provide a means to control the situation. However, there was some speculation about whether COVID-19 vaccines could be developed in a reasonable timeline, with some predicting that it could take several years until effective vaccines would be available worldwide [141].

Remarkably, however, within one year, two highly effective COVID-19 mRNA vaccines were independently developed by Pfizer–BioNTech and Moderna, demonstrating the power of RNA technologies. Recently, it has been argued that, without the previous two decades of basic research surrounding mRNA and modified mRNA, the breakthrough achieved by Pfizer–BioNTech and Moderna would not have been possible [128, 142]. However, the importance of LNP formulations as enabling technologies [143] for the RNA technology platform cannot be overstated. LNPs, based on ionizable lipids, functioned as delivery vehicles, without which mRNA would not have been appropriately expressed in the target cells [133]. LNPs also acted as an adjuvant that promoted strong immune cellular responses [144]. The outstanding contribution of LNP formulation is beyond the scope of this chapter and is discussed elsewhere [145]. Nevertheless, since the clinical trial results obtained so far with unmodified mRNA COVID-19 vaccines (but similarly LNP formulated) fell short of the expectations of many in the field (discussed in Section 3.6.3), it is safe to say that modification of the mRNA with N1-methyl-Ψ played a crucial role in developing COVID-19 mRNA vaccines at a record time speed.

Two LNP-formulated N1-methyl-Ψ mRNA COVID-19 vaccines were developed in less than a year, both offering protection against severe disease and death at a rate higher than 90%. Pfizer–BioNTech's Comirnaty® (also known as BNT162b2) was the first approved. Moderna's Spikevax® (previously known as mRNA-1273) followed shortly [146, 147]. Both vaccines coded for S (spike) protein, a target that had already been identified as the antigen for vaccines against a similar coronavirus, SARS-CoV, more than a decade ago [148] for its immunogenicity and ability to induce a neutralizing antibody response. This protein, well conserved among human coronavirus in general (including COVID-19 virus SARS-CoV-2), mediates host receptor recognition and the fusion with the target cells [149]. This fusion process is mediated by a host protease known as Furin, which cleaves the S protein into S1 and S2 subunits at the interface between the two. The mRNA of both Comirnaty (Pfizer–BioNTech) and Spikevax (Moderna) codes for the Spike protein and has two mutations (K986P and V987P) that stabilize the prefusion conformation of the Spike protein to improve its antigenicity [150–153]. Further, Comirnaty and Spikevax mRNA vaccines were prepared via *in vitro* transcription, with the uridine triphosphate component in the rNTP mix replaced by N1-methyl-Ψ triphosphate [154]. Kim et al. confirmed that the N1-methyl-Ψ-modified mRNA encoding the COVID-19 S protein is translated faithfully [14]. Nevertheless, Mulroney et al. recently observed that this RNA modification could potentially cause ribosome stalling, which could in turn lead to a frameshifting phenomenon during the translation process, although to a small extent [155]. This translational +1 frameshifting could lead to the synthesis of a small amount of out-of-frame peptides that could be immunogenic. Despite the potential advantages of this outcome in a vaccine setting, this phenomenon should be studied in more detail to fully understand if codon optimization strategies can mitigate this effect to increase fidelity, which would be especially relevant for future protein replacement therapeutic applications of N1-methyl-Ψ-modified mRNA, where redosing will be required.

Finally, it is worth noting that instead of a single stop codon, both vaccines have consecutive stop codons: Comirnaty has two (ΨGAΨGA), while Spikevax has three contiguous stop codons (ΨGAΨAAΨAG). This has been suggested to prevent a potential read-through (an extension of translation that would occur beyond the stop codons) and a possible +1 frameshifting [128, 154]. This hypothesis warrants further study.

3.6.3 Unmodified mRNA COVID-19 vaccines

In the early days of therapeutic mRNA research, following Karikó/Weissman's work on pseudouridylated mRNA, there was the belief that unmodified mRNA, with its immunostimulatory nature capable of boosting its coadjuvant activity, could become an essential tool as a vaccine platform technology for infectious diseases [156]. In fact, several studies over the following years showed evidence that unmodified mRNA could perform as competitively as Ψ-modified mRNA *in vitro* and in small mammals [157, 158]. Despite this, as of today, unmodified mRNA COVID-19 vaccines have underperformed their Ψ-modified counterparts and have, thus, failed to meet expectations [159]. While the reasons for this are not yet entirely clear [128], it is plausible to assume that N1-methyl-Ψ plays an important role. Here, we will describe some examples of preclinical and clinical trial results obtained with unmodified mRNA vaccines.

One example was CureVac's first attempt at developing a COVID-19 mRNA vaccine, CVnCoV, lacking Ψ or N1-methyl-Ψ and encoding for the S-protein [160]. CVnCoV showed an efficacy of only 48% in preventing any severity of COVID-19 disease in phase III trials [161]. Since CVnCoV was encapsulated in an almost identical LNP formulation to the one used in Comirnaty, namely Acuitas ALC-0315 [162], some found this surprising. While one could argue that the poor efficacy could have been caused by the simultaneous presence of several variants at the time of the CVnCoV's clinical trial, the fact that N1-methyl-Ψ-modified mRNA vaccines were still effective against the same variants favors the argument that N1-methyl-Ψ-modification contributed significantly to the effectiveness of the approved vaccines [163, 164]. Moreover, another potential explanation for the different efficacy outcomes of modified and unmodified mRNA vaccines is related to the vaccine dose.

CureVac's CVnCoV dose (12 μg) was significantly smaller than Comirnaty (30 μg) or Spikevax (100 μg) [165] because higher doses of CVnCoV were generally intolerable to patients [166, 167]. This was not unexpected because of the effect of N1-methyl-Ψ in decreasing mRNA's inflammatory and reactogenic character. Therefore, it is likely that the incorporation of N1-methyl-Ψ in Comirnaty and Spikevax enabled a higher dose, potentially needed for sufficient translation of the S-protein in the target (dendritic) cells. Instead of relying on Ψ or N1-methyl-Ψ to reduce mRNA's intrinsic reactogenicity, CureVac scientists attempted a different strategy but oriented for the same goal. CureVac performed intensive codon optimization to minimize the number of uridines in the mRNA. The company pursued this strategy by taking advantage of the degeneracy of the genetic code (codon redundancy). This approach, which has been applied for several years in different *in vivo* applications [168], would still render therapeutic mRNA that could be used in repetitive treatments, with good protein expression *in vitro* and *in vivo* [169].

However, this codon optimization procedure could have several drawbacks explaining the less-than-expected efficacy of CureVac's unmodified mRNA COVID-19 vaccine. First, it could increase the overall GC content in the mRNA to an excessive level. Since eight amino acid codons have at least one uridine, reducing U-containing codons while maintaining the same coding sequence ultimately leads to more GC-rich codons. Second, heavy sequence engineering that avoids uridines in the coding sequence could lead to the loss of valuable out-of-frame ORF viral epitopes [170]. In this regard, a recent analysis of the HLA-I immunopeptidome of human cells infected with COVID-19 showed some out-of-frame epitopes derived from the S-protein, inducing a more robust T-cell response than the canonical ORF epitopes in a mouse model [170]. In fact, it could be that the residual ribosomal frameshifting phenomenon caused by the presence of the N1-methyl-Ψ modification in Comirnaty and Spikevax could have slightly contributed to a positive effect in efficacy of these vaccines [155]. Third, codon optimization strategies could introduce unwanted cryptic epitopes responsible for increasing mRNA's reactogenicity [171]. Finally, when performing heavy codon optimization of the mRNA to reduce uridines, the outcome might not be optimal considering the natural tRNA abundance in the target cells, with a potential impact on protein expression [172, 173].

Following the disappointing CvnCoV trial results, CureVac has discontinued its clinical development to focus on its second-generation COVID-19 mRNA vaccine platform technology. The company decided this time to assess, in parallel, both the pseudouridine-modified and unmodified versions of the backbone. CureVac initially expected the second generation of unmodified mRNA vaccines to perform better from a safety and efficacy point of view after encouraging data obtained in cell culture and rats [174] and nonhuman primates [175]. From the sequence alone, the second-generation COVID-19 mRNA vaccines differ from CVnCoV in their noncoding region, particularly the inclusion of a 5′ untranslated region UTR (inexistent in CVnCoV) from the human hydroxysteroid 17-beta dehydrogenase 4 gene (HSD17B4) and a 3′UTR derived from human proteasome 20S subunit beta 3 gene (PSMB3) [175]. Further, CureVac's second-generation COVID-19 mRNA vaccines and CVnCoV have the same LNPs and a GC-enriched ORF encoding the COVID-19 Spike protein with the K986P and V987P mutations. Finally, CureVac decided to test mRNA vaccines encoding new variants such as Omicron BA.1 (CV0501, a pseudouridine-modified mRNA vaccine).

The company recently announced encouraging phase 1 trials for their CV0501 vaccine, developed in collaboration with GlaxoSmithKline plc (GSK) [176]. In this study, the company assessed CV0501 reactogenicity, safety, and immunogenicity as a booster vaccine, with doses ranging from 12 to 200 μg. The company showed that, with the lowest dose of this pseudouridine-modified mRNA vaccine, patients generated significant levels of neutralizing antibodies with a good tolerability profile, better than the unmodified counterpart, when assessed in parallel [177]. Some in the field have argued that this head-to-head comparison puts to rest the discussion between modified versus unmodified mRNA vaccines for COVID-19 [178]. In fact, CureVac recognized that it will use modified mRNA for its new COVID-19 programs. In addition, CureVac is currently running clinical trials testing both an unmodified multivalent and a modified monovalent mRNA vaccine against influenza (Flu-SV-mRNA, doses ranging from 2 to 54 μg). Based on the data obtained so far, it is shown that at the lowest dose, the modified Flu-SV-mRNA vaccine boosted antibody titers and was tolerated well [177]. Accordingly, the company decided to pursue the modified mRNA from now on for its influenza program as well.

There are other ongoing efforts for unmodified mRNA COVID-19 vaccines. For example, Walvax Biotechnology and Suzhou Abogen Biosciences recently reported a good safety and tolerability profile in phase 1 clinical trials with their

LNP-encapsulated unmodified mRNA (AWcorna or ARCoV) vaccine (15 μg dose). This vaccine, encoding the Receptor-Binding Domain (RBD) of the wild-type COVID-19 Spike protein, elicited neutralizing antibodies against COVID-19 and a Th1-biased cellular response, in mice and nonhuman primates, following intramuscular injection [179]. Treated patients had a twofold higher titer of neutralizing antibodies than convalescent COVID-19 patients [180]. Data from the larger-scale phase 3 clinical trial (NCT04847102) is still expected [181], and AWcorna was the first Chinese COVID-19 mRNA vaccine to get approval [182] so far, only in Indonesia [183].

Another unmodified mRNA COVID-19 vaccine, initially developed by Translate Bio (now a Sanofi company) and later Sanofi, was discontinued in phase ½ clinical trials [184]. Worth noting that Sanofi, in their recent presentation of the clinical trial results of their LNP-formulated flu-unmodified mRNA vaccine, indicated comparable immunogenicity to a similar N1-methyl-Ψ-modified mRNA vaccine in NHPs [185]. Therefore, the company decided to develop the modified version of their flu mRNA vaccine instead as a strategy to reduce the reactogenicity observed in the unmodified mRNA COVID-19 vaccine (60% of grade 3 adverse events with the first dose of 15 or 45 μg [185]). This would also support the hypothesis that the N1-methyl-Ψ modification played a critical role in decreasing the intrinsic reactogenicity of unmodified mRNA.

Low doses of unmodified mRNA could be a way to tackle excessive reactogenicity. Recently, CureVac has presented promising results for an experimental rabies vaccine, also known as CV7202, consisting of LNP-encapsulated unmodified mRNA expressing rabies virus glycoprotein (RABV-G). In a phase 1 trial (NCT03713086), the company presented data in subjects treated with 1 and 2 μg doses, namely good tolerability and induction of an immune response consisting of neutralizing antibodies, while subjects treated with 5 μg presented excessive reactogenicity [186], as expected.

Beyond the (nonreplicating) mRNA vaccine platform technology described so far, synthetic replicating mRNA vaccines are under intense development. This novel approach, known as the self-amplifying mRNA vaccines, would theoretically enable much lower administered mRNA vaccine doses and provide a more durable immune response effect of the mRNA vaccines. In nonreplicating mRNA vaccines (e.g. Comirnaty and Spikevax), the number of antigen molecules translated is directly proportional to the dose, i.e. the number of mRNA copies administered per injection. Because self-amplifying mRNA vaccines carry, in addition to the antigen coding sequence, a set of instructions for the mRNA to replicate in the cell, this platform technology enables the generation of multiple mRNA copies from lower administered doses. Such instructions are usually derived from viral-engineered RNA replicons (replicative factors), including an RNA-dependent RNA polymerase [187]. In an initial study, the self-amplifying mRNA vaccine approach developed by Arcturus Therapeutics showed an efficacy of 55% against COVID-19 symptoms and 95% protection against severe illness and death [188]. Subjects were treated with two doses of ARCT-021 (28 days apart) consisting of 5 μg of the self-amplifying mRNA. More recently, a complete analysis of Arcturus Therapeutics phase I/II trials with ARCT-021 was published [189]. This self-amplifying mRNA vaccine is formulated with proprietary lipid nanoparticles (LUNAR®) and does not include the Ψ or the N1-methyl-Ψ modification. An RNA-based self-amplifying RNA vaccine platform cannot be, in principle, Ψ-modified, as protein expression has been shown to decrease as a result of the incorporation of this modification [190]. Recently, however, Azizi et al. suggested that 5-methylcytidine and 5-methyluridine can be used in self-amplifying RNAs as a means to improve protein expression and the immunogenicity profile, which could be relevant in the context of protein replacement therapies [191].

3.6.4 Cancer mRNA Vaccines

The idea of treating cancer using our immune system's arsenal is not novel [192]. Theoretically, cells from our immune system could be engineered to recognize and destroy cancer cells. However, in most tumors, the immune system is weakened precisely to avoid this [193]. With the development of the mRNA platform and several of its enabling technologies (formulations, nucleoside modifications, etc.), many are pursuing this goal by using mRNA to deliver specific genetic instructions that would activate our immune system against cancer cells [194]. This effort is currently being accelerated by the success of mRNA COVID-19 vaccines [195]. While the approved vaccines, so far, rely on N1-methyl-Ψ-modified mRNA, there are reasons to believe that the extra reactogenicity of unmodified mRNA could become an advantage in the process of activating cold tumors (tumors that are not likely to induce an immune response) into hot ones [196, 197]. There are several examples of unmodified mRNA cancer vaccines currently in clinical development, and some will be briefly discussed here.

For example, CureVac is developing an unmodified noncoding single-stranded RNA, CV8102, a TLR7/8/RIG-1 agonist [198], currently in phase 1 for the treatment of advanced melanoma, skin, neck, and head squamous cell carcinomas, and adenoid cystic carcinoma (NCT03291002). CV8102 is an RNA-based adjuvant that contains polyU repeats, where the RNA is complexed with a polymeric carrier. The combination of unmodified RNA and the carrier was designed to provide an immunostimulatory activity to induce a systemic immune response and modulate the tumor's microenvironment. The current CV8102 trial is being executed as both a single agent and an anti-PD-1 antibody [199]. The company has recently announced that the noncoding CV8102 will become a complementary platform technology for cancer mRNA vaccines [200].

Etherna Immunotherapies NV, a Belgium biotech company, has also developed an unmodified mRNA-based adjuvant consisting of mRNAs expressing three proteins: CD70, CD40L, and caTLR4. The three immune activator proteins that stimulate dendritic cells have been used alone or combined with other mRNAs in cancer clinical trials [201].

BioNTech, despite the massive success of its nucleoside-modified mRNA technology platform (COVID-19 vaccines), is also developing LNP-encapsulated unmodified mRNA vaccines for different types of cancer [202]. For example,

BNT122, encoding up to 20 patient-specific tumor neoantigens, and BNT111, encoding a fixed set of four melanoma-associated antigens, are being tested as potential treatments for melanoma. In parallel, BioNTech is also developing an mRNA cancer vaccine for head and neck squamous cell carcinoma (HNSCC), focusing on BNT113, an unmodified mRNA encoding E6 and E7, two oncoproteins often found in HPV16+ solid cancers. Further, the company is also running phase 1 trials in non-small cell lung cancer (NSCLC) patients with BNT116, an unmodified mRNA vaccine encoding antigens often expressed in these tumors.

Nevertheless, the recent results in a randomized phase 2 clinical trial of a personalized modified mRNA cancer vaccine developed by Moderna and Merck Co. point to the hypothesis that the modified mRNA platform technology might be crucial for developing new cancer treatments. The modified mRNA administered in combination with a checkpoint inhibitor (Keytruda®, a humanized antibody targeting PD-1) significantly lowered the risk of death or cancer recurrence (by 44%) when compared to the checkpoint-inhibitor monotherapy (control group) [203].

3.7 Conclusions

There is no doubt that the encapsulation of mRNA vaccines in LNPs was of critical importance for the success of the mRNA platform. Without LNPs, the IVT mRNA would be much more likely to be degraded, more challenging to be taken up by the cells, and harder to be released into the cytosol from the endosomes due to the endosome-entrapment problem. In addition, LNPs act as coadjuvants in the vaccine. Still, the formulation of mRNA in LNPs is a necessary but insufficient condition for successfully developing COVID-19 mRNA vaccines with high efficacy and low reactogenicity – at least judging from the clinical data generated so far.

The debate thus continues regarding which enabling technologies (LNPs versus Ψ-modified mRNA) were most critical in the success of the mRNA vaccine platform. For example, it was recently argued that the effectiveness of nucleoside modifications such as Ψ and N1-methyl-Ψ in LNP-formulated mRNAs could be somehow dependent upon factors beyond the modified mRNA itself [204]. Melamed et al. showed that while modifications such as N1-methyl-Ψ do improve the translation in spleen and immune system cells, the contribution of RNA modifications also depends on the chemical composition of the LNPs used, the type of cells targeted, as well as the organ where the LNP-delivered mRNA is delivered to express therapeutic/antigenic proteins. How these variables can impact successful modified/unmodified mRNA strategies warrants further study.

On the other hand, unmodified mRNA and Ψ-modified IVT mRNA COVID-19 vaccines have led so far to different clinical outcomes, with the former having higher reactogenicity (at comparable doses of Ψ-modified mRNA) and lower vaccine efficacy and protection. The uridines in the unmodified IVT mRNA contribute to the activation of RNA sensors such as TLR3, TLR7, TLR8, and RIG-I, which ultimately lead to the production of type-I interferon, proinflammatory cytokines,

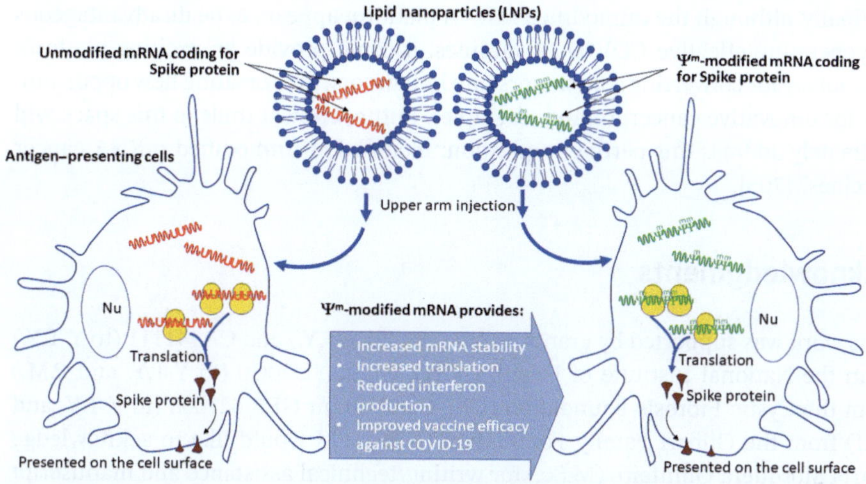

Figure 3.4 Unmodified and Ψ^{m}-modified mRNA COVID-19 vaccines lead to different outcomes. Both can encode the Spike protein with the two mutations that stabilize the pre-fusion conformation of the protein (K986P and V987P). Likewise, both can be formulated in lipid nanoparticles (LNPs) and injected into the upper arm, where they carry the cargo to the lymph nodes and are internalized by dendritic cells (antigen-presenting cells). The LNPs enable both the unmodified or the Ψ-modified (or N1-methyl-Ψ) mRNA to escape endosome entrapment. Finally, the mRNA vaccine is released into the cytoplasm for ribosomal translation. However, the uridines in the unmodified mRNA can activate RNA sensors during this process (TLR3, TLR7, TLR8, and RIG-I), ultimately leading to type-I interferon production and significant inflammatory response. On the other hand, Ψ-modified IVT mRNA can trick the cell's immune response, enabling more antigenic protein production while generating less reactogenicity than unmodified mRNA. Nu, nucleus.

and inflammatory response (Figure 3.4). Further, unmodified mRNA contributes to two important processes. First is the activation of PKR, which inhibits translation. Second, the unmodified mRNA is more prone to activate OAS (2′-5′-oligoadenylate synthetase), which induces RNase L-mediated rRNA degradation, ultimately leading to reduced protein expression and antigen production.

By avoiding the detection by RNA sensors and PKR, Ψ-modified IVT mRNA can trick the cell's immune response against exogenous IVT mRNA. Thus, the cell produces fewer interferon and proinflammatory cytokines, and less inflammatory response is mounted. Further, more antigenic protein is produced, thus optimizing the mRNA immunogenicity and producing less reactogenicity. Consequently, it leads to overall better COVID-19 vaccine protection.

It is possible that higher doses of unmodified IVT mRNA (similar to the ones used in Ψ-modified IVT mRNA) could produce enough antigenic protein, but unfortunately, this could come with more adverse effects for patients. Moreover, it is clear that both Ψ and N1-methyl-Ψ provide a means for IVT mRNA to trick the immune system. Since both nucleosides share the freely rotatable covalent glycosidic C—C bond, further empirical data is needed to understand better the biophysical consequences of such flexibility in the RNA recognition processes.

Finally, although the unmodified mRNA platform appears to be disadvantageous in generating effective COVID-19 vaccines, it could provide an exciting platform technology for converting cold tumors into hot tumors, thus creating new opportunities for innovative cancer immunotherapies. Future clinical trials in this space will ultimately address this pertinent question: modified or unmodified mRNA cancer vaccines? [205].

Acknowledgments

This work was supported by grants GM138387 (to Y-T.Y.) and CA241111 (to Y-T.Y.) from the National Institute of Health (NIH), Grant YU20G0 (to Y-T.Y. and P.M.) from the Cystic Fibrosis Foundation (CFF), and Grant GFF 521008 (to Y-T.Y. and P.M) from the Gilbert Family Foundation (GFF). PM would like to acknowledge Marta Mosquera Quinteiro (M.Sc.) for writing/technical assistance and manuscript proofreading.

Conflict of Interest

Y-T.U. and P.M. (and others) have filled a patent application on nucleic acid molecules for pseudouridylation using guide RNAs (WO/2019/191232). Until September 30, 2022, P.M. was a ProQR Therapeutics (The Netherlands) employee, and since then, he has been working at Bayer Pharmaceuticals (Germany).

References

1 Helm, M. and Motorin, Y. (2017). Detecting RNA modifications in the epitranscriptome: predict and validate. *Nat. Rev. Genet.* 18: 275–291. https://doi.org/10.1038/nrg.2016.169.

2 Ontiveros, R.J., Stoute, J., and Liu, K.F. (2019). The chemical diversity of RNA modifications. *Biochem. J.* 476: 1227–1245. https://doi.org/10.1042/BCJ20180445.

3 Ge, J. and Yu, Y.-T. (2013). RNA pseudouridylation: new insights into an old modification. *Trends Biochem. Sci.* 38: 210–218. https://doi.org/10.1016/j.tibs.2013.01.002.

4 Furuse, Y. (2021). RNA modifications in genomic RNA of influenza A virus and the relationship between RNA modifications and viral infection. *Int. J. Mol. Sci.* 22: 9127. https://doi.org/10.3390/ijms22179127.

5 McIntyre, W., Netzband, R., Bonenfant, G. et al. (2018). Positive-sense RNA viruses reveal the complexity and dynamics of the cellular and viral epitranscriptomes during infection. *Nucleic Acids Res.* 46: 5776–5791. https://doi.org/10.1093/nar/gky029.

6 Fleming, A.M., Mathewson, N.J., Howpay Manage, S.A., and Burrows, C.J. (2021). Nanopore dwell time analysis permits sequencing and conformational

assignment of pseudouridine in SARS-CoV-2. *ACS Cent. Sci.* 7: 1707–1717. https://doi.org/10.1021/acscentsci.1c00788.

7 Cohn, W.E. and Volkin, E. (1951). Nucleoside-5′-phosphates from ribonucleic acid. *Nature* 167: 483–484. https://doi.org/10.1038/167483a0.

8 Davis, F.F. and Allen, F.W. (1957). Ribonucleic acids from yeast which contain a fifth nucleotide. *J. Biol. Chem.* 227: 907–915. https://doi.org/10.1016/S0021-9258(18)70770-9.

9 Adler, M. and Gutman, A.B. (1959). Uridine isomer (5-ribosyluracil) in human urine. *Science* 130: 862–863. https://doi.org/10.1126/science.130.3379.862.

10 Adams, W.S., Davis, F., and Nakatani, M. (1960). Purine and pyrimidine excretion in normal and leukemic subjects. *Am. J. Med.* 28: 726–734. https://doi.org/10.1016/0002-9343(60)90130-3.

11 Veerareddygari, G.R., Singh, S.K., and Mueller, E.G. (2016). The pseudouridine synthases proceed through a glycal intermediate. *J. Am. Chem. Soc.* 138: 7852–7855. https://doi.org/10.1021/jacs.6b04491.

12 Davis, D.R. (1995). Stabilization of RNA stacking by pseudouridine. *Nucleic Acids Res.* 23: 5020–5026. https://doi.org/10.1093/nar/23.24.5020.

13 Westhof, E. (2019). Pseudouridines or how to draw on weak energy differences. *Biochem. Biophys. Res. Commun.* 520: 702–704. https://doi.org/10.1016/j.bbrc.2019.10.009.

14 Kim, K.Q., Burgute, B.D., Tzeng, S.-C. et al. (2022). N1-methylpseudouridine found within COVID-19 mRNA vaccines produces faithful protein products. *Cell Rep.* 40: 111300. https://doi.org/10.1016/j.celrep.2022.111300.

15 Kierzek, E., Malgowska, M., Lisowiec, J. et al. (2014). The contribution of pseudouridine to stabilities and structure of RNAs. *Nucleic Acids Res.* 42: 3492–3501. https://doi.org/10.1093/nar/gkt1330.

16 Naylor, R., Ho, N.W.Y., and Gilham, P.T. (1965). Selective chemical modifications of uridine and pseudouridine in polynucleotides and their effect on the specificities of ribonuclease and phosphodiesterases. *J. Am. Chem. Soc.* 87: 4209–4210. https://doi.org/10.1021/ja01096a050.

17 Leppek, K., Byeon, G.W., Kladwang, W. et al. (2022). Combinatorial optimization of mRNA structure, stability, and translation for RNA-based therapeutics. *Nat. Commun.* 13: 1536. https://doi.org/10.1038/s41467-022-28776-w.

18 Arnez, J.G. and Steitz, T.A. (1994). Crystal structure of unmodified tRNAGln complexed with glutaminyl-tRNA synthetase and ATP suggests a possible role for pseudo-uridines in stabilization of RNA structure. *Biochemistry* 33: 7560–7567. https://doi.org/10.1021/bi00190a008.

19 Newby, M.I. and Greenbaum, N.L. (2001). A conserved pseudouridine modification in eukaryotic U2 snRNA induces a change in branch-site architecture. *RNA* 7: 833–845. https://doi.org/10.1017/S1355838201002308.

20 Newby, M.I. and Greenbaum, N.L. (2002). Sculpting of the spliceosomal branch site recognition motif by a conserved pseudouridine. *Nat. Struct. Biol.* 9: 958–965. https://doi.org/10.1038/nsb873.

21 Goldwasser, E. and Heiniukson, R.L. (1966). The biochemistry of pseudouridine. *Prog. Nucleic Acid Res. Mol. Biol.* 5, Elsevier: 399–416. https://doi.org/10.1016/S0079-6603(08)60241-X.

22 Johnson, L. and Söll, D. (1970). In vitro biosynthesis of pseudouridine at the polynucleotide level by an enzyme extract from *Escherichia coli*. *Proc. Natl. Acad. Sci.* 67: 943–950. https://doi.org/10.1073/pnas.67.2.943.

23 Borchardt, E.K., Martinez, N.M., and Gilbert, W.V. (2020). Regulation and function of RNA pseudouridylation in human cells. *Annu. Rev. Genet.* 54: 309–336. https://doi.org/10.1146/annurev-genet-112618-043830.

24 Li, X., Zhu, P., Ma, S. et al. (2015). Chemical pulldown reveals dynamic pseudouridylation of the mammalian transcriptome. *Nat. Chem. Biol.* 11: 592–597. https://doi.org/10.1038/nchembio.1836.

25 Carlile, T.M., Martinez, N.M., Schaening, C. et al. (2019). mRNA structure determines modification by pseudouridine synthase 1. *Nat. Chem. Biol.* 15: 966–974. https://doi.org/10.1038/s41589-019-0353-z.

26 Rintala-Dempsey, A.C. and Kothe, U. (2017). Eukaryotic stand-alone pseudouridine synthases – RNA modifying enzymes and emerging regulators of gene expression? *RNA Biol.* 14: 1185–1196. https://doi.org/10.1080/15476286.2016.1276150.

27 De Zoysa, M.D. and Yu, Y.-T. (2017). Posttranscriptional RNA pseudouridylation. *Enzymes* 41, Elsevier: 151–167. https://doi.org/10.1016/bs.enz.2017.02.001.

28 Kiss, D.J., Oláh, J., Tóth, G. et al. (2022). The structure-derived mechanism of Box H/ACA pseudouridine synthase offers a plausible paradigm for programmable RNA editing. *ACS Catal.* 12: 2756–2769. https://doi.org/10.1021/acscatal.1c04870.

29 Yu, Y.-T. and Meier, U.T. (2014). RNA-guided isomerization of uridine to pseudouridine—pseudouridylation. *RNA Biol.* 11: 1483–1494. https://doi.org/10.4161/15476286.2014.972855.

30 Kiss, A.M., Jády, B.E., Bertrand, E., and Kiss, T. (2004). Human box H/ACA pseudouridylation guide RNA machinery. *Mol. Cell. Biol.* 24: 5797–5807. https://doi.org/10.1128/MCB.24.13.5797-5807.2004.

31 Morais, P., Adachi, H., Chen, J.L., and Yu, Y.-T. (2021). Mechanisms and clinical applications of RNA pseudouridylation. In: *Epitranscriptomics*, vol. 12 (ed. S. Jurga and J. Barciszewski), 505–526. Cham: Springer International Publishing https://doi.org/10.1007/978-3-030-71612-7_19.

32 De Zoysa, M.D., Wu, G., Katz, R., and Yu, Y.-T. (2018). Guide-substrate base-pairing requirement for box H/ACA RNA-guided RNA pseudouridylation. *RNA* 24: 1106–1117. https://doi.org/10.1261/rna.066837.118.

33 Kelly, E.K., Czekay, D.P., and Kothe, U. (2019). Base-pairing interactions between substrate RNA and H/ACA guide RNA modulate the kinetics of pseudouridylation, but not the affinity of substrate binding by H/ACA small nucleolar ribonucleoproteins. *RNA* 25: 1393–1404. https://doi.org/10.1261/rna.071043.119.

34 Duan, J., Li, L., Lu, J. et al. (2009). Structural mechanism of substrate RNA recruitment in H/ACA RNA-guided pseudouridine synthase. *Mol. Cell* 34: 427–439. https://doi.org/10.1016/j.molcel.2009.05.005.

35 Li, L. and Ye, K. (2006). Crystal structure of an H/ACA box ribonucleoprotein particle. *Nature* 443: 302–307. https://doi.org/10.1038/nature05151.

36 Rashid, R., Liang, B., Baker, D.L. et al. (2006). Crystal structure of a Cbf5-Nop10-Gar1 complex and implications in RNA-guided pseudouridylation and dyskeratosis congenita. *Mol. Cell* 21: 249–260. https://doi.org/10.1016/j.molcel.2005.11.017.

37 Majumder, M., Bosmeny, M.S., and Gupta, R. (2016). Structure–function relationships of archaeal Cbf5 during in vivo RNA-guided pseudouridylation. *RNA* 22: 1604–1619. https://doi.org/10.1261/rna.057547.116.

38 Li, S., Duan, J., Li, D. et al. (2011). Reconstitution and structural analysis of the yeast box H/ACA RNA-guided pseudouridine synthase. *Genes Dev.* 25: 2409–2421. https://doi.org/10.1101/gad.175299.111.

39 Goldberg, I.H. and Rabinowitz, M. (1961). The incorporation of 5-ribosyluracil triphosphate into RNA in nuclear extracts of mammalian cells. *Biochem. Biophys. Res. Commun.* 6: 394–398. https://doi.org/10.1016/0006-291X(61)90152-8.

40 Karijolich, J. and Yu, Y.-T. (2015). The new era of RNA modification. *RNA* 21: 659–660. https://doi.org/10.1261/rna.049650.115.

41 Spenkuch, F., Motorin, Y., and Helm, M. (2014). Pseudouridine: still mysterious, but never a fake (uridine)! *RNA Biol.* 11: 1540–1554. https://doi.org/10.4161/15476286.2014.992278.

42 Huang, C., Karijolich, J., and Yu, Y.-T. (2016). Detection and quantification of RNA 2′-O-methylation and pseudouridylation. *Methods* 103: 68–76. https://doi.org/10.1016/j.ymeth.2016.02.003.

43 Pardi, N., Muramatsu, H., Weissman, D., and Karikó, K. (2013). In vitro transcription of long RNA containing modified nucleosides. In: *Synthetic Messenger RNA and Cell Metabolism Modulation*, vol. 969 (ed. P.M. Rabinovich), 29–42. Totowa, NJ: Humana Press https://doi.org/10.1007/978-1-62703-260-5_2.

44 Potapov, V., Fu, X., Dai, N. et al. (2018). Base modifications affecting RNA polymerase and reverse transcriptase fidelity. *Nucleic Acids Res.* 46: 5753–5763. https://doi.org/10.1093/nar/gky341.

45 Ma, X., Yang, C., Alexandrov, A. et al. (2005). Pseudouridylation of yeast U2 snRNA is catalyzed by either an RNA-guided or RNA-independent mechanism. *EMBO J.* 24: 2403–2413. https://doi.org/10.1038/sj.emboj.7600718.

46 Xiao, M., Yang, C., Schattner, P., and Yu, Y.-T. (2009). Functionality and substrate specificity of human box H/ACA guide RNAs. *RNA* 15: 176–186. https://doi.org/10.1261/rna.1361509.

47 Adachi, H., Chen, J.L., Yin, Q. et al. (2023). In vitro reconstitution of pseudouridylation catalyzed by human box H/ACA ribonucleoprotein particles. In: *RNA-Protein Complexes Interact*, vol. 2666 (ed. R.-J. Lin), 177–191. New York, NY: Springer US https://doi.org/10.1007/978-1-0716-3191-1_14.

48 Krieg, P.A. and Melton, D.A. (1984). Functional messenger RNAs are produced by SP6 *in vitro* transcription of cloned cDNAs. *Nucleic Acids Res.* 12: 7057–7070. https://doi.org/10.1093/nar/12.18.7057.

49 Melton, D.A., Krieg, P.A., Rebagliati, M.R. et al. (1984). Efficient *in vitro* synthesis of biologically active RNA and RNA hybridization probes from plasmids containing a bacteriophage SP6 promoter. *Nucleic Acids Res.* 12: 7035–7056. https://doi.org/10.1093/nar/12.18.7035.

50 Milligan, J.F., Groebe, D.R., Witherell, G.W., and Uhlenbeck, O.C. (1987). Oligoribonucleotide synthesis using T7 RNA polymerase and synthetic DNA templates. *Nucleic Acids Res.* 15: 8783–8798. https://doi.org/10.1093/nar/15.21.8783.

51 Steitz, T.A. (2004). The structural basis of the transition from initiation to elongation phases of transcription, as well as translocation and strand separation, by T7 RNA polymerase. *Curr. Opin. Struct. Biol.* 14: 4–9. https://doi.org/10.1016/j.sbi.2004.01.006.

52 Beckert, B. and Masquida, B. (2011). Synthesis of RNA by in vitro transcription. In: *RNA*, vol. 703 (ed. H. Nielsen), 29–41. Totowa, NJ: Humana Press https://doi.org/10.1007/978-1-59745-248-9_3.

53 Chen, C., Zhao, X., Kierzek, R., and Yu, Y.-T. (2010). A flexible RNA backbone within the polypyrimidine tract is required for U2AF 65 binding and pre-mRNA splicing in vivo. *Mol. Cell. Biol.* 30: 4108–4119. https://doi.org/10.1128/MCB.00531-10.

54 Karikó, K., Buckstein, M., Ni, H., and Weissman, D. (2005). Suppression of RNA recognition by toll-like receptors: the impact of nucleoside modification and the evolutionary origin of RNA. *Immunity* 23: 165–175. https://doi.org/10.1016/j.immuni.2005.06.008.

55 Karikó, K., Muramatsu, H., Welsh, F.A. et al. (2008). Incorporation of pseudouridine into mRNA yields superior nonimmunogenic vector with increased translational capacity and biological stability. *Mol. Ther.* 16: 1833–1840. https://doi.org/10.1038/mt.2008.200.

56 Padilla, R. and Sousa, R. (2002). A Y639F/H784A T7 RNA polymerase double mutant displays superior properties for synthesizing RNAs with non-canonical NTPs. *Nucleic Acids Res.* 30: 138e–138e. https://doi.org/10.1093/nar/gnf138.

57 Yu, Y.-T. (1998). Modifications of U2 snRNA are required for snRNP assembly and pre-mRNA splicing. *EMBO J.* 17: 5783–5795. https://doi.org/10.1093/emboj/17.19.5783.

58 Andries, O., Mc Cafferty, S., De Smedt, S.C. et al. (2015). N1-methylpseudouridine-incorporated mRNA outperforms pseudouridine-incorporated mRNA by providing enhanced protein expression and reduced immunogenicity in mammalian cell lines and mice. *J. Control. Release* 217: 337–344. https://doi.org/10.1016/j.jconrel.2015.08.051.

59 Fleming, A.M. and Burrows, C.J. (2023). Nanopore sequencing for N1-methylpseudouridine in RNA reveals sequence-dependent discrimination of the modified nucleotide triphosphate during transcription. *Nucleic Acids Res.* gkad044. https://doi.org/10.1093/nar/gkad044.

60 Karikó, K., Muramatsu, H., Ludwig, J., and Weissman, D. (2011). Generating the optimal mRNA for therapy: HPLC purification eliminates immune activation and improves translation of nucleoside-modified, protein-encoding mRNA. *Nucleic Acids Res.* 39: e142. https://doi.org/10.1093/nar/gkr695.

61 Baiersdörfer, M., Boros, G., Muramatsu, H. et al. (2019). A facile method for the removal of dsRNA contaminant from in vitro-transcribed mRNA. *Mol Ther Nucleic Acids* 15: 26–35. https://doi.org/10.1016/j.omtn.2019.02.018.

62 Kis, Z., Kontoravdi, C., Shattock, R., and Shah, N. (2020). Resources, production scales and time required for producing RNA vaccines for the global pandemic demand. *Vaccine* 9: 3. https://doi.org/10.3390/vaccines9010003.

63 Kellner, S., Burhenne, J., and Helm, M. (2010). Detection of RNA modifications. *RNA Biol.* 7: 237–247. https://doi.org/10.4161/rna.7.2.11468.

64 Zhang, L.-S., Dai, Q., and He, C. (2023). BID-seq: the quantitative and base-resolution sequencing method for RNA pseudouridine. *ACS Chem. Biol.* 18: 4–6. https://doi.org/10.1021/acschembio.2c00881.

65 Bakin, A. and Ofengand, J. (1993). Four newly located pseudouridylate residues in *Escherichia coli* 23S ribosomal RNA are all at the peptidyltransferase center: analysis by the application of a new sequencing technique. *Biochemistry* 32: 9754–9762. https://doi.org/10.1021/bi00088a030.

66 Ofengand, J., Del Campo, M., and Kaya, Y. (2001). Mapping pseudouridines in RNA molecules. *Methods* 25: 365–373. https://doi.org/10.1006/meth.2001.1249.

67 Carlile, T.M., Rojas-Duran, M.F., Zinshteyn, B. et al. (2014). Pseudouridine profiling reveals regulated mRNA pseudouridylation in yeast and human cells. *Nature* 515: 143–146. https://doi.org/10.1038/nature13802.

68 Lovejoy, A.F., Riordan, D.P., and Brown, P.O. (2014). Transcriptome-wide mapping of pseudouridines: pseudouridine synthases modify specific mRNAs in *S. cerevisiae*. *PLoS One* 9: e110799. https://doi.org/10.1371/journal.pone.0110799.

69 Nakamoto, M.A., Lovejoy, A.F., Cygan, A.M., and Boothroyd, J.C. (2017). mRNA pseudouridylation affects RNA metabolism in the parasite *Toxoplasma gondii*. *RNA* 23: 1834–1849. https://doi.org/10.1261/rna.062794.117.

70 Schwartz, S., Bernstein, D.A., Mumbach, M.R. et al. (2014). Transcriptome-wide mapping reveals widespread dynamic-regulated pseudouridylation of ncRNA and mRNA. *Cell* 159: 148–162. https://doi.org/10.1016/j.cell.2014.08.028.

71 Marinov, G.K. (2017). On the design and prospects of direct RNA sequencing. *Brief. Funct. Genomics* 16: 326–335. https://doi.org/10.1093/bfgp/elw043.

72 Wang, Y., Zhao, Y., Bollas, A. et al. (2021). Nanopore sequencing technology, bioinformatics and applications. *Nat. Biotechnol.* 39: 1348–1365. https://doi.org/10.1038/s41587-021-01108-x.

73 Workman, R.E., Tang, A.D., Tang, P.S. et al. (2019). Nanopore native RNA sequencing of a human poly(A) transcriptome. *Nat. Methods* 16: 1297–1305. https://doi.org/10.1038/s41592-019-0617-2.

74 Sun, X., Song, L., Yang, W. et al. (2020). Nanopore sequencing and its clinical applications. In: *Precis. Med.*, vol. 2204 (ed. T. Huang), 13–32. New York, NY: Springer US https://doi.org/10.1007/978-1-0716-0904-0_2.

75 Smith, A.M., Jain, M., Mulroney, L. et al. (2019). Reading canonical and modified nucleobases in 16S ribosomal RNA using nanopore native RNA sequencing. *PLoS One* 14: e0216709. https://doi.org/10.1371/journal.pone.0216709.

76 Liu, H., Begik, O., Lucas, M.C. et al. (2019). Accurate detection of m6A RNA modifications in native RNA sequences. *Nat. Commun.* 10: 4079. https://doi.org/10.1038/s41467-019-11713-9.

77 Furlan, M., Delgado-Tejedor, A., Mulroney, L. et al. (2021). Computational methods for RNA modification detection from nanopore direct RNA sequencing data. *RNA Biol.* 18: 31–40. https://doi.org/10.1080/15476286.2021.1978215.

78 Hassan, D., Acevedo, D., Daulatabad, S.V. et al. (2022). Penguin: a tool for predicting pseudouridine sites in direct RNA nanopore sequencing data. *Methods* 203: 478–487. https://doi.org/10.1016/j.ymeth.2022.02.005.

79 Morais, P., Adachi, H., and Yu, Y.-T. (2021). Spliceosomal snRNA epitranscriptomics. *Front. Genet.* 12: 652129. https://doi.org/10.3389/fgene.2021.652129.

80 Roca, X., Sachidanandam, R., and Krainer, A. (2005). Determinants of the inherent strength of human 5' splice sites. *RNA* 11: 683–698. https://doi.org/10.1261/rna.2040605.

81 Roca, X., Akerman, M., Gaus, H. et al. (2012). Widespread recognition of 5' splice sites by noncanonical base-pairing to U1 snRNA involving bulged nucleotides. *Genes Dev.* 26: 1098–1109. https://doi.org/10.1101/gad.190173.112.

82 Wu, G., Adachi, H., Ge, J. et al. (2016). Pseudouridines in U2 snRNA stimulate the ATPase activity of Prp5 during spliceosome assembly. *EMBO J.* 35: 654–667. https://doi.org/10.15252/embj.201593113.

83 Zhao, X. and Yu, Y.-T. (2004). Pseudouridines in and near the branch site recognition region of U2 snRNA are required for snRNP biogenesis and pre-mRNA splicing in Xenopus oocytes. *RNA* 10: 681–690. https://doi.org/10.1261/rna.5159504.

84 Martinez, N.M., Su, A., Burns, M.C. et al. (2022). Pseudouridine synthases modify human pre-mRNA co-transcriptionally and affect pre-mRNA processing. *Mol. Cell* 82: 645–659.e9. https://doi.org/10.1016/j.molcel.2021.12.023.

85 Ofengand, J. (2002). Ribosomal RNA pseudouridines and pseudouridine synthases. *FEBS Lett.* 514: 17–25. https://doi.org/10.1016/S0014-5793(02)02305-0.

86 Decatur, W.A. and Fournier, M.J. (2003). RNA-guided nucleotide modification of ribosomal and other RNAs. *J. Biol. Chem.* 278: 695–698. https://doi.org/10.1074/jbc.R200023200.

87 Charette, M. and Gray, M. (2000). Pseudouridine in RNA: what, where, how, and why. *IUBMB Life Int. Union Biochem. Mol. Biol. Life* 49: 341–351. https://doi.org/10.1080/152165400410182.

88 Penzo, M. and Montanaro, L. (2018). Turning uridines around: role of rRNA pseudouridylation in ribosome biogenesis and ribosomal function. *Biomolecules* 8: 38. https://doi.org/10.3390/biom8020038.

89 Zhao, Y., Rai, J., Yu, H., and Li, H. (2022). CryoEM structures of pseudouridine-free ribosome suggest impacts of chemical modifications on

ribosome conformations. *Structure* 30 (7): 983–992.e5. https://doi.org/10.1016/j.str.2022.04.002.

90 Tomita, K. (1999). The presence of pseudouridine in the anticodon alters the genetic code: a possible mechanism for assignment of the AAA lysine codon as asparagine in echinoderm mitochondria. *Nucleic Acids Res.* 27: 1683–1689. https://doi.org/10.1093/nar/27.7.1683.

91 Beier, H., Barciszewska, M., and Sickinger, H.-D. (1984). The molecular basis for the differential translation of TMV RNA in tobacco protoplasts and wheat germ extracts. *EMBO J.* 3: 1091–1096. https://doi.org/10.1002/j.1460-2075.1984.tb01934.x.

92 Zerfass, K. and Beier, H. (1992). Pseudouridine in the anticodon GΨA of plant cytoplasmic $tRNA^{Tyr}$ is required for UAG and UAA suppression in the TMV-specific context. *Nucleic Acids Res.* 20: 5911–5918. https://doi.org/10.1093/nar/20.22.5911.

93 Zerfass, K. and Beier, H. (1992). The leaky UGA termination codon of tobacco rattle virus RNA is suppressed by tobacco chloroplast and cytoplasmic tRNAs(Trp) with CmCA anticodon. *EMBO J.* 11: 4167–4173. https://doi.org/10.1002/j.1460-2075.1992.tb05510.x.

94 Karijolich, J. and Yu, Y.-T. (2011). Converting nonsense codons into sense codons by targeted pseudouridylation. *Nature* 474: 395–398. https://doi.org/10.1038/nature10165.

95 Fernández, I.S., Ng, C.L., Kelley, A.C. et al. (2013). Unusual base pairing during the decoding of a stop codon by the ribosome. *Nature* 500: 107–110. https://doi.org/10.1038/nature12302.

96 Adachi, H., Pan, Y., He, X. et al. (2023). Targeted pseudouridylation: an approach for suppressing nonsense mutations in disease genes. *Mol. Cell* 83 (4): 637–651.e9. https://doi.org/10.1016/j.molcel.2023.01.009.

97 Morais, P., Adachi, H., and Yu, Y.-T. (2020). Suppression of nonsense mutations by new emerging technologies. *Int. J. Mol. Sci.* 21: 4394. https://doi.org/10.3390/ijms21124394.

98 Song, J., Dong, L., Sun, H. et al. (2023). CRISPR-free, programmable RNA pseudouridylation to suppress premature termination codons. *Mol. Cell* 83: 139–155.e9. https://doi.org/10.1016/j.molcel.2022.11.011.

99 Dai, Q., Zhang, L.-S., Sun, H.-L. et al. (2022). Quantitative sequencing using BID-seq uncovers abundant pseudouridines in mammalian mRNA at base resolution. *Nat. Biotechnol.* https://doi.org/10.1038/s41587-022-01505-w.

100 Nir, R., Hoernes, T.P., Muramatsu, H. et al. (2022). A systematic dissection of determinants and consequences of snoRNA-guided pseudouridylation of human mRNA. *Nucleic Acids Res.* 50: 4900–4916. https://doi.org/10.1093/nar/gkac347.

101 Mort, M., Ivanov, D., Cooper, D.N., and Chuzhanova, N.A. (2008). A meta-analysis of nonsense mutations causing human genetic disease. *Hum. Mutat.* 29: 1037–1047. https://doi.org/10.1002/humu.20763.

102 Peltz, S.W., Morsy, M., Welch, E.M., and Jacobson, A. (2013). Ataluren as an agent for therapeutic nonsense suppression. *Annu. Rev. Med.* 64: 407–425. https://doi.org/10.1146/annurev-med-120611-144851.

103 Eyler, D.E., Franco, M.K., Batool, Z. et al. (2019). Pseudouridinylation of mRNA coding sequences alters translation. *Proc. Natl. Acad. Sci.* 116: 23068–23074. https://doi.org/10.1073/pnas.1821754116.

104 Fujita, Y., Kameda, T., Singh, C.R. et al. (2022). Translational recoding by chemical modification of non-AUG start codon ribonucleotide bases. *Sci. Adv.* 8: eabm8501. https://doi.org/10.1126/sciadv.abm8501.

105 Anderson, B.R., Muramatsu, H., Nallagatla, S.R. et al. (2010). Incorporation of pseudouridine into mRNA enhances translation by diminishing PKR activation. *Nucleic Acids Res.* 38: 5884–5892. https://doi.org/10.1093/nar/gkq347.

106 Karikó, K., Muramatsu, H., Keller, J.M., and Weissman, D. (2012). Increased erythropoiesis in mice injected with submicrogram quantities of pseudouridine-containing mRNA encoding erythropoietin. *Mol. Ther.* 20: 948–953. https://doi.org/10.1038/mt.2012.7.

107 Qin, W., Scicluna, B.P., and van der Poll, T. (2021). The role of host cell DNA methylation in the immune response to bacterial infection. *Front. Immunol.* 12: 696280. https://doi.org/10.3389/fimmu.2021.696280.

108 Tong, J., Zhang, W., Chen, Y. et al. (2022). The emerging role of RNA modifications in the regulation of antiviral innate immunity. *Front. Microbiol.* 13: 845625. https://doi.org/10.3389/fmicb.2022.845625.

109 Krieg, A.M. (1996). Lymphocyte activation by CpG dinucleotide motifs in prokaryotic DNA. *Trends Microbiol.* 4: 73–77. https://doi.org/10.1016/0966-842X(96)81515-0.

110 Petryk, N., Bultmann, S., Bartke, T., and Defossez, P.-A. (2021). Staying true to yourself: mechanisms of DNA methylation maintenance in mammals. *Nucleic Acids Res.* 49: 3020–3032. https://doi.org/10.1093/nar/gkaa1154.

111 Alexopoulou, L., Holt, A.C., Medzhitov, R., and Flavell, R.A. (2001). Recognition of double-stranded RNA and activation of NF-κB by Toll-like receptor 3. *Nature* 413: 732–738. https://doi.org/10.1038/35099560.

112 Weissman, D., Ni, H., Scales, D. et al. (2000). HIV Gag mRNA transfection of dendritic cells (DC) delivers encoded antigen to MHC Class I and II molecules, causes DC maturation, and induces a potent human in vitro primary immune response. *J. Immunol.* 165: 4710–4717. https://doi.org/10.4049/jimmunol.165.8.4710.

113 Kumar, M. and Carmichael, G.G. (1998). Antisense RNA: function and fate of duplex RNA in cells of higher eukaryotes. *Microbiol. Mol. Biol. Rev.* 62: 1415–1434. https://doi.org/10.1128/MMBR.62.4.1415-1434.1998.

114 Karikó, K., Ni, H., Capodici, J. et al. (2004). mRNA is an endogenous ligand for toll-like receptor 3. *J. Biol. Chem.* 279: 12542–12550. https://doi.org/10.1074/jbc.M310175200.

115 Ferré-D'Amaré, A.R. (2003). RNA-modifying enzymes. *Curr. Opin. Struct. Biol.* 13: 49–55. https://doi.org/10.1016/S0959-440X(02)00002-7.

116 Anderson, B.R., Muramatsu, H., Jha, B.K. et al. (2011). Nucleoside modifications in RNA limit activation of 2′-5′-oligoadenylate synthetase and increase resistance to cleavage by RNase L. *Nucleic Acids Res.* 39: 9329–9338. https://doi.org/10.1093/nar/gkr586.

117 Heil, F., Hemmi, H., Hochrein, H. et al. (2004). Species-specific recognition of single-stranded rna via toll-like receptor 7 and 8. *Science* 303: 1526–1529. https://doi.org/10.1126/science.1093620.

118 Diebold, S.S., Massacrier, C., Akira, S. et al. (2006). Nucleic acid agonists for toll-like receptor 7 are defined by the presence of uridine ribonucleotides. *Eur. J. Immunol.* 36: 3256–3267. https://doi.org/10.1002/eji.200636617.

119 Huang, S., Zhang, W., Katanski, C.D. et al. (2021). Interferon inducible pseudouridine modification in human mRNA by quantitative nanopore profiling. *Genome Biol.* 22: 330. https://doi.org/10.1186/s13059-021-02557-y.

120 Warren, L., Manos, P.D., Ahfeldt, T. et al. (2010). Highly efficient reprogramming to pluripotency and directed differentiation of human cells with synthetic modified mRNA. *Cell Stem Cell* 7: 618–630. https://doi.org/10.1016/j.stem.2010.08.012.

121 Rosa, A. and Brivanlou, A.H. (2010). Synthetic mRNAs: powerful tools for reprogramming and differentiation of human cells. *Cell Stem Cell* 7: 549–550. https://doi.org/10.1016/j.stem.2010.10.002.

122 Zangi, L., Lui, K.O., von Gise, A. et al. (2013). Modified mRNA directs the fate of heart progenitor cells and induces vascular regeneration after myocardial infarction. *Nat. Biotechnol.* 31: 898–907. https://doi.org/10.1038/nbt.2682.

123 McKenzie, R., Fried, M.W., Sallie, R. et al. (1995). Hepatic failure and lactic acidosis due to fialuridine (FIAU), an investigational nucleoside analogue for chronic hepatitis B. *N. Engl. J. Med.* 333: 1099–1105. https://doi.org/10.1056/NEJM199510263331702.

124 Sahin, U., Karikó, K., and Türeci, Ö. (2014). mRNA-based therapeutics—developing a new class of drugs. *Nat. Rev. Drug Discov.* 13: 759–780. https://doi.org/10.1038/nrd4278.

125 Wurm, J.P., Meyer, B., Bahr, U. et al. (2010). The ribosome assembly factor Nep1 responsible for Bowen–Conradi syndrome is a pseudouridine-N1-specific methyltransferase. *Nucleic Acids Res.* 38: 2387–2398. https://doi.org/10.1093/nar/gkp1189.

126 Brand, R.C., Klootwijk, J., Planta, R.J., and Maden, B.E.H. (1978). Biosynthesis of a hypermodified nucleotide in *Saccharomyces carlsbergensis* 17S and HeLa-cell 18S ribosomal ribonucleic acid. *Biochem. J.* 169: 71–77. https://doi.org/10.1042/bj1690071.

127 Boccaletto, P., Machnicka, M.A., Purta, E. et al. MODOMICS: a database of RNA modification pathways. 2017 update. *Nucleic Acids Res.* 2018 (46): D303–D307. https://doi.org/10.1093/nar/gkx1030.

128 Morais, P., Adachi, H., and Yu, Y.-T. (2021). The critical contribution of pseudouridine to mRNA COVID-19 vaccines. *Front. Cell Dev. Biol.* 9: 789427. https://doi.org/10.3389/fcell.2021.789427.

129 Svitkin, Y.V., Cheng, Y.M., Chakraborty, T. et al. (2017). N1-methyl-pseudouridine in mRNA enhances translation through eIF2α-dependent and independent mechanisms by increasing ribosome density. *Nucleic Acids Res.* 45: 6023–6036. https://doi.org/10.1093/nar/gkx135.

130 Parr, C.J.C., Wada, S., Kotake, K. et al. (2020). N 1-Methylpseudouridine substitution enhances the performance of synthetic mRNA switches in cells. *Nucleic Acids Res.* 48: e35. https://doi.org/10.1093/nar/gkaa070.

131 Nelson, J., Sorensen, E.W., Mintri, S. et al. (2020). Impact of mRNA chemistry and manufacturing process on innate immune activation. *Sci. Adv.* 6: eaaz6893. https://doi.org/10.1126/sciadv.aaz6893.

132 Chen, T.-H., Potapov, V., Dai, N. et al. (2022). N1-methyl-pseudouridine is incorporated with higher fidelity than pseudouridine in synthetic RNAs. *Sci. Rep.* 12: 13017. https://doi.org/10.1038/s41598-022-17249-1.

133 Pardi, N., Tuyishime, S., Muramatsu, H. et al. (2015). Expression kinetics of nucleoside-modified mRNA delivered in lipid nanoparticles to mice by various routes. *J. Control. Release* 217: 345–351. https://doi.org/10.1016/j.jconrel.2015.08.007.

134 Pardi, N., Hogan, M.J., Pelc, R.S. et al. (2017). Zika virus protection by a single low-dose nucleoside-modified mRNA vaccination. *Nature* 543: 248–251. https://doi.org/10.1038/nature21428.

135 Richner, J.M., Himansu, S., Dowd, K.A. et al. (2017). Modified mRNA vaccines protect against zika virus infection. *Cell* 168: 1114–1125.e10. https://doi.org/10.1016/j.cell.2017.02.017.

136 Krienke, C., Kolb, L., Diken, E. et al. (2021). A noninflammatory mRNA vaccine for treatment of experimental autoimmune encephalomyelitis. *Science* 371: 145–153. https://doi.org/10.1126/science.aay3638.

137 Meyer, M., Huang, E., Yuzhakov, O. et al. (2018). Modified mRNA-based vaccines elicit robust immune responses and protect guinea pigs from Ebola virus disease. *J. Infect. Dis.* 217: 451–455. https://doi.org/10.1093/infdis/jix592.

138 Pardi, N., Hogan, M.J., Naradikian, M.S. et al. (2018). Nucleoside-modified mRNA vaccines induce potent T follicular helper and germinal center B cell responses. *J. Exp. Med.* 215: 1571–1588. https://doi.org/10.1084/jem.20171450.

139 Svitkin, Y.V., Gingras, A.-C., and Sonenberg, N. (2021). Membrane-dependent relief of translation elongation arrest on pseudouridine- and *N* 1-methyl-pseudouridine-modified mRNAs. *Nucleic Acids Res.* gkab1241. https://doi.org/10.1093/nar/gkab1241.

140 Hayashi, C.T.H., Cao, Y., Clark, L.C. et al. (2022). mRNA-LNP expressing PfCSP and Pfs25 vaccine candidates targeting infection and transmission of *Plasmodium falciparum*. *NPJ Vaccines* 7: 155. https://doi.org/10.1038/s41541-022-00577-8.

141 Hanney, S.R., Wooding, S., Sussex, J., and Grant, J. (2020). From COVID-19 research to vaccine application: why might it take 17 months not 17 years and what are the wider lessons? *Health Res. Policy Syst.* 18: 61. https://doi.org/10.1186/s12961-020-00571-3.

142 Nance, K.D. and Meier, J.L. (2021). Modifications in an emergency: the role of N1-methylpseudouridine in COVID-19 vaccines. *ACS Cent. Sci.* 7: 748–756. https://doi.org/10.1021/acscentsci.1c00197.

143 Adachi, H., Hengesbach, M., Yu, Y.-T., and Morais, P. (2021). From antisense RNA to RNA modification: therapeutic potential of RNA-based technologies. *Biomedicine* 9: 550. https://doi.org/10.3390/biomedicines9050550.

144 Alameh, M.-G., Tombácz, I., Bettini, E. et al. (2021). Lipid nanoparticles enhance the efficacy of mRNA and protein subunit vaccines by inducing robust T follicular helper cell and humoral responses. *Immunity* 54: 2877–2892.e7. https://doi.org/10.1016/j.immuni.2021.11.001.

145 Labouta, H.I., Langer, R., Cullis, P.R. et al. (2022). Role of drug delivery technologies in the success of COVID-19 vaccines: a perspective. *Drug Deliv. Transl. Res.* https://doi.org/10.1007/s13346-022-01146-1.

146 Baden, L.R., El Sahly, H.M., Essink, B. et al. (2021). Efficacy and safety of the mRNA-1273 SARS-CoV-2 vaccine. *N. Engl. J. Med.* 384: 403–416. https://doi.org/10.1056/NEJMoa2035389.

147 Haynes, B.F. (2021). A new vaccine to battle COVID-19. *N. Engl. J. Med.* 384: 470–471. https://doi.org/10.1056/NEJMe2035557.

148 Du, L., He, Y., Zhou, Y. et al. (2009). The spike protein of SARS-CoV—a target for vaccine and therapeutic development. *Nat. Rev. Microbiol.* 7: 226–236. https://doi.org/10.1038/nrmicro2090.

149 Huang, Y., Yang, C., Xu, X. et al. (2020). Structural and functional properties of SARS-CoV-2 spike protein: potential antivirus drug development for COVID-19. *Acta Pharmacol. Sin.* 41: 1141–1149. https://doi.org/10.1038/s41401-020-0485-4.

150 Hsieh, C.-L., Goldsmith, J.A., Schaub, J.M. et al. (2020). Structure-based design of prefusion-stabilized SARS-CoV-2 spikes. *Science* 369: 1501–1505. https://doi.org/10.1126/science.abd0826.

151 Kyriakidis, N.C., López-Cortés, A., González, E.V. et al. (2021). SARS-CoV-2 vaccines strategies: a comprehensive review of phase 3 candidates. *NPJ Vaccines* 6: 28. https://doi.org/10.1038/s41541-021-00292-w.

152 Pallesen, J., Wang, N., Corbett, K.S. et al. (2017). Immunogenicity and structures of a rationally designed prefusion MERS-CoV spike antigen. *Proc. Natl. Acad. Sci.* 114: E7348–E7357. https://doi.org/10.1073/pnas.1707304114.

153 Wrapp, D., Wang, N., Corbett, K.S. et al. (2020). Cryo-EM structure of the 2019-nCoV spike in the prefusion conformation. *Science* 367: 1260–1263. https://doi.org/10.1126/science.abb2507.

154 Xia, X. (2021). Detailed dissection and critical evaluation of the Pfizer/BioNTech and modern mRNA vaccines. *Vaccine* 9: 734. https://doi.org/10.3390/vaccines9070734.

155 Mulroney, T.E., Pöyry, T., Yam-Puc, J.C. et al. (2024). N^1-methylpseudouridylation of mRNA causes +1 ribosomal frameshifting. *Nature* 625: 189–194. https://doi.org/10.1038/s41586-023-06800-3.

156 Ishii, K.J. and Akira, S. (2005). Innate immune recognition of nucleic acids: beyond toll-like receptors. *Int. J. Cancer* 117: 517–523. https://doi.org/10.1002/ijc.21402.

157 Kauffman, K.J., Mir, F.F., Jhunjhunwala, S. et al. (2016). Efficacy and immunogenicity of unmodified and pseudouridine-modified mRNA delivered systemically with lipid nanoparticles in vivo. *Biomaterials* 109: 78–87. https://doi.org/10.1016/j.biomaterials.2016.09.006.

158 Lutz, J., Lazzaro, S., Habbeddine, M. et al. (2017). Unmodified mRNA in LNPs constitutes a competitive technology for prophylactic vaccines. *NPJ Vaccines* 2: 29. https://doi.org/10.1038/s41541-017-0032-6.

159 Cohen, J. (2021). What went wrong with CureVac's mRNA vaccine? *Science* 372: 1381. https://doi.org/10.1126/science.372.6549.1381.

160 Rauch, S., Roth, N., Schwendt, K. et al. (2021). mRNA-based SARS-CoV-2 vaccine candidate CVnCoV induces high levels of virus-neutralising antibodies and mediates protection in rodents. *NPJ Vaccines* 6: 57. https://doi.org/10.1038/s41541-021-00311-w.

161 Kremsner, P.G., Ahuad Guerrero, R.A., Arana-Arri, E. et al. (2022). Efficacy and safety of the CVnCoV SARS-CoV-2 mRNA vaccine candidate in ten countries in Europe and Latin America (HERALD): a randomised, observer-blinded, placebo-controlled, phase 2b/3 trial. *Lancet Infect. Dis.* 22: 329–340. https://doi.org/10.1016/S1473-3099(21)00677-0.

162 Buschmann, M.D., Carrasco, M.J., Alishetty, S. et al. (2021). Nanomaterial delivery systems for mRNA vaccines. *Vaccine* 9: 65. https://doi.org/10.3390/vaccines9010065.

163 Abu-Raddad, L.J., Chemaitelly, H., and Butt, A.A. (2021). Effectiveness of the BNT162b2 COVID-19 vaccine against the B.1.1.7 and B.1.351 variants. *N. Engl. J. Med.* 385: 187–189. https://doi.org/10.1056/NEJMc2104974.

164 Sheikh, A., McMenamin, J., Taylor, B., and Robertson, C. (2021). SARS-CoV-2 delta VOC in Scotland: demographics, risk of hospital admission, and vaccine effectiveness. *Lancet* 397: 2461–2462. https://doi.org/10.1016/S0140-6736(21)01358-1.

165 Pascolo, S. (2021). Synthetic messenger RNA-based vaccines: from Scorn to Hype. *Viruses* 13: 270. https://doi.org/10.3390/v13020270.

166 Cohen, J. (2021). What went wrong with CureVac's highly anticipated new mRNA vaccine for COVID-19? *Science* https://www.science.org/content/article/what-went-wrong-curevac-s-highly-anticipated-new-mrna-vaccine-covid-19.

167 Dolgin, E. (2021). CureVac COVID vaccine let-down spotlights mRNA design challenges. *Nature* 594: 483. https://doi.org/10.1038/d41586-021-01661-0.

168 Mauro, V.P. and Chappell, S.A. (2014). A critical analysis of codon optimization in human therapeutics. *Trends Mol. Med.* 20: 604–613. https://doi.org/10.1016/j.molmed.2014.09.003.

169 Thess, A., Grund, S., Mui, B.L. et al. (2015). Sequence-engineered mRNA without chemical nucleoside modifications enables an effective protein therapy in large animals. *Mol. Ther.* 23: 1456–1464. https://doi.org/10.1038/mt.2015.103.

170 Weingarten-Gabbay, S., Klaeger, S., Sarkizova, S. et al. (2021). Profiling SARS-CoV-2 HLA-I peptidome reveals T cell epitopes from out-of-frame ORFs. *Cell* 184: 3962–3980.e17. https://doi.org/10.1016/j.cell.2021.05.046.

171 Lorenz, F.K.M., Wilde, S., Voigt, K. et al. (2015). Codon optimization of the human papillomavirus E7 oncogene induces a CD8+ T cell response to a cryptic epitope not harbored by wild-type E7. *PLoS One* 10: e0121633. https://doi.org/10.1371/journal.pone.0121633.

172 Hanson, G. and Coller, J. (2018). Codon optimality, bias and usage in translation and mRNA decay. *Nat. Rev. Mol. Cell Biol.* 19: 20–30. https://doi.org/10.1038/nrm.2017.91.

173 Linares-Fernández, S., Lacroix, C., Exposito, J.-Y., and Verrier, B. (2020). Tailoring mRNA vaccine to balance innate/adaptive immune response. *Trends Mol. Med.* 26: 311–323. https://doi.org/10.1016/j.molmed.2019.10.002.

174 Roth, N., Schön, J., Hoffmann, D. et al. (2022). Optimised non-coding regions of mRNA SARS-CoV-2 vaccine CV2CoV improves homologous and heterologous neutralising antibody responses. *Vaccine* 10: 1251. https://doi.org/10.3390/vaccines10081251.

175 Gebre, M.S., Rauch, S., Roth, N. et al. (2022). Optimization of non-coding regions for a non-modified mRNA COVID-19 vaccine. *Nature* 601: 410–414. https://doi.org/10.1038/s41586-021-04231-6.

176 CureVac (2022).CureVac Starts Phase 1 Clinical Study of Modified, Omicron-Targeting COVID-19 Vaccine Candidate. https://www.curevac.com/en/curevac-starts-phase-1-clinical-study-of-modified-omicron-targeting-covid-19-vaccine-candidate/ (accessed 11 July 2024).

177 CureVac (2023). CureVac Announces Positive Data on Joint COVID-19 and Flu mRNA Vaccine Development Programs. https://www.curevac.com/en/curevac-announces-positive-data-on-joint-covid-19-and-flu-mrna-vaccine-development-programs/ (accessed 11 July 2024).

178 Dolgin, E. (2023). Trial settles debate over best design for mRNA in COVID vaccines. *Nature* 613: 419–420. https://doi.org/10.1038/d41586-023-00042-z.

179 Zhang, N.-N., Li, X.-F., Deng, Y.-Q. et al. (2020). A thermostable mRNA vaccine against COVID-19. *Cell* 182: 1271–1283.e16. https://doi.org/10.1016/j.cell.2020.07.024.

180 Chen, G.-L., Li, X.-F., Dai, X.-H. et al. (2022). Safety and immunogenicity of the SARS-CoV-2 ARCoV mRNA vaccine in Chinese adults: a randomised, double-blind, placebo-controlled, phase 1 trial. *Lancet Microbe* 3: e193–e202. https://doi.org/10.1016/S2666-5247(21)00280-9.

181 Zhang, N.-N., Zhang, R.-R., Zhang, Y.-F. et al. (2022). Rapid development of an updated mRNA vaccine against the SARS-CoV-2 Omicron variant. *Cell Res.* 32: 401–403. https://doi.org/10.1038/s41422-022-00626-w.

182 Ye, Y. (2022). China's first mRNA vaccine is close—will that solve its COVID woes? *Nature*:d41586-022-01690–3. https://doi.org/10.1038/d41586-022-01690-3.

183 A Chinese mRNA COVID vaccine is approved for the first time – in Indonesia 2022. https://www.reuters.com/business/healthcare-pharmaceuticals/indonesia-drug-agency-approves-chinas-walvax-mrna-vaccine-emergency-use-2022-09-29/ (accessed 11 July 2024).

184 Sanofi (2021).Sanofi announces positive Phase 1/2 study interim results for its first mRNA-based vaccine candidate 2021. https://www.sanofi.com/en/media-room/press-releases/2021/2021-09-28-06-00-00-2304069 (accessed 11 July 2024).

185 Sanofi (2021). Vaccines Investor Event Part 2021. https://www.sanofi.com/en/investors/financial-results-and-events/investor-presentations/Vaccines-Day-2021 (accessed 11 July 2024).

186 Aldrich, C., Leroux-Roels, I., Huang, K.B. et al. (2021). Proof-of-concept of a low-dose unmodified mRNA-based rabies vaccine formulated with lipid nanoparticles in human volunteers: A phase 1 trial. *Vaccine* 39: 1310–1318. https://doi.org/10.1016/j.vaccine.2020.12.070.

187 Borah, P., Deb, P.K., Al-Shar'i, N.A. et al. (2021). Perspectives on RNA vaccine candidates for COVID-19. *Front. Mol. Biosci.* 8: 635245. https://doi.org/10.3389/fmolb.2021.635245.

188 Cohen, J. (2022). An mRNA vaccine with a twist—it copies itself—protects against COVID-19. *Science* https://www.science.org/content/article/mrna-vaccine-twist-it-copies-itself-protects-against-covid-19 (accessed 11 July 2024).

189 Low, J.G., de Alwis, R., Chen, S. et al. (2022). A phase I/II randomized, double-blinded, placebo-controlled trial of a self-amplifying Covid-19 mRNA vaccine. *NPJ Vaccines* 7: 161. https://doi.org/10.1038/s41541-022-00590-x.

190 Erasmus, J.H., Archer, J., Fuerte-Stone, J. et al. (2020). Intramuscular delivery of replicon RNA encoding ZIKV-117 human monoclonal antibody protects against zika virus infection. *Mol. Ther. Methods Clin. Dev.* 18: 402–414. https://doi.org/10.1016/j.omtm.2020.06.011.

191 Azizi, H., Renner, T.M., Agbayani, G. et al. (2024). Self-amplifying RNAs generated with the modified nucleotides 5-methylcytidine and 5-methyluridine mediate strong expression and immunogenicity *in vivo*. *NAR Mol. Med.* 1 (2): ugae004. https://doi.org/10.1093/narmme/ugae004.

192 Overwijk, W.W. and Restifo, N.P. (2000). Autoimmunity and the immunotherapy of cancer: targeting the "self" to destroy the "other". *Crit. Rev. Immunol.* 20: 18. https://doi.org/10.1615/CritRevImmunol.v20.i6.10.

193 Gouttefangeas, C. and Rammensee, H.-G. (2000). Problem solving for tumor immunotherapy. *Nat. Biotechnol.* 18: 491–492. https://doi.org/10.1038/75343.

194 He, Q., Gao, H., Tan, D. et al. (2022). mRNA cancer vaccines: advances, trends and challenges. *Acta Pharm. Sin. B* 12 (7): 2969–2989. https://doi.org/10.1016/j.apsb.2022.03.011.

195 Barbier, A.J., Jiang, A.Y., Zhang, P. et al. (2022). The clinical progress of mRNA vaccines and immunotherapies. *Nat. Biotechnol.* 40: 840–854. https://doi.org/10.1038/s41587-022-01294-2.

196 Duan, Q., Zhang, H., Zheng, J., and Zhang, L. (2020). Turning cold into hot: firing up the tumor microenvironment. *Trends Cancer* 6: 605–618. https://doi.org/10.1016/j.trecan.2020.02.022.

197 Ruffell, D. (2021). The future in an RNA molecule: from mRNA vaccines to therapeutics – An interview with Drew Weissman. *FEBS Lett.* 595: 2305–2309. https://doi.org/10.1002/1873-3468.14190.

198 Ziegler, A., Soldner, C., Lienenklaus, S. et al. (2017). A new RNA-based adjuvant enhances virus-specific vaccine responses by locally triggering TLR- and RLH-dependent effects. *J. Immunol.* 198: 1595–1605. https://doi.org/10.4049/jimmunol.1601129.

199 Zawit, M., Swami, U., Awada, H. et al. (2021). Current status of intralesional agents in treatment of malignant melanoma. *Ann. Transl. Med.* 9: 1038. https://doi.org/10.21037/atm-21-491.

200 CureVac (2022). CureVac Presents Preliminary Data from Phase 1 Study Expansion of Oncology Candidate CV8102. https://www.curevac.com/en/curevac-presents-preliminary-data-from-phase-1-study-expansion-of-oncology-candidate-cv8102/ (accessed 11 July 2024).

201 Jansen, Y., Kruse, V., Corthals, J. et al. (2020). A randomized controlled phase II clinical trial on mRNA electroporated autologous monocyte-derived dendritic cells (TriMixDC-MEL) as adjuvant treatment for stage III/IV melanoma patients who are disease-free following the resection of macrometastases. *Cancer Immunol. Immunother.* 69: 2589–2598. https://doi.org/10.1007/s00262-020-02618-4.

202 BioNTech (2023). Pipeline and Products 2023. https://www.biontech.com/int/en/home/pipeline-and-products/pipeline.html (accessed 11 July 2024).

203 Moderna and Merck Announce mRNA-4157/V940, an Investigational Personalized mRNA Cancer Vaccine, in Combination With KEYTRUDA® (pembrolizumab), Met Primary Efficacy Endpoint in Phase 2b KEYNOTE-942 Trial 2022. https://www.merck.com/news/moderna-and-merck-announce-mrna-4157-v940-an-investigational-personalized-mrna-cancer-vaccine-in-combination-with-keytruda-pembrolizumab-met-primary-efficacy-endpoint-in-phase-2b-keynote-94 (accessed 11 July 2024).

204 Melamed, J.R., Hajj, K.A., Chaudhary, N. et al. (2022). Lipid nanoparticle chemistry determines how nucleoside base modifications alter mRNA delivery. *J. Control. Release* 341: 206–214. https://doi.org/10.1016/j.jconrel.2021.11.022.

205 Lowe D. (2023). Curevac Comes Around. https://www.science.org/content/blog-post/curevac-comes-around (accessed 11 July 2024).

4

Self-Replicating RNA Viruses for Vaccine Development

Kenneth Lundstrom

PanTherapeutics, Route de Lavaux 49, Lutry 1095, Switzerland

4.1 Introduction

Viral vectors have been frequently used for vaccine development targeting both infectious diseases and different cancers [1]. Not surprisingly, self-replicating RNA viruses have been engineered as vectors for the expression of surface antigens from viruses, bacteria, and parasites, tumor-associated antigens (TAAs), and cytotoxic, anti-tumor, and immunostimulatory genes. The special feature of self-replicating RNA viruses, which has made them attractive as therapeutic and vaccine vectors, relates to their efficient self-replication in the cytoplasm of infected cells. It has been estimated that approximately 10^6 copies of subgenomic RNA are accumulated per host cell [2]. The self-amplification provides the means for potentially enhancing the immune responses of delivered RNA and/or application of reduced doses for immunization. Recent mRNA vaccines developed against severe-acute respiratory syndrome-coronavirus-2 (SARS-CoV-2) have demonstrated good vaccine efficacy [3, 4], which suggests that taking advantage of the RNA amplification feature can provide further improvement.

In this review, expression systems for self-replicating RNA viruses are described. Their applications for vaccine development against infectious diseases and cancers are presented through examples from preclinical studies and clinical trials.

4.2 Expression Systems For Self-Replicating RNA Viruses

Self-replicating alphaviruses, flaviviruses, measles viruses (MVs), and rhabdoviruses all possess a single-stranded RNA (ssRNA) genome with an envelope protein structure [5]. However, the genomes of alphaviruses and flaviviruses are of positive polarity, while MVs and rhabdoviruses possess negative-strand RNA genomes. For this reason, the application of positive- and negative-strand RNA viruses as expression systems differs as illustrated in Figure 4.1. More specifically, expression systems for

Trends in mRNA Vaccine Research, First Edition. Edited by Gabor Tamas Szabo and Norbert Pardi.

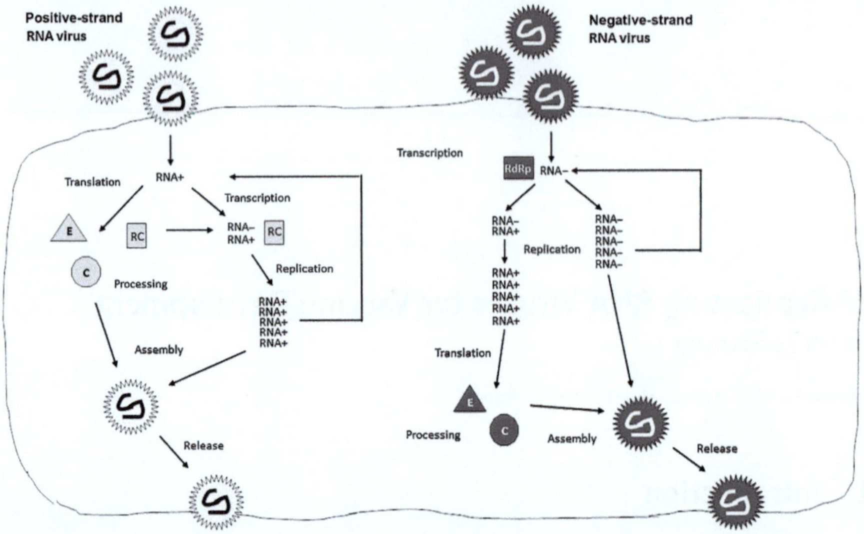

Figure 4.1 Schematic presentation of the lifecycles of positive and negative strand self-replicating RNA viruses. Left: steps involved in replication, translation, processing of structural proteins, assembly, and release of mature viral particles for positive-strand RNA viruses. Right: the corresponding steps for negative strand self-replicating RNA viruses. C, capsid protein; E, envelope protein; RC, replication complex; RdRp, RNA-dependent RNA polymerase.

alphaviruses have mainly been engineered for Semliki Forest virus (SFV) [6], Sindbis virus (SIN) [7], and Venezuelan equine encephalitis virus (VEE) [8]. The basic alphavirus expression vector contains the four nonstructural protein (nsP1-4) genes and the gene of interest (GoI), which is expressed from the 26S subgenomic promoter located at the 3′ end of the nsP4 gene (Figure 4.2a). The helper vector carries the alphavirus structural protein genes, providing the capsid and envelope proteins. *In vitro* transcribed RNA for expression and helper vectors is electroporated or transfected into baby hamster kidney (BHK) cells for the production of recombinant particles. As the RNA packaging signal is located in the nsP2 and nsP1 genes in the SFV and SIN genomes [9], respectively, only RNA from the expression vector will be introduced into nucleocapsids for the production of mature replication-deficient particles. The generated particles are capable of infecting host cells, but the lack of structural protein genes in replication-deficient particles prevents further production of virus progeny. However, due to the efficient self-replication of RNA combined with the strong 26S subgenomic promoter, extreme levels of transient expression of the GoI can be obtained in infected host cells [10].

Replication-proficient expression vectors have been engineered by the introduction of a second subgenomic promoter either upstream or downstream of the structural protein genes for the expression of the GoI (Figure 4.2b). In this case, transfection of *in vitro* transcribed RNA generates new replication-proficient

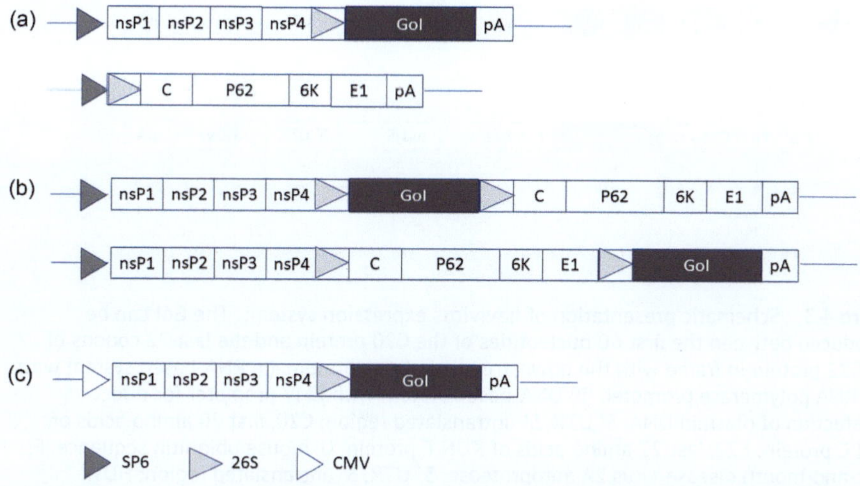

Figure 4.2 Schematic presentation of alphavirus expression systems. (a) Replication deficient system with the gene of interest (GoI) on the expression vector and the viral structural genes on the helper vector. (b) Replication proficient system with the GoI introduced either downstream of the nsP4 gene or the structural protein genes. (c) DNA replicon system with CMV promoter for direct transfection of plasmid DNA. C, capsid protein; E1, envelope protein 1; nsP, nonstructural protein; p62, a precursor for E2 and E3 proteins; pA, polyadenylation signal; SP6, SP6 RNA polymerase promoter; 26S, SFV subgenomic promoter; CMV, cytomegalovirus promoter.

alphavirus particles and expression of the GoI. This approach presents certain advantages for *in vivo* applications, where both extended transgene expression in time and space can be accomplished. In addition to recombinant virus particles, naked or liposome nanoparticle-encapsulated RNA can be used for vaccine development. Alphavirus-based expression can also be applied using plasmid DNA vectors, where the SP6 or T7 RNA polymerase promoter has been replaced by a CMV promoter (Figure 4.2c). In this context, the alphavirus DNA replicon vector containing the GoI is transfected into host cells or delivered *in vivo* applying standard DNA transfection or delivery methods. In contrast to ssRNA delivery, the double-stranded DNA (dsDNA) needs to be transported to the cell nucleus for *in vivo* RNA transcription to occur before self-replication of RNA can take place in the cytoplasm. The drawbacks of using DNA replicon vectors are inferior DNA delivery compared to viral infections and the inefficient step of delivery to the nucleus. On the other hand, the production of plasmid DNA is cheaper and faster than viral production, and no safety concerns related to viral infections need to be addressed [11].

Expression vector systems have also been engineered for different flaviviruses. For example, Kunjin virus (KUN) expression systems have been constructed, where the GoI has been inserted between the first 60 nucleotides of the core protein (C20) and the last 22 codons of the envelope protein (E22) in frame with the downstream KUN polyprotein (Figure 4.3) [12]. However, the expression of the GoI as a fusion to the

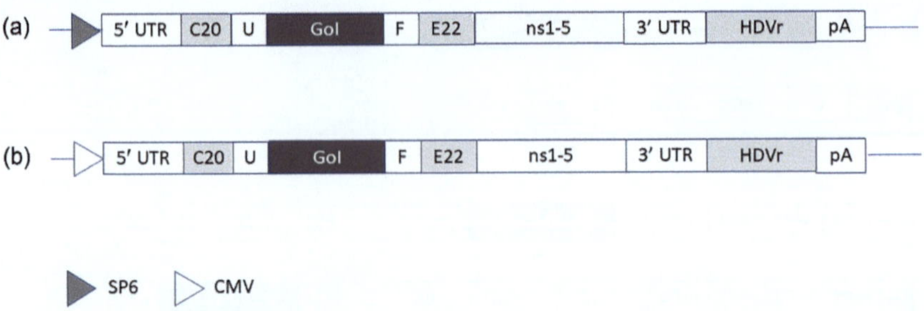

Figure 4.3 Schematic presentation of flavivirus expression systems. The GoI can be introduced between the first 60 nucleotides of the C20 protein and the last 22 codons of the E22 protein in frame with the downstream viral polyprotein. (a) RNA-based system with SP6 RNA polymerase promoter. (b) DNA-based system with CMV promoter for direct transfection of plasmid DNA. 5′ UTR, 5′ untranslated region; C20, first 20 amino acids of KUN C protein; E22, last 22 amino acids of KUN E protein; U, mouse ubiquitin sequence; F, Foot-and-mouth disease virus 2A autoprotease; 3′ UTR, 3′ untranslated region; HDVr, Hepatitis delta virus ribozyme; pA, polyadenylation signal; SP6, SP6 RNA polymerase promoter; CMV, cytomegalovirus promoter.

KUN polyprotein has required the introduction of an FMDV-2A protein sequence into the vector to provide the removal of viral sequences from the recombinant protein [13]. To facilitate the application of KUN vectors, a packaging system has been engineered in the tetKUNCprMEC cell line [14]. Expression systems have also been developed for West Nile virus (WNV) [15], yellow fever virus (YFV) [16], Dengue virus (DENV) [17], and tick-borne encephalitis virus (TBEV) [18].

Despite the more complicated manipulation of negative-strand RNA viruses, both MV- [19] and rhabdovirus-based [20, 21] expression systems have been engineered (Figure 4.4). Packaging systems have been generated for MV by transfection of the full-length MV genome carrying the GoI into HEK293 cells stably expressing MV-N (nucleocapsid), MV-P (phosphoprotein), and T7 polymerase [22]. Alternatively, HEK293 cells expressing the MV-N, MV-P, and the MV genome have been super-infected with vaccinia virus [23]. Also, CMV-based expression of the MV genome and the RNA-dependent RNA polymerase (RdRp) has allowed the rescue of MV particles [24]. The GoI can be inserted either between the phosphoprotein (P) and the matrix protein (M) genes or between the hemagglutinin (HA) and the large protein (L) genes (Figure 4.4) in MV vectors.

Rhabdovirus expression systems are mainly based on rabies virus (RABV) [25], vesicular stomatitis virus (VSV) [21], and to some extent on Maraba virus [26]. For RABV, the GoI can be introduced into the RABV genome between the nucleoprotein (N) and the P protein [25] (Figure 4.4a). Two different approaches have been pursued for VSV vectors. Engineering of VSV pseudoviruses has been achieved by replacing the VSV glycoprotein (G) gene with another envelope protein gene [20] (Figure 4.4b). Alternatively, the GoI can be introduced between the G and L genes [21] (Figure 4.4c). In the case of the Maraba virus, the GoI is also inserted between the G and L genes [26] (Figure 4.4c).

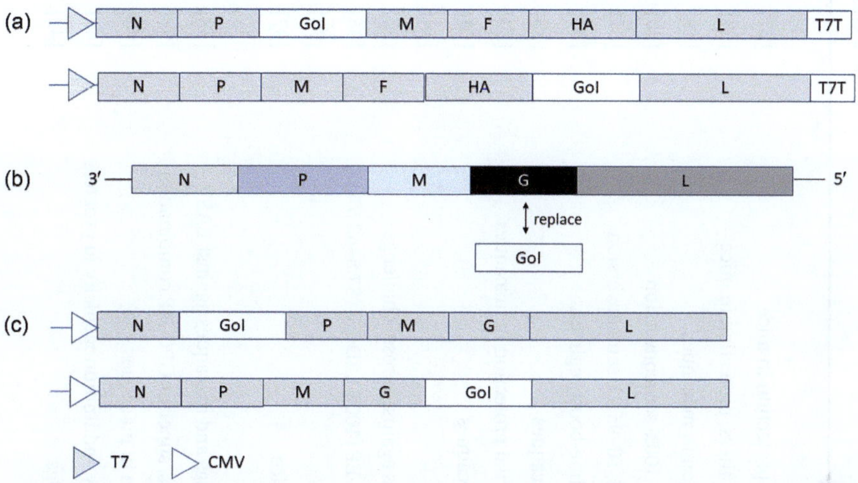

Figure 4.4 Schematic presentation of negative-strand RNA virus expression systems. (a) Measles virus system. The GoI is inserted either between the phosphoprotein (P) and the matrix protein (M) or the hemagglutinin (HA) and the large protein (L). T7, T7 RNA polymerase promoter; T7T, T7 terminator. (b) VSV system. The VSV glycoprotein (G) gene is replaced by the GoI. (c) RABV system. The GoI can be introduced either between the nucleoprotein (N) and the phosphoprotein (P) or the glycoprotein (G) and the large protein (L). CMV, cytomegalovirus promoter.

4.3 Vaccines Against Infectious Diseases

Both positive- and negative-strand self-replicating RNA viruses have been frequently used for vaccine development against infectious diseases. Examples from preclinical studies and clinical trials are described below and summarized in Table 4.1.

Alphaviruses have not only been engineered as expression vector systems but can also cause epidemics. For example, Chikungunya virus (CHIKV) [131, 132] and VEE [133] have been responsible for outbreaks in Africa, Polynesia, and South America. In this context, immunization of mice with a VSV vector, where the VSV G protein envelope was replaced by the CHIKV envelope polyprotein (E3-E3-6K-E1) elicited neutralizing antibodies and protected A129 mice against CHIKV challenges [27]. An attenuated MV strain has been utilized for the expression of the CHIKV capsid and envelope proteins, inducing high CHIKV antibody titers and protection of mice against CHIKV after a single immunization [28]. Moreover, a prime-boost regimen with the MV–CHIKV vaccine candidate was carried out in nine cynomolgus macaques [29]. The immunization was well tolerated, elicited strong neutralizing antibody responses, and protected macaques against viremia after challenges with a CHIKV strain from La Reunion. The MV–CHIKV vaccine candidate has also been subjected to clinical evaluation. In the first-in-man phase I trial, healthy volunteers were immunized with low, medium, or high doses of MV–CHIKV, which showed seroconversion rates of 44%, 92%, and 90%, respectively, after a single immunization and 100% seroconversion for all doses after a second vaccination [30]. In a

Table 4.1 Self-replicating RNA viruses against infectious diseases.

Disease	Expression System	Target	Response	References
Alphaviruses				
CHIKF	VSV–CHIKV Env	E3-E2-6K-E1	Strong nAb responses, protection in mice	[27]
CHIKF	MV–CHIKV Capsid/Env	C-E3-E2-6K-E1	High-CHIKV antibody titers, protection in mice	[28]
CHIKF	MV–CHIKV Capsid/Env	C-E3-E2-6K-E1	Well tolerated, protection in macaques	[29]
CHIKF	MV–CHIKV Capsid/Env	C-E3-E2-6K-E1	Phase I: well tolerated, 100% seroconversion	[30]
CHIKF	MV–CHIKV Capsid/Env	C-E3-E2-6K-E1	Phase II: well tolerated, 50–95.9% seroconversion	[31]
CHIKF	MV–CHIKV Capsid/Env	C-E3-E2-6K-E1	Phase II: prime and prime-boost regimen	[32]
EEE	EEE-E2-E3 furin mutant	E3-E2-6K-E1	Protection in mice, macaques	[33]
WEE	WEE-E2-E3 furin mutant	E3-E2-6K-E1	Protection in mice, partial protection in macaques	[33]
VEE	VEE-E2-E3 furin mutant	E3-E2-6K-E1	Protection in mice, macaques	[33]
VEE	VEE V4020 DNA	VEE-TC-83	Protection in mice	[34]
VEE	VEE V4020 DNA	VEE TC-83	Protection in macaques against aerosol challenge	[35]
VEE	VEE DNA	E3-E2-6K-E1	Phase I: nAbs after IM-EP (100%), ID-EP (87.5–62.5%)	[36]
VEE	VEE-LAV RNA-CNE	VEE ΔTC-83	Protection in mice	[37]
VEE	VEE-IAV RNA-CNE	VEE TC-83 C	Partial protection in mice	[37]
Arenaviruses				
LHF	VSV-LASFV-GPC	GPC	Protection in guinea pigs and macaques against LASV	[38]
LHF	MV-LASV-GPC-NP	GPC, NP	Protection in macaques, superior GPC-NP combination	[39]
LHF	MV-LASV-GPC-NP	GPC, NP	Long-lasting protection in macaques	[40]
LHF	MV-LASV-GPC-NP	GPC, NP	Phase I: study on safety and immunogenicity in progress	[41]
LHF	YFV-LASV-GPC	GPC	Protection in guinea pigs	[42]

LHF	YFV-LASV-GP1/GP2	GP1/GP2	Specific $CD8^+$ T-cell responses, protection in guinea pigs	[43]
LHF	VEE-LASV-GPC/NP	GPC/NP	Protection in guinea pigs against LASV	[44]
LHF	VEE-LASV-GPCwt/ΔGPfib	GPCwt/ΔGPfib	Strong immunogenicity, protection in mice	[45]
AHF	VEE-JUNV/MACV-GPC	GPC	Protection of guinea pigs against JUNV	[46]
BHF	VEE-JUNV/MACV-GPC	GPC	Protection of guinea pigs against MACV	[46]
Filoviruses				
EVD	KUN-EBOV-GP/D637L	GP/D637L	Protection in guinea pigs against EBOV	[47]
EVD	KUN-EBOV-GP/D637L	GP/D637L	Protection in three of four primates against EBOV	[48]
EVD	VSV-EBOV-GP	GP	Complete protection in primates against EBOV	[49]
EVD	ΔVSV-ZEBOV-GP	GP	Protection in BALB/c mice after intraperitoneal injection	[50]
EVD	ΔVSV-ZEBOV-GP	GP	Protection in macaques after intramuscular injection	[16]
EVD	ΔVSV-ZEBOV-GP	GP	Protection in macaques after intramuscular injection	[51]
EVD	ΔVSV-ZEBOV-GP	GP	Protection in mice after intranasal injection	[50]
EVD	ΔVSV-ZEBOV-GP	GP	Protection in macaques after oral injection	[52]
MHF	ΔVSV-MARV-GP	GP	Protection in macaques, also after re-challenge at day 113	[50]
MHF	ΔVSV-MARV-GP	GP	Cross-protection against Ravn and Angola MARV strains	[53]
MHF	VEE-MARV-GP	GP	Protection in macaques against MARV	[54]
EVD	VEE-SUDV-GP	GP	Protection in primates against SUDV	[54]
EVD	VEE-SUDV-GP	GP	Partial protection against EBOV	[54]
EVD	VEE-SUDV-GP/VEE-EBOV-GP	GP	Protection against both SUDV and EBOV	[54]
EVD	VSV-ZEBOV	GP	Phase III: 100% EBOV vaccine efficacy	[55]
EVD	VSV-ZEBOV	GP	Phase III: EBOV vaccine efficacy confirmed	[56]
EVD	VSV-ZEBOV (Ervebo)	GP	Approval by the FDA, EMA for EVD	[57]

(Continued)

Table 4.1 (Continued)

Disease	Expression System	Target	Response	References
Flaviviruses				
DF	LIV-VEE-DENV-E85	E85	T-cell and nAb responses, protection in mice	[58]
DF	VEE-DENV-prME + pDNA	prME	Superior protection in macaques for VEE + pDNA	[59]
DF	MV-DENV-ED3	ED3	Strong immunogenicity, partial protection in mice	[60]
DF	Tetravalent YFV-DENV	prME	Good safety and tolerability in macaques	[61]
DF	Tetravalent YFV-DENV	prME	Phase IIb: good safety and tolerability, 30.2% efficacy	[62]
DF	Tetravalent YFV-DENV	prME	Phase III: good safety, 56.5% efficacy	[63]
DF	Tetravalent YFV-DENV	prME	Phase III: 42.3–77.7% depending on DENV serotype	[64]
ZVD	VEE-ZIKV RNA-NLCs	prME	Protection in mice with 10 ng RNA–NLCs	[65]
ZVD	VSV-ZIKV-prME	prME	Protection in mice against ZIKV	[27]
ZVD	MV-ZIKV-E2	E	Protection in mice against ZIKV	[66]
ZVD	MV-ZIKV-E/MV-ZIKV-NS1	E, NS1	ZIKV clearance from the reproductive tract	[66]
ZVD	MV-ZIKA	E	Phase I: study completed; no results available	[67]
ZVD	MV-ZIKA-RSP	RSP, E	Phase I: study in process	[68]
LIV	SFV-LIV-prME/NS1	LIV-prME/NS1	Partial/complete protection in sheep depending on the route	[69]
LIV	SFV-LIV-prME/NS1 RPs/DNA	LIV-prME/NS1	Superior protection from RPs compared to DNA	[70]
LIV	SFV-LIV-prME RNA	LIV-prME	Protection of 70% of mice	[71]
Hepatotropic Viruses				
HB	MV-HBsAg	HBsAg	Humoral immune responses in mice	[72]
HB	MV-HBsAg	HBsAg	Protective HBsAg antibodies in two out of four primates	[73]
HB	SFV-MHB-VLVs	MHB	T-cell responses, protection in mice	[74]

HB	SFV-HBcAg-VLVs	HBcAg	No T-cell response or protection in mice	[74]
Lentiviruses				
AIDS/HIV	MV-HIV gp160	HIV gp160	Cellular and humoral responses in mice	[75]
AIDS/HIV	VSV-HIV-1 Env	HIV-1 Env	Anti-Env antibody responses in mice	[76]
AIDS/HIV	VSV-HIV-1 Env	HIV-1 Env	Protection in 67% of primates	[77]
AIDS/HIV	VSV-HIV gp160/SIV Gag gp55	HIV-Env/SIV-Gag	Immunogenicity, protection in primates	[78]
AIDS/HIV	VSV-HIV Env gp140	HIV-Env gp140	Env gp140-specific immune responses in mice	[79]
AIDS/HIV	RABV-HIV Env gp160	HIV-Env gp160	Strong immunogenicity after boost with rec gp120	[80]
AIDS/HIV	SFV-HIV-Env	HIV Env	Superior immunogenicity to DNA and Env protein	[81]
AIDS/HIV	SIN-HIV-1 Env	HIV-1 Env	Env-specific humoral immune response in mice	[82]
AIDS/HIV	SFV-HIV Env RNA	HIV Env	Env-specific response in mice, 12H2 mAb production	[83]
AIDS/HIV	SFV-HIV particles/RNA	HIV-Env/Gag/PolRT	Stronger immune response of particles compared to RNA	[84]
AIDS/HIV	VEE-HIV gp160 DNA	HIV Envgp160	10–100-fold less DNA per dose compared to con-DNA	[85]
AIDS/HIV	SFV-HIV Env/Gag-Pol-Nef	HIV Env/GPN	Efficient priming of replicon DNA with MVA boost	[86]
AIDS/HIV	VEE-HIV gp140 RNA-CNE	HIV gp140	Superior to VEE particles and recombinant HIV gp140	[87]
AIDS/HIV	VEE-HIV Gag	HIV Gag	Phase I: vaccine stability problems, early termination	[88]
Influenza Viruses				
IFVA	MV-AIK-C-HA	IFVA HA	Protection in cotton rats against IFVA	[89]
IFVA	VSVΔG-H5N1	HA, NA	Attenuated replication, protection in mice	[90]
IFVA	VSV-HAfl	HAfl (H5N1)	Protection and cross-protection in mice	[91]
IFVA	VEE-HA	HA	HA-specific antibodies, protection in chickens	[92]
IFVA	SFV-HA RNA	HA	Protection in 90% of mice against IFVA	[71]

(Continued)

Table 4.1 (Continued)

Disease	Expression System	Target	Response	References
IFVA	VEE-HA RNA	HA	64-fold less replicon RNA for protection	[93]
IFVA	SFV-HA taRNA	HA	50 ng of taRNA elicited nAbs and protected mice	[94]
IFVA	SIN-E2S1-M2e	M2e	Protection against IFVA challenges in mice	[95]
IFVA	CSFV-HA/NP VRPs/PEI RNA	HA/NP	Superior immunogenicity of VRPs over PEI RNA in pigs	[96]
IFVA	VEE-HA (AVX502)	HA	Phase I/II: immunogenicity in 80–86% of participants	[97]
IFVA	VEE-HA (AVX502)	HA	Phase I/II: immunogenicity in 50% of participants	[98]
Orthopneumoviruses				
RSV	SFV-RSV F RNA	RSV F	32% reduction in RSV titers in mouse lung	[71]
RSV	VEE-RSV F LNP-RNA	RSV F	Superior to RNA or particles in mice	[99]
RSV	VEE-RSV F LNP-RNA	RSV F	Superior to RNA, particles and subunits in cotton rats	[100]
Coronaviruses				
SARS	VEE-SARS-CoV S	SARS-CoV S	Protection against SARS-CoV in mice	[101]
MERS	VSVΔG-MERS-CoV S	MERS-CoV S	Strong nAb and T-cell responses in macaques	[102]
PED	BVDV-PEDV S	PEDV S	BVDV- and PEDV-specific Ab responses in mice	[103]
COVID-19	MV-SARS-CoV-2 S	SARS-CoV-2 S	Th1-biased Ab and T-cell responses in mice	[104]
COVID-19	MV-SARS-CoV-2 S (TMV-083)	SARS-CoV-2 S	Phase I: weak response, early termination of trial	[105]
COVID-19	VSV-SARS-CoV-2 S	SARS-CoV-2 S	Strong immune responses, protection in mice	[106]
COVID-19	VSV-SARS-CoV-2 S (V590)	SARS-CoV-2 S	Phase I: weaker response than in COVID patients	[107]
COVID-19	VSVΔG-SARS-CoV-2 S	SARS-CoV-2 S	Strong nAb responses, protection in hamsters	[108]
COVID-19	VSVΔG-SARS-CoV-2 S	SARS-CoV-2 S	Good safety, robust binding and nAb titers	[109]
COVID-19	VSVΔG-SARS-CoV-2 S (IIBR100)	SARS-CoV-2 S	Phase I/II: study in progress	[110]

COVID-19	VSVΔG-SARS-CoV-2 S (IIBR100)	SARS-CoV-2 S	Phase IIb/III: study initiated	[111]
COVID-19	VEE-SARS-CoV-2 S LNP-RNA	SARS-CoV-2 S	Strong dose-dependent Ab responses in mice	[112]
COVID-19	VEE-SARS-CoV-2 S LNP RNA	SARS-CoV-2 S	Phase I: safe and tolerable, dose-related response	[113]
COVID-19	VEE-repRNA-CoV2S-LION	SARS-CoV-2 S	nAbs and T-cell responses in mice and macaques	[65]
COVID-19	repRNA-COV2S-LION (Gemcov-19)	SARS-CoV-2 S	Phase II/III: safety, tolerability and immunogenicity	[114]
COVID-19	repRNA-COV2S-LION (Gemcov-19)	SARS-CoV-2 S	EUA in India	[115]
COVID-19	VEE LUNAR-COV19 RNA LNP	SARS-CoV-2 S	nAb responses, protection in mice	[116]
COVID-19	LUNAR-COV19 (ARCT-021)	SARS-CoV-2 S	Phase I/II: safety and immunogenicity	[117]
COVID-19	LUNAR-COV19 (ARCT-021)	SARS-CoV-2 S	Phase I/II: ascending vaccine dose	[118]
COVID-19	LUNAR-COV19 (ARCT-021)	SARS-CoV-2 S	Phase II: safety and vaccine efficacy	[119]
COVID-19	LUNAR-COV19 (ARCT-021)	SARS-CoV-2 S	Phase II: safety and long-term immunogenicity	[120]
COVID-19	LUNAR-COV19 (ARCT-021)	SARS-CoV-2 S	Phase III: 95% efficacy against severe COVID-19	[121]
COVID-19	SIN-SARS-CoV-2 S + αOX40	SARS-CoV-2 S	nAb responses, protection in mice	[122]
COVID-19	LNP-saRNA + ChAdOx1 nCoV-19	SARS-CoV-2 S	Superior immunogenicity after heterologous regimen	[123]
COVID-19	VEE-SARS-CoV-2 S-LNPs (oral)	SARS-CoV-2 S	nAbs against SARS-CoV-2 alpha and delta variants	[124]
Bacterial				
Anthrax	SIN-PA	*B. anthracis* PA	Protection in mice with co-administered ciprofloxacin	[125]
Anthrax	SFV-PA VRPs, DNA	*B. anthracis* PA	Superior to conventional DNA, protection in mice	[126]
Brucellosis	SFV-IF3	*B. abortus* IF3	Antibody and T-cell responses, protection in mice	[127]

(Continued)

Table 4.1 (Continued)

Disease	Expression System	Target	Response	References
Parasitic				
Malaria	SFV-Pf332 VRPs, RNA, DNA	*P. falciparum* Pf332	Th1-biased immune responses in mice for VRPs and DNA	[128]
Malaria	SIN-SYVPSAEQI-CS	*P. yoelii* CS epitope	Immunogenicity, protection against malaria in mice	[129]
Leishmaniasis	SFV-PpSP15-LmSTI1 RNA, DANN	PpSP15-LmSTI1	Superior replicon RNA responses compared to DNA	[130]

AHF, Argentine hemorrhagic fever; BHF, Bolivian hemorrhagic fever; BVDV, bovine viral diarrhea virus; con-DNA, conventional plasmid DNA; CHIKF, Chikungunya fever; CHIKV, Chikungunya virus; CNE, cationic nanoemulsion; CS, circumsporozoite; DENV, Dengue virus; DF, Dengue fever; EBOV, Ebola virus; ED3, DENV envelope protein domain III; EUA, Emergency Use Authorization; EVD, Ebola virus disease; GPC. Glycoprotein; GPN, Gag-Pol-Nef; HB, Hepatitis B; HBcAg, Hepatitis B core antigen; HBsAg, Hepatitis B surface antigen; IAV, irreversibly attenuated VEE; ID-EP, intradermal administration + electroporation; IFVA, influenza virus A; IM-EP. Intramuscular injection + electroporation; JUNV, Junín virus; LASV, Lassa virus; LAV, live-attenuated VEE; LHF, Lassa hemorrhagic fever; LION, lipid inorganic nanoparticles; LIV, louping ill virus; LNPs, lipid nanoparticles; M2e, the 23-amino acid external domain of IFVA M protein; mAb, monoclonal antibody; MACV, Machupo virus; MARV, Marburg virus; MHB, HBV middle surface envelope glycoprotein; MHF, Marburg hemorrhagic fever; MV, measles virus; MVA, Modified Vaccinia Ankara virus; nAbs, neutralizing antibodies; NP, nucleoprotein; pDNA, plasmid DNA; PED, porcine epidemic diarrhea; PEDV, porcine epidemic diarrhea virus; prME, premembrane-envelope protein of DENV; RSV, respiratory syncytial virus; saRNA, self-amplifying RNA; SFV. Semliki Forest virus; SIN, Sindbis virus; taRNA, trans-amplifying RNA; VEE, Venezuelan equine encephalitis virus; VLVs, virus-like vesicles; VRPs, viral replicon particles; YFV, yellow fever virus; ZIKV, Zika virus; Z-ME. ZIKV membrane-envelope polyprotein; ZVD, Zika virus disease.

phase II study, doses of 5×10^4 $TCID_{50}$ and 5×10^5 $TCID_{50}$ of MV–CHIKV were intramuscularly administered to healthy volunteers [31]. No serious adverse events were demonstrated, strong neutralizing antibody responses were obtained, and the seroconversion rates were 50% for the lower dose and 95.9% for the higher dose. Moreover, in a phase II trial, participants received the MV–CHIKV vaccine candidate either as a prime or prime-boost regimen [32]. Although both strategies elicited robust immune responses, the prime-boost immunization resulted in significantly stronger immune responses. However, in the prime-boost approach, the antibodies decreased rapidly over time and at six months both vaccine strategies displayed similar antibody profiles. These findings suggested that the prime-boost immunization was more appropriate for CHIKV-endemic regions, whereas the prime approach should be sufficient for the vaccination of travelers.

Among alphaviruses, VEE, western equine encephalitis (WEE) virus, and eastern equine encephalitis (EEE) virus vectors have been engineered, where the Furin cleavage site between the corresponding E2 and E3 envelope proteins has been removed [33]. Mice immunized with the combination of VEE, WEE, and EEV or individually with each type of alphavirus vector elicited strong neutralizing antibody responses and provided protection against challenges with lethal viruses [33]. However, although strong antibody responses and protection were obtained after immunizations with the three alphavirus vectors and individual immunizations with VEE and EEE particles in primates, immunization with WEE particles resulted only in partial protection in macaques [33]. VEE DNA replicon vectors have been engineered based on the attenuated TC-83 strain by expressing the VEE capsid gene from a second subgenomic promoter inserted downstream of the envelope genes [34]. The vaccine candidate, named V4020, showed no adverse effects, elicited strong neutralizing antibodies, and protected mice from VEE challenges after a single immunization [34]. Intramuscular administration of V4020 in cynomolgus macaques elicited robust immune responses and provided protection against aerosol challenges with VEE [35]. VEE DNA replicons expressing the E3-E2-6K-E1 polyprotein have been subjected to a phase I clinical trial [36]. VEE DNA replicons were administered by intramuscular (IM-EP) (0.5 or 2.0 mg) or intradermal (ID-EP) (0.08 or 0.3 mg) electroporation. No vaccine- or device-related serious adverse events were recorded, and neutralizing antibody responses were induced for both low and high doses of IM-EP administration in all participants. In contrast, seven out of eight individuals receiving the high ID-EP dose elicited neutralizing antibodies, whereas after low-dose administration neutralizing antibody responses were detected in five out of eight participants. VEE RNA replicon vectors have also been subjected to vaccine formulation of live-attenuated VEE particles (VEE-LAV) and irreversibly attenuated VEE particles (VEE-IAV) with synthetic cationic nanoemulsion (CNE) [37]. The replication-proficient VEE-LAV carries the full-length VEE TC-83 genome, while the deletion of the capsid gene in VEE-IAV renders it replication-deficient. Immunization of mice with LAV-CNE RNA replicons elicited strong immune responses and provided 100% protection against VEE challenges. Although IAV-CNE RNA replicons induced immune responses, only partial protection was achieved in mice.

Among arenaviruses, VSV particles expressing the Lassa virus (LASV) glycoprotein (GPC) provided complete protection against challenges with LASV isolates from Liberia, Mali, and Nigeria in immunized guinea pigs and macaques [38]. Furthermore, a single immunization of macaques with MV–LASV–GPC elicited robust secondary T-cell and antibody responses and protected against challenges with LASV [39]. However, the MV vector co-expressing LASV–GPC and LASV nucleoprotein (NP) was superior in comparison to the administration of MV–LASV–GPC alone. The acquired immune response was long-lasting, as demonstrated by the protection of primates against LASV challenges one year after the immunization [40]. In the context of clinical evaluation, two doses of the MV–LASV vaccine candidate V182-001 are administered to healthy volunteers in a phase I trial [41]. The safety, tolerability, and immunogenicity are validated in the study currently in progress. The LASV–GPC gene has also been introduced into a replication-competent YFV flavivirus vector between the envelope (E) and nonstructural protein 1 (NS1) genes [42]. Immunization of guinea pigs with YFV–LASV–GPC elicited LASV-specific antibodies and provided protection against LASV challenges despite poor replication of the virus. Engineering of shorter LASV–GPC inserts consisting of the GP1 and GP2 subunits enhanced the stability of recombinant YFV, induced specific $CD8^+$ T-cell responses in mice, and protected guinea pigs against LASV challenges [43]. However, although rodents were efficiently protected by YFV–LASV–GPC immunizations, this was not the case for marmosets illustrating the challenge of reproducibility of vaccination efficacy in larger animals [134]. Immunization of guinea pigs with an attenuated VEE strain expressing either the LASV–GPC or NP resulted in protection against LASV challenges [44]. Moreover, a bicistronic VEE vector simultaneously expressing the wild-type GPC (VEE–LASV–GPCwt and a modified noncleavable version with a C-terminal deletion (ΔGPfib) from two subgenomic 26S promoters was engineered [45]. Immunization of mice with biscistronic VEE particles expressing both GPCwt and ΔGPfib resulted in the accumulation of ΔGPfib trimers in the endoplasmic reticulum (ER), induction of apoptosis, and promotion of antigen cross-priming. Robust immune responses and protection against LASV were obtained in immunized mice. Replication-restricted VEE particles have also been applied for vaccine development against Junín virus (JUNV) and Machupo virus (MACV) by co-expression of JUNV and MACV GPCs from a bicistronic vector [46]. Robust humoral immune responses were induced after immunization of guinea pigs with VEE–JUNV/MACV–GPC particles, which also protected against challenges with both JUNV and MACV.

Ebola virus (EBOV) is the most prominent filovirus, which has been the target for vaccine development because of several serious outbreaks in Africa [135]. For example, the D637L mutant EBOV glycoprotein (GP) was expressed from a KUN vector showing superior cleavability and shedding compared to the wild-type EBOV GP [47]. Immunization of guinea pigs with KUN–EBOV–GP/D637L generated dose-dependent protection against EBOV challenges. Two subcutaneous injections of KUN–EBOV–GP/D637L protected three out of four nonhuman primates against EBOV challenges [48]. VSV vectors have been frequently used for targeting Ebola virus disease (EVD). For example, complete protection against the

EBOV–Makona strain was achieved in macaques immunized with VSV–EBOV–GP particles seven days prior to the challenge [49]. In contrast, if the immunization took place only three days prior to the challenge, only partial protection could be established. In another approach, the VSV G protein was replaced by the GP from the EBOV Zaire strain (ZEBOV), the Sudan virus (SUDV) strain (SEBOV), and the Marburg virus (MARV), respectively [136]. Immunization of BALB/c mice with a single intraperitoneal injection of ΔVSV–ZEBOV GP resulted in complete protection [50]. Similarly, intramuscular immunization of cynomolgus macaques elicited strong humoral and cellular immune responses and provided protection against ZEBOV challenges [16]. In contrast, no cross-protection was detected in ΔVSV–ZEBOV GP-immunized macaques challenged with SEBOV, resulting in fatal disease [16]. Moreover, a single intramuscular administration of ΔVSV–ZEBOV GP protected macaques against aerosol challenges with ZEBOV [51]. Furthermore, either intranasal or oral administration of ΔVSV–ZEBOV GP generated complete protection against ZEBOV challenges in BALB/c mice and macaques [50, 52]. In the context of MARV, a single immunization of macaques with ΔVSV–MARV GP resulted in complete protection against MARV challenges [16]. Moreover, immunized macaques showed protection when rechallenged after 113 days with a MARV strain [16]. Cross-protection was also achieved for the most disparate Ravn MARV strain and the most virulent Angola MARV strain [53]. Immunization of macaques with VEE particles expressing MARV–GP showed protection against MARV challenges [54]. Intramuscular administration of VEE–SUDV–GP particles protected cynomolgus macaques against challenges with SUDV [54]. In addition, it was demonstrated that macaques immunized with VEE–SUDV–GP could provide partial protection against challenges with EBOV [54]. However, co-immunization with VEE–SUDV–GP and VEE–EBOV–GP protected macaques against both SUDV and EBOV challenges [54].

VSV–ZEBOV particles have been subjected to several clinical trials. In a phase III trial, 4123 individuals were immediately vaccinated, and 3528 participants received a delayed vaccination after 21 days in Guinea, west Africa [55]. Interim results revealed 43 cases of serious adverse events, of which only one case could be causally associated with the vaccination. Among the immediately vaccinated participants, no cases of EDV were detected, and among those receiving delayed vaccination only 16 cases were recorded [55] confirming the 100% vaccine efficacy. In another phase III study in Guinea and Sierra Leone, no cases of EVD were detected in either immediately vaccinated individuals or in those where the vaccination was delayed by 21 days [56]. Among the 80 cases of serious adverse events, one febrile reaction and one case of anaphylaxis were suggested to be associated with the vaccination. The encouraging results from the clinical evaluation resulted in the approval of the VSV–ZEBOV vaccine by the FDA and the EMA [57]. Moreover, a systematic data review on phases I–III trials comprising 17 600 adults and 234 children confirmed a good risk–benefit balance in adults, children, pregnant and lactating women, and patients with HIV [137].

The recent DENV [138] and Zika virus (ZIKV) [139] outbreaks have triggered vaccine development against flaviviruses. For example, VEE vectors have been utilized for the expression of the ectodomain (E85) of the DENV envelope protein [58]. Immunization of mice with VEE-DENV-E85 elicited neutralizing antibody and T-cell responses and resulted in protective immunity. In an immunization study in macaques, VEE particles expressing the DENV type 1 pre-membrane and envelope proteins (prME) were compared to plasmid DNA-based delivery of prME [59]. The immunization strategy comprised three doses of VEE-prME (VVV), three doses of conventional plasmid DNA-prME (DDD), or two doses of plasmid DNA-prME followed by a third dose of VEE-prME (DDV). The results demonstrated superior DENV-specific IgG antibody responses and complete protection against DENV challenges for the DDV regimen. In contrast, both the DDD and VVV strategies reduced the viremia only partially. Immunization of mice with MV particles expressing the DENV envelope protein domain III (ED3) elicited strong immune responses and showed partial protection against DENV challenges [60]. Moreover, the tetravalent vaccine based on the chimeric live-attenuated YFV–DENV vector expressing four DENV prME serotypes [140] showed good tolerance and no cytotoxicity when administered to cynomolgus macaques [61]. In the context of clinical evaluation, the YFV–DENV showed no safety issues, was well tolerated, and reached a 30.2% vaccine efficacy in a phase IIb clinical study in Thailand [62]. In a large Southeast Asian phase III study, a good safety profile was seen, and a 56.5% vaccine efficacy was achieved [63]. Moreover, a good safety profile was established, and 42.3–77.7% vaccine efficacy was obtained in a phase III trial in 20 869 children in Latin America [64]. The variation in vaccine efficacy depended on the DENV serotype. In any case, a vaccine efficacy of 80.3% against hospitalization due to Dengue fever (DF) was obtained. Self-replicating RNA virus vectors have also been applied for vaccine development against ZIKV. For example, VEE RNA replicons have been introduced into nanocarrier lipids (NLCs) for the expression of ZIKV prME [65]. Immunization of C57BL/6 mice provided complete protection against ZIKV challenges after a single administration of 10 ng VEE-ZIKV prME RNA–NLCs [65]. Moreover, immunization of mice with VSV–ZIKV prME particles induced strong ZIKV-specific immune responses and provided protection against ZIKV challenges [27]. Also, mice were immunized with MV vectors expressing the ZIKV E gene (MV-E2), which resulted in protection against challenges with the nonlethal ZIKV Asian strain PRVABC59 and the lethal African strain MR766 [66]. Although immunized mice showed 100% protection against ZIKV, the virus remained in the brain and the reproductive tract. However, co-immunization with MV–ZIKV-NS1 contributed to viral clearance and provided fetal protection [66]. In the context of clinical evaluation, a phase I study in healthy volunteers was conducted with the MV–ZIKA (V186-001) vaccine candidate to verify safety, immunogenicity, and tolerability [67]. The study has been conducted, but no results have been published so far. Another phase I trial applying the MV–ZIKA–RSP (V187-001) vaccine has been conducted in healthy adult volunteers [68]. In the case of looping ill virus (LIV), sheep were immunized intramuscularly with SFV particles expressing the LIV prME and NS1 proteins [69]. Partial protection of sheep was established after intranasal LIV challenges, and complete protection was achieved when the challenge was through the subcutaneous route. Moreover, the SFV–LIV–prME/NS1 vaccine candidate was administered as recombinant particles or DNA replicons and compared with a commercial chemically inactivated whole particle vaccine [70]. All three evaluated vaccines elicited humoral immune responses but showed various levels of protection against challenges with LIV. Only for the recombinant SFV particle vaccine full protection against LIV could be established. Both the SFV DNA replicon and whole particle vaccines managed to provide only partial protection. In another approach, 10 μg of SFV–LIV–prME RNA was injected intramuscularly into BALB/c mice, which elicited significant LIV-specific antibody titers and provided protection in 70% of immunized animals [71].

Although Engerix and Recombivax HB have been approved as vaccines against hepatitis B virus (HBV) [72], activities related to self-replicating RNA virus vectors have been conducted. For example, MV vectors have provided expression of the hepatitis B surface antigen (HBsAg), eliciting humoral immune responses in mice [73]. Moreover, immunization of rhesus macaques induced protective levels of HBsAg antibodies in two out of four animals [73]. In another approach, SFV replicon RNA molecules containing the HBV middle surface envelope glycoprotein (MHB) and the HBV core antigen (HBcAg) were encapsulated by the VSV-G protein resulting in virus-like vesicles (VLVs), which were used for immunization of mice [74]. A single intramuscular administration of C57BL/6 mice with VLV–MHB elicited functional $CD8^+$ T-cell responses and protected mice against challenges with HBV. In contrast, neither immune responses nor protection against HBV was achieved for immunization with VLV–HBcAg.

The AIDS/HIV pandemic has naturally accelerated the interest in vaccine development. For instance, strong cellular and humoral responses were obtained in mice immunized with a live-attenuated MV vector expressing the HIV gp160 envelope protein [75]. VSV vectors have been engineered for optimized immunogenicity of the HIV envelope glycoprotein (Env) [141]. For example, one strategy has involved the selection of Env for optimized antibody engineering, antibody-dependent cell-mediated cytotoxicity (ADCC), and broad neutralization/inhibition of most HIV-1 strains [142, 143]. In the context of VSV, immunization of mice with pseudotyped VSV particles carrying the HIV-1 Env protein induced anti-Env binding antibodies and cell-mediated immune responses [76]. Furthermore, immunization of nonhuman primates with VSV-HIV-1 Env provided protection against HIV-1 challenges in 67% of animals [77]. Co-immunization of rhesus macaques with VSV vectors expressing the HIV Env gp160 and simian immunodeficiency virus (SIV) Gag p55 proteins induced strong immune responses and provided protection against HIV challenges and AIDS [78]. Moreover, mice immunized with three HIV-Env-based vaccine candidates (rVSV-B6-NL4.3Env/SIVtm, rVSV-B6-NL4.3Env/Ebtm, and rVSV-B6-A74Env (PN6)/SIVtm) elicited HIV gp140-specific immune responses in immunized mice [79]. In another approach, prime immunization with RABV particles expressing the HIV-1 Env gp160 protein followed by boost vaccination with recombinant gp120 protein induced HIV-1 neutralizing antibodies in mice [80]. In the case of alphaviruses, SFV particles expressing HIV Env protein showed superior antibody responses in immunized mice compared to a plasmid DNA vaccine and a recombinant Env protein-based vaccine [81]. SIN-HIV-1 Env particles elicited

Env-specific humoral immune responses in mice, which were superior compared to immunization with recombinant Env protein [82]. Moreover, intramuscular administration of SFV–HIV Env replicon RNA induced Env-specific immune responses in four out of five immunized mice [83]. It was also possible to quickly generate the 12H2 monoclonal antibody (mAb) against the gp41 protein [83]. In another study, SFV particles and replicon RNA containing the Indian HIV-1C Env-Gag-PolRT genes were administered to BALB/c mice resulting in significant HIV-specific immune responses for both individual and prime-boost immunization strategies [84]. In this case, the immune responses were stronger for immunization with SFV particles in comparison to replicon RNA. Alphavirus DNA replicons have also been utilized for HIV gp160 expression [85]. Immunization of mice with VEE–HIV gp160 DNA replicons generated a significantly stronger humoral immune response compared to conventional plasmid DNA vaccines [85]. Moreover, 10–100-fold lower doses of DNA replicons induced the same immune responses as seen for immunization with conventional plasmid DNA. Encouraging results have also been obtained from prime-boost vaccinations with VEE particles and VEE DNA replicons [85]. Moreover, the SFV–HIV Env and SFV-HIV Gag-Pol-Nef DNA replicon vectors have been used in a heterologous prime-boost regimen together with the Modified Vaccinia Ankara (MVA) virus expressing HIV-Env and HIV-Gag-Pol-Nef, showing robust immune responses in BALB/c mice [86]. Efficient priming with SFV DNA replicons was achieved with only 0.2 μg of DNA. In the context of VEE-based RNA delivery, stronger immune responses were observed for CNE formulations of VEE-HIV-1 gp140 RNA compared to immunization of rhesus macaques with VEE particles or recombinant HIV gp140 protein combined with the MF59 adjuvant [87]. In clinical settings, the vaccine candidate AVX101 based on replication-deficient VEE–HIV Gag particles was subjected to safety and immunogenicity evaluation in a phase I trial in the United States and South Africa [88]. Disappointingly the study was terminated early due to instability issues of the vaccine candidate.

The seasonal influenza virus outbreaks have made vaccine development an important part of prophylactic treatment. For instance, immunization of cotton rats with MV particles expressing the HA gene from the influenza virus A/Sapporo/107/2013 (H1N1pdm) strain elicited strong immune responses and protected against challenges with lethal doses of influenza virus A (IFVA) [89]. Moreover, pseudotyped VSV particles expressing the HA gene from the highly pathogenic avian influenza virus (HPAIV) A/Vietnam/1203/04 (VN1203) strain and the neuraminidase (NA) gene from the mouse-adapted H1N1 influenza virus A/Puerto Rico/8/34 (PR8) were intramuscularly or intranasally administered to mice, which profoundly attenuated *in vivo* replication and protected animals against challenges with the H5N1 virus [90]. In another approach, a pan-influenza vaccine has been engineered based on a VSV-H5N1 vector [91]. Immunization with a single dose of VSV particles expressing the full-length HA (HAfl) showed 100% protection in mice against the homologous H5 clade 1 virus. Similarly, cross-protective H5-specific antibodies were elicited, and mice were protected against challenges with various H5 clade 2 viruses [91]. Immunization of chicken with VEE particles expressing the HA gene from the Hong Kong Influenza A isolate (A/HK/156/97) elicited HA-specific antibody responses and provided protection against IFVA challenges [92]. RNA-based immunization of BALB/c mice with 10 μg of SFV-HA RNA replicons generated 90% protection against IFVA challenges [71]. It has also been demonstrated that substantially less replicon RNA is needed for successful immunization compared to conventional synthetic mRNA, where only 1.25 μg of VEE-HA RNA was sufficient to protect mice against influenza virus challenges compared to 80 μg of synthetic mRNA [93]. In another approach, an SFV-based bipartite trans-amplifying RNA (taRNA) system has been established, where the GoI is introduced as a trans-replicon from an SFV RNA vector with the nsP1-4 genes deleted [94]. The replicase activity can be provided by either a standard self-replicating RNA vector or an engineered optimized nonreplicating (nrRNA) vector. Application of the nrRNA vector demonstrated 10–100-fold higher transgene expression, probably due to higher transfection efficacy and lack of interference with cellular translation [94]. Immunization of mice with only 50 ng of SFV-HA taRNA elicited neutralizing antibodies and provided protection against IFVA challenges [94]. Chimeric SIN–IFVA particles have been engineered, where a 23-residue external domain of the IFVA M2 protein (M2e) was introduced at the N-terminal of the SIN E2 protein [95]. Mice immunized intranasally with SIN-E2S1-M2e particles were protected against IFVA challenges [95]. The flavivirus Classic Swine Fever virus (CSFV) has been engineered as a vaccine vector [96]. Pigs have been immunized with CSFV particles and polyethyleneimine (PEI)-CSFV RNA replicon complexes expressing the IFVA NP and HA genes. Immunization with CSFV-HA/NP particles elicited superior HA- and NP-specific humoral immune responses compared to immunization with CSFV-HA/NP PEI-RNA [96]. However, the latter still induced strong immune responses, while naked CSFV-HA/NP RNA elicited only weak immunogenicity. VEE-HA particles (AVX502) have been evaluated in two phase I/II clinical trials [144]. In one study in vaccinated 18–40-year-old healthy volunteers, one and two doses of AVX502 elicited robust antibody titers in 80% and 86% of vaccinees, respectively [97]. Moreover, T-cell immune responses remained high for more than four months. In the other trial, conducted in 65-year-old or older volunteers, the AVX502 vaccine candidate demonstrated relatively poor immunogenicity, showing a fourfold increase in 50% of the participants after two vaccinations [98].

In the case of Orthopneumoviruses, expression of the fusion envelope of the respiratory syncytial virus (RSV F) from SFV RNA replicons reduced RSV lung titers by 32% in immunized mice [71]. Moreover, VEE-RSV F RNA replicons encapsulated in lipid nanoparticles (LNPs) significantly enhanced the RSV F-specific immunogenicity [99]. A comparison of naked RNA and VEE–RSV F LNP-RNA showed that a 10-fold reduction in the dose to 0.1 μg of the encapsulated RNA was significantly more immunogenic and equivalent to the administration of 1×10^6 IU of VEE–RSV F particles [99]. Moreover, a single dose of 0.01 μg of VEE–RSV F LNP–RNA was sufficient to establish seroconversion in mice compared to the need for two immunizations of 1 μg of naked RNA. A comparative study of naked VEE–RSV F RNA, VEE–RSV F LNP–RNA, recombinant VEE–RSV F particles, and an RSV F subunit vaccine was carried out in cotton rats [100]. All tested vaccine candidates protected cotton rats against RSV challenges. However, the VEE–RSV F LNP–RNA induced approximately eightfold higher F-specific IgG titers and 10-fold higher neutralizing antibody titers than naked VEE–RSV F RNA [100].

Although vaccine development has been conducted for years, the recent COVID-19 pandemic certainly accelerated the efforts in the field. Encouragingly, Emergency Use Approval (EUA) for both RNA- and adenovirus-based vaccines [145], and the FDA approval of the BNT162b2 and mRNA-1273 vaccines [3] represent important milestones. Self-replicating RNA viruses have also been used for vaccine development against coronaviruses [146]. Related to the SARS epidemic, VEE particles expressing the SARS-CoV Spike (S) protein showed protection against SARS-CoV challenges in immunized mice [101]. Likewise, immunization of rhesus macaques with chimeric VSVΔG particles, where the VSV G protein was replaced by the Middle East respiratory syndrome (MERS)-CoV S protein elicited strong neutralizing antibody and T cell responses [102]. In another approach, a fragment of the spike antigen of the porcine epidemic diarrhea virus (PEDV) was introduced into the flavivirus bovine viral diarrhea virus (BVDV) vector [103]. Immunization of BALB/c mice with chimeric BVDV-PEDV S particles induced BVDV- and PEDV-specific antibody responses.

In the context of COVID-19, different self-replicating RNA virus vectors have been utilized for vaccine development, most commonly targeting the SARS-CoV-2 S protein. For example, immunization of mice with MV particles expressing SARS-CoV-2 S elicited strong Th1-biased antibody and T-cell responses [104]. A phase I clinical trial has also been conducted with the MV-SARS-CoV-2 S vaccine candidate TMV-083 [105]. Disappointingly, the weak immune response seen in the interim assessment of vaccinated volunteers led to an early termination of the study. Using a VSV-based approach, immunization of mice with replication-competent VSV-SARS-CoV-2 particles induced strong antibody responses and provided protection against SARS-CoV-2 challenges [106]. The VSV-SARS-CoV-2 S vaccine candidate (V590) was administered to healthy volunteers in a phase I study showing good safety and tolerability profiles [107]. However, the trial was prematurely terminated because the immune responses were weaker than those recorded in recovered COVID-19 patients [107]. Furthermore, a single immunization of Syrian golden hamsters with replication-competent VSVΔG particles expressing the SARS-CoV-2 S protein elicited strong neutralizing antibodies and protected hamsters against challenges with SARS-CoV-2 [108]. Moreover, New Zealand white rabbits were intramuscularly immunized with VSVΔG-SARS-CoV-2 S particles for the evaluation of toxicity, local tolerance, biodistribution, and immunogenicity [109]. The immunization caused only minimal myofiber necrosis at the injection site and enhanced lymphocytic cellularity in lymph nodes and in the spleen. The binding and neutralizing antibody titers were significantly increased. In summary, the safety and immunogenicity of the vaccine candidate supported the clinical evaluation. In a phase I/II clinical trial, VSVΔG-SARS-CoV-2 S particles (IIBR-100) are administered to 18–55-year-old volunteers at an escalating single dose in the phase I part and as either one or two injections in elderly individuals in the phase II part [110]. In addition, a phase IIb/III trial for IIBR-100 to demonstrate noninferiority to approved COVID-19 vaccines has been initiated [111].

In the context of RNA-based delivery, VEE RNA replicons expressing the prefusion-stabilized SARS-CoV-2 S gene were encapsulated in LNPs showing strong dose-dependent specific antibody responses in immunized BALB/c mice, which were superior to those seen in convalescent COVID-19 patients [112]. The first-in-human phase I trial comprised two intramuscular injections at six doses from 0.1 to 10 μg of LNP-nCoV saRNA (VEE-SARS-CoV-2 S) in healthy 18–45-year-old volunteers [113]. Safe and well-tolerated administration caused no serious adverse events. Neutralization of SARS-CoV-2 was seen in 15–48% of vaccinated individuals depending on the dose applied. Despite achieving immune responses with low vaccine doses, it is desired to optimize humoral responses for improved vaccine efficacy.

The repRNA-CoV2S vaccine candidate comprising lipid inorganic nanoparticle (LION)-encapsulated VEE RNA replicons expressing the SARS-CoV-2 S protein elicited strong Th1-biased immune responses in mice after a single immunization [65]. Moreover, modest T-cell and robust antibody responses were detected in pigtail macaques after a single or prime-boost administration of repRNA-CoV2S-LION [65]. The immunogenicity persisted for at least 70 days and SARS-CoV-2 neutralizing antibody titers were similar to those found in convalescent COVID-19 patients. The repRNA-CoV2S-LION vaccine candidate (Gemcovac-19) has been subjected to a randomized phase II clinical trial followed by a phase III study for the evaluation of safety, tolerability, and immunogenicity [114]. Furthermore, it has been granted EUA in India [115]. The RNA (STARR)-based LUNAR-COV19 vaccine comprises the encapsulation of VEE RNA replicons expressing the full-length SARS-CoV-2 gene in LNPs [116]. A single dose of only 2 μg of the LUNAR-COV19 vaccine elicited strong neutralizing antibody responses and protected transgenic humanized ACE2 mice against SARS-CoV-2 challenges. The LUNAR-COV19 vaccine candidate (ARCT-021) has been subjected to several phase I and phase II clinical trials [117–120]. Recently, interim results from phase III studies in Vietnam showed 95% vaccine efficacy for protection against severe COVID-19 and 55% overall protection against symptomatic disease, where both delta and omicron variants were dominant [121]. In addition to VEE, SIN particles expressing SARS-CoV-2 in combination with the OX40 immunostimulatory antibody (αOX40) elicited long-lasting neutralizing antibody and T-cell responses and provided protection against SARS-CoV-2 challenges in immunized mice [122].

The vaccine efficacy and granting of EUA for COVID-19 vaccines has triggered the evaluation of the so-called "mix-and-match" approach, including heterologous vaccine strategies for the adenovirus-based ChAdOx1 nCoV-19 vaccine and the LNP-nCoVsaRNA vaccine candidate [123]. It was demonstrated that a two-dose heterologous immunization regimen elicited stronger antibody responses than single immunizations. In addition, heterologous administration induced similar or higher neutralizing antibody titers in comparison to prime-boost vaccination with ChAdOx1 nCoV-19 alone. Oral delivery of VEE-SARS-CoV-2 S RNA replicons encapsulated in LNPs elicited high quantities of specific IgG and IgA antibodies in

BALB/c mice [124]. Th1/Th2-biased immune responses were obtained. Moreover, neutralization of both SARS-CoV-2 alpha and delta variants was achieved.

Bacteria and parasites have also been targets for vaccine development using self-replicating RNA viruses. For example, expression of the *Bacillus anthracis* protective antigen from SIN particles elicited PA-specific IgG and neutralizing antibody responses in immunized Swiss Webster mice, and synergized protection was achieved with ciprofloxacin [125]. In another approach, the *B. anthracis* PA was expressed from either SFV particles or SFV DNA replicons in comparison to conventional plasmid DNA [126]. Mice immunized with SFV particles or SFV DNA replicons induced stronger PA-specific immune responses than conventional plasmid DNA and provided protection against challenges with the *B. anthracis* A16R strain with low vaccine doses. Moreover, SFV particles expressing the *Brucella abortus* translation initiation factor 3 (IF3) have been subjected to immunization of BALB/c mice [127]. The vaccination elicited IF3-specific IgM antibody and T-cell proliferative responses and protected mice against challenges with *B. abortus*.

Among parasites, SFV particles and SFV RNA and DNA replicons expressing the *Plasmodium falciparum* Pf332 antigen were compared to conventional plasmid DNA immunizations in BALB/c mice [128]. Both plasmid DNA-based immunizations and SFV RNA and particles elicited relatively weak immune responses. However, the SFV vaccinations generated Th1-biased responses, while the conventional DNA immunization resulted in Th2-biased responses [128]. It was also suggested that due to the induction of immunological memory, booster immunizations with the corresponding protein could provide efficient activation of immunogenicity. In the context of malaria, the *Plasmodium yoelii* circumsporozoite (CS) protein class I major histocompatibility complex-restricted-9-mer epitope SYVPSAEQI was expressed from SIN particles (SIN-MAL) [129]. Subcutaneous immunization of BALB/c mice with SIN-MAL particles induced robust epitope-specific $CD8^+$ T-cell responses and protected immunized mice against malaria. Leishmaniasis has been evaluated for vaccine development by expression of the fusion of *Plebotomus papatasi* SP15 (PpSP15) and the *Leishmania major* stress-inducible protein 1 (LmSTI1) from an SFV vector [130]. The expression of PpSP15-LmSTI1 in mammalian cell lines was significantly higher when SFV RNA replicons were utilized compared to SFV DNA replicons or conventional plasmid DNA transfection [130], which needs to be confirmed in suitable animal models.

4.4 Vaccines Against Cancers

In addition to infectious diseases, self-replicating RNA virus vectors have also been used for vaccine development against various cancers. Not only the overexpression of TAAs but also the delivery of cytotoxic, anti-tumor, and immunostimulatory genes have been utilized for cancer therapy and cancer immunotherapy [147]. As self-replicating RNA viruses, particularly alphaviruses, have been demonstrated to induce apoptosis in host cells. Cell killing by plain viral vectors carrying no therapeutic gene has been confirmed and illustrated by the expression of reporter genes. In addition, oncolytic viruses characterized by replication in and killing of tumor cells have been efficiently used for cancer virotherapy [148]. Examples of utilization of self-replicating RNA virus vectors for different types of cancers using reporter genes, TAAs, cytotoxic and anti-tumor genes, immunostimulatory genes, and oncolytic viruses are presented below and summarized in Table 4.2.

4.4.1 Reporter Gene Expression

The utilization of reporter genes has served the purpose of providing easy live monitoring of delivery and gene expression levels in cell lines and animal models. However, particularly alphaviruses induce caspase activation leading to prominent apoptosis of infected host cells [227, 228]. For example, replication-deficient SFV particles expressing EGFP showed growth inhibition and killing of human H358a nonsmall cell lung cancer (NSCLC) cells and H358a spheroids [149]. Complete tumor regression was achieved in three out of seven nu/nu mice implanted with H358a xenografts after intratumoral administration of SFV–EGFP. In the case of using alphavirus RNA replicons, a single intramuscular immunization of mice implanted with CT26 colon tumors with 0.1 μg of SFV-LacZ RNA induced strong immune responses and provided protection against challenges with CT26 tumor cells [150]. MV vectors have also been used for reporter gene expression evaluations. For example, MV–GFP was transduced into glioma stem cells (GSCs) showing cytotoxic effects due to the oncolytic nature of the MV vector [151]. When GSCs transduced with MV–GFP were implanted into the right caudate nucleus of nude mice carrying glioblastomas a significant extension of survival was observed [151].

4.4.2 Tumor-associated Antigens

Self-replicating vector-based delivery of TAAs has been a common approach for cancer therapy and cancer vaccine development. In this context, SIN DNA replicons expressing the HER2/neu gene generated tumor growth inhibition in mice only when SIN-HER2/neu DNA replicons were administered before challenges with A2L2 breast tumor cells [152]. Moreover, prime immunization with SIN-HER2/neu DNA replicons followed by a booster with adenovirus-based neu expression prolonged the survival of mice significantly [152]. In another study, SIN-HER2/neu DNA replicons were compared to conventional plasmid DNA vectors, showing that robust antibody responses and protection of BALB/c mice against challenges with tumor cells were achieved with 80% less DNA replicons [153]. VEE particles have been utilized for the expression of the extracellular domain (ECD) and transmembrane (TM) domains of HER2 [154]. Immunization of mice with VEE-HER2-ECD/TM particles showed complete protection against challenges with HER2/neu tumors. In clinical evaluation, VEE-HER2-ECD/TM particles administered to stage IV HER2 overexpressing breast cancer patients, good tolerance, partial response (PR), and stable disease (SD) were reported from a phase I study [155]. VEE-HER2-ECD/TM particles have also been subjected to combination therapy with pembrolizumab in HER2-positive breast cancer patients

Table 4.2 Examples of preclinical and clinical cancer therapy.

Cancer	Expression System	Target	Response	References
Reporter Genes				
Lung H358a	SFV-EGFP	EGFP	Complete tumor regression in 43% of mice	[149]
Colon CT26	SFV-LacZ RNA	LacZ	Tumor regression, protection against tumors	[150]
GBM	GSC-MV-GFP	GFP	Prolonged survival in mice	[151]
Tumor-associated Antigens				
Breast A2L2	SIN-HER2/neu DNA	HER2/neu	Inhibition of tumor growth in mice	[152]
Breast A2L2	SIN-HER2/neu DNA + Ad-neu	HER2/neu	Prime-boost significantly prolonged survival	[152]
Breast A2L2	SIN-HER2/neu DNA	HER2/neu	80% less replicon DNA compared to con DNA	[153]
Breast A2L2	VEE-HER2-ECD/TM	HER2-ECD/TM	Complete protection against tumors in mice	[154]
Breast HER2	VEE-HER2-ECD/TM	HER2-ECD/TM	Phase I: good safety, PR and SD	[155]
Breast HER2	VEE-HER2-ECD/TM	HER2-ECD/TM	Phase II: study in progress	[156]
GBM	MV-CEA/MV-NIS	CEA, NIS	Cytotoxic effect in GSCs	[151]
HPV	VEE-HPV-E7	HPV16- E7	Robust immune responses, protection in mice	[157]
HPV	SFVenh-HPV E6-E7	HPV E6-E7	Complete eradication of established tumors	[158]
HPV	SFVenh-HPV E6-E7 (Vvax001)	HPV E6-E7	Phase I: good safety, immunogenicity in all pts	[159]
HPV	SFV-sHELP-E7SH	HPV E6-E7	Tumor regression, protection in mice	[160]
HPV	SFV-HPV E6-E7 DNA	HPV E6-E7	85% tumor-free mice with 0.05 μg replicon DNA	[161]
HPV	MV-HPV-L1	HPV-L1	Strong immune responses in mice	[162]
HPV	MV-HPV-L1 + rec L1	HPV-L1	HPV-specific Abs. Superior prime-boost	[163]
HPV	VSV-HPV16-E7	HPV16-E7	10-fold reduced tumor volume	[164]

CRPV	VSV-CRPV-E1/E2/E3/E6/E7	CRPV E1-E7	96,9% reduced tumor volume	[165]
CT26 colon	SFV-VEGFR-2	VEGFR-2	Tumor regression, prolonged survival in mice	[166]
CRC	VEE-CEA	CEA	Phase I: Ab responses, long-term survival	[167]
CT26 colon	KUN-GM-CSF	GM-CSF	Tumor regression, cure of 50% of mice	[168]
MC38a colon	MV-GM-CSF	GM-CSF	Prolonged survival, remission in 33% of mice	[169]
A549/H2009 lung	MV Edmonston-CEA	CEA	Tumor regression in nude mice	[170]
B16 melanoma	VEE-TRP-2	TRP-2	Anti-tumor activity, prolonged survival	[171]
B16 melanoma	VEE-TRP-2	TRP-2 + CTLA-4	Tumor regression in 50% of mice	[172]
B16 melanoma	VEE-TRP-2	TRP-2-GITR	Tumor regression in 90% of mice	[172]
B16 melanoma	SFV-VEGFR-2/IL-12 DNA+	VEGFR-2/IL-12+	Superior tumor growth inhibition, survival from combination therapy	[173]
	SFV-Survivin//β-hCG Ag	Survivin//β-hCG Ag		
B16-OVA	KUN-GM-CSF	GM-CSF	Tumor regression, cure of >50% of mice	[168]
B16-OVA	YFV-SIINFEKL	SIINFEKL epitope	Protection in mice	[174]
MOSEC ovarian	SFV-OVA	OVA + VV-OVA	Superior activity after prime (SFV)-boost (VV)	[175]
SKOV3.ip.1	MV-CEA + MV-NIS	CEA + NIS	Superior activity of MV-CEA + MV-NIS	[176]
RROC	MV-CEA	CEA	Phase I: dose-dependent activity, SD in 14/21 pts	[177]
MePC	VEE-CEA	CEA	Phase I: Ab responses, prolonged overall survival	[178]
TRAMP	VEE-PSMA	PSMA	Th-1 biased, CTL activity, IgG2a/2b in mice	[179]
CRPC	VEE-PSMA	PSMA	Phase I: good safety, weak immunogenicity	[180]
TRAMP-C	VEE-mSTEAP	mSTEAP + DNA	STEAP-specific response, tumor protection	[181]
TRAMP	VEE-PSCA	PSCA	Long-term survival in 90% of mice	[182]
PC-3	MV-CEA	CEA	Tumor suppression, prolonged survival	[183]

(Continued)

Table 4.2 (Continued)

Cancer	Expression System	Target	Response	References
Cytotoxic and Anti-tumor Genes				
GBM	SFV-Endostatin	Endostatin	Superior tumor inhibition to retrovirus, SFV-LacZ	[184]
GL261	GLESS-FAST-VSV	FAST	Significantly improved survival in mice	[185]
RG5	GLESS-FAST-VSV	FAST	Significantly improved survival in rats	[185]
Immunostimulatory Genes				
GBM	SFV-IL-18 in DCs	IL-18 + IL-12	Anti-tumor activity, protective immunity	[186]
RG2	SFV-IL-12	IL-12	Dose-dependent tumor regression	[187]
B16	SIN-gp100/IL-12 DNA	gp100, IL-12	Therapeutic activity, prolonged survival in mice	[188]
MC38-CEA	VEE-IL-12/VEE-CEA	IL-12, CEA	Superior immunogenicity for combination	[189]
MC38	SFV-IL-12/SFVeng-IL-12	IL-12	Complete tumor regression in mice	[190]
4T1	SFV-IL-12 + LVR01	IL-12 + LVR01	Prolonged survival in 90% of mice	[191]
A549, H2009	VSV-IFNβ	IFNβ	Tumor growth inhibition in mice	[192]
LM2	VSV-IFNβ	IFNβ	Tumor regression, cure in 30% of mice	[192]
ES2 ovarian	SIN-IL-12	IL-12 + irinotecan	Long-term survival in 35% of mice	[193]
Melanoma III-IV	LSFV-IL-12	IL-12	Phase I: good safety. Tenfold IL-12 increase	[194]
Oncolytic Viruses				
GBM	SFV VA-GFP	Oncolytic SFV	Oncolytic activity, prolonged survival in 16/17 mice	[195]
CT-2A	SFV4-miRT124	Oncolytic SFV	Reduced neurotropism, tumor inhibition	[196]
GBM	ZIKV	Oncolytic ZIKV	Potential vector for treatment of GBM	[197]
GBM	VSVΔG-CHIKV Env	CHIKV Env	Prolonged survival in mice	[198]
ICM	VSVΔG-CHIKV Env	CHIKV Env	Tumor targeting and killing	[198]

G62	Semi-repl. VSV	VSVΔG/VSVΔL	Long-term tumor regression in mice	[199]
TNBC	M1	oM1 + Dox	100-fold oncolytic effect, reduced tumor growth	[200]
TNBC	VSV(M51R)/TNBC ICV	VSV ICV	Enhanced NK and CD8$^+$ T-cell activity *ex vivo*	[201]
4T1	VSV(M51R)-LacZ	oVSV	Metastasis targeting, prolonged survival in mice	[202]
MCF7	MV Edm	MV + DoX + IR	No radio- and chemoresistance in mice	[203]
MCF7	rMV-SLAMblind	SLAMblind	Superior oncolytic activity in mice	[204]
MCF7	rMV-SLAMblind	SLAMblind	Safe delivery in primates, no cytotoxicity	[204]
HeLaS3, C33A	SIN AR339	oSIN	Cytotoxic effect, apoptosis *in vitro*	[205]
Cervical	SIN AR339	oSIN	Strong tumor regression in mice	[205]
HOC-1, OMC-3	SIN AR339	oSIN	Cytotoxic effect, apoptosis *in vitro*	[205]
Ovarian	SIN AR339	oSIN	Ascites formation in metastatic ovarian cancer	[205]
PC	Maraba MG1-IL-12	Maraba, IL-12	Reduced tumors, 100% long-term survival in mice	[206]
MIOC	Maraba MG1-OVA	Maraba-OVA, PD-1	Immunological changes in tumors in mice	[207]
Sarcoma	Maraba MG1-GFP	Maraba-GFP	Efficacy *in vitro*, *ex vivo*, long-term survival in mice	[208]
NA	Maraba MG1-MAGE-A3	Ad/MG1 MAGE-A3	Safe, well tolerated in macaques	[209]
Solid tumors	Maraba MG1-MAGE-A3	Ad/MG1 MAGE-A3	Phase I: study in progress	[210]
NSCLC	MAraba MG1-MAGE-A3	MAGE-A3 + Pem	Phase I/II: study in progress	[211]
CRC	VSV-NDV/F(L289A)	oVSV-NDV/F	Long-term survival in rats with the liver metastases	[212]
A549	SFV VA-GFP	oSFV	Superior survival in mice compared to Ad	[213]
CT26.CL25	SIN-LacZ	oSIN	Complete tumor regression, prolonged survival	[214]
LLC	MV-Hu191	oMV	Tumor growth inhibition, prolonged survival in mice	[215]
Adenocarcinoma	MV Schwarz	oMV	Inhibition of tumor growth in mice	[216]

(Continued)

Table 4.2 (Continued)

Cancer	Expression System	Target	Response	References
Mel Z	MV L-16	oMV	Inhibition of tumor growth in mice	[217]
B16-OVA	VSV-LCMP	oVSV	Tumor and metastase reduction, prolonged survival	[218]
A2780, SKOV6	VSV-LCMV-GP	LCMV-GP	Efficient killing of ovarian cancer cell lines	[219]
SKOV3.ip.1	VSV-LCMV-GP	LCMV-GP + Rux	Enhanced tumor regression in mice	[219]
LAPC	MV-αFR	scFv-αFR	Reduced tumors, prolonged survival in mice	[220]
LAPC	M1	oM1 + IRE	Killing of pancreatic cancer cell lines	[221]
LAPC	M1	oM1 + IRE	Tumor inhibition, prolonged survival	[221]
PADC	VSV	oVSV	Superior oncolytic activity to Sendai virus and RSV	[222]
PADC	VSV-GFP, VSV-ΔM51-GFP	oVSV + Gem	Superior oncolytic activity of oVSV with Gem	[223]
KLM1	MV SLAMBlind	SLAMBlind	Reduced tumor growth in mice	[224]
Capan-2	MV SLAMBlind	SLAMBlind	Reduced tumor growth in mice	[224]
DU145, PC-3	VSV-ΔM51-GFP	oVSV	Apoptosis, the killing of prostate tumor cells	[225]
DU145	VSV-ΔM51-GFP	oVSV	Eradication of tumors in nude mice	[225]
Du145, 22Rv1	VSV-LCMV-GP	LCMV-GP	Long-term remission in mice	[226]
PC-3	oMV + MuV	oMV + MuV	Superior combination of oMV and MuV	

CEA, carcinoembryonic antigen; CHIKV, Chikungunya virus; con DNA, conventional plasmid DNA; CRC, colorectal cancer; CRPC, castration resistant metastatic prostate cancer; CTLA-4, CTL antigen-4 monoclonal antibody; Dox, doxorubicin; GBM, glioblastoma multiforme; GITR, glucocorticoid-induced tumor necrosis factor receptor monoclonal antibody; GM-CSF, granular macrophage-colony stimulating factor; ICM, intracranial melanoma; ICV, infected cell vaccine; IFNβ, interferon-β; IR, ionizing radiation; IRE, irreversible electroporation; KUN, Kunjin virus; LAPC, locally advanced pancreatic cancer; LLC, Lewis lung carcinoma; LSFV, liposome encapsulated SFV; MIII-IV, stages III-IV melanoma; MePC, metastatic prostate cancer; MOSEC, murine ovarian surface epithelial carcinoma; MV, measles virus; MuV, mumps virus; mSTEAP, mouse six-transmembrane epithelial antigen of the prostate; NA, not applicable; NSCLC, nonsmall cell lung cancer; OMC, ovarian metastatic carcinoma; PC, peritoneal carcinomatosis; Pem, Pembrolizumab; PSCA, prostate stem cell antigen; PSMA, prostate-specific membrane antigen; RROC, refractory recurrent ovarian cancer; Rux, ruxolitinib; SFV. Semliki Forest virus; SIN, Sindbis virus; TNBC, triple-negative breast cancer; TRAMP, transgenic adenocarcinoma of the prostate; TRP-2, tyrosine-related protein-2; VEE, Venezuelan equine encephalitis virus; VEGFR-2, vascular endothelial growth factor receptor-2; VV, vaccinia virus; YFV, yellow fever virus; ZIKV, Zika virus.

in a phase II trial [156]. In the case of MV vectors, expression of the carcinoembryonic antigen (CEA) and sodium iodide symporter (NIS) genes generated cytotoxic effects in GSCs [151]. Pseudotyped VSV vectors were engineered, in which the VSV G protein was replaced by the SIN surface glycoprotein (gp) containing the Fc-binding domain of the *Staphylococcus aureus* protein A (Sindbis-ZZ) [229]. In human SKBR3 breast cancer cells, the VSV-Sindbis-ZZ titers were less than 1% of pseudotyped VSV particles coated with wild-type SIN (Sindbis-gp). Conjugation of the 4D5 mAb against the HER2/neu receptor with the VSV-Sindbis-ZZ increased the titer 50-fold. Moreover, the titer was increased 36-fold in the human MCF7/H2 cell line, which is known to possess a lower concentration of cell surface HER2/neu receptors. This approach showed the feasibility of engineering VSV vectors with a restricted host cell range.

Self-replicating RNA viruses have also been used for cervical cancer targeting human papillomavirus (HPV). VEE particles expressing the HPV E7 protein elicited strong T-cell responses and protected immunized C57BL/6 mice from tumor challenges [157]. Moreover, expression of an HPV E6-E7 fusion protein from the SFVenh vector provided enhanced expression levels due to the presence of the translation enhancer signal from the SFV capsid gene [158]. Immunization of C57BL/6 mice with SFVenh-HPV E6-E7 elicited robust immune responses and completely eradicated established cervical tumors. The SFVenh-HPV E6-E7 (Vvax001) has been subjected to the first-in-human clinical phase I trial in patients with cervical intraepithelial neoplasia [159]. The intramuscular immunization procedure was safe and elicited immune responses in all 12 patients. SFV-sHELP-E7SH particles containing helper T-cell epitopes and an ER targeting signal fused to the HPV E6 and E7 proteins were administered to C57BL/6JOlaHsd mice leading to substantial tumor regression and protection against tumor challenges [160]. In the context of DNA replicons, intradermal administration of SFV-HPV E6-E7 DNA replicons combined with electroporation prevented tumor growth in C57BL/6 mice, and 85% of treated mice were tumor-free [161]. In comparison to conventional plasmid DNA, 200-fold lower doses, equivalent to 0.05 μg of DNA were required. MV particles expressing the HPV-16 L1 capsid protein induced strong immune responses in transgenic mice [162]. In a comparative study, HPV-16 L1 and HPV-18 L1 recombinant proteins produced in *Pichia pastoris* yeast showed similar HPV-specific total IgG and neutralizing antibodies to MV HPV-16 L1 particles [163]. However, a prime-boost strategy showed enhanced immunogenicity. In the case of VSV, VSV-HPV-16 E7 particles elicited E7-specific immune responses, anti-tumor activity, and a 10-fold decrease in tumor volume in immunized C57BL/6 mice with implanted TC-1 tumors [164]. Moreover, VSV-based expression of cottontail rabbit papillomavirus (CRPV) E1, E2, E6, and E7 proteins resulted in a significant reduction in tumor size in immunized rabbits [165]. Particularly, VSV-CRPV E7 was efficient, reducing the tumor volume by 96.9% and eradicating tumors. Significant inhibition of tumor growth and prevention of metastatic spread was achieved in mice with CT26 colon tumor xenografts immunized with SFV particles expressing the vascular endothelial growth factor receptor-2 (VEGFR-2) [166]. Evaluation of combination therapy with SFV vectors expressing cytokines revealed that SFV-VEGFR-2 and SFV-IL-12 particles did neither affect antibody responses nor anti-tumor activity, whereas co-administration of SFV-IL-4 particles increased VEGFR-2-specific antibody titers and extended the survival time of mice. In the case of VEE particles expressing CEA, antigen-specific immune responses and long-term survival were achieved in a phase I clinical trial of patients with stages III and IV colorectal cancer (CRC) [167]. In another approach, noncytopathic KUN particles expressing the granulocyte–macrophage colony-stimulating factor (GM–CSF) elicited $CD8^+$ T-cell responses, generated tumor regression, and cured 50% of immunized BALB/c mice carrying CT26 colon tumors [168]. MV vectors expressing GM–CSF elicited adaptive immune responses in immunized mice carrying MC38a colon tumors [169]. Intratumoral MV–GM–CSF administration delayed tumor progression and extended the survival time, resulting in complete remission in one-third of the mice. Moreover, expression of CEA from the MV Edmonston strain induced regression of A549 and H2009 lung tumors in nude mice [170]. VEE particles expressing the tyrosine-related protein-2 (TRP-2) showed a humoral response, anti-tumor activity, and extended survival in a B16 mouse melanoma model [171]. Combination of VEE-TRP-2 particles with antagonist anti-CTL antigen-4 (CTLA-4) or agonist anti-glucocorticoid-induced tumor necrosis factor receptor (GITR) mAbs, provided superior tumor regression in mice [172]. Tumor regression of 50% was achieved by combining VEE-TRP-2 with CTLA-4 and 90% for co-administration with GITR. Furthermore, the combination of one SFV DNA replicon vector expressing VEGFR-2 and IL-12 and another expressing survivin and β-hCG antigen provided superior inhibition of tumor growth and survival in mice than immunization with either of the SFV DNA replicons alone [173].

Administration of KUN-GM-CSF particles to C57BL/6 mice implanted with B16-OVA melanoma xenografts resulted in significant tumor regression, and more than half of the immunized animals were cured [168]. In another study, immunization of C57BL/6 mice with the YFV flavivirus expressing the chicken OVA CTL epitope SIINFEKL rendered protection against challenges with B16-OVA and B16FO melanoma cells [174]. Moreover, a prime-boost combination of SFV-OVA and vaccinia virus, VV-OVA, particles elicited OVA-specific $CD8^+$ T-cell responses and superior tumor activity in C57BL/6 mice grafted with murine ovarian surface epithelial carcinoma (MOSEC) [175]. The combination of MV-CEA and MV-NIS particles has been subjected to immunization studies in the SKOV3.ip.1 mouse ovarian model showing superior therapeutic activity compared to either MV-CEA or MV-NIS administration alone [176]. In a phase I trial in patients with refractory recurrent ovarian cancer (RROC), MV-CEA was safe and well tolerated [177]. The dose-dependent activity resulted in SD in 14 out of 21 patients. As VEE-CEA particles have previously demonstrated efficacy in preclinical studies [189], a phase I clinical trial was conducted in patients with metastatic pancreatic cancer [178]. Intramuscular VEE-CEA administration elicited clinically relevant T-cell and antibody response, tumor cell killing, and prolonged survival [178]. VEE particles have also been used for the expression of the prostate-specific membrane antigen (PSMA) [179]. Immunization studies in the transgenic adenocarcinoma of the prostate (TRAMP) mouse model showed strong immune responses and CTL activity. In a phase I clinical trial in patients with castration-resistant metastatic prostate cancer (CRPC), VEE-PSMA particles showed good safety and tolerance, but the weak PSMA-specific immune responses need to be addressed by optimization of dosing and expression [180]. In another approach, VEE-based expression of the mouse six-transmembrane epithelial antigen of the prostate (mSTEAP) was combined with a gene gun-based booster immunization with gold-coated conventional pcDBA-3-mSTEAP plasmid DNA, which elicited mSTEAP-specific immune responses and protected mice against tumor cell challenges [181]. Moreover, VEE particles expressing the prostate stem cell antigen (PSCA) generated long-term survival for at least 12 months in 90% of immunized mice [182]. In the case of MV, immunization with MV-CEA particles resulted in delayed tumor growth and prolonged survival in a prostate PC-3 mouse model [183].

4.4.3 Cytotoxic and Anti-tumor Genes

As endostatin can specifically inhibit endothelial proliferation, angiogenesis, and tumor growth it has been used for SFV-based cancer therapy [184]. Compared to SFV-LacZ particles and a retrovirus vector, SFV-endostatin showed superior inhibition of tumor growth and reduced intratumoral vascularization [184]. In a brain tumor approach, VSV particles where the VSV G protein was replaced by the fusion-associated small transmembrane (FAST) gene (GLESS-FAST-VSV) were intratumorally injected into F344 and C57BL/6 mice with rat RG2 and mouse GL261 implanted brain tumors [185]. The treatment was well tolerated and significantly prolonged the survival of animals compared to control rats and mice.

4.4.4 Immunostimulatory Genes

Different types of cancers have been targeted by vector-based delivery of immunostimulatory genes. For example, dendritic cells (DCs) transduced with SFV-IL-18 particles were evaluated in a mouse B16 brain tumor model [186]. Administration of SFV-IL-18/DCs together with recombinant IL-12 protein was superior in relation to Th1 responses, anti-tumor activity, and protective immunity compared to systemic delivery of IL-12 alone. In another study, dose-dependent therapeutic effects were demonstrated for SFV-IL-12 in a syngeneic RG2 rat glioma model [187]. SIN DNA replicons expressing the human gp100 and mouse IL-18 were administered intramuscularly to mice with implanted B16-gp100 brain tumors, which showed strong therapeutic activity and prolonged survival [188]. Moreover, VEE-IL-12 and VEE-CEA particles were administered to C57BL/6 mice carrying MC38-CEA-2 mouse tumors [189]. VEE-IL-12 particles elicited superior immune responses compared to recombinant IL-12 protein. Moreover, the combination of VEE-IL-12 and VEE-CEA particles induced stronger tumor activity and prolonged survival of mice compared to either VEE-IL-12 or VEE-CEA particles alone [189]. In another approach, SFV-IL-12 and SFVenh-IL-12 particles were evaluated in the poorly immunogenic MC38 colon adenocarcinoma mouse model [190]. Although eight-fold higher IL-12 levels and superior anti-tumor activity were associated with SFVenh-IL-12 immunization compared to SFV-IL-12, both provided complete tumor regression and prolonged tumor-free survival in mice with MC38 tumors. Furthermore, SFV-IL-12 particles were co-administered with the *Salmonella typhimurium* aroC strain (LVR01) in BALB/c mice with implanted 4T1 mammary tumors, which resulted in complete inhibition of lethal lung metastasis formation and long-term survival in 90% of animals [191]. Intratumoral immunization of mice implanted with A549 and H2009 lung tumors with VSV particles expressing interferon-β (VSV-IFNβ) resulted in significant inhibition of tumor growth [192]. Moreover, immunization with VSV-IFNβ particles provided prolonged survival and cure in 30% of mice with LM2 lung tumors [192]. In another approach, SIN-IL-12 particles combined with irinotecan, a CPT-11 topoisomerase inhibitor, provided long-term survival in 35% of SCID mice implanted with highly aggressive human ES2 ovarian tumors [193]. In a clinical setting, a phase I study in stage III and stage IV metastasizing melanoma and renal carcinoma patients was conducted with liposome-encapsulated SFV particles expressing IL-12 (LSFV-IL-12) [193]. Intravenous administration of LSFV-IL-12 particles did not cause any major toxicity, only mild inflammatory reactions, in any of the 18 patients. The IL-12 concentrations were 10-fold increased after LSFV-IL-12 administration. However, the IL-12 expression was transient and lasted for three to four days. Most importantly, repeated administration of LSFV-IL-12 did not induce any toxic reactions or antibody responses against SFV particles or liposomes.

4.4.5 Oncolytic Viruses

Intravenous administration of replication-proficient SFV VA-EGFP particles showed complete inhibition of stably expressed firefly luciferase in BALB/c mice with subcutaneous orthotopic tumors [195]. Moreover, it also led to the long-term survival of 16 out of 17 immunized mice. The neurotropism of alphaviruses has, however, caused some concern for their therapeutic use [230]. One approach has been to introduce neuron-specific micro-RNA (miRT124) sequences into the replication-proficient SFV4 vector, which normally causes lethal encephalitis in mice, resulting in replication in glioblastoma cells [196]. Moreover, significant inhibition of tumor growth and prolonged survival were achieved in C57BL/6 mice carrying CT-2A orthotopic gliomas immunized with SFV4-miRT124 particles.

Among flaviviruses, ZIKV has shown the potential as a vector for glioblastoma treatment [197]. In another approach, immunization of mice carrying glioblastoma xenografts with a chimeric VSV vector with the VSV G protein replaced by the CHIKV E3-E2-6K-E1 polyprotein prolonged the survival of mice for more than 100 days [198]. Tumor killing and minor effects on normal cells were observed for VSVΔG-CHIKV Env-immunized mice with intracranial primary patient-derived melanoma xenografts. Moreover, two trans-complementing, propagation-deficient VSV vectors were used for the engineering of a semi-replication-competent VSV system [199]. For example, deletion mutants for the VSV polymerase proteins P and L (VSVΔP and VSVΔL) efficiently lysed glioblastoma cells after *in vitro* or *in vivo* co-propagation. Administration of VSVΔG/VSVΔL did not cause neurotoxicity but resulted in long-term regression in mice with subcutaneous xenografts [199].

The oncolytic M1 alphavirus has been shown to efficiently kill triple-negative breast cancer (TNBC) cells [200]. Moreover, co-administration of M1 with doxorubicin enhanced the oncolytic effect of M1 100-fold in TNBC cells *in vitro* and significantly slowed down TNBC tumor growth in mice. In another promising study on TNBC, the oncolytic VSV(M51R) vector with the M51R mutation in the matrix (M) protein was transduced into TNBC cells *ex vivo* resulting in enhanced functionality of natural killer cells and $CD8^+$ T-cells [201]. In another study, VSV(M51R)-LacZ particles were intravenously administered to BALB/c mice implanted with syngeneic 4T1 breast tumors [202]. Repeated injections of VSV(M51R)-LacZ into the tail vein of mice significantly prolonged the survival time and did not induce any cytotoxicity. Combination therapy of the MV Edmonston strain, doxorubicin, and ionizing radiation provided a synergistic effect in breast cancer resistant to radio- or chemotherapy in mice with MCF7 tumors [203]. In the context of breast cancer, the introduction of the signaling lymphocyte activation molecule (SLAM) into the MV vector prevented infection of SLAM-positive lymphoid cells while breast cancer cells remained susceptible [204]. Administration of rMV-SLAMBlind particles to immunodeficient mice with human breast cancer xenografts resulted in anti-tumor activity and significantly greater oncolytic activity compared to the MV Edmonston strain. Moreover, no clinical symptoms of MV were detected in monkeys seronegative for MV [204]. In another approach, the oncolytic SIN AR339 strain generated cytopathic effects and apoptosis in the human HeLaS3 and C33A cervical cancer cells and HOC-1, HAC-2, and OMC-3 ovarian cancer cells [205]. Intratumoral and intravenous administration of SIN AR339 resulted in substantial tumor regression in mice with implanted cervical tumors. In a mouse model of metastatic ovarian cancer, ascites formation was suppressed [205]. Oncolytic Maraba MG1 viral particles expressing IL-12 have been utilized as an infected cell vaccine (ICV) by transduction of colon cancer cells *ex vivo* [206]. Intraperitoneal administration of the ICV showed migration of activated NK cells, reduced tumor burden, and improved survival in a mouse colon cancer model of peritoneal carcinomatosis (PC) [206]. Even in mice with bulky tumors larger than 8 mm, 100% long-term survival was achieved. Furthermore, the Maraba virus expressing OVA was used for a booster vaccination in C57BL/6 mice with metastatic intraperitoneal ovarian cancer prime-vaccinated with OVA protein mixed with MIS416 adjuvant [207]. The heterologous vaccination regimen elicited strong tumor-specific $CD8^+$ T-cell responses resulting in unique immunological changes in the tumors. However, as the treatment was not curative and the T-cells in the tumor microenvironment were suppressed, it was partially overcome by adding the checkpoint PD-1 blockade to the prime/boost strategy. In a comparative study, the Maraba MG1 virus was evaluated in parallel with reovirus, VV, and herpes simplex virus (HSV) for the ability to infect and kill human and canine sarcoma cell lines, human sarcoma samples *ex vivo*, and therapeutic and protective efficacy *in vivo* [208]. *In vitro*, Maraba MG1-GFP showed the highest potency and infected more than 80% of human sarcoma tissue *ex vivo*. Moreover, a significant increase in long-lasting cure in sarcoma-bearing BALB/c mice was seen. In preparation for clinical trials, the safety and immunogenicity of Maraba MG1 expressing the melanoma-associated antigen 3 (MAGE-A3) was evaluated as a booster immunization in macaques prime-vaccinated with a replication-deficient adenovirus expressing MAGE-A3 [209]. The vaccination caused no severe adverse events. The Maraba MG1-MAGE-A3 boost elicited robust remarkable levels of hMAGE-A3-specific $CD4^+$ and $CD8^+$ T-cell and humoral responses, contributing to clinical evaluation of Maraba MG1-MAGE-A3 in a phase I study in patients with solid tumors [210] and in combination with pembrolizumab in a phase I/II trial in patients with NSCLC [211]. VSV particles (VSV-NDV/F(L289A)) expressing a mutant Newcastle disease virus (NDV) fusion protein were administered to rats with multiple CRC lung metastases and multifocal CRC liver metastases [212]. VSV–NDV/F(L289A) significantly prolonged the survival for more than 100 days in the liver metastasis model. In contrast, although prolonged survival was detected in the lung metastasis model, none of the immunized rats survived long term.

In the case of lung cancer, oncolytic SFV VA-GFP particles showed superior efficacy and survival in nude mice with implanted A549 lung adenocarcinomas in comparison to a conditionally replicating adenovirus (Ad-Delta24TK-GFP) [213]. Furthermore, SIN-LacZ particles administered to mice implanted with CT26.CL25 lung tumors demonstrated complete tumor regression and prolonged survival [214]. In another pre-clinical lung cancer study, C57BL/6 mice carrying Lewis lung carcinomas (LLC) were immunized with the oncolytic MV Hu-191 strain causing strong suppression of tumor growth and significantly prolonged survival [215]. In addition, nude mice with implanted lung tumor xenografts showed inhibition of tumor growth after immunization with the oncolytic MV Schwarz strain [216]. Another oncolytic MV strain, MV Leningrad-16 (L-16), provided efficient inhibition of tumor growth in a MelZ mouse melanoma model after subcutaneous immunization [217]. In another melanoma study, the VSV G protein was replaced by the lymphocytic choriomeningitis virus (LCMV) glycoprotein in a pseudotyped VSV vector used for immunization in a subcutaneous A375 xenograft model and a B16-OVA syngeneic mouse tumor model, which led to tumor regression, reduction in lung metastases and prolonged survival [218]. Moreover, the pseudotyped VSV-LCMV-GP particles showed efficient killing of ovarian A2780, HOC7, and SKOV6 cancer cell lines [219]. Immunization studies with VSV-LCMV-GP particles showed tumor regression in the A2780 ovarian mouse tumor model, which was further enhanced in combination with ruxolitinib [219]. In another ovarian cancer study, a tumor-targeting MV vector was engineered by the introduction of a single-chain antibody (scFv) sequence for the alpha-folate receptor (αFR) [220]. Immunization of mice with ovarian SKOV3ip.1 xenografts with MV-αFR resulted in reduction of tumor volumes and prolongation of overall survival [220].

In the case of pancreatic cancer, the oncolytic M1 alphavirus has shown therapeutic efficacy in the treatment of locally advanced pancreatic cancer (LAPC), which was further enhanced by combination with irreversible electroporation (IRE) [221]. *In vivo*, the combination of MI and IRE showed synergistic effects resulting in inhibition of tumor proliferation and prolonged survival in immunocompetent mice with orthotopic pancreatic tumors [221]. In another pancreatic cancer study, oncolytic VSV particles were compared to Sendai virus and RSV in aggressive pancreatic ductal adenocarcinoma (PADC) cell lines [222]. The oncolytic activity provided by VSV was superior to that seen for Sendai and RSV. Wild-type VSV, VSV-GFP, and oncolytic VSV-ΔM51-GFP particles were evaluated for oncolytic activity in PADC cell lines, which demonstrated the superiority of VSV-ΔM51-GFP compared to the other VSV particles [223]. The oncolytic activity was further enhanced by combination therapy with gemcitabine [223]. Moreover, SCID mice carrying pancreatic KLM1 and Capan-2 xenografts were immunized with MV-SLAMBlind particles, which resulted in significant tumor suppression [224].

Furthermore, oncolytic self-replicating viruses have also been evaluated for prostate cancer. For example, modified VSV-ΔM51-GFP particles showed induction of apoptosis and efficient killing of human DU-145 and PC-3 prostate cancer cells and also eradicated tumor cells without affecting normal cells in immunized mice with implanted DU-145 xenografts [225]. Intratumoral and intravenous immunization with oncolytic VSV-LCMV-GP particles resulted in long-term remission of subcutaneous tumors and bone metastases in mice with implanted DU-145 and 22Rv1 prostate tumors [226]. Finally, in a combination approach, oncolytic MV and mumps virus (MuV) particles were evaluated in the PC-3 prostate cancer mouse model [231]. Co-immunization with MV and MuV resulted in superior anti-tumor activity and longer survival than immunization with either MV or MuV alone [231].

4.5 Conclusions and Future Aspects

Self-replicating RNA viruses have been evaluated both in preclinical animal models and clinical trials for vaccine development against infectious diseases and cancers. Robust immune responses and protection against challenges with pathogenic viruses, bacteria, and parasites have been obtained. Likewise, prophylactic and therapeutic activity against tumor challenges have been demonstrated. Although progress has been made in clinical trials and the VSV-based vaccine Ervebo has been approved by the FDA and the EMA for vaccination against EVD, optimization of vector delivery and gene expression is still required.

In the case of infectious diseases, viral and bacterial surface proteins have been demonstrated as feasible vaccine targets. Related to cancers, TAA, cytotoxic and anti-tumor, and immunostimulatory genes have been successfully evaluated. Moreover, oncolytic viruses and especially alphaviruses inducing apoptosis have been valuable in providing tumor regression and eradication.

In comparison to other vaccine approaches, self-replicating RNA virus-based vaccines provide certain advantages. The greatest asset is the extreme RNA self-replication occurring in the host cell cytoplasm, which permits the production of superior levels of antigen and/or administration of significantly reduced doses. Another advantage is the flexibility of using recombinant viral particles, naked or encapsulated RNA replicons, and DNA replicons. In the context of RNA and

DNA replicons, the required doses are 100–1000 times lower compared to synthetic mRNA and conventional DNA plasmids, respectively. Manufacturing of RNA and DNA replicons is easy, rapid and inexpensive and packaging cell lines engineered for self-replicating RNA viruses are further assets. However, improvements are still needed in some areas of vaccine development based on self-replicating RNA viruses. For example, delivery of both DNA and RNA can be enhanced by polymer- and liposome-based formulations. Moreover, RNA stability is an important issue to address, not only related to delivery but also to the storage and transport of the RNA end-point product. Another issue of urgency is to improve the transition of vaccine efficacy seen in preclinical studies especially in rodents to humans in clinical trials. Recent success in vaccine development against COVID-19 for both viral vector-based and mRNA-based vaccines is very encouraging and bodes well for self-replicating RNA viruses as vehicles for vaccine development against infectious diseases and cancers.

References

1 Lundstrom, K. (2022). Application of viruses for gene therapy and vaccine development. In: *The Biological Role of a Virus. Advances in Environmental Microbiology*, 9e (ed. C.J. Hurst), 285–341. Switzerland: Springer Nature.

2 Frolov, I., Hoffman, T.A., Pragal, B.M. et al. (1996). Alphavirus-based expression vectors: strategies and applications. *Proc. Natl. Acad. Sci. USA* 93: 11371–11377.

3 Lamb, Y.N. (2021). BNT162b2 mRNA COVID-19 vaccine: first approval. *Drugs* 81: 495–501.

4 Oliver, S.E., Gargano, J.W., Marin, M. et al. (2021). The advisory committee on immunization practices' interim recommendation for use of Moderna COVID-19 vaccine – United States, December 2020. *MMWR Morb. Mortal Wkly. Rep.* 69: 1653–1656.

5 Strauss, J.H. and Strauss, E.G. (1994). The alphaviruses: gene expression, replication and evolution. *Microbiol. Rev.* 58: 491–562.

6 Liljestrom, P. and Garoff, H. (1991). A new generation of animal cell expression vectors based on the Semliki Forest virus replicon. *Bio/Technology* 9: 1356–1361.

7 Xiong, C., Levis, R., Shen, P. et al. (1989). Sindbis virus: an efficient, broad host range vector for gene expression in animal cells. *Science* 243: 1188–1191.

8 Davis, N.L., Willis, L.V., Smith, J.F., and Johnston, R.F. (1989). In vitro synthesis of infectious Venezuelan equine encephalitis virus RNA from a cDNA clone: analysis of a viable deletion mutant. *Virology* 171: 189–204.

9 Frolova, E., Frolov, I., and Schlesinger, S. (1997). Packaging signals in alphaviruses. *J. Virol.* 71: 248–258.

10 Lundstrom, K. (2003). Semliki forest virus vectors for rapid and high-level expression of integral membrane protein. *Biochim. Biophys. Acta* 1610: 90–96.

11 DiCiommo, P.D. and Bremner, R. (1998). Rapid, high level protein production using DNA-based Semliki Forest virus vectors. *J. Biol. Chem.* 273: 18060–18066.

12 Pijlman, G.P., Suhrbier, A., and Khromykh, A.A. (2006). Kunjin virus replicons: an RNA-based non-cytopathic viral vector system for protein production, vaccine and gene therapy applications. *Expert. Opin. Biol. Ther.* 6: 134–145.

13 De Felipe, F. (2004). Skipping the co-expression problem: the new 2A 'CHYSEL' technology. *Genet. Vaccines Ther.* 2: 13.

14 Khromykh, A.A., Varnavski, A.N., and Westaway, E.G. (1998). Encapsidation of the flavivirus Kunjin replicon RNA by using a complementation system providing Kunjin virus structural proteins in trans. *J. Virol.* 72: 5967–5977.

15 Scholle, I., Girard, Y.A., Zhao, Q. et al. (2004). Trans-packaged West Nile virus-like particles: infectious properties in vitro and in infected mosquito vectors. *J. Virol.* 78 (21): 11605–11614.

16 Jones, S.M., Feldmann, J., Strober, U. et al. (2005). Live attenuated recombinant vaccine protects nonhuman primates against Ebola ad Marburg viruses. *Nat. Med.* 11: 786–790.

17 Pang, X., Zhang, M., and Dayton, A.I. (2001). Development of dengue virus type 2 replicons capable of prolonged expression in host cells. *BMC Microbiol.* 1: 18.

18 Hayasaka, D., Yoshii, K., Ueki, T. et al. (2004). Sub-genomic replicons of tick-borne encephalitis virus. *Arch. Virol.* 149: 1245–1256.

19 Radecke, F., Spielhofer, P., Schneider, H. et al. (1995). Rescue of measles viruses from cloned DNA. *EMBO J.* 14: 5773–5784.

20 Li, Q., Liu, Q., Huang, W. et al. (2018). Current status on the development of pseudoviruses for enveloped viruses. *Rev. Med. Virol.* 28: e1963.

21 Schnell, M.J., Buonocore, L., Kretzschmar, E. et al. (1996). Foreign glycoproteins expressed from recombinant vesicular stomatitis viruses are incorporated efficiently into virus particles. *Proc. Natl. Acad. Sci. USA* 93: 11359–11365.

22 Mühlebach, M.D. (2017). Vaccine platform recombinant measles virus. *Virus Genes* 53: 733–740.

23 Schneider, H., Spielhofer, P., Kaelin, K. et al. (1997). Rescue of measles virus using a replication-deficient vaccinia-T7 vector. *J. Virol. Methods* 64: 57–64.

24 Martin, A., Staeheli, P., and Schneider, U. (2006). RNA polymerase II-controlled expression of antigenomic RNA enhances the rescue efficacies of two different members of the Mononegavirales independently of the site of viral genome replication. *J. Virol.* 80: 5708–5715.

25 Osakada, F. and Callaway, E.M. (2013). Design and generation of recombinant rabies virus vectors. *Nat. Protoc.* 8: 1583–1601.

26 Pol, J.G., Zhang, L., Bridle, B.W. et al. (2014). Maraba virus as a potent oncolytic vaccine vector. *Mol. Ther.* 22: 420–429.

27 Chattopadhyay, A., Aquilar, P.V., Bopp, N.E. et al. (2018). A recombinant virus vaccine that protects both against Chikungunya and Zika virus infections. *Vaccine* 36: 3894–3900.

28 Brandler, S., Ruffié, C., Combredet, C. et al. (2013). A recombinant measles vaccine expressing chikungunya virus-like particles is strongly immunogenic and protects mice from lethal challenge with chikungunya virus. *Vaccine* 31: 3718–3725.

29 Rossi, S.L., Comer, J.E., Wang, E. et al. (2019). Immunogenicity and efficacy of a measles virus-vectored chikungunya vaccine in nonhuman primates. *J. Infect. Dis.* 220: 735–742.

30 Ramsauer, K., Schwameis, M., Firbas, C. et al. (2015). Immunogenicity, safety, and tolerability of a recombinant measles virus-based chikungunya vaccine: a randomised, double-blind, placebo controlled, active-comparator, first-in-man trial. *Lancet Infect. Dis.* 15: 519–527.

31 Reisinger, E.C., Tschismarov, R., Beubler, E. et al. (2018). Immunogenicity, safety, and tolerability of the measles-vectored chikungunya virus vaccine MV-CHIK: a double-blind, randomised, placebo-controlled and active-controlled phase 2 trial. *Lancet* 392: 2718–2727.

32 Tschismarov, R., Zellweger, R.M., Koh, M.J. et al. (2021). Antibody effector analysis of prime versus prime-boost immunizations with a recombinant measles-vectored chikungunya virus vaccine. *JCI Insight* 6: e151095.

33 Reed, D.S., Glass, P.J., Bakken, R.R. et al. (2014). Combined alphavirus replicon particle vaccine induces durable and cross-protective immune responses against equine encephalitis virus. *J. Virol.* 88: 12077–12086.

34 Tretyakova, I., Tibbens, A., Jokinen, J.D. et al. (2019). Novel DNA-launched Venezuelan equine encephalitis virus vaccine with rearranged genome. *Vaccine* 37: 3317–3325.

35 Tretyakova, I., Plante, K.S., Rossi, S.L. et al. (2020). Venezuelan equine encephalitis vaccine with rearranged genome resists reversion and protects non-human primates from viremia after aerosol challenge. *Vaccine* 38: 3378–3386.

36 Hannaman, D., Dupuy, L.C., Ellefsen, B., and Schmaljohn, C.S. (2016). A Phase 1 clinical trial of a DNA vaccine for Venezuelan equine encephalitis delivered by intramuscular or intradermal electroporation. *Vaccine* 34: 3607–3612.

37 Samsa, M.M., Dupuy, L.C., Beard, C.W. et al. (2019). Self-amplifying RNA vaccines for Venezuelan equine encephalitis virus induce robust protective immunogenicity in mice. *Mol. Ther.* 27: 850–865.

38 Safronetz, D., Mire, C., Rosenke, K. et al. (2015). A recombinant vesicular stomatitis virus-based Lassa fever vaccine protects guinea pigs and macaques against challenge with geographically and genetically distinct Lassa viruses. *PLoS Negl. Trop. Dis.* 9: e0003736.

39 Mateo, M., Reynard, S., Carnec, X. et al. (2019). Vaccines inducing immunity to Lassa fever glycoprotein and nucleoprotein protect macaques after a single shot. *Sci. Transl. Med.* 11: eaaw3163.

40 Mateo, M., Reynard, S., Carnec, X. et al. (2021). A single-shot Lassa vaccine induces long-term immunity and protects cynomolgus monkeys against heterologous strains. *Sci. Transl. Med.* 13: eabf6348.

41 A Trial to Evaluate the Optimal Dose of MV-LASV (V182-001). https://clinicaltrials.gov/ct2/show/NCT04055454 (accessed 20 June 2022).

42 Bredenbeek, P.J., Molenkamp, R., Spaan, W.J.M. et al. (2006). A recombinant Yellow Fever 17D expressing Lassa virus glycoproteins. *Virology* 345: 299–304.

43 Jiang, X., Dalebout, T.J., Bredenbeck, P.J. et al. (2011). Yellow fever 17D-vectored vaccines expressing LASV GP1 and GP2 glycoproteins provide protection against fatal disease in guinea pigs. *Vaccine* 29: 1248–1257.

44 Pushko, P., Geisbert, J., Parker, M. et al. (2001). Individual and bivalent vaccines based on alphavirus replicons protect guinea pigs against infection with Lassa and Ebola virus. *J. Virol.* 75: 11677–11685.

45 Wang, M., Jokinen, J., Tretyakova, I. et al. (2018). Alphavirus-based replicon particles expressing multivalent cross-protective Lassa virus glycoproteins. *Vaccine* 36: 683–690.

46 Johnson, D.M., Jokinen, J.D., Wang, M. et al. (2020). Bivalent Junin and Machupo experimental vaccine based on alphavirus RNA replicon vector. *Vaccine* 38: 2949–2959.

47 Reynard, O., Mokhonov, V., Mokhonova, E. et al. (2011). Kunjin virus replicon-based vaccines expressing Ebola virus glycoprotein GP protect the guinea pig against lethal Ebola virus infection. *J. Infect. Dis.* 204: S1060–S1065.

48 Pyankov, O.V., Bodnev, S.A., Pyankova, O.G. et al. (2015). A Kunjin replicon virus-like vaccine provides protection against Ebola virus infection in nonhuman primates. *J. Infect. Dis.* 212: S368–S371.

49 Marzi, A., Robertson, S.J., Haddock, E. et al. (2015). Ebola vaccine. VSV-EBOV rapidly protects macaques against infection with the 2014/2015 Ebola virus outbreak strain. *Science* 349: 739–742.

50 Jones, S.M., Stroher, U., Fernando, L. et al. (2007). Assessment of a vesicular stomatitis virus-based vaccine by use of the mouse model of Ebola virus hemorrhagic fever. *J. Infect. Dis.* 196: 5404–5412.

51 Geisbert, T.W., Daddario-DiCaprio, K.M., Geisbert, J.B. et al. (2008). Vesicular stomatitis virus-based vaccines protect nonhuman primates against aerosol challenge with Ebola and Marburg viruses. *Vaccine* 26: 6894–6900.

52 Qiu, X., Fernando, L., Alimonti, J.B. et al. (2009). Mucosal immunization of cynomolgus macaques with the VSVDeltaG/ZEBOV GP vaccine stimulates strong Ebola GP-specific immune responses. *PLoS One* 4: e5447.

53 Daddario-DiCaprio, K.M., Geisbert, T.W., Geisbert, J.B. et al. (2006). Cross-protection against Marburg virus strains using a live, attenuated recombinant vaccine. *J. Virol.* 80: 9659–9666.

54 Herbert, A.S., Kuehne, A.I., Barth, J.F. et al. (2013). Venezuelan equine encephalitis virus replicon particle vaccine protects nonhuman primates from intramuscular and aerosol challenge with ebolavirus. *J. Virol.* 87: 4852–4964.

55 Henao-Restrepo, A.M., Longini, I.M., Egger, M. et al. (2015). Efficacy and effectiveness of an rVSV-vectored vaccine expressing Ebola surface glycoprotein: Interim results from the Guinea ring vaccination cluster-randomised trial. *Lancet* 386: 857–866.

56 Henao-Restrepo, A.M., Camacho, A., Longini, I.M. et al. (2017). Efficacy and effectiveness of an rVSV-vectored vaccine in preventing Ebola virus disease: final results from the Guinea ring vaccination, open-label, cluster-randomised trial (Ebola Ca Suffit!). *Lancet* 389: 505–518.

57 Maxmen, A. (2017). Ebola vaccine approved for use in ongoing outbreak. *Nature* https://doi.org/10.1038/nature.2017.22024.

58 Khalil, S.M., Tonkin, D.R., Mattocks, M.D. et al. (2014). A tetravalent alphavirus-vector based dengue vaccine provides effective immunity in an early life mouse model. *Vaccine* 32: 4068–4074.

59 Chen, L., Ewing, D., Subramanian, H. et al. (2007). A heterologous DNA prime-Venezuelan equine encephalitis virus replicon particle boost dengue vaccine regimen affords complete protection from virus challenge in cynomolgus macaques. *J. Virol.* 81: 11634–11639.

60 Hu, H.M., Chen, H.W., Hsiao, Y. et al. (2016). The successful induction of T-cell and antibody responses by a recombinant measles virus-vectored tetravalent dengue vaccine provides partial protection against dengue-2 infection. *Hum. Vaccin. Immunother.* 12: 1678–1689.

61 Ravel, G., Mantel, N., Silvano, J. et al. (2017). Biodistribution and safety of a live and attenuated tetravalent dengue vaccine in the cynomolgus monkey. *Vaccine* 35: 5918–5923.

62 Sabchareon, A., Wallace, D., Sirivichayakul, C. et al. (2012). Protective efficacy of the recombinant, live-attenuated, CYD tetravalent dengue vaccine in Thai schoolchildren: a randomised, controlled phase 2b trial. *Lancet* 380: 1559–1567.

63 Capeding, M.R., Tran, N.H., Hadinegoro, S.R. et al. (2014). Clinical efficacy and safety of a novel tetravalent dengue vaccine in healthy children in Asia: a phase 3, randomised, observer-masked, placebo-controlled trial. *Lancet* 384: 1358–1365.

64 Villar, L., Dayan, G.H., Arredondo-Garcia, J.L. et al. (2015). Efficacy of a tetravalent dengue vaccine in children in Latin America. *New Engl. J. Med.* 372: 113–123.

65 Erasmus, J.H., Khandhar, A.P., Guderian, J. et al. (2018). A nanostructured lipid carrier for delivery of a replicating viral RNA provides single, low-dose protection against Zika. *Mol. Ther.* 26: 2507–2522.

66 Kurup, D., Wirblich, C., Lambert, R. et al. (2022). Measles-based Zika vaccine induces long-term immunity and requires NS1 antibodies to protect the female reproductive tract. *NPJ Vaccines* 7: 43.

67 Zika-Vaccine Dose Finding Study Regarding Safety, Immunogenicity and Tolerability (V186-001). https://clinicaltrials.gov/ct2/show/NCT02996890 (accessed 22 June 2022).

68 Safety and Immunogenicity of a Novel Vaccine Formulation MV-ZIKA-RSP (V187-001) (MV-ZIKA-RSP). https://clinicaltrials.gov/ct2/show/NCT04033068 (accessed 22 June 2022).

69 Morris-Downes, M.M., Sheahan, B.J., Fleeton, M.N. et al. (2001). A recombinant Semliki Forest virus particle vaccine encoding the prME and NS1 proteins of louping ill virus is effective in a sheep challenge model. *Vaccine* 19: 3877–3884.

70 Fleeton, M.N., Liljeström, P., Sheahan, B.J., and Atkins, G.J. (2000). Recombinant Semliki Forest virus particles expressing louping ill virus antigens induce a better protective response than plasmid-based DNA vaccines or an inactivated whole particle vaccine. *J. Gen. Virol.* 81: 749–758.

71 Fleeton, M.N., Chen, M., Berglund, P. et al. (2001). Self-replicative RNA vaccines elicit protection against influenza A virus, respiratory syncytial virus, and a tickborne encephalitis virus. *J. Infect. Dis.* 183: 1395–1398.

72 Roldão, A., Mellado, M.C., Castilho, L.R. et al. (2010). Virus-like particles in vaccine development. *Expert Rev. Vaccines* 9: 1149–1176.

73 Del Valle, J.R., Devaux, P., Hodge, G. et al. (2007). A vectored measles virus induces hepatitis B surface antigen antibodies while protecting macaques against virus challenge. *J. Virol.* 81: 10597–10605.

74 Reynolds, T.D., Buonocore, L., Rose, N.F. et al. (2015). Virus-like vesicle-based therapeutic vaccine vectors for chronic hepatis B virus infection. *J. Virol.* 89: 10407–10415.

75 Lorin, C., Mollet, L., Delebecque, F. et al. (2004). A single injection of recombinant measles virus vaccine expressing human immunodeficiency virus (HIV) type 1 clade B envelope glycoproteins induces neutralizing antibodies and cellular immune responses to HIV. *J. Virol.* 78: 146–157.

76 Rabinovich, S., Powell, R.I.R., Lindsay, R.W.B. et al. (2014). A novel, live-attenuated vesicular stomatitis virus vector displaying conformationally intact, functional HIV-1 envelope trimers that elicits potent cellular and humoral responses in mice. *PLoS One* 9: e106597.

77 Parks, C.L. (2017). Mucosal vaccination with a replication-competent VSV-HIV chimera delivering Env trimers protects rhesus macaques from rectal SHIV infection. *J. Acquir. Immune Defic. Syndr.* 2017: 74.

78 Rose, N.F., Marx, P.A., Luckay, A. et al. (2001). An effective AIDS vaccine based on live attenuated vesicular stomatitis virus recombinants. *Cell* 106: 539–549.

79 Mangion, M., Gélinas, J.-F., Zadeh Gashti, A.B. et al. (2020). Evaluation of novel HIV vaccine candidates using recombinant vesicular stomatitis virus vector produced in serum-free Vero cell cultures. *Vaccine* 38: 7949–7955.

80 Schnell, M.J., Foley, H.D., Siler, C.A. et al. (2000). Recombinant rabies virus as potential live-viral vaccines for HIV-1. *Proc. Natl. Acad. Sci. USA* 97: 3544–3549.

81 Brand, D., Lemiale, F., Turbica, I. et al. (1998). Comparative analysis of humoral immune responses to HIV type 1 envelope glycoproteins in mice immunized with a DNA vaccine, recombinant Semliki Forest virus RNA, or recombinant Semliki Forest virus particles. *AIDS Res. Hum. Retrovir.* 14: 1369–1377.

82 Center, R.J., Miller, A., Wheatley, A.K. et al. (2013). Utility of the Sindbis replicon system as an Env-targeted HIV vaccine. *Vaccine* 31: 2260–2266.

83 Giraud, A., Ataman-Onal, Y., and Battail, N. (1999). Generation of monoclonal antibodies to native human immunodeficiency virus type 1 envelope glycoprotein by immunization of mice with naked RNA. *J. Virol. Methods* 79: 75–84.

84 Ajbani, S.P., Velhal, S.M., Kadam, R.B. et al. (2017). Immunogenicity of virus-like Semliki Forest virus replicon particles expressing Indian HIV-1C gag, env and pol RT genes. *Immunol. Lett.* 190: 221–232.

85 Ljungberg, K., Whitmore, A.C., Fluet, M.E. et al. (2007). Increased immunogenicity of a DNA-launched Venezuelan equine encephalitis virus-based replicon DNA vaccine. *Virology* 81: 13412–13423.

86 Knudsen, M.L., Ljungberg, K., Tatoud, R. et al. (2015). Alphavirus replicon DNA expressing HIV antigens is an excellent prime for boosting with recombinant modified vaccinia Ankara (MVA) or with HIV gp140 protein antigen. *PLoS One* 10: e0117042.

87 Bogers, W.M., Oostermeijer, H., Mooij, P. et al. (2015). Potent immune responses in *Rhesus macaques* induced by nonviral delivery of self-amplifying RNA vaccine expressing HIV type 1 envelope with a cationic emulsion. *J. Infect. Dis.* 211: 947–955.

88 Wecker, M., Gilbert, P., Russell, N. et al. (2020). Phase I safety and immunogenicity evaluations of an alphavirus replicon HIV-1 subtype C gag vaccine in healthy HIV-1-uninfected adults. *Clin. Vaccine Immunol.* 19: 1651–1660.

89 Ito, T., Kumagai, T., Yamaji, Y. et al. (2020). Recombinant measles AIK-C vaccine strain expressing influenza HA protein. *Vaccine* 8: 149.

90 Ryder, A.B., Buonocore, L., Vogel, L. et al. (2015). A viable recombinant rhabdovirus lacking its glycoprotein gene and expressing influenza virus hemagglutinin and neuraminidase is a potent influenza vaccine. *J. Virol.* 89: 2820–2830.

91 Furuyama, W., Reynolds, P., Haddock, E. et al. (2020). A single dose of a vesicular stomatitis virus-based influenza vaccine confers rapid protection against H5 viruses from different clades. *NPJ Vaccines* 5: 4.

92 Schultz-Cherry, S., Dybing, J.K., Davis, N.L. et al. (2000). Influenza virus (A/HK/156/97) hemagglutinin expressed by an alphavirus replicon system protects against lethal infection with Hong Kong-origin H5N1 viruses. *Virology* 278: 55–59.

93 Vogel, A.B., Lambert, L., Kinnear, E. et al. (2018). Self-amplifying RNA vaccines give equivalent protection against influenza to mRNA vaccines but at much lower doses. *Mol. Ther.* 26: 446–455.

94 Beissert, T., Perkovic, M., Vogel, A. et al. (2020). A trans-amplifying RNA vaccine strategy for induction of potent protective immunity. *Mol. Ther.* 28: 119–128.

95 Krishnavajhala, H.R., Willimas, J., and Heidner, H. (2018). An Influenza A virus vaccine based on an M2e-modified alphavirus. *Arch. Virol.* 163: 483–488.

96 Démoulins, T., Ruggli, N., Gerber, M. et al. (2021). Self-amplifying pestivirus replicon RNA encoding influenza virus nucleoprotein and hemagglutinin promote humoral and cellular immune responses in pigs. *Front. Immunol.* 11: 622385.

97 A Phase 1/2 Clinical Trial on an Alphavirus Replicon Vaccine for Influenza. https://clinicaltrials.gov/ct2/show/ NCT00440362 (accessed 28 June 2022).

98 A Safety and Immunogenicity Trial in Adults 65 Years of Age or Over to Prevent Influenza (AVX502-003). https://clinicaltrials.gov/ct2/show/ NCT00706732 (accessed 28 June 2022).

99 Geall, A.J., Verma, A., Otten, G.R. et al. (2012). Non-viral delivery of self-amplifying RNA vaccines. *Proc. Natl. Acad. Sci. USA* 109: 14604–14609.

100 Prince, G.A., Horswood, R.L., and Chanock, R.M. (1985). Quantitative aspects of passive immunity to respiratory syncytial virus infection in infant cotton rats. *J. Virol.* 55: 517–520.

101 Sheahan, T., Whitmore, A., Long, K. et al. (2011). Successful vaccination strategies that protect aged mice from lethal challenge from influenza virus and heterologous severe acute respiratory syndrome coronavirus. *J. Virol.* 85: 217–230.

102 Liu, R., Wang, J., Shao, Y. et al. (2018). A recombinant VSV-vectored MERS-CoV vaccine induces neutralizing antibody and T cell responses in rhesus monkeys after single dose immunization. *Antivir. Res.* 150: 30–38.

103 Tao, J., Li, B., Shi, Y. et al. (2020). Attenuated porcine-derived type 2 bovine viral diarrhea virus as vector stably expressing viral gene. *J. Virol. Methods* 279: 113842.

104 Hörner, C., Schürmann, C., Auste, A. et al. (2020). A highly immunogenic and effective measles virus-based Th1-biased COVID-19 vaccine. *Proc. Natl. Acad. Sci. USA* 117: 32657–32666.

105 Clinical Trial to Evaluate the Safety and Immunogenicity of the COVID-19 Vaccine (COVID-19-101). https://clinicaltrials.gov/ct2/show/NCT04497298 (accessed 29 June 2022).

106 Case, J.B., Rothlauf, P.W., Chen, R.E. et al. (2020). Replication-competent vesicular stomatitis virus vaccine vector protects against SARS-CoV-2-mediated pathogenesis in mice. *Cell Host Microbe* 28: 465–474.

107 Dose Ranging Trial to Assess Safety and Immunogenicity of V590 (COVID-19 Vaccine) in Healthy Adults (V590-001) https://clinicaltrials.gov/ct2/show/NCT04569786 (accessed 29 June 2022).

108 Yahalom-Ronen, Y., Tamir, H., Melamed, S. et al. (2020). A single dose of recombinant VSV-ΔG-spike provides protection against SARS-CoV-2 challenge. *Nat. Commun.* 11: 6402.

109 Rosner, A., Steiner, M., Melamed, S. et al. (2022). rVSV-ΔG-SARS-CoV-2-S vaccine, repeated intramuscular (IM) toxicity, local tolerance, immunogenicity and biodistribution study in NZW rabbits. *Arch. Toxicol.* 96: 2329–2339.

110 Evaluate the Safety, Immunogenicity and Potential Efficacy of an rVSV-SARS-CoV-2-S Vaccine. https://clinicaltrials.gov/ct2/show/ NCT04608305 (accessed 1 July 2022).

111 Phase 2b/3 Trial of VSV-ΔG SARS-CoV-2 Vaccine (BRILIFE) Against Approved Comparator Vaccine. (BRILIFE002). https://clinicaltrials.gov/ct2/show/NCT04990466 (accessed 1 July 2022).

112 McKay, P.F., Hu, K., Blakney, A.K. et al. (2020). Self-amplifying RNA SARS-CoV-2 lipid nanoparticle vaccine candidate induces high neutralizing antibodies in mice. *Nat. Commun.* 11: 3523.

113 Pollock, K.M., Cheeseman, H.M., Szubert, A.J. et al. (2022). Safety and immunogenicity of a self-amplifying RNA vaccine against COVID-19: COVAC1, a Phase I dose-ranging trial. *E Clin. Med.* 44: 101262.

114 Safety, Tolerability and Immunogenicity of the candidate GEMCOVAC-19 (COVID-19) vaccine in healthy pediatric subjects of 5 to less than 18 years. www.ctri.nic.in/Clinicaltrials/pmaindet2.php?trialid=66638 (accessed 1 July 2022).

115 HDT Bio receives Emergency Use Approval for Covid-19 vaccine in India. www.pharmaceutical-technology.com/news/hdt-bio-vaccine-india-approval/ (accessed 1 July 2022).

116 De Alwis, R., Gan, E.S., Chen, S. et al. (2021). A single dose of self-transcribing and replicating RNA-based SARS-CoV-2 vaccine produces protective adaptive immunity in mice. *Mol. Ther.* 29: 1970–1983.

117 A Trial Evaluating the Safety and Immunogenicity of 3 COVID-19 SARS-CoV-2 RNA Vaccines in Healthy Adults. https://clinicaltrials.gov/ct2/show/NCT05037097 (accessed 4 July 2022).

118 Ascending Dose Study of Investigational SARS-CoV-2 Vaccine ARCT-021 in Healthy Adult Subjects. https://clinicaltrials.gov/ct2/show/NCT0448095 (accessed 4 July 2022).

119 A Trial Evaluating the Safety and Effects of an RNA Vaccine ARCT-021 in Healthy Adults. https://clinicaltrials.gov/ct2/show/NCT04668339 (accessed 4 July 2022).

120 Open Label Extension Study to Assess the Safety and Long-Term Immunogenicity of ARCT-021. https://clinicaltrials.gov/ct2/show/NCT04728347 (accessed 4 July 2022).

121 Arthur, R. 2022. Arcturus' self-amplifying COVID-19 mRNA vaccine meets Phase 3 primary end points. Biopharma-reporter.com.

122 Scaglione, A., Opp, S., Hurtado, A. et al. (2021). Combination of a Sindbis-SARS-CoV-2 spike vaccine and αOX40 antibody elicits protective immunity against SARS-CoV-2 induced disease and potentiates long-term SARS-CoV-2-specific humoral and T-cell immunity. *Front. Immunol.* 12: 719077.

123 Spencer, A., McKay, P.F., Beilij-Rammerstorfer, S. et al. (2021). Heterologous vaccination regimens with self-amplifying RNA and adenoviral COVID vaccines induce robust immune responses in mice. *Nat. Commun.* 12: 2893.

124 Mohammadi, G., Sotoudehnia Koranni, Z., and Jebali, A. (2021). The oral vaccine based on self-replicating RNA lipid nanoparticles can simultaneously neutralize bot SARS-CoV-2 variants alpha and delta. *Int. Immunopharmacol.* 101: 108231.

125 Thomas, J.M., Moen, S.T., Gnade, B.T. et al. (2009). Recombinant Sindbis virus vectors designed to express protective antigen of *Bacillus anthracis* protect animals from anthrax and display synergy with ciprofloxacin. *Clin. Vaccine Immunol.* 16: 1696–1699.

126 Wang, H.C., An, H.J., Yu, Y.Z., and Xu, Q. (2015). Potentiation of anthrax vaccines using protective antigen-expressing viral replicon vectors. *Immunol. Lett.* 163: 206–213.

127 Cabrera, A., Saez, D., Cespedes, S. et al. (2009). Vaccination with recombinant Semliki Forest virus particles expressing translation initiation factor 3 of Brucella abortus induces protective immunity in BALB/c mice. *Immunobiology* 214: 467–474.

128 Andersson, C., Vasconcelos, N.M., Sievertzon, M. et al. (2001). Comparative immunization study using RNA and DNA constructs encoding a part of the *Plasmodium falciparum* antigen Pf332. *Scand. J. Immunol.* 54: 117–124.

129 Tsuji, M., Bergmann, C.C., Takita-Sonoda, Y. et al. (1998). Recombinant Sindbis viruses expressing a cytotoxic T-lymphocyte epitope of a malaria parasite or of influenza virus elicit protection against the corresponding pathogen in mice. *J. Virol.* 72: 6907–6910.

130 Savar, N.S., Vallet, T., Azizi, M. et al. (2021). Quantitative evaluation of PpSP15- LmSTI1 fusion gene expression following transfection with an alphavirus-derived self-amplifying mRNA and conventional DNA vaccine platforms. *Mol. Cell. Probes* 59: 101749.

131 Kelvin, A.A. (2011). Outbreak of Chikungunya in the Republic of Congo and the global picture. *J. Infect. Dev. Ctries.* 5: 441–444.

132 Jansen, K.A. (2013). The 2005–2007 Chikungunya epidemic in Reunion: ambiguous etiologies, memories, and meaning-making. *Med. Anthropol.* 32: 174–189.

133 Weaver, S.C., Salas, R., Rico-Hesse, R. et al. (1996). Re-emergence of epidemic Venezuelan equine encephalomyelitis in South America VEE Study Group. *Lancet* 348: 436–440.

134 Lukashevich, I.S. and Pushko, P. (2016). Vaccine platforms to control Lassa fever. *Exp. Rev. Vaccines* 15: 1135–1150.

135 Coltart, C.E., Lindsey, B., Ghinai, I. et al. (2017). The Ebola outbreak 2013-2016: old lessons for new epidemics. *Philos. Trans. R. Soc. Lond. Ser. B Biol. Sci.* 372: 20160297.

136 Geisbert, T.W. and Feldmann, H. (2011). Recombinant vesicular stomatitis virus-based vaccines against Ebola and Marburg infections. *J. Infect. Dis.* 204: S1075–S1081.

137 Bache, B.E., Grobusch, M.P., and Agnandji, S.T. (2020). Safety, immunogenicity and risk-benefit analysis of rVSV-ΔG-ZEBOV-GP (V920) Ebola vaccine in Phase I-III clinical trials across regions. *Fut. Microbiol.* 15: https://doi.org/10.2217/fmb-2019-0237.

138 Guo, C., Zhou, Z., Wen, Z. et al. (2017). Global epidemiology of dengue outbreaks in 1990-2015: a systematic review and meta-analysis. *Front. Cell. Infect. Microbiol.* 7: 317.

139 Pielnaa, P., Al-Saadawe, M., Saro, A. et al. (2020). Zika virus spread, epidemiology, genome, transmission cycle, clinical manifestation, associated challenges, vaccine and antiviral drug development. *Virology* 543: 34–42.

140 Guy, B., Saville, M., and Lang, J. (2010). Development of Sanofi Pasteur tetravalent dengue vaccine. *Hum. Vaccines* 6: 696–705.

141 Racine, T., Kobinger, G.P., and Arts, E.J. (2017). Development of an HIV vaccine using a vesicular stomatitis virus vector expressing designer HIV-1 envelope glycoproteins to enhance humoral responses. *AIDS Res. Ther.* 14: 55.

142 McCoy, L.E., van Gils, M.J., Ozorowski, G. et al. (2016). Holes in the glycan shield of the native HIV envelope are a target of trimer-elicited neutralizing antibodies. *Cell Rep.* 16: 2327–2338.

143 Kong, L., Ju, B., Chen, Y. et al. (2016). Key gp120 glycans pose roadblocks to the rapid development of VRC01-class antibodies in an HIV-1-infected Chinese donor. *Immunity* 44: 939–950.

144 Sebastian, S. and Lambe, T. (2018). Clinical advances in viral-vectored influenza vaccines. *Vaccine* 6: 29.

145 Lythgoe, M.P. and Middleton, P. (2021). Comparison of COVID-19 vaccine approvals at the US Food and Drug Administration, European Medicines Agency, and Health Canada. *JAMA Netw. Open* 4: e2114531.

146 Lundstrom, K. (2021). Self-replicating RNA viruses for vaccine development against infectious diseases and cancer. *Vaccine* 9: 1187.

147 Lundstrom, K. (2022). Self-replicating vehicles based on negative strand RNA viruses. *Cancer Gene Ther.* 30 (6): 771–784. https://doi.org/10.1038/s41417-022-00436-7.

148 Fukuhara, H., Ino, Y., and Todo, T. (2016). Oncolytic virus therapy: a new era of cancer treatment at dawn. *Cancer Sci.* 107: 1373–1379.

149 Murphy, A.M., Morris-Downes, M.M., Sheahan, B.J., and Atkins, G.J. (2000). Inhibition of human lung carcinoma cell growth by apoptosis induction using Semliki Forest virus recombinant particles. *Gene Ther.* 7: 1477–1482.

150 Ying, H., Zaks, T.Z., Wang, R.-F. et al. (1999). Cancer therapy using a self-replicating RNA vaccine. *Nat. Med.* 5: 823–827.

151 Allen, C., Opyrchal, M., Aderca, I. et al. (2013). Oncolytic measles virus strains have a significant antitumor activity against glioma stem cells. *Gene Ther.* 2: 444–449.

152 Wang, X., Wang, J.P., Rao, X.M. et al. (2005). Prime-boost vaccination with plasmid and adenovirus gene vaccines control HER2/neu+ metastatic breast cancer in mice. *Breast Cancer Res.* 7: R580–R588.

153 Lachman, L.B., Rao, X.M., Kremer, R.H. et al. (2001). DNA vaccination against neu reduces breast cancer incidence and metastasis in mice. *Cancer Gene Ther.* 8: 259–268.

154 Wang, X., Wang, J.-P., Maughan, M.F., and Lachman, L.B. (2005). Alphavirus replicon particles containing the gene for HER2/neu inhibit breast cancer growth and tumorigenesis. *Breast Cancer Res.* 7: R145–R155.

155 A Study to Evaluate Concurrent VRP-HER2 Vaccination and Pembrolizumab for Patients With Breast Cancer. https://clinicaltrials.gov/ct2/show/NCT03632941 (accessed on 18 August 2022).

156 Crosby, E.J., Gwin, W., Blackwell, K. et al. (2019). Vaccine-induced memory $CD8^+$ T cells provide clinical benefit in HER2 expressing breast cancer: a mouse to human translational study. *Clin. Cancer Res.* 25: 2723–2736.

157 Velders, M.P., McElhiney, S., Cassetti, M.C. et al. (2001). Eradication of established tumors by vaccination with Venezuelan equine encephalitis virus replicon particles delivering human papillomavirus 16 E7 RNA. *Cancer Res.* 61: 7861–7867.

158 Daemen, T., Riezebos-Brilman, A., Bungener, L. et al. (2003). Eradication of established HPV16-transformed tumours after immunisation with recombinant Semliki Forest virus expressing a fusion protein of E6 and E7. *Vaccine* 21: 1082–1088.

159 Komdeur, F.L., Singh, A., Van de Wall, S. et al. (2021). First-in-human phase I clinical trial of an SFV based RNA replicon cancer vaccine against HPV-induced cancers. *Mol. Ther.* 29: 611–625.

160 Ip, P.P., Boerma, A., Walczak, M. et al. (2015). Antigen design enhances the immunogenicity of Semliki Forest virus-based therapeutic human papillomavirus vaccines. *Gene Ther.* 22: 560–567. https://doi.org/10.1038/gt.2015.24.

161 Van de Wall, S., Ljungberg, K., Ip, P.P. et al. (2018). Potent therapeutic efficacy of an alphavirus replicon DNA vaccine expressing human papilloma virus E6 and E7 antigens. *Onco Targets Ther* 7: e1487913.

162 Cantarella, G., Liniger, M., Zuniga, A. et al. (2009). Recombinant measles virus-HPV vaccine candidates for prevention of cervical carcinoma. *Vaccine* 27: 3386–3390.

163 Gupta, G., Giannino, V., Rishi, N., and Glueck, R. (2016). Immunogenicity of next-generation HPV vaccines in non-human primates: measles-vectored HPV vaccine versus *Pichia pastoris* recombinant protein vaccine. *Vaccine* 34: 4724–4731.

164 Liao, J.B., Publicover, J., Rose, J.K., and DiMaio, D. (2008). Single-dose, therapeutic vaccination of mice with vesicular stomatitis virus expressing human papillomavirus type 16 E7 protein. *Clin. Vaccine Immunol.* 15: 817–824.

165 Brandsma, J.L., Shylankevich, M., Su, Y. et al. (2007). Vesicular stomatitis virus-based therapeutic vaccination targeted to the E1, E2, E6, and E7 proteins of cottontail rabbit papillomavirus. *J. Virol.* 81: 5749–5758.

166 Lyons, J.A., Sheahan, B.J., Galbraith, S.E. et al. (2007). Inhibition of angiogenesis by a Semliki Forest virus vector expressing VEGFR-2 reduces tumour growth and metastasis in mice. *Gene Ther.* 14: 503–513.

167 Crosby, E.J., Hobeika, A.C., Niedzweicki, D. et al. (2020). Long-term survival of patients with stage III colon cancer treated with VRP-CEA(6D), an alphavirus vector that increases the $CD8^+$ effector memory T cell to Treg ration. *J. Immunother. Cancer* 8: e001662.

168 Hoang-Le, D., Smeenk, L., Anraku, I. et al. (2009). A Kunjin replicon vector encoding granulocyte macrophage colony-stimulating factor for intra-tumoral gene therapy. *Gene Ther.* 16: 190–199.

169 Grossardt, C., Engeland, C.E., Bossow, S. et al. (2013). Granulocyte-macrophage colony-stimulating factor-armed oncolytic measles virus is an effective therapeutic cancer vaccine. *Hum. Gene Ther.* 24: 644–654.

170 Patel, M.R., Jacobson, B.A., Belgum, H. et al. (2014). Measles vaccine strains for virotherapy of non-small cell lung carcinoma. *J. Thorac. Oncol.* 9: 1101–1110.

171 Avogadri, F., Merghoub, T., Maughan, M.F. et al. (2010). Alphavirus replicon particles expressing TRP-2 provide potent therapeutic effect on melanoma through activation of humoral and cellular immunity. *PLoS One* 5: e12670.

172 Avogadri, F., Zappasodi, R., Yang, A. et al. (2014). Combination of alphavirus replicon particle-based vaccination with immunomodulatory antibodies: therapeutic activity in the B16 melanoma mouse model and immune correlates. *Cancer Immunol. Res.* 2: 448–458.

173 Yin, X., Wang, W., Zhu, X. et al. (2015). Synergistic antitumor efficacy of combined DNA vaccines targeting tumor cells and angiogenesis. *Biochem. Biophys. Res. Commun.* 465: 239–244.

174 McAllister, A., Arbetman, A.E., Mandl, S. et al. (2000). Recombinant yellow fever viruses are effective therapeutic vaccines for treatment of murine solid tumors and pulmonary metastases. *J. Virol.* 74: 9197–9205.

175 Zhang, Y.Q., Tsai, Y.C., Monie, A. et al. (2010). Enhancing the therapeutic effect against ovarian cancer through a combination of viral oncolysis and antigen-specific immunotherapy. *Mol. Ther.* 18: 692–699.

176 Hasegawa, K., Pham, L., O'Connor, M.K. et al. (2006). Dual therapy of ovarian cancer using measles viruses expressing carcinoembryonic antigen and sodium iodide symporter. *Clin. Cancer Res.* 12: 1868–1875.

177 Galanis, E., Hartmann, L.C., Cliby, W.A. et al. (2010). Phase I trial of intraperitoneal administration of an oncolytic measles virus strain engineered to express carcinoembryonic antigen for recurrent ovarian cancer. *Cancer Res.* 70: 875–882.

178 Morse, M.A., Hobeika, A.C., Osada, T. et al. (2010). An alphavirus vector overcomes the presence of neutralizing antibodies and elevated numbers of Tregs to induce immune responses in humans with advanced cancer. *J. Clin. Invest.* 120: 3234–3241.

179 Durso, R.J., Andjelic, S., Gardner, J.P. et al. (2007). A novel alphavirus vaccine encoding prostate-specific membrane antigen elicits potent cellular and humoral immune responses. *Clin. Cancer Res.* 13: 3999–4008.

180 Slovin, S.F., Kehoe, M., Durso, R. et al. (2013). A phase I dose escalation trial of vaccine replicon particles (VRP) expressing prostate-specific membrane antigen (PSMA) in subjects with prostate cancer. *Vaccine* 31: 943–949.

181 Garcia-Hernandez, M.L., Gray, A., Hubby, B., and Kast, W.M. (2007). In vivo effects of vaccination with six-transmembrane epithelial antigen of the prostate: A candidate antigen for treating prostate cancer. *Cancer Res.* 67: 1344–1351.

182 Garcia-Hernandez, M.L., Gray, A., Hubby, B. et al. (2008). Prostate stem cell antigen vaccination induces a long-term protective immune response against prostate cancer in the absence of autoimmunity. *Cancer Res.* 68: 861–869.

183 Msaouel, P., Iankov, I.D., Allen, C. et al. (2009). Engineered measles virus as a novel oncolytic therapy against prostate cancer. *Prostate* 69: 82–91.

184 Yamanaka, R., Zullo, S.A., Ramsey, J. et al. (2001). Induction of therapeutic antitumor anti-angiogenesis by intratumoral injection of genetically engineered endostatin-producing Semliki Forest virus. *Cancer Gene Ther.* 8: 796–802.

185 Jiang, B., Huang, D., He, W. et al. (2021). Inhibition of glioma using a novel non-neurotoxic vesicular stomatitis virus. *Neurosurg. Focus.* 50: E9. https://doi.org/10.3171/2020.11.FOCUS20839.

186 Yamanaka, R., Tsuchiya, N., Yajima, N. et al. (2003). Induction of an antitumor immunological response by an intratumoral injection of dendritic cells pulsed with genetically engineered Semliki Forest virus to produce interleukin-18 combined with the systemic administration of interleukin-12. *J. Neurosurg.* 99: 746–753.

187 Roche, F.P., Sheahan, B.J., O'Mara, S.M., and Atkins, G.J. (2010). Semliki Forest virus-mediated gene therapy the RG2 rat glioma. *Neuropathol. Appl. Neurobiol.* 36: 648–660. https://doi.org/10.1111/j.1365-2990.2010.01110.x.

188 Yamanaka, R. and Xanthopoulos, K.G. (2005). Induction of antigen-specific immune responses against malignant brain tumors by intramuscular injection of sindbis DNA encoding gp100 and IL-18. *DNA Cell Biol.* 24: 317–324.

189 Osada, T., Berglund, P., Morse, M.A. et al. (2012). Co-delivery of antigen and IL-12 by Venezuelan equine encephalitis virus replicon particles enhances antigen-specific immune responses and anti-tumor effects. *Cancer Immunol. Immunother.* 61: 1941–1951. https://doi.org/10.1007/s00262-012-1248-y.

190 Rodriguez-Madoz, J.R., Prieto, J., and Smerdou, C. (2005). Semliki forest virus vectors engineered to express higher IL-12 levels induce efficient elimination of murine colon adenocarcinomas. *Mol. Ther.* 12: 153–163.

191 Kramer, M.G., Masner, M., Casales, E. et al. (2015). Neoadjuvant administration of Semliki Forest virus expressing interleukin-12 combined with attenuated Salmonella eradicates breast cancer metastasis and achieves long-term survival in immunocompetent mice. *BMC Cancer* 15: 620.

192 Patel, M.R., Jacobson, B.A., Ji, Y. et al. (2015). Vesicular stomatitis virus expressing interferon-β is oncolytic and promotes antitumor immune responses in a syngeneic murine model of non-small cell lung cancer. *Oncotarget* 6: 33165–33177.

193 Granot, T. and Meruelo, D. (2012). The role of natural killer cells in combinatorial anti-cancer therapy using Sindbis viral vector and irinotecan. *Cancer Gene Ther.* 19: 588–591.

194 Ren, H., Boulikas, T., Lundstrom, K. et al. (2003). Immunogene therapy of recurrent glioblastoma multiforme with a liposomally encapsulated replication-incompetent Semliki Forest virus vector carrying the human interleukin-12 gene – a phase I/II clinical protocol. *J. Neuro-Oncol.* 64: 147–154. https://doi.org/10.1007/BF02700029.

195 Heikkilä, J.E., Vähä-Koskela, M.J., Ruotsalainen, J.J. et al. (2010). Intravenously administered alphavirus vector VA7 eradicates orthotopic human glioma xenografts in nude mice. *PLoS One* 5: e8603.

196 Martikainen, M., Niittykoski, M., von und zu Frauenberg, M. et al. (2015). MicroRNA attenuated clone of virulent Semliki Forest virus overcomes antiviral type I interferon in resistant mouse CT-2A glioma. *J. Virol.* 89: 10637–10647.

197 Su, K.Y. and Balasubramaniam, V.R.M.T. (2019). Zika virus as oncolytic therapy for brain cancer: myth or reality? *Front. Microbiol.* 10: 2715.

198 Zhang, X., Mao, G., and Van den Pol, A.N. (2018). Chikungunya-vesicular stomatitis chimeric virus targets and eliminates brain tumors. *Virology* 522: 244–259.

199 Muik, A., Dold, C., Geiß, Y. et al. (2012). Semireplication-competent vesicular stomatitis virus as a novel platform for oncolytic therapy. *J. Mol. Med. (Berl)* 90: 959–970.

200 Zhang, J., Liu, Y., Tan, J. et al. (2021). Necroptotic virotherapy of oncolytic alphavirus M1 cooperated with Doxorubicin displays promising therapeutic efficacy in TNBC. *Oncogene* 40: 4783–4795.

201 Niavarani, S.R., Lawson, C., Boudaud, M. et al. (2020). Oncolytic vesicular stomatitis virus-based cellular vaccine improves triple-negative breast cancer outcome by enhancing natural killer and CD8(+) T-cell functionality. *J. Immunother. Cancer* 8: e000465. https://doi.org/10.1136/jitc-2019-000465.

202 Ebert, O., Harbaran, S., Shinozaki, K., and Woo, S.L. (2005). Systemic therapy of experimental breast cancer metastases by mutant vesicular stomatitis virus in immune-competent mice. *Cancer Gene Ther.* 12: 350–358.

203 Yang, B., Shi, J., Sun, Z. et al. (2020). Attenuated measles virus overcomes radio- and chemoresistance in human breast cancer cells by inhibiting the non-homologous end joining pathway. *Oncol. Rep.* 44: 2253–2264.

204 Sugiyama, T., Yoneda, M., Kuraishi, T. et al. (2013). Measles virus selectively blind to signaling lymphocyte activation molecule as a novel oncolytic virus for breast cancer treatment. *Gene Ther.* 20: 338–347.

205 Unno, Y., Shino, Y., Kondo, F. et al. (2005). Oncolytic virotherapy for cervical and ovarian cancer cells by Sindbis virus strain AR339. *Clin. Cancer Res.* 11: 4553–4560.

206 Alkayyal, A.A., Tai, L.-H., Kennedy, M.A. et al. (2017). NK-Cell recruitment is necessary for eradication of peritoneal carcinomatosis with an IL12-expressing Maraba virus cellular vaccine. *Cancer Immunol. Res.* 5: 211–221.

207 McGray, A.J.R., Huang, R.Y., Battaglia, S. et al. (2019). Oncolytic Maraba virus armed with tumor antigen boosts vaccine priming and reveals diverse therapeutic response patterns when combined with checkpoint blockade in ovarian cancer. *J. Immunother. Cancer* 7: 189. https://doi.org/10.1186/s40425-019-0641-x.

208 Le Boeuf, F., Selman, M., Son, H.H. et al. (2017). Oncolytic Maraba virus MG1 as a treatment for sarcoma. *Int. J. Cancer* 141: 1257–1264. https://doi.org/10.1002/ijc.30813.

209 Pol, J.G., Acuna, S.A., Yadollahi, B. et al. (2018). Preclinical evaluation of a MAGE-A3 vaccination utilizing the oncolytic Maraba virus currently in first-in-human trials. *Onco Targets Ther* 8: e1512329. https://doi.org/10.1080/2162402X.2018.1512329.

210 MG1 Maraba/MAGE-A3, With and Without Adenovirus Vaccine With Transgenic MAGE-A3 Insertion in Incurable MAGE-A3-Expressing Solid Tumours. https://clinicaltrials.gov/ct2/show/NCT02285816 (accessed 25 August 2022).

211 Oncolytic MG1-MAGEA3 With Ad-MAGEA3 Vaccine in Combination With Pembrolizumab for Non-Small Cell Lung Cancer Patients. https://clinicaltrials.gov/ct2/show/NCT02879760 (accessed 25 August 2022).

212 Yamaki, M., Shinozaki, K., Sakaguchi, T. et al. (2013). The potential of recombinant vesicular stomatitis virus-mediated virotherapy against metastatic colon cancer. *Int. J. Mol. Med.* 31: 299–306.

213 Määttä, A.M., Mäkinen, K., Ketola, A. et al. (2008). Replication competent Semliki Forest virus prolongs survival in experimental lung cancer. *Int. J. Cancer* 123: 1704–1711.

214 Granot, T., Yamanashi, Y., and Meruelo, D. (2014). Sindbis viral vectors transiently deliver tumor-associated antigens to lymph nodes and elicit diversified antitumor $CD8^+$ T-cell immunity. *Mol. Ther.* 22: 112–122.

215 Zhao, D., Chen, P., Yang, H. et al. (2013). Live attenuated measles virus vaccine induces apoptosis and promotes tumor regression in lung cancer. *Oncol. Rep.* 29: 199–204.

216 Boisgerault, N., Guillerme, J.B., Pouliquen, D. et al. (2013). Natural oncolytic activity of live-attenuated measles virus against human lung and colorectal adenocarcinomas. *Biomed. Res. Int.* 2013: 387362.

217 Ammour, Y., Ryabaya, O., Shchetinina, Y. et al. (2020). The susceptibility of human melanoma cells to infection with the Leningrad-16 vaccine strain of measles virus. *Viruses* 12: 173.

218 Kimpel, J., Urbiola, C., Koske, I. et al. (2018). The Oncolytic virus VSV-GP is effective against malignant melanoma. *Viruses* 10: 108.

219 Dold, C., Rodriguez Urbiola, C., Wollmann, G. et al. (2016). Application of interferon modulators to overcome partial resistance to ovarian cancers to VSV-GP oncolytic viral therapy. *Mol. Ther. Oncolytics* 3: 16021.

220 Hasegawa, K., Nakamura, T., Harvey, M. et al. (2006). The use of a tropism-modified measles virus in folate receptor-targeted virotherapy of ovarian cancer. *Clin. Cancer Res.* 12: 6170–6178.

221 Sun, S., Liu, Y., He, C. et al. (2021). Combining Nanoknife with M1 oncolytic virus enhances anticancer activity in pancreatic cancer. *Cancer Lett.* 502: 9–24. https://doi.org/10.1016/j.canlet.2020.12.1018.

222 Murphy, A.M., Besmer, D.M., Moerdyk-Schauwecker, M. et al. (2012). Vesicular stomatitis virus as an oncolytic agent against pancreatic ductal adenocarcinoma. *J. Virol.* 86: 3073–3087.

223 Hastle, E., Besmer, D.M., Shah, N.R. et al. (2013). Oncolytic vesicular stomatitis virus in an immunocompetent model of MUC1-positive or MUC1-nulll pancreatic ductal adenocarcinoma. *J. Virol.* 87: 10283–10294.

224 Awano, M., Fujiyuki, T., Shoji, K. et al. (2016). Measles virus selectively blind to signaling lymphocyte activity molecule has oncolytic efficacy against nectin-4-expressing pancreatic cancer cells. *Cancer Sci.* 107: 1647–1652. https://doi.org/10.1111/cas.13064.

225 Zhao, X., Huang, S., Luo, H. et al. (2014). Evaluation of vesicular stomatitis virus mutant as an oncolytic agent against prostate cancer. *Int. J. Clin. Exp. Med.* 7: 1204–1213.

226 Urbiola, C., Santer, F.R., Petersson, M. et al. (2018). Oncolytic activity of the rhabdovirus VSV-GP against prostate cancer. *Int. J. Cancer* 143: 1786–1796.

227 Barry, G., Fragkoudis, R., Ferguson, M.C. et al. (2010). Semliki forest virus-induced endoplasmic reticulum stress accelerates apoptotic death of mammalian cells. *J. Virol.* 84: 7369–7377. https://doi.org/10.1128/JVI.02310-09.

228 Urban, C., Rhême, C., Maerz, S. et al. (2008). Apoptosis induced by Semliki Forest virus is RNA replication dependent and mediated via Bak. *Cell Death Differ.* 15: 1396–1407. https://doi.org/10.1038/cdd.2008.61.

229 Bergman, I., Whitaker-Dowling, P., Gao, Y. et al. (2003). Vesicular stomatitis virus expressing a chimeric Sindbis glycoprotein containing an Fc antibody binding domain target to Her2/neu overexpressing breast cancer cells. *Virology* 316: 337–347.

230 Griffin, D.E. (2016). Neurotropic alphaviruses. In: *Neurotropic Viral Infections* (ed. C. Reiss and E. Springer), 175–204. Switzerland: Cham.

231 Son, H.A., Zhang, L., Cuong, B.K. et al. (2018). Combination of vaccine-strain measles and mumps viruses enhances oncolytic activity against human solid malignancies. *Cancer Investig.* 7: 106–117.

5

Circular RNA Therapeutics and Vaccines

Xiang Liu and Guizhi Zhu

University of Michigan, Biointerfaces Institute, College of Pharmacy, Department of Pharmaceutical Sciences, 428 Church Street, Ann Arbor, MI 48109, USA

5.1 Introduction

Due to the success of recent messenger RNA (mRNA) COVID vaccines [1, 2], mRNA therapeutics and vaccines have experienced significant and broad interest not only for infectious diseases such as SARS-CoV-2, Zika virus, and influenza virus [3] but also for various types of cancers [4–6], genetic disorders [7, 8], and autoimmune diseases [9, 10]. Moreover, nonviral delivery technologies (e.g. lipid nanoparticle [LNP]) for mRNA therapeutics and vaccines bypass some concerns associated with conventional pathogen-based vaccines, such as poor pharmacokinetics and the safety risk of genomic integration or virulent reversion [11, 12]. Yet, the suboptimal stability of mRNA indicates room to improve its efficiency and duration of protein expression and therapeutic/prophylactic efficacies [13, 14]. Moreover, the extensive nucleotide modifications during manufacturing [15] as well as the costly cold-chain storage and transportation pose particular challenges to the implementation of mRNA vaccines, especially in developing countries [16]. Circular RNA (circRNA) has emerged as an attractive type of RNA to partially address these issues due to its high stability [17]. This chapter will discuss natural circRNAs [18], the design and synthesis of engineered circRNA, and their biomedical applications [19].

The natural circRNA was once known as the rare by-product of aberrant splicing of a 5′ splice site to an upstream 3′ splice site [20, 21]. Recently, with the advancements of RNA sequencing technologies, such as high-throughput deep sequencing of RNA and the recent single-cell universal polyA-independent RNA sequencing (SUPeR-seq) using fixed anchor sequences with random primers, circRNA transcripts have been identified in various biological samples [22, 23]. So far, circRNA has been found pervasive within metazoan cells ranging from protists [24], fungi [25], and plants [26] to fruit flies [27], mice [22], and humans [28]. The increasing number of discoveries on the physiological functions of circRNA, ranging from protein and gene sponges and cell activity modulators to protein translation templates [29], has aroused interest in developing technologies for synthetic circRNA as novel therapeutics and vaccines [17].

Trends in mRNA Vaccine Research, First Edition. Edited by Gabor Tamas Szabo and Norbert Pardi.

5.2 The Biogenesis and Physiological Functions of Natural circRNA

5.2.1 The Biogenesis of Natural circRNA

Natural circRNAs typically arise from RNA canonical linear-splicing or back-splicing processes (Figure 5.1). A small fraction of circRNA derives from the canonical linear splicing of which an upstream donor splice site joins forces with a downstream acceptor splice site, generating an intronic lariat in some mammalian cells [30, 31]. The predominant mechanism involves back splicing, which requires the connection of a 5′ donor splice site to a 3′ acceptor splice site, resulting in the formation of a 3′–5′ phosphodiester bond at the junction site and the generation of an exon-containing circRNA [25]. Since numerous circRNAs have been identified in various tissues, there has been a growing recognition of the involvement of endogenous circRNAs in versatile biological processes encompassing cell proliferation, gene transcription, tumorigenesis, protein expression, and the regulation of immune response [29].

5.2.2 The Physiological Functions of Natural circRNA

Though the physiological functions of biogenic circRNAs have not been fully elucidated, recent discoveries uncovered their versatile biological roles as, for instance, molecular sponges. As sponges, circRNAs can bind with microRNA (miRNA) as well as proteins. For example, by sequestering miRNAs, circHIPK2, originating from the homeodomain interacting protein kinase 2 (*HIPK2*) gene, can free the target mRNAs and consequently increase the transcription of these mRNA [32]. Similarly, the overexpression of circHIPK3 accelerates the progression of multiple malignancies through the sponge effect [33, 34]. It is worth noting that the covalently closed structure of circRNA contributes to its long half-life compared to linear RNA counterparts, which extended its stability as sponges compared to linear RNA sponges. Moreover, these characteristics allow circRNA to be utilized as potential cancer diagnostic tools. Additionally, when bound to proteins, circRNAs can inhibit or promote the physiological functions of the cognate proteins. For example, circRNA can be an antagonist for cyclic GMP–AMP (cGAMP) synthase (cia-cGAS) in the nucleus of long-term hematopoietic stem cells (LT-HSCs) [35]. cGAMP synthase functions as a cytosolic sensor for double-stranded DNA and can subsequently generate cGAMP, which activates the stimulator of interferon genes (STING) pathway, triggering the production of type I interferons [36]. Cia-cGAS can sequester nuclear cGAS from self-DNA, thus reducing the production of type I Interferon and protecting LT-HSCs from immune exhaustion [37]. In contrast, a class of exon–intron circRNAs (ElciRNAs) acts as scaffolds in the nucleus, which could help the proteins regulate gene expression [38]. As another physiological function, natural circRNA may be translated to proteins or peptides. Despite the lack of 5′ cap and untranslated regions (UTRs), some natural circRNAs can be translated into protein mediated by the internal ribosome entry site (IRES) [39].

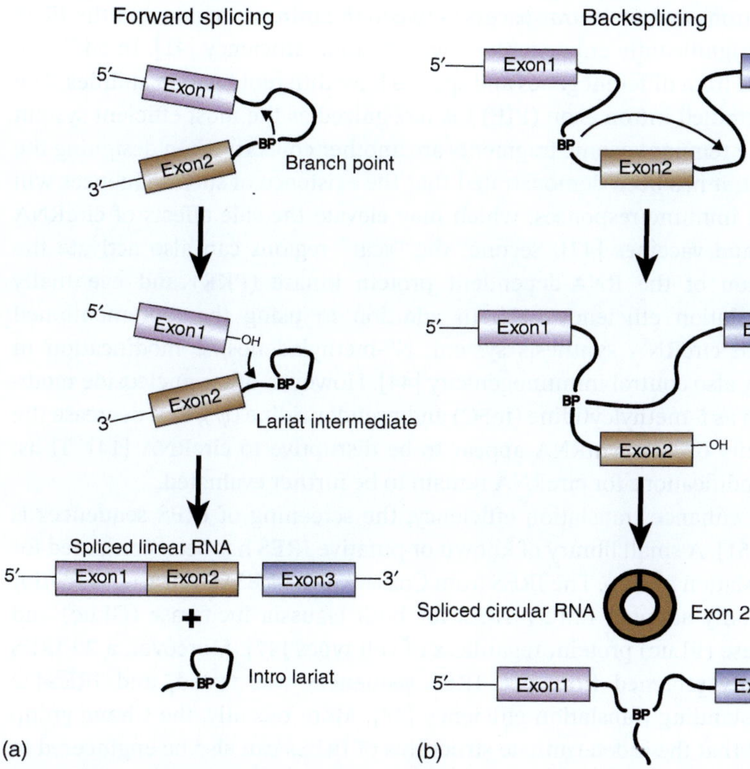

Figure 5.1 The biogenesis processes of natural intronic circRNA and exonic circRNA. (a) Intronic circRNA is produced during forward splicing, where an upstream donor splice site joins forces with a downstream acceptor splice site. (b) Exonic circRNA is produced by back splicing, where a downstream donor splice site connects with an upstream acceptor. Source: Liu et al. [17]/with permission of Elsevier.

The structurally diverse IRES sequences initiate protein translation via various mechanisms [40].

5.3 The Design and Synthesis of Synthetic circRNA

Synthetic circRNAs have garnered increasing interest in the development of RNA therapeutics, vaccines as well as diagnostic or analytic tools. The design and optimization of circRNA constructs have been the subject of the investigation to enhance circRNA circularization and improve the efficiency of protein and peptide translation.

5.3.1 Design Considerations of Synthetic circRNAs for Vaccines

The circularization and protein/peptide translation efficiency are vital for circRNA therapeutics and vaccines. As described above, the "homology arm" at the 5′ and 3′

ends of the introns and the extra spacers between the intronic region and the IRES structure can significantly enhance the circularization efficiency [41]. In addition, introns derived from different genes and species have different ligation abilities. The Anabaena permuted intron exon (PIE) I is recognized as the most efficient system so far [19]. The remnant exonic fragments are another concern when designing the circRNA. First, it has been demonstrated that the existence of such sequences will induce innate immune responses, which may elevate the side effects of circRNA therapeutics and vaccines [42]. Second, the "scar" regions can also activate the phosphorylation of the RNA-dependent protein kinase (PKR) and eventually decrease translation efficiency [43]. In addition to using the aforementioned "scar-less" PIE circRNA synthesis system, N^6-methyladenosine modification in circRNAs may also control immunogenicity [44]. However, other nucleoside modifications, such as 5-methylcytidine (m5C) and pseudouridine (ψ), that decrease the immunogenicity of linear mRNA appear to be disruptive to circRNA [14]. Thus, nucleoside modifications for circRNA remain to be further evaluated.

In order to enhance translation efficiency, the screening of IRES sequences is essential [45–51]. A small library of known or putative IRES has been compared for circRNA translation *in vitro*. The IRES from Coxsackievirus B3 (CVB3) was superior to the commonly adopted EMCV IRES for both Gaussia luciferase (GLuc) and firefly luciferase (FLuc) protein, regardless of cell types [47]. Moreover, a 20-IRES library virtually screened from 600 IRES sequences was tested, and IRES422 exhibited outstanding translation efficiency [48]. More recently, the Chang group demonstrated that the indeterminate structures of IRESs can also be engineered to enhance translation efficiency [50]. With the insertion of eukaryotic initiation factor 4G aptamer to IRES derived from human rhinovirus B3 (HRVB3), the circRNA can achieve a higher protein expression level than its counterpart linear mRNA in some cases [50]. Nonetheless, though the translation efficiency can be improved by sequence engineering, the length of the virus-derived IRESs (typically 500–800 nucleotides) is much longer than the combination of 5′ UTR and 3′ UTR, which are about 200 or 300 nucleotides in the two COVID-19 mRNA vaccines (mRNA-1273 and BNT162b2) approved for humans [49, 52]. Some truncated versions of IRES can be screened for circRNA [53]. Similar to mRNA, optimizing the open reading frame (ORF) sequence further enhances both the stability and translatability of circRNA [54]. An artificial intelligence-assisted approach has been developed to facilitate the screening for lead circRNA (with optimal structural stability and codon usage) among a large number of synonymous circRNA candidates [55]. Further investigation of the interaction between the inalterable IRES structure and the ORF region should be conducted as well.

5.3.2 Approaches to circRNA Synthesis

Typically, current methods of circRNA synthesis involve the production of one or multiple precursor linear RNAs, which are then circularized through chemical or enzymatic ligation. Those precursor RNAs are synthesized by either chemical or enzymatic approaches depending on the circularization methods [56, 57]. The current approach of chemical oligonucleotide synthesis uses phosphoramidate for solid phase synthesis [58]. The oligonucleotides raw products are detached from the solid supports (controlled pore glass and macroporous polystyrene) [58]. Combined with postsynthesis purification, chemical synthesis can generate oligonucleotides with high purity. However, the length of chemically synthesized RNA is limited by the pore size of the solid support as well as the limited yields of stepwise chemical reactions [19]. This limitation can be circumvented by ligating multiple oligonucleotides to one large circRNA with a length of about 300 nucleotides [46]. For larger circRNA (>500 nucleotides), the synthesis is often conducted in two steps: *in vitro* transcription (IVT) followed by circularization. IVT uses RNA polymerases derived from bacteriophages such as T7, SP6, or T3 [59], as well as DNA templates, usually amplified or directly cut off from the corresponding bacteria-amplified plasmids or enzymatically synthesized DNA templates. The purity and amount of the DNA templates and the incubation time of the polymerase-containing system impact the yield and purity of the mRNA product.

There are also multiple approaches to RNA circularization via chemical, enzymatic, and ribozymatic ligation (Figure 5.2). For example, chemical circularization approaches use condensing agents such as cyanogen bromide (BrCN) or water-soluble 1-ethyl-3-(3-dime-thylaminopropyl) carbodiimide (EDC) to facilitate the ligation of 5′-end phosphate with 3′-end hydroxyl on linear RNA (Figure 5.2a) [60]. This method's notable challenge is forming 2′,5′-phosphodiester bonds. 2′-Deoxynucleotides at the 3′-end of oligonucleotides to be ligated or circularized can be employed as a solution [61]. However, the yields of natural phosphodiester bond formation are often unsatisfactory. More efficient circularization can be achieved by alternative chemistries such as ligation of a 3′-thiophosphate with a tosylate 5′-end or iodinated 5′ end, ligation of a 3′-aldehyde with a 5′ oxoamine, and ligation of a 5′- or 3′-azide with a 3′- or 5′-alkyne [61]. Although these chemistries allow high yield and specificity, introducing the functional groups is costly, and the safety and toxicity of the resulting unnatural linkages remain to be comprehensively evaluated.

Protein enzymatic RNA circularization typically has high efficiency (Figure 5.2b). RNA ligases derived from T4 bacteriophage, such as T4 RNA ligases 1 and 2, are commonly utilized to ligate monophosphate-terminated linear RNAs [62]. It is reported that T4 RNA ligase 1 prefers ligating single-stranded RNAs with cytidine and adenosine at the ligation site ($A > G \geq C > U$ for the 3′-terminal nucleotide acceptor and $pC > pU > pA > pG$ for the 5′-terminal nucleotide donor) [59, 63]. In contrast, the T4 RNA ligase 2 prefers the junction in a double-stranded region [59]. The preference of the type of nucleotides at the ligation site of T4 RNA ligase 2 is yet to be validated. Besides, both T4 RNA ligase 1 and 2 can achieve the ligation of single-stranded RNA with the help of a splint nucleic acid [64]. This splint is a single-stranded DNA/RNA oligonucleotide partially complementary to the RNA of interest and can bring the two termini into proximity. This approach essentially enhanced the circularization efficiency and ligate up to four oligonucleotides, generating a mini circRNA vaccine [53]. However, it is also possible for this method to produce dimeric or multimeric RNA via undesired intermolecular RNA

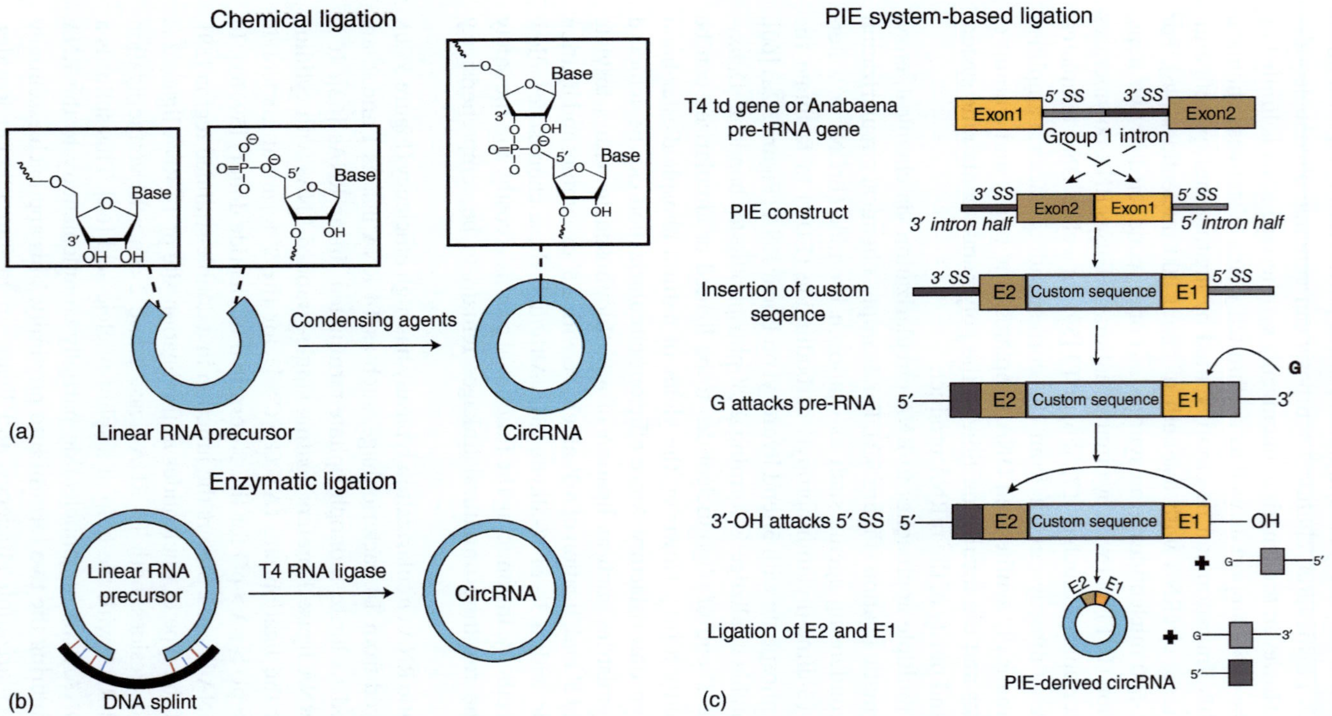

Figure 5.2 Schematic illustration of RNA circularization methods. (a) Chemical RNA ligation by the conjugation of 5′-end phosphate with 3′-end hydroxyl. (b) Enzymatic RNA ligation is catalyzed by T4 RNA ligase using DNA splints that bring the ends of RNA into close proximity to facilitate site-specific ligation. (c) PIE system-based RNA ligation. Permutation of a native group I intron and insertion of a custom RNA into the exonic region generate a PIE construct, which is then spontaneously circularized in the presence of free guanosine to form circRNA of the native exonic RNA. Source: Liu et al. [17]/with permission of Elsevier.

ligation [53]. Rational design of the precursor RNA enabling the formation of a few intramolecular base pairs at the terminal may reduce the output of intermolecular products, but this has only been validated in short precursor RNAs (less than 30 nt) thus far [65]. It is also worth noting that the enzymatic methods only function when the nucleotides have monophosphates. When using RNA products from IVT, which have 5′ triphosphates, dephosphorylation and rephosphorylation may be needed to cleave 5′ triphosphate and attach a 5′ monophosphate [19]. Alternatively, enzymes such as RNA 5′ pyrophosphohydrolase (RppH) can eliminate β and γ phosphates, which may be helpful for the above preprocessing of RNA before circularization [66].

Ribozymes, a class of RNA enzymes, can also synthesize circRNA by catalyzing the ligation of precursor linear RNAs through PIE systems (Figure 5.2c). The Anabaena and Tetrahymena pre-tRNA group I intron was first used to construct the PIE system by transferring the 5′ half to the tail of the exon but keeping the 3′ half of the intron at the head [67]. They can generate circRNA with a short-defined sequence within the exonic region [67]. Other backbones, such as group I intron from the phage T4 (thymidylate synthase) td gene and group II introns, have also been used to synthesize circRNAs [68, 69]. However, long insertion sequences (>1 kb) may reduce the splicing efficiency due to the interference with the splicing sites from forming a stable complex [41]. Wesselhoeft et al. added perfectly complementary "homology arms" at the 5′ and 3′ ends of the precursor RNA to bring the 5′ and 3′ splice sites into proximity [47]. In order to reduce the interactions between PIE and IRES structures, RNA spacers were inserted between them and increased the circularization efficiency to over 80% [47]. With the advanced PIE system, they have achieved the synthesis of multiple protein-coding circRNAs, including FLuc (2384 nt) and Cas9 endonuclease (4934 nt) [47]. Later, Wang and coworkers developed a PIE II-mediated circRNA synthesis platform that can introduce a short "scar" sequence of 12 nt, in contrast to the "scar" sequence of 80 nt generated by the PIE I system [70]. Though truncated, the "scar" sequence remains in the final circRNA product and may induce undesired immunogenicity, which in turn not only aggravates the side effects of the products but also circumvents the biostability and translation efficiency of circRNA [42]. More recently, two "scar-less" systems have reduced such concerns and achieved precise circRNA synthesis. One is using optimized *Tetrahymena thermophila* group I intron with inserted antisense region at both ends that can subsequently fall off, and the other is concealing the exon sequences into the ORF based on synonymous codon usage [48, 71]. Large-scale manufacturing of circRNAs via the PIE strategy has been evidenced by the successful circularization of the IVT products from 1 L transcription reaction with 4 g final circRNA products [48]. However, the manufacturing is still limited by a required high-pressure liquid chromatography (HPLC) purification process to rule out by-products like introns or uncircularized RNA precursors [47, 48, 70, 71].

5.4 The Applications of Synthetic circRNA as Novel Therapeutics and Vaccines

As sequence design and synthesis techniques continue to progress, more synthetic circRNA have been engineered to explore their applications for cancer and infectious diseases [13, 53, 55, 72–75]. Synthetic circRNAs containing foreign introns have been demonstrated to trigger robust immune signaling and effectively hinder viral infection through a mechanism involving retinoic acid-inducible gene I (RIG-I) [76]. Also, the immunogenicity of circRNA was found to be related to its secondary structures and the methods used for circRNA synthesis as well as administered dosage [42, 76]. A foreign intron-derived engineered circRNA vaccine encoding severe acute respiratory syndrome 2 (SARS-CoV-2) receptor-binding domain (RBD) antigen was reported [13] with efficient and long-lasting RBD translation (Figure 5.3a) [13]. After one-month storage at 4 °C or fortnight at room temperature, the circRNA-encapsulated LNPs showed the same antigen expression levels as the fresh prepared ones, suggesting the great stability of these formulations under these conditions (Figure 5.3b). The enhanced thermostability of circRNA partially overcomes the stringent storage and transportation requirement for mRNA counterparts [12]. The vaccines induced the production of interleukin-6 (IL-6) and monocyte chemoattractant protein-1 (MCP-1), indicating the activation of innate immune responses (Figure 5.3c) [13]. Interestingly, the animals showed steady body temperature after vaccine administration, suggesting that this vaccine has a promising safety profile (Figure 5.3d) [13]. Further, the testing of circRNA vaccines against multiple infectious diseases such as rabies virus and varicella-zoster virus further leverages the capability of circRNA as next-generation prophylactic vaccines [55].

CircRNA vaccines can be designed to elicit not only humoral responses [13, 55] but also cytotoxic T-cell responses [74, 75]. In mice, circRNA-LNP vaccines triggered potent antigen-specific T-cell responses in multiple tumor models and displayed comparable prophylactic and therapeutic effects to modified-mRNA LNP [75]. Interestingly, in a late-stage syngeneic melanoma mouse model, the circRNA showed a synergic antitumor effect with adoptive T-cell therapy, which explores the application of circRNA in tumor therapy [75]. The adjuvanticity of circRNA is demonstrated by the enhanced cytokine release in myeloid cells by codelivery of peptide antigens and irrelevant circRNA, supporting the synergic antitumor effect of circRNA with other immune therapies [74].

In addition to encoding antigen proteins/peptides, circRNA can also be used for the expression of cytokines (interferon-alpha 2b, interleukin-12 single chain, and active interleukin-12), which can, in turn, modulate the intratumoral and systematic antitumor immune responses [73]. Besides, circRNA was designed to express proteolysis targeting chimera (PROTAC) containing the binding domain of the protein of interest and an E3 ligase [72]. The proliferating cell nuclear antigen-targeting degradation induced by circRNA PROTAC caused immunogenic cell death and exhibited tumor suppression effect *in vivo* [72]. Taken together, these studies highlight the great potential of synthetic protein/peptide-encoding circRNAs as prophylactic and therapeutic vaccines.

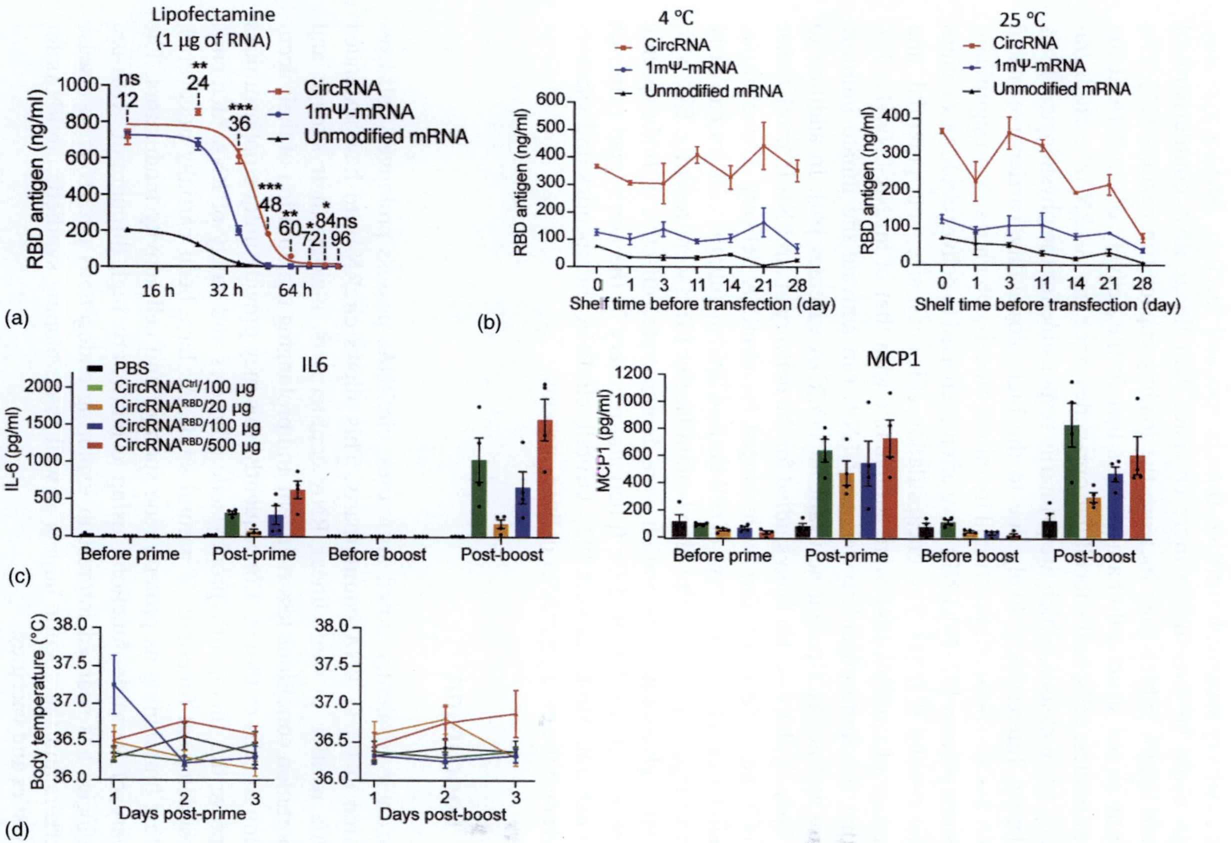

Figure 5.3 A circRNA vaccine encoding SARS-CoV-2 RBD antigen. (a) Measurements of RBD antigen expression in the supernatant of HEK293T cells transfected with circRNA^{RBD} and 1mΨ-mRNA^{RBD} through Lipofectamine MessengerMax. (b) Measurement of RBD antigen expression in the supernatant of HEK293T cells transfected with LNP-circRNA^{RBD}, LNP-1mΨ-mRNA^{RBD}, and LNP-unmodified-mRNA^{RBD} that were stored at 4 °C (left) and 25 °C (right) for the indicated duration, prior to transfection into cells. (c) IL-6 and MCP-1 levels in the plasma of circRNA-immunized rhesus macaques. (d) Body temperature of circRNA-immunized rhesus macaques. Source: Qu et al. [13]/with permission of Elsevier.

5.5 The Delivery Systems of Synthetic circRNA

Synthetic circRNAs have been primarily delivered using well-established viral and nonviral delivery systems for mRNA therapeutics and vaccines. Besides, typically, circRNA could be structurally more compact than linear RNA counterparts of the same length, which may increase the loading capacity in carriers [17]. The covalently closed structural characteristics benefit the delivery of circRNA at the levels of tissues, cells, and subcellular organelles since the circRNAs resist degradation by exonucleases, which are primarily responsible for the physiological RNA degradation. Interestingly, likely due to the high biostability, carrier-free naked circRNA has also been administrated in animal models, which results in significant therapeutic efficacy [77–79]. LNPs have often been used to deliver circRNA vaccines and therapeutics [13, 14]. The encapsulation efficiency, size, zeta potential, and morphology of circRNA-LNP were comparable with that of mRNA-LNP [13, 75]. Note that the immunogenicity of many LNPs can activate the innate immune response and act as a potent adjuvant for circRNA vaccines [80]. In addition to LNPs, lipopolyplex has also been studied for the delivery of circRNA [55, 74]. Other types of nanocarriers can also be leveraged for circRNA delivery. For example, extracellular vesicles (EVs), a type of cell-derived lipid membrane vesicles, can carry circRNA cargo to penetrate the blood–brain barrier [81]. More recently, EVs with rabies virus glycoprotein decoration were demonstrated effective in brain-specific delivery of circRNA designed for functional recovery in the nonhuman primates (NHP) ischemic stroke models [82]. Overall, circRNA therapeutics and vaccines may leverage the existing mRNA delivery systems.

5.6 Conclusion

Due to their covalently closed structures, circRNAs possess prolonged half-lives compared to linear RNA counterparts. This allows circRNAs to have extended shelf-life relative to their linear RNA counterparts, making their storage and transportation conditions less stringent and prolonging the duration of their accumulation in cells or tissues. Consequently, this may provide unique opportunities to improve the therapeutic/prophylactic efficacies and safety of RNA medicine. The physiological functions of natural circRNAs have been partially uncovered, including functioning as protein/gene sponges and cell activity modulators. The discovery of versatile functions using evolutionary high-throughput RNA-seq technologies has sparked interest in exploring endogenous circRNAs as disease biomarkers and therapeutic targets as well as developing synthetic circRNAs for theranostics and vaccines.

Synthetic circRNAs have been designed and synthesized as noncoding or protein-coding therapeutics and vaccines. Compared to conventional vaccines based on pathogens, DNA, and proteins/peptides, circRNA may offer great thermostability and biostability with minimal safety concerns associated with genomic integration or virulent reversion. However, current circRNA synthesis approaches still have some limitations, such as suboptimal circularization efficiency and the purification of circRNA. It is envisioned that technological advancement in these fields can address these limitations and advance the development of circRNA therapeutics and vaccines. Lastly, delivery systems, such as EVs and LNPs, have demonstrated the potential for efficient circRNA delivery with minimal side effects. In conclusion, circRNA represents an emerging class of RNA therapeutics and vaccines with exciting potential for biomedical applications.

References

1 Baden, L.R., El Sahly, H.M., Essink, B. et al. (2021). Efficacy and safety of the mRNA-1273 SARS-CoV-2 vaccine. *N. Engl. J. Med.* 384 (5): 403–416.

2 Vogel, A.B., Kanevsky, I., Che, Y. et al. (2021). BNT162b vaccines protect rhesus macaques from SARS-CoV-2. *Nature* 592 (7853): 283–289.

3 Alameh, M.G., Weissman, D., and Pardi, N. (2020). Messenger RNA-based vaccines against infectious diseases. In: *mRNA Vaccines*, Current Topics in Microbiology and Immunology, vol. 440 (ed. D. Yu and B. Petsch), 111–145. Cham: Springer International Publishing. https://link.springer.com/10.1007/82_2020_202 (accessed 30 June 2023).

4 Sahin, U., Oehm, P., Derhovanessian, E. et al. (2020). An RNA vaccine drives immunity in checkpoint-inhibitor-treated melanoma. *Nature* 585 (7823): 107–112.

5 Oberli, M.A., Reichmuth, A.M., Dorkin, J.R. et al. (2017). Lipid nanoparticle assisted mRNA delivery for potent cancer immunotherapy. *Nano Lett.* 17 (3): 1326–1335.

6 Huang, P., Jiang, L., Pan, H. et al. (2023). An integrated polymeric mRNA vaccine without inflammation side effects for cellular immunity mediated cancer therapy. *Adv. Mater.* 35 (3): 2207471.

7 Liu, J., Chang, J., Jiang, Y. et al. (2019). Fast and efficient CRISPR/Cas9 genome editing in vivo enabled by bioreducible lipid and messenger RNA nanoparticles. *Adv. Mater.* 31 (33): 1902575.

8 Zhang, X., Zhao, W., Nguyen, G.N. et al. (2020). Functionalized lipid-like nanoparticles for in vivo mRNA delivery and base editing. *Sci. Adv.* 6 (34): eabc2315.

9 Kato, Y., Morita, T., and Kumanogoh, A. (2023). Efficacy and risk of mRNA vaccination in patients with autoimmune inflammatory rheumatic diseases. *Inflamm. Regen.* 43 (1): 1.

10 Krienke, C., Kolb, L., Diken, E. et al. (2021). A noninflammatory mRNA vaccine for treatment of experimental autoimmune encephalomyelitis. *Science* 371 (6525): 145–153.

11 Hou, X., Zaks, T., Langer, R., and Dong, Y. (2021). Lipid nanoparticles for mRNA delivery. *Nat. Rev. Mater.* 6: 1078–1094. https://www.nature.com/articles/s41578-021-00358-0 (accessed 10 August 2021).

12 Pardi, N., Hogan, M.J., Porter, F.W., and Weissman, D. (2018). mRNA vaccines - a new era in vaccinology. *Nat. Rev. Drug Discov.* 17 (4): 261–279.

13 Qu, L., Yi, Z., Shen, Y. et al. (2022). Circular RNA vaccines against SARS-CoV-2 and emerging variants. *Cell* 185 (10): 1728–1744.e16.

14 Wesselhoeft, R.A., Kowalski, P.S., Parker-Hale, F.C. et al. (2019). RNA circularization diminishes immunogenicity and can extend translation duration in vivo. *Mol. Cell* 74 (3): 508–520.e4.

15 Gilbert, W.V., Bell, T.A., and Schaening, C. (2016). Messenger RNA modifications: form, distribution, and function. *Science* 352 (6292): 1408–1412.

16 Wouters, O.J., Shadlen, K.C., Salcher-Konrad, M. et al. (2021). Challenges in ensuring global access to COVID-19 vaccines: production, affordability, allocation, and deployment. *Lancet* 397 (10278): 1023–1034.

17 Liu, X., Zhang, Y., Zhou, S. et al. (2022). Circular RNA: an emerging frontier in RNA therapeutic targets, RNA therapeutics, and mRNA vaccines. *J. Control. Release* 348: 84–94.

18 Zhang, Y., Xue, W., Li, X. et al. (2016). The biogenesis of nascent circular RNAs. *Cell Rep.* 15 (3): 611–624.

19 Obi, P. and Chen, Y.G. (2021). The design and synthesis of circular RNAs. *Methods* 196: 85–103. https://www.sciencedirect.com/science/article/pii/S1046202321000657 (accessed 12 December 2021) .

20 Pasman, Z., Been, M.D., and Garcia-Blanco, M.A. (1996). Exon circularization in mammalian nuclear extracts. *RNA* 2 (6): 603–610.

21 Nigro, J.M., Cho, K.R., Fearon, E.R. et al. (1991). Scrambled exons. *Cell* 64 (3): 607–613.

22 Fan, X., Zhang, X., Wu, X. et al. (2015). Single-cell RNA-seq transcriptome analysis of linear and circular RNAs in mouse preimplantation embryos. *Genome Biol.* 16: 148.

23 Westholm, J.O., Miura, P., Olson, S. et al. (2014). Genome-wide analysis of drosophila circular RNAs reveals their structural and sequence properties and age-dependent neural accumulation. *Cell Rep.* 9 (5): 1966–1980.

24 Broadbent, K.M., Broadbent, J.C., Ribacke, U. et al. (2015). Strand-specific RNA sequencing in *Plasmodium falciparum* malaria identifies developmentally regulated long non-coding RNA and circular RNA. *BMC Genomics* 16: 454.

25 Barrett, S.P., Wang, P.L., and Salzman, J. (2015). Circular RNA biogenesis can proceed through an exon-containing lariat precursor. *elife* 4: e07540.

26 Lu, T., Cui, L., Zhou, Y. et al. (2015). Transcriptome-wide investigation of circular RNAs in rice. *RNA* 21 (12): 2076–2087.

27 Kramer, M.C., Liang, D., Tatomer, D.C. et al. (2015). Combinatorial control of Drosophila circular RNA expression by intronic repeats, hnRNPs, and SR proteins. *Genes Dev.* 29 (20): 2168–2182.

28 Veno, M.T., Hansen, T.B., Veno, S.T. et al. (2015). Spatio-temporal regulation of circular RNA expression during porcine embryonic brain development. *Genome Biol.* 16: 245.

29 Chen, L.L. (2020). The expanding regulatory mechanisms and cellular functions of circular RNAs. *Nat. Rev. Mol. Cell Biol.* 21 (8): 475–490.

30 Qian, L., Vu, M.N., Carter, M., and Wilkinson, M.F. (1992). A spliced intron accumulates as a lariat in the nucleus of T cells. *Nucleic Acids Res.* 20 (20): 5345–5350.

31 Talhouarne, G.J. and Gall, J.G. (2014). Lariat intronic RNAs in the cytoplasm of *Xenopus tropicalis* oocytes. *RNA* 20 (9): 1476–1487.

32 Huang, R., Zhang, Y., Han, B. et al. (2017). Circular RNA HIPK2 regulates astrocyte activation via cooperation of autophagy and ER stress by targeting MIR124-2HG. *Autophagy* 13 (10): 1722–1741.

33 Liu, D.C., Song, L.L., Li, X.Z. et al. (2021). Circular RNA circHIPK3 modulates prostate cancer progression via targeting miR-448/MTDH signaling. *Clin. Transl. Oncol.* 23 (12): 2497–2506.

34 Luo, N., Liu, S., Li, X. et al. (2021). Circular RNA circHIPK3 promotes breast cancer progression via sponging MiR-326. *Cell Cycle* 20 (13): 1320–1333.

35 Chen, Q., Sun, L., and Chen, Z.J. (2016). Regulation and function of the cGAS-STING pathway of cytosolic DNA sensing. *Nat. Immunol.* 17 (10): 1142–1149.

36 Zhang, Y., Shen, T., Zhou, S. et al. (2020). pH-Responsive STING-activating DNA nanovaccines for cancer immunotherapy. *Adv. Therap.* 3 (9): 2000083.

37 Xia, P., Wang, S., Ye, B. et al. (2018). A circular RNA protects dormant hematopoietic stem cells from DNA sensor cGAS-mediated exhaustion. *Immunity* 48 (4): 688–701.e7.

38 Li, Z., Huang, C., Bao, C. et al. (2015). Exon-intron circular RNAs regulate transcription in the nucleus. *Nat. Struct. Mol. Biol.* 22 (3): 256–264.

39 Chen, C.Y. and Sarnow, P. (1995). Initiation of protein synthesis by the eukaryotic translational apparatus on circular RNAs. *Science* 268 (5209): 415–417.

40 Filbin, M.E. and Kieft, J.S. (2009). Toward a structural understanding of IRES RNA function. *Curr. Opin. Struct. Biol.* 19 (3): 267–276.

41 Vicens, Q., Paukstelis, P.J., Westhof, E. et al. (2008). Toward predicting self-splicing and protein-facilitated splicing of group I introns. *RNA* 14 (10): 2013–2029.

42 Liu, C.X., Guo, S.K., Nan, F. et al. (2022). RNA circles with minimized immunogenicity as potent PKR inhibitors. *Mol. Cell* 82 (2): 420–434.e6.

43 Kariko, K., Muramatsu, H., Welsh, F.A. et al. (2008). Incorporation of pseudouridine into mRNA yields superior nonimmunogenic vector with increased translational capacity and biological stability. *Mol. Ther.* 16 (11): 1833–1840.

44 Chen, Y.G., Chen, R., Ahmad, S. et al. (2019). N6-methyladenosine modification controls circular RNA immunity. *Mol. Cell* 76 (1): 96–109.e9.

45 Vimberg, V., Tats, A., Remm, M., and Tenson, T. (2007). Translation initiation region sequence preferences in *Escherichia coli*. *BMC Mol. Biol.* 8 (1): 100.

46 Abe, N., Matsumoto, K., Nishihara, M. et al. (2015). Rolling circle translation of circular RNA in living human cells. *Sci. Rep.* 5 (1): 16435.

47 Wesselhoeft, R.A., Kowalski, P.S., and Anderson, D.G. (2018). Engineering circular RNA for potent and stable translation in eukaryotic cells. *Nat. Commun.* 9 (1): 2629.

48 Qiu, Z., Hou, Q., Zhao, Y. et al. (2022). Clean-PIE: a novel strategy for efficiently constructing precise circRNA with thoroughly minimized immunogenicity to direct potent and durable protein expression. *BioRxiv* http://biorxiv.org/lookup/doi/10.1101/2022.06.20.496777 (accessed 14 July 2023).

49 Fan, X., Yang, Y., Chen, C., and Wang, Z. (2022). Pervasive translation of circular RNAs driven by short IRES-like elements. *Nat. Commun.* 13 (1): 3751.

50 Chen, R., Wang, S.K., Belk, J.A. et al. (2023). Engineering circular RNA for enhanced protein production. *Nat. Biotechnol.* 41 (2): 262–272.

51 Kozak, M. (1987). An analysis of 5′-noncoding sequences from 699 vertebrate messenger RNAs. *Nucleic Acids Res.* 15 (20): 8125–8148.

52 Fang, E., Liu, X., Li, M. et al. (2022). Advances in COVID-19 mRNA vaccine development. *Signal Transduct. Target. Ther.* 7 (1): 94.

53 Zhu, G. and Zhang, Y. (2022). Mini circular RNA therapeutics and vaccines and methods of use thereof. WO2022173730A1.

54 Zhang, H., Zhang, L., Lin, A. et al. (2023). Algorithm for optimized mRNA design improves stability and immunogenicity. *Nature* 621: 396–403. https://www.nature.com/articles/s41586-023-06127-z (accessed 21 July 2023).

55 Xu, C., Zhang, L., Wang, W. et al. (2023). Improving the circularization efficiency, stability and translatability of circular RNA by circDesign. *BioRxiv* http://biorxiv.org/lookup/doi/10.1101/2023.07.09.548293 (accessed 21 July 2023).

56 Rong, M., He, B., McAllister, W.T., and Durbin, R.K. (1998). Promoter specificity determinants of T7 RNA polymerase. *Proc. Natl. Acad. Sci. USA* 95 (2): 515–519.

57 Usman, N. and Cedergren, R. (1992). Exploiting the chemical synthesis of RNA. *Trends Biochem. Sci.* 17 (9): 334–339.

58 Glazier, D.A., Liao, J., Roberts, B.L. et al. (2020). Chemical synthesis and biological application of modified oligonucleotides. *Bioconjug. Chem.* 31 (5): 1213–1233.

59 Petkovic, S. and Muller, S. (2018). Synthesis and engineering of circular RNAs. *Methods Mol. Biol.* 1724: 167–180.

60 Nakamoto, K., Abe, N., Tsuji, G. et al. (2020). Chemically synthesized circular RNAs with phosphoramidate linkages enable rolling circle translation. *Chem. Commun. (Camb.)* 56 (46): 6217–6220.

61 Muller, S. and Appel, B. (2017). In vitro circularization of RNA. *RNA Biol.* 14 (8): 1018–1027.

62 Romaniuk, E., McLaughlin, L.W., Neilson, T., and Romaniuk, P.J. (1982). The effect of acceptor oligoribonucleotide sequence on the T4 RNA ligase reaction. *Eur. J. Biochem.* 125 (3): 639–643.

63 Chen, X. and Lu, Y. (2021). Circular RNA: biosynthesis in vitro. *Front. Bioeng. Biotechnol.* 9: 787881.

64 Lang, K. and Micura, R. (2008). The preparation of site-specifically modified riboswitch domains as an example for enzymatic ligation of chemically synthesized RNA fragments. *Nat. Protoc.* 3 (9): 1457–1466.

65 Chen, H., Cheng, K., Liu, X. et al. (2020). Preferential production of RNA rings by T4 RNA ligase 2 without any splint through rational design of precursor strand. *Nucleic Acids Res.* 48 (9): e54.

66 Deana, A., Celesnik, H., and Belasco, J.G. (2008). The bacterial enzyme RppH triggers messenger RNA degradation by 5′ pyrophosphate removal. *Nature* 451 (7176): 355–358.

67 Puttaraju, M. and Been, M.D. (1992). Group I permuted intron-exon (PIE) sequences self-splice to produce circular exons. *Nucleic Acids Res.* 20 (20): 5357–5364.

68 Jarrell, K.A. (1993). Inverse splicing of a group II intron. *Proc. Natl. Acad. Sci. USA* 90 (18): 8624–8627.

69 Ford, E. and Ares, M. (1994). Synthesis of circular RNA in bacteria and yeast using RNA cyclase ribozymes derived from a group I intron of phage T4. *Proc. Natl. Acad. Sci. U. S. A.* 91 (8): 3117–3121.

70 Chen, C., Wei, H., Zhang, K. et al. (2022). A flexible, efficient, and scalable platform to produce circular RNAs as new therapeutics. *BioRxiv* http://biorxiv.org/lookup/doi/10.1101/2022.05.31.494115 (accessed 14 July 2023).

71 Cui, J., Zhang, L., Zhang, Z. et al. (2023). A precise and efficient circular RNA synthesis system based on a ribozyme derived from *Tetrahymena thermophila*. *Nucleic Acids Res.* 51 (14): e78.

72 Yang, J., Sun, J., Zhu, J. et al. (2022). Circular mRNA encoded PROTAC (Ribo-PROTAC) as a new platform for the degradation of intracellular therapeutic targets. *BioRxiv* http://biorxiv.org/lookup/doi/10.1101/2022.04.22.489232 (accessed 21 July 2023).

73 Yang, J., Zhu, J., Sun, J. et al. (2022). Intratumoral delivered novel circular mRNA encoding cytokines for immune modulation and cancer therapy. *Mol. Ther. Nucleic Acids* 30: 184–197.

74 Amaya, L., Grigoryan, L., Li, Z. et al. (2023). Circular RNA vaccine induces potent T cell responses. *Proc. Natl. Acad. Sci. U. S. A.* 120 (20): e2302191120.

75 Li, H., Peng, K., Yang, K. et al. (2022). Circular RNA cancer vaccines drive immunity in hard-to-treat malignancies. *Theranostics* 12 (14): 6422–6436.

76 Chen, Y.G., Kim, M.V., Chen, X. et al. (2017). Sensing self and foreign circular RNAs by intron identity. *Mol. Cell* 67 (2): 228–238.e5.

77 Zhang, L., Liang, D., Chen, C. et al. (2018). Circular siRNAs for reducing off-target effects and enhancing long-term gene silencing in cells and mice. *Mol. Ther. Nucleic Acids.* 10: 237–244.

78 Wang, Z., Ma, K., Cheng, Y. et al. (2019). Synthetic circular multi-miR sponge simultaneously inhibits miR-21 and miR-93 in esophageal carcinoma. *Lab. Investig.* 99 (10): 1442–1453.

79 Zhang, L., Liang, D., Wang, Y. et al. (2018). Caged circular siRNAs for photomodulation of gene expression in cells and mice. *Chem. Sci.* 9 (1): 44–51.

80 Verbeke, R., Hogan, M.J., Loré, K., and Pardi, N. (2022). Innate immune mechanisms of mRNA vaccines. *Immunity* 55 (11): 1993–2005.

81 Zhang, Z.G., Buller, B., and Chopp, M. (2019). Exosomes - beyond stem cells for restorative therapy in stroke and neurological injury. *Nat. Rev. Neurol.* 15 (4): 193–203.

82 Yang, L., Han, B., Zhang, Z. et al. (2020). Extracellular vesicle-mediated delivery of circular RNA SCMH1 promotes functional recovery in rodent and nonhuman primate ischemic stroke models. *Circulation* 142 (6): 556–574.

6

Good Manufacturing Practices and Upscaling of mRNA Vaccine Production

Eleni Stamoula[1,2], Theofanis Vavilis[3,4], Ioannis Dardalas[2], and Georgios Papazisis[2,5]

[1] *Biomedical Research Foundation of the Academy of Athens, Centre of Basic Research, Department of Biotechnology, 4 Soranou Ephessiou St., 11527 Athens, Greece*
[2] *Aristotle University of Thessaloniki, School of Medicine, Department of Clinical Pharmacology, University Campus, 54124 Thessaloniki, Greece*
[3] *Aristotle University of Thessaloniki, School of Medicine, Laboratory of Biology and Genetics, University Campus, 54124 Thessaloniki, Greece*
[4] *European University Cyprus, Department of Dentistry, 6 Diogenous Str., Egkomi, Nicosia 2404, Cyprus*
[5] *Aristotle University of Thessaloniki, School of Medicine, Special Unit for Biomedical Research and Education, Clinical Research Unit, University Campus, 54124 Thessaloniki, Greece*

6.1 Introduction

The severe acute respiratory syndrome coronavirus 2 (SARS-CoV-2) pandemic brought into spotlight a new type of vaccine candidate once considered impractical for clinical use due to several challenges associated with messenger ribonucleic acid (mRNA) technology [1]. These challenges included the inherent instability of mRNA, making it susceptible to degradation by RNases, its propensity to trigger immune responses upon administration, and the difficulty in effectively delivering naked mRNA molecules *in vivo*, which limited its therapeutic potential [1]. However, these challenges were largely overcome through technological advancements in RNA modifications such as structural optimization and nucleoside modifications alongside with advancements in formulations, enabling mRNA vaccines to meet the demands of the pandemic and assume a prominent defensive role against the virus [2]. The characteristics that allowed this "unlikely" candidate to be swiftly drafted against the pandemic were the ease, speed, and adaptability that theoretically characterized its manufacturing as well, since it was faster and more flexible than previously elaborated and widely used vaccines and vaccine development strategies [3–5].

mRNA technology cleverly shifted the arduous task of antigen production from the industrial complex to the natural expert, the cell, bypassing many complicated steps required for traditional vaccine developments. The laboratory-scale production of an mRNA therapeutic product is straightforward [6]. The DNA template encoding for the desired protein is designed and incorporated in a suitable vector, e.g. a plasmid. After transfection into a bacterial culture, the plasmid is harvested, linearized,

Trends in mRNA Vaccine Research, First Edition. Edited by Gabor Tamas Szabo and Norbert Pardi.

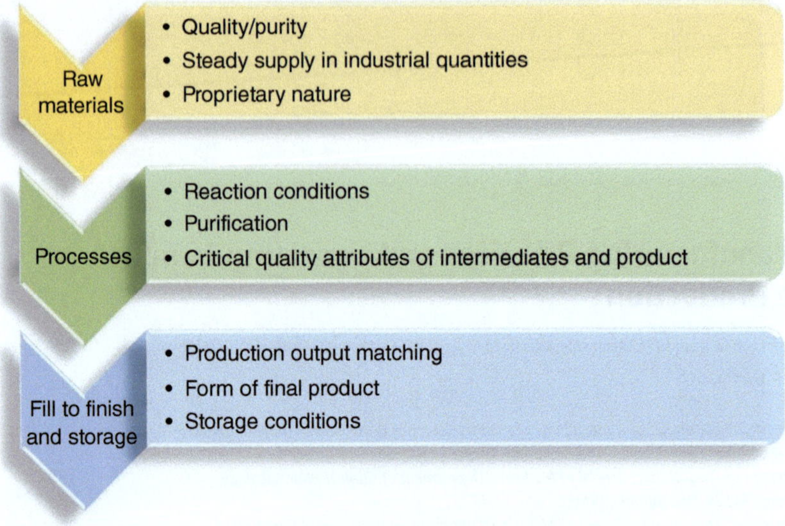

Figure 6.1 Considerations during GMP-compliant scale-up of mRNA vaccines/products.

and subjected to *in vitro* transcription (IVT). During IVT, the DNA template gets transcribed into the respective mRNA, in a cell-free system using high-fidelity RNA polymerase enzymes. At this stage, RNA modifications such as the incorporation of modified nucleosides (e.g. 1-methylpseudourine) can be used to make the functional mRNA "invisible" to the cell's innate immunity [7–9]. In the last stage, mRNA encapsulation is performed to protect it from the hostile extracellular environment and facilitate cellular uptake [10].

While the knowledge and the tools exist, the worldwide demand for an mRNA vaccine soon proved to be a formidable exercise in the emergency scale-up of a novel biopharmaceutical. Industrial processes had to be developed and a continuous supply of raw – sometimes proprietary – materials had to be secured. Furthermore, the storage and later the distribution and shipment of the final product under special conditions have to be solved as well (Figure 6.1). In this chapter, we show the upscaling considerations, challenges, and bottlenecks of good manufacturing practice (GMP) mRNA product manufacturing step by step.

6.2 Plasmid Production

The first step for mRNA vaccine production is to provide DNA plasmid coding for the selected antigen, which will be used after linearization as a template for the IVT process. Processes concerning DNA production via cloning and plasmid manufacturing are widely used in the industry for a long time and as such the upscaling methods are validated and approved [11–13].

Plasmid DNA (pDNA), the circular DNA molecule of bacterial origin which is capable of independent replication from the host's genetic material, is engineered to carry the inserted template for mRNA IVT [14].

As a general rule, a small volume of a preculture of the plasmid-transfected *Escherichia coli* is set up, before using it to inoculate industrial bioreactors of increased capacity [12]. During the industrial cultivation procedure, synthetic, chemically defined media are used and the oxygenation, temperature, pH, and stirring parameters are tightly controlled. After cultivation, the cells will be collected before lysis and clarification can be employed. Centrifugation and microfiltration-tangential flow filtration (MF-TFF) are two methods used for the isolation of the product. Centrifugation is the most cost-effective in either small or large volumes [15, 16].

Lysis of the cells can be achieved by a chemical or physicomechanical method. Chemical methods include alkaline lysis, the use of appropriate enzymes or detergents, and various protocols employing osmotic shock to lyse the cells [17–19]. Physicomechanical handling can be performed in several ways, namely application of heat, agitation or ultrasonification, and freeze-thawing. After this step, purification is performed by filtration to remove unwanted genomic DNA and bacterial RNA, proteins, and endotoxins [15].

The most widespread method is the alkaline method in combination with the use of detergents. The most widely used protocol employs alkalization at pHs 12–12.5 achieved by the addition of NaOH and the detergent sodium dodecyl sulfate (SDS). During the alkaline method, the incubation time and the pH should be carefully monitored [17]. Cell lysis using the alkaline technique can result in the formation of solid aggregates. To address this issue, clarification should be performed where any solid impurities will be removed using filters, most frequently depth filters [20]. Purification of the pDNA is challenging since many impurities share the same physicochemical characteristics with it, including size, charge, and hydrophobicity. Anion exchange chromatography (AEX) and hydrophobic interaction chromatography (HIC) or their combination are established as high-performance methods for pDNA purification [18]. Before sterilization, ultrafiltration (UF) or diafiltration (DF) is performed and the pDNA is resuspended in the final buffer. At an industrial scale, tangential flow filtration (TFF) is preferred since it is highly efficient and cost-effective.

Following the purification of the pDNA, circular DNA must be linearized [6], which takes place in a bioreactor, utilizing restriction enzymes. After the linearization process, DNA has to be purified using chromatographic methods like AEX, HIC, or size exclusion chromatography (SEC) [21].

The linearization step can probably be avoided by initially utilizing linear plasmids such as plasmid extended variable length (pEVL) [22]. Another alternative would be the chemically synthesized DNA such as the GMP-compliant "doggybone" DNA (dbDNA), which is also available at a higher scale [23]. dbDNA is a linear, closed-end DNA molecule that is produced in a cell-free enzymatic process [24–29], classified by the regulatory agencies as nonbiological, in contrast with biological plasmids originating from bacterial cultivation procedures [23]. Another alternative approach to generate IVT template is the employment of polymerase chain reaction (PCR) [30]. While this option avoids the linearization stage and the more laborious clean-up utilized with bacterial lysates, it is more suitable when low amounts of mRNA are required and when the template does not contain repetitions, hence limiting its scalability under GMP conditions [30, 31].

6.3 Considerations of *In Vitro Transcription* Stage

IVT is the cell-free process through which the mRNA is produced from template DNA carrying the gene of interest. This process takes place in bioreactors under tightly controlled conditions.

6.3.1 The *In Vitro Transcription* Reaction

For the IVT reaction, the following ingredients are required: linear(ized) DNA template, DNA-dependent RNA polymerase (e.g. T7,T3, or SP6 RNA polymerases), nucleoside triphosphates (NTPs), appropriate buffers, and in the case of cotranscriptional capping, cap analog [6]. Auxiliary reagents are also added to increase product yields by prolonging and protecting enzymatic action (dithiothreitol, DTT), enhancing transcription (spermidine or other polyamines), preventing Mg ion precipitation (pyrophosphatase, PPase), or inhibiting degradation of the mRNA product (RNase inhibitors) [32–35].

One of the main challenges when scaling up IVT for mass production is deciphering the exact reaction conditions with the objective to achieve the maximum yield, with the minimum formation of by-products that can decrease the yield and require an extensive purification step and can lead to unwanted biological consequences. RNA yields can be doubled or even tripled when nucleotides are supplemented in surplus during the IVT reaction, which also translates into prolonged reaction times that can compromise the RNA integrity [32]. Contaminants such as double-strand RNA (dsRNA) species can also be minimized by optimizing IVT conditions, since the polymerase and Mg ion concentration, reaction temperature, pH, process time, fed-batch cycles, final concentrations of the nucleotides and cap analogs, or the length of the mRNA all influence the final quality [32, 36]. Recently, RNA polymerases are engineered to be thermotolerant allowing for higher than 48 °C reaction temperatures in order to effectively minimize dsRNA formation by the inhibition of the unintended 3′ extension of the transcript that occurs at lower temperatures [21, 37, 38].

Another decision that can lead to further challenges is the employed 5′ capping method. The 5′ cap is an essential mRNA structure that confers translatability and stability to the molecule, preventing it from early degradation and contributing to translation initiation [39, 40]. One strategy is the cotranscriptional capping during IVT, whereas another approach favors the addition of the 5′ cap in a separate step. Cotranscriptional capping can employ antireverse cap (ARCA, 3′-*O*-Me-m7G(5′)ppp(5′)G), Cap 1(m7GpppNm), or Cap 2 (m7GpppNmNm) analogs [41–43]. Utilization of ARCAs incorporates a Cap 0 to the transcribed mRNA and while the resulting mRNA is translatable, this method suffers from drawbacks such as suboptimal capping efficiency (~70%) and the inherent immunogenicity of the Cap 0 toward the mRNA itself [44]. Cap 1 analogs can be incorporated by T7 RNA polymerase to the 5′ end of the transcript [45]. Cotranscriptional capping using the CleanCap analog is employed for the manufacture of Pfizer-BioNTech COVID-19 vaccines (BNT162b2) [46]. While the use of CleanCap technology has some prerequisites as far as the starting sequence of the mRNA is concerned, there are options offered for capping both nonreplicating and self-replicating RNAs [47].

As an alternative, post-IVT capping requires a separate reaction where a Vaccinia virus capping enzyme adds the necessary structure to the RNA transcript [48]. This approach was chosen for the manufacture of Moderna's mRNA-1713 vaccines [6]. When comparing cotranscriptional capping to post-transcriptional capping, the latter results in a capping efficiency reaching nearly 100%, whereas with the former method a capping efficiency of at least 90% is achievable [45, 49]. The higher efficiency of the post-transcription approach comes at the cost of adding another step in the manufacture of the product. The disadvantages of post-transcriptional capping are as follows: it adds an extra filtration step of the IVT mixture, it necessitates the addition of a second reaction vessel to the manufacturing array, and consequently it can also affect the yields [32].

6.3.2 Purification of the *In Vitro* Transcribed RNA

Industrial GMP manufacturing of biopharmaceuticals employs workup stages to remove unwanted components such as reactants, enzymes, solvents, by-products, unreacted substrates, and undesirable artifacts from the product. Purifying the *in vitro* transcribed mRNA becomes necessary in all upstream manufacturing processes, prior to its downstream delivery for final product formulation. Impurities in mRNA production can arise in a process-dependent and/or in a product-dependent manner and pose a serious concern that can affect the final product's quality by impacting translatability and immunogenicity as well as introducing batch-to-batch variations [50].

Process-dependent contaminants include residual pDNA or its fragments, various enzymes (RNA polymerases, DNases, restriction enzymes, and capping enzymes), unused triphosphate nucleosides or cap analogs, salts, and solvents. Product-dependent contaminants typically include short-truncated mRNAs, DNA–RNA hybrids, and dsRNAs.

pDNA and its fragments can complicate purification procedures since DNA remnants are practically the main source of DNA–RNA hybrid formation [51]. Residual enzymes can act as antigens inducing inflammatory reactions in the recipient [52]. Triphosphate nucleotides as well as cap analogs are also undesirable in the final product, given that they exhibit pharmacological activity in humans through interactions with purinergic receptors (P2X,P2Y) [53, 54]. Finally, the presence of residual salts and solvents, apart from raising toxicity issues, can interfere with downstream mRNA encapsulation procedures such as the subsequent formulation of mRNA–LNP (lipid nanoparticle) [55, 56].

All product-dependent contaminants such as dsRNAs, DNA–RNA hybrids, and truncated RNAs can have a wide range of unwanted biological side effects. They carry a sizable risk of activation of the cellular innate immune response leading to rapid intracellular degradation of the mRNA, inhibition of the translation, can mimic viral infections contributing to the incidence of cytokine storms in the product recipient, or lead the target cell to an apoptotic death canceling its role as an antigen/protein-producing factory [57–60]. Currently, it is considered acceptable if dsRNA content is less than 0.5% and truncated RNA content does not exceed 1% of the total mass [61, 62].

Purification of IVT mRNA in a laboratory- or a small-scale production environment suitable for preclinical use is achievable by utilization of a cornucopia of methods [63]. Unfortunately, scaling up those procedures to the industrial level can be challenging because it must be technically feasible to upgrade them, which ultimately depends on the method's physicochemical modus operandi and the feasibility of avoidance of human-use prohibited reagents and solvents. The purification method should also account for the sensitivity of large mRNA molecules to shear forces and consequent degradation. Additionally, the hazards of the required reagents and solvents as well as the waste after purification should be taken into account regarding the cost and legislative requirements of proper storage and waste disposal of hazardous materials.

An illustrative example of the upscaling difficulties is the common laboratory purification of mRNA from the IVT mixture, utilizing hazardous and expensive reagents. In a laboratory setting, after IVT has taken place, the DNA template would be degraded via DNase I digestion, and the nucleic acids would be precipitated from the solution using the lithium chloride method [58, 64]. This isolation method would require a further step since it removes proteins and nucleotides but coprecipitates product-dependent contaminants. The next step would be an advanced chromatography technique, such as reverse phase ion pairing high-performance liquid chromatography (HPLC) (or equivalents), which uses a poorly scalable acetonitrile as a solvent [65–67].

The exact specifications of post-IVT purification at a commercial scale are usually not disclosed by the industry [32, 38]. However, many published workflows on scaled-up production of mRNA tend to employ a setup where a chromatography step is "sandwiched" between two TFF stages [21, 32, 33, 58, 61, 68]. TFF, also known as crossflow filtration, is a scalable technique where the filtration of the product through a membrane is driven by transmembrane pressure as the feed passes laterally on its surface [69]. This allows not only the separation of the product from smaller impurities but can also concentrate, ultrafilter, and diafilter mRNA [70, 71]. For example, TFF could utilize a polyethersulfone (PESU) membrane or hollow fiber-modified PESU membranes (m-PES) and 4-(2-hydroxyethyl)-1-piperazineethanesulfonic acid (HEPES) as the equilibration buffer [61]. The chromatography step utilizes affinity chromatography (AC), anion exchange/ion

Table 6.1 Chromatography methods utilized for RNA purification.

Chromatography method	Advantages	Disadvantages	Notes
Affinity chromatography (AC)	• High product purity • Use of aqueous solutions	• Low binding capacity • Some dsRNA binding	• Follow-up with AEX/IEC • ±1.8 mg RNA/resin ml dynamic binding capacity
Anion/ion exchange chromatography (AEX/IEC)	• Cost-effective scale-up • High binding capacity	• Requires denaturing conditions to release product (85 °C or chaotropes)	• Suitable also for longer RNAs (saRNAs) • RNAs <500 bp elute at RT • >10 mg RNA/ml dynamic binding capacity
Ion-pair reverse chromatography (IPC)	• Rapid and efficient	• Limited scalability • Lower binding capacity compared to AEX/IEC • Prone to fouling by proteins and aggregates • Requires use of toxic/flammable solvents (acetonitrile)	• Follow-up with diafiltration • Better reserved for polishing • <10 mg RNA/ml dynamic binding capacity
Hydrophobic interaction chromatography (HIC)	• Use of aqueous solutions and salt • Can remove metal ions and pyrophosphate	• Prone to fouling by proteins	• Better reserved for "polishing"
Mixed-mode/ multimodal chromatography (MMC)	• High load capacity • High binding capacity • Variable	• Variable	• Advantages and disadvantages depend on modes combined and physicochemical characteristics of the beads

exchange chromatography (AEX/IEC), ion-pair reverse chromatography (IPC), HIC, and mixed-mode (multimodal) chromatography (MMC). Table 6.1 summarizes the advantages and disadvantages of each method.

AC used in mRNA purification utilizes an oligo-dT functionalized resin to capture and purify the IVT mRNA by forming hydrogen bonds with the poly(A) tail [70]. It can efficiently remove contaminants such as enzymes, buffer components, and DNA but might also capture dsRNA alongside the main single-stranded mRNA product. Given those limitations, AC can be followed by other chromatographic techniques like AEX/IEC to remove residual impurities. AC offers high product purity using aqueous solutions, although it might not be the most cost-effective option due to its low binding capacity [72, 73].

AEX/IEC operates on the principle of charge differences to distinguish impurities from products [74]. Resins utilized in this method carry positively charged ions that can attract and bind negatively charged mRNA molecules. AEX/IEC is cost-effective and scalable with a higher binding capacity to AC [75]. However, a major drawback of AEX/IEC is that the elution of the product requires denaturing conditions such as heating at 85 °C or the use of chaotropic agents. The length of the mRNA can be a limitation, since mRNAs shorter than 500 nts can elute at ambient temperature [75, 76].

IPC is another form of high-yield chromatography, but with a lower binding capacity compared to AEX/IEC [58, 74, 75, 77]. During IPC, mRNA is retained in the hydrophobic/lipophilic stationary phase, after its charged sugar-phosphate backbone has been neutralized by quaternary ammonium-carrying eluent. IPC is a rapid and efficient method that offers good separation of products, although its scalability can be limited due to several constraints such as the use of flammable solvents, the easy fouling by the presence of proteins and aggregates, and the requirement of a postchromatography DF step. This renders IPC more suitable for polishing purposes rather than the main purification method.

HIC can be considered an alternative to IPC, alleviating some of the limitations of the latter [33, 78]. HIC operates by utilizing high salt concentrations to precipitate mRNA on the stationary phase. Instead of organic solvents, it uses aqueous buffers and with minor manipulations can effectively remove metal ions and pyrophosphate remnants among other impurities. Still, it retains the sensitivity of IPC toward protein fouling.

Finally, MMC takes a combinatorial approach, utilizing more than one form of interaction of the stationary phase and the flowthrough, making it suitable for multiple types of RNA. An example of MMC is the Captocore columns that utilize core bead technology offering a high load capacity and robust binding performance [79].

The scale-up industrial approach could benefit from the adoption of novel methods and advancements in the field of material science. Chromatography methods employing cellulose resins or electrospinned cellulose fibers that could be a scalable option offer high binding capacity and quick elution of the product [80, 81]. Other approaches focus on improvements of AEX or the introduction of hydrogen bonding chromatography [78]. A notable mention is also the switch from AEX, AC, HIC, and MMC bead/resin chromatography to the equivalent monolith technology [82, 83]. Monoliths come as hollow cylinder structures that are formed from a single block of polymer run through by continuous interconnected channels. Their structure allows for longer RNAs to elute much faster compared to resins [82]. Purification of larger RNAs, such as self-amplifying RNAs (saRNAs), could probably benefit from such an approach, given that the monolith's structure allows for a low turbulence flow that exerts milder shear forces compared to resins. The specifics of the purification methods of saRNAs used in current clinical trials are not publicly disclosed [84].

6.4 Considerations of Lipid Nanoparticles (LNPs)

To overcome one of the main obstacles of mRNA for immunization, different formulations including RNA conjugates, viral vectors, polymers, lipid-like and protein derivatives, microparticles, and nanoparticles were developed that can shield the mRNA from degradation and can facilitate its delivery to the cells [10, 85, 86]. In this context, LNPs serve as the primary subject of scrutiny, since conjugates can possibly bind to serum proteins leading to aggregates and viral vectors can result in higher immunogenicity and pose challenges during industrial production. [87–90]. To date, LNPs have found extensive applications, with a particular emphasis on their pivotal role in the development of COVID-19 vaccines.

There are four main classes of LNPs: liposomes, solid lipid nanoparticles (SLNs), nanostructured lipid carriers (NLCs), and hybrid lipid-polymeric nanoparticles [91]. LNPs consist of a lipid shell by nonidentical mildly cationic lipids, encapsulating the negatively charged RNA [92–94]. Besides these ionizable cationic lipids, cholesterol and lipid-anchored polyethylene glycol (PEG) are also employed to enhance the properties of the LNPs and facilitate receptor-mediated endocytosis or micropinocytosis by the cells. PEG is connected to the lipid head and influences particle size also averting their aggregation during storage, contributing to colloidal stability. The pivotal role of PEG remains relevant even after administration of the product, as it protects the lipid particles from the host's immune system response by decreasing complement activation [95]. PEGylation should be carefully considered since on one hand it can enhance lymphatic drainage while on the other hand overPEGylation reduces endocytosis and LNP circulation for extended periods of time in the blood [96, 97]. Special consideration should be given to PEGylating products designed for multiple administrations as PEG can lead to the formation of anti-PEG antibodies that can drastically augment its clearance or induce allergic reactions [98].

LNP formulation itself can act as an adjuvant, increasing the efficacy of the vaccines [99, 100]. This increases their immunogenicity, which is favorable if the product is intended for vaccination. LNP-triggered immunogenicity can be a double-edged sword: while it can prove beneficial for an mRNA vaccine, increased LNP-triggered immunogenicity toward a product that would require multiple or chronic administration, such as a gene therapy mRNA biopharmaceutical or mRNA-based anticancer medication, would make subsequent treatments less effective due to an increased immune response against the therapeutic formulation [99, 101, 102].

6.4.1 Synthesis of LNP and mRNA Encapsulation

The common formulation method is based on dissolving the lipids in an organic solvent such as ethanol and then mixing with the aqueous RNA solution [55, 56, 103]. While the first synthesis attempts were based on sonication to suspended lipids in water, this method presented certain limitations such as molecular degradation, contamination, and lack of scalability [85]. Molecular degradation may arise as a consequence of heightened kinetic energy imparted to the molecules during the process. Concurrently, issues such as contamination and limited scalability could be attributed to inherent equipment characteristics, energy demands associated with industrial-scale sonicators, and potential reductions in efficiency or LNP uniformity when processing larger volumes.

More modern approaches use a T-shaped mixing chamber to merge the laminar flows of the two solutions in a tightly controlled manner, where temperature, flow, and mixing rate can be adjusted [104].

A technique of LNP synthesis that employs fast mixing rates of the aqueous phase and ethanol is the use of a "Staggered herringbone mixer," a device inducing rotational chaotic advection in the laminar flow or in other words a turbulent flow ensuring rapid mixing of the two phases [105]. In this method, LNP size can be adjusted by manipulating the flow rate. The advantages of this technique mainly include the high encapsulation efficiency and the capability of small particle generation [85].

6.4.2 Scaling Up Production of LNPs to Industrial Standards

Solvent-based technology employs solvents in order to mix the components of the LNP but requires the removal of the solvent by evaporation, displacement, or diffusion. Low temperatures make it suitable for nanoencapsulation of thermosensitive active substances. A main drawback of this method is its inability to fully remove the solvents, making it inappropriate for utilization with solvents displaying appreciable toxicity even as residues [106]. For large-scale production of LNPs, static mixers have been created in various forms (tubes, columns, or reactors) that can provide controlled tortuous flows, which offer fast and highly homogeneous results [91].

Nonsolvent-based technology can be performed either by the high-pressure homogenization (HPH) method or microemulsion [107]. In the HPH method, the lipids are melted at 5–10 °C above their melting temperature and form an emulsion with the molecule to be encapsulated under HPH [91]. Homogenization and sonication durations, the concentration of the drug, and the nature of the lipids and the surfactants have to be tightly controlled. The desired drug concentration might pose a limit as excessive concentration may result in uncapsulated, exposed material [108].

Microemulsion formation at an industrial level employs precision temperature-controlled tanks allowing for better control of the process [108]. Limitations of these two similar methods include the extensive use of surfactants in microemulsion, the energy-intensive procedures required by the HPH method, and the heating manipulation of lipids in both methods that may damage the encapsulated drug of interest [91].

The last stage of LNP products usually incorporates their purification, sterile filtration, and dilution to the appropriate concentration before proceeding to the fill-to-finish processes [109].

6.5 Considerations of Fill-to-Finish and Storage

The final stage of mRNA vaccine production is the "fill-to-finish" stage, where the product is filled into vials, subjected to quality control, sealed, and finally labeled and packaged. The whole process must guarantee the sterility of the final product and should be carried out under GMP conditions. The sterility aspect can be addressed in modern terms, by the incorporation of closed, automated production process, to reduce the risk of any contamination [110].

Fill-to-finish procedures can be divided into two essential components. The first is the solution preparation, where dilution of the product or solution formulation takes place. The second component includes the procedures required for filling the formulated mRNA solutions into vials or alternative containers, performing vial capping or sealing, inspecting the product, affixing labels, and packaging of the final product. These operations also include the transfer steps between each stage of the chain. The fill-to-finish procedure can become a bottleneck when the drug product (DP) is produced faster than predicted in the initial analysis of process development or when the production is forced to meet a pandemic-scale demand [111].

In the case of mRNA–LNP products, the storage and subsequent transport procedures can be challenging due to the product's stringent storage temperature requirements [112]. A probable factor compromising mRNA–LNP stability that pertains to fill-to-finish procedures is the inclusion of up to 1/5 water into LNPs, which primes the encapsulated mRNA toward destruction through hydrolysis [93, 113]. This should not be the case since LNPs, contrary to liposomes, are supposed to minimize RNA–water contact at their core, a distinctive property that makes them suitable for efficient RNA delivery.

A scalable solution to mRNA degradation due to co-encapsulation with water is utilizing techniques such as lyophilization. During lyophilization, the product to be preserved is frozen and the water is driven off through sublimation under vacuum [114, 115]. Compared to other methods of drying, such as ones utilizing increased temperatures, this method retains an intact LNP morphology [116]. So far, lyophilization has provided excellent preliminary results in stabilizing mRNA–LNP complexes. Lyophilized complexes managed to concurrently retain both their physicochemical properties and *in vivo* potency, for 12 and 24 weeks at room temperature (25 °C) and 4 °C, respectively [116]. It should be kept in mind that the lyophilization procedure, apart from GMP industrial-size equipment procurement, might call for changes in final formulation of the product as well as in the specifics of the fill-to-finish procedure. For example, as freezing requires cryoprotectants, lyophilization makes use of lyoprotectants such as sugars (glucose, trehalose, and mannitol), hyaluronic acid, or γ-cyclodextrin [117]. Furthermore, the product's shelf life can be extended by storing the lyophilized mRNA–LNPs under inert atmosphere. This would translate into a fill-to-finish procedure of flushing the vials before sealing with an inert gas such as nitrogen [116].

6.6 mRNA and mRNA–LNP Critical Quality Attribute Analysis

Critical quality attributes (CQAs) are defined as those chemical, biological, or physical characteristics of a product that must fall within a predefined and acceptable range [32]. At this level, a general consideration would be the specifics of their

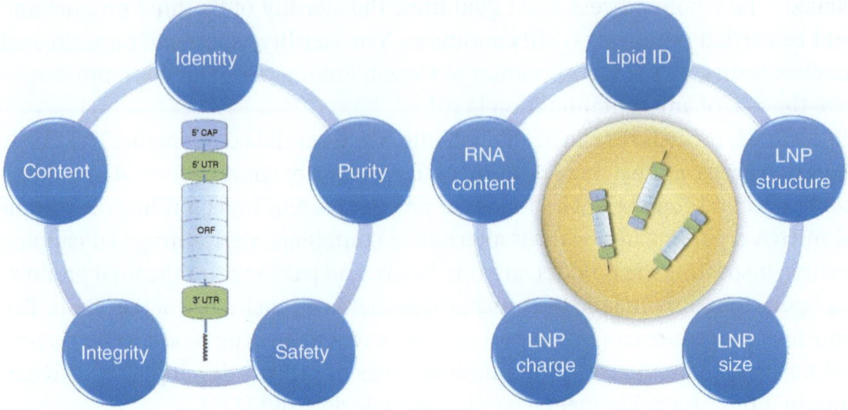

Figure 6.2 CQA categories for mRNA (right) and mRNA–LNPs (left).

offline, online, or inline implementation at each manufacturing stage. For mRNA and mRNA–LNP products, analytical tools to assess their CQAs in the context of large-scale production have been established [32, 118]. Figure 6.2 displays the basic CQA categories for mRNA and mRNA–LNPs.

mRNA is analyzed for its content/quantity, identity, purity (dsRNA, DNA residues, and product-related impurities), safety (sterility, bioburden, and endotoxins), and integrity (mRNA integrity, fragmentation, capping efficiency, and length of poly-A tail). mRNA–LNPs are analyzed for the RNA content (mRNA encapsulated), lipid identity (content, relevant impurities), structure, size alongside with polydispersity, stability, and charge.

mRNA identity can be verified by sequencing methods, whereas real-time PCR and ultraviolet (UV) spectroscopy provide information on the quantity of mRNA received from IVT; additionally, electrophoresis methods, such as capillary gel electrophoresis, can be employed to confirm mRNA size. Length of poly(A) tail and capping efficiency (capped versus uncapped mRNA percentages) can be monitored using HPLC methods. 5′ cap efficiency can also be evaluated by ribozyme cleavage assays [119]. Purity can be assayed on grounds of residual DNA template and dsRNA presence, utilizing quantitative polymerase chain reaction (qPCR) and immunoblotting, respectively. Finally, mRNAs bioburden, endotoxin content, and sterility can be evaluated as per the established United States Pharmacopeia – National Formulary criteria [118].

The resulting mRNA–LNPs, as a single finalized entity, are also subject to quality control [120]. The encapsulation rate of mRNA in the resulting particles can be verified using HPLC methods, Ribogreen assay, UV–vis or Raman spectrometry, and cryo-electron microscopy (cryoEM). Dynamic light scattering, multiangle light scattering, and refractive index methods can be used to assess the size of LNPs, their polydispersity, and their stability. The lipid identity and related impurities can be assessed using charged aerosol detectors coupled with HPLC or liquid chromatography–mass spectrometry (LC-MS) and the morphology of the resulting LNPs can be evaluated by means of cryoEM, nuclear magnetic resonance, and small-angle neutron scattering. Lastly, electrophoretic light scattering, phase-analysis light scattering, and capillary electrophoresis can provide valuable insight into the LNP's charge.

6.7 General Remarks and Further Considerations

The lack of a generally enforced guideline framework for RNA mass production, both from a manufacturer and from a quality/analytic point of view, creates an interesting situation [121–123]. It is challenging for the newly founded mRNA pharmaceutical companies to coordinate process development effort, while at the same time it provides an opportunity for the early adoption or even development of innovative technologies. One of the major considerations is raw material quality and procurement [38, 61, 124, 125]. In the case of mRNA–LNP products, the raw materials novelty and often limited supply adds significantly to the production cost and procurement intricacies [126]. It is of utmost importance not only to secure a steady supply of industrially relevant quantities but also to ensure that each batch procured equally fulfills the quality standards. The innovative and proprietary nature of some of the reagents, such as 5′ caps and lipids, can limit the suppliers that can guarantee to provide a steady supply of the relevant non-animal-origin GMP-grade material [38, 58, 126]. In this regard, upscaling would require extensive audits before choosing a supplier and could benefit from employing either a third-party or an in-house testing of the inbound reagents.

State-of-the-art quality in raw materials calls for special considerations pertaining to the sensitive nature of the product manufactured. Two major concerns are the presence of RNases and the presence of endotoxins [61]. mRNA is prone to degradation and very sensitive against the omnipresent RNases, so even slight contamination could degrade the product. Endotoxin's presence in raw materials could pose many downstream issues. The most common introduction points of such contaminants are in the IVT step as well as every purification step where large amounts of buffers are used [61]. The use of enzymes, such as T7 polymerase, should also be tightly regulated to avoid any variability between suppliers [127]. Ideally, the scale-up should utilize the exact enzymes used in preliminary laboratory-scale experiments for process streamlining, since variations in enzymatic activity under the given reaction conditions can seriously impact product quality. It would be prudent to acquire enzyme samples to experimentally verify their enzymatic activity under the current operation conditions, before committing to a different supplier.

An illustrative example of the complexity involved and the intertwinement of factors at play would be switching from a nonreplicating RNA to an saRNA. Due to the latter's potentially lower requirements of mRNA per dose, increased production rates are achievable compared to the nonamplifying producing counterparts [126]. An assessment would have to follow on the efficiency of "scaling out" employing smaller parallel LNP formulation devices versus scaling up by increasing the capacity of one LNP formulator. Then, a rollover of the "strain" toward "fill-to-finish" operations is to be expected, affecting choices like utilizing multidose or single-dose packaging and whether to recruit off-site packaging partners [128]. Furthermore, changes in the size of the RNA produced, given that saRNA is always longer, could require different TFF membrane characteristics during filtration and "gentler" chromatographic methods exerting less pronounced shear forces [82, 129].

Another important consideration is the mode of operation of the production processes that is whether a batch, a fed-batch, or a continuous approach is implemented, while remaining GMP compliant. At the time of writing, there is a shift of interest toward the continuous approach [21, 103, 127, 130, 131]. A continuous approach can increase productivity and even reduce the cost of operation, because it can accommodate *in situ* product acquisition while at the same time enabling recycling of raw materials. The latter is important since raw materials such as 5′ caps and polymerase enzymes are (i) expensive, (ii) used in excess during the IVT reaction, and (iii) 99% of their quantity gets discarded in batch operations, making them the main cost factor in RNA vaccine synthesis [131]. Issues can arise when switching from batch to continuous, which could mandate changes in equipment [32, 58]; hence, other options such as aqueous two-phase systems or single-pass TFF might be preferable.

Regarding quality control, implementation of the quality by design (QbD) model and design of experiments (DoE) are worth considering, since not only they are capable of streamlining process design and cutting costs but they can also safeguard product quality [21, 32, 61, 103, 110, 123, 130–134]. DoE, the main component of QbD, is a method used to establish a mathematical model of the relationships between processes or their outputs and the influencing variables. The QbD concept transcends reliance on increased testing as a means of quality assurance and proposes that product quality should be ingrained in the production procedure itself. It reduces the need for excessive testing of mRNA products, which can also be a bottleneck, by identifying and producing mathematical models on critical process parameters and CQAs for each step [32]. Such an approach also offers a great opportunity for shifting from simple GMP compliance to current good manufacturing practices (cGMP) standards. So far, no mRNA vaccines following the QbD paradigm have been developed.

Compared to the above, a simpler scenario would be the production of a single, well-defined product (such as a specific mRNA COVID-19 vaccine) and/or a "one-off" production of such a vaccine to support a developing country. The infrastructural and process development challenges can be side-stepped by utilization of ready-made and Mobile on Demand models [135, 136]. In one of these models, a one unit portable GMP-compliant mRNA factory is described [135]. Each unit comprises of two containers and has a single-use capacity of producing one million doses of Moderna's COVID-19 vaccines. In this example, the employment of single-use equipment, such as reactors and filtration devices, offers the benefit of sterility and minimizes maintenance.

Another more advanced multiuse multiproduct GMP-compliant example is BioNTainer modular factory developed by BioNTech [136]. BioNTainers are ergonomic and portable ISO-sized containers, which follow a modular approach of "plug and play" philosophy: they can be shipped to the target region and assembled to form a fully functional GMP-compliant mRNA production facility. Each "portable" factory is a two-module construction comprised of 12 containers, with six containers forming a module. BioNTainer's two modules are the drug substance (DS) module and the drug product (DP) module. The DS module is where the mRNA production through IVT takes place alongside with the required mRNA purification and concentration. The DP formulation, in this specific case the manufacture of the LNP–mRNA complexes, is carried out in the DP module, while local partners can carry out the fill-and-finish procedures. The construct is characterized by technical autonomy. The modularity and portability of BioNTainers can bestow countries in challenging socioeconomic environments such as in Africa with the capacity to develop self-reliance in mRNA production without compromises in quality.

References

1 Pardi, N., Hogan, M.J., Porter, F.W., and Weissman, D. (2018). mRNA vaccines — a new era in vaccinology. *Nat. Rev. Drug Discov.* 17 (4): 261–279.

2 Bok, K., Sitar, S., Graham, B.S., and Mascola, J.R. (2021). Accelerated COVID-19 vaccine development: milestones, lessons, and prospects. *Immunity* 54 (8): 1636–1651.

3 Schlake, T., Thess, A., Fotin-Mleczek, M., and Kallen, K.J. (2012). Developing mRNA-vaccine technologies. *RNA Biol.* 9 (11): 1319–1330.

4 Walsh, G. (2015). Large-scale protein production. In: *Proteins*, 141–176. Wiley https://onlinelibrary.wiley.com/doi/abs/10.1002/9781119117599.ch5 (accessed 30 August 2022).

5 Tripathi, N.K. and Shrivastava, A. (2019). Recent developments in bioprocessing of recombinant proteins: expression hosts and process development. *Front. Bioeng. Biotechnol.* 7: 420. https://www.frontiersin.org/articles/10.3389/fbioe.2019.00420 (accessed 30 August 2022).

6 Ouranidis, A., Vavilis, T., Mandala, E. et al. (2021). mRNA therapeutic modalities design, formulation and manufacturing under pharma 4.0 principles. *Biomedicines* 10 (1): 50.

7 Chabanovska, O., Galow, A.M., David, R., and Lemcke, H. (2021). mRNA - a game changer in regenerative medicine, cell-based therapy and reprogramming strategies. *Adv. Drug Deliv. Rev.* 179: 114002.

8 Karikó, K., Buckstein, M., Ni, H., and Weissman, D. (2005). Suppression of RNA recognition by Toll-like receptors: the impact of nucleoside modification and the evolutionary origin of RNA. *Immunity* 23 (2): 165–175.

9 Karikó, K., Muramatsu, H., Welsh, F.A. et al. (2008). Incorporation of pseudouridine into mRNA yields superior nonimmunogenic vector with increased translational capacity and biological stability. *Mol. Ther.* 16 (11): 1833–1840.

10 Hou, X., Zaks, T., Langer, R., and Dong, Y. (2021). Lipid nanoparticles for mRNA delivery. *Nat. Rev. Mater.* 6 (12): 1078–1094.

11 Prather, K.J., Sagar, S., Murphy, J., and Chartrain, M. (2003). Industrial scale production of plasmid DNA for vaccine and gene therapy: plasmid design, production, and purification. *Enzym. Microb. Technol.* 33 (7): 865–883.

12 Schmeer, M. and Schleef, M. (2014). Pharmaceutical grade large-scale plasmid DNA manufacturing process. *Methods Mol. Biol.* 1143: 219–240.

13 Chartrain, M., Bentley, L.K., Krulewicz, B.A. et al. (2011). Process for large scale production of plasmid DNA by *E. coli* fermentation. US7998732B2. https://patents.google.com/patent/US7998732B2/en (accessed 28 August 2022).

14 Gagnon, P. (2020). *Purification of Nucleic Acids: A Handbook for Purification of DNA Plasmids and mRNA for Gene Therapy and Vaccines*, 1st electronice. Ajdovščina: BIA Separations.

15 Ruiz, O., Limonta, M., Valdés, J. et al. (2011). Scalable technology to produce pharmaceutical grade plasmid DNA for gene therapy. In: *Gene Therapy - Developments and Future Perspectives* (ed. C. Kang). InTech http://www.intechopen.com/books/gene-therapy-developments-and-future-perspectives/scalable-technology-to-produce-pharmaceutical-grade-plasmid-dna-for-gene-therapy (accessed 26 August 2022).

16 Raghunath, B., Bin, W., Pattnaik, P., and Janssens, J. (2012). Best practices for optimization and scale-up of microfiltration TFF processes. *Bioprocess. J.* 11 (1): 30–40.

17 Meacle, F.J., Lander, R., Ayazi Shamlou, P., and Titchener-Hooker, N.J. (2004). Impact of engineering flow conditions on plasmid DNA yield and purity in chemical cell lysis operations. *Biotechnol. Bioeng.* 87 (3): 293–302.

18 Urthaler, J., Buchinger, W., and Necina, R. (2005). Industrial scale cGMP purification of pharmaceutical grade plasmid-DNA. *Chem. Eng. Technol.* 28 (11): 1408–1420.

19 Zhu, K., Jin, H., He, Z. et al. (2006). A continuous method for the large-scale extraction of plasmid DNA by modified boiling lysis. *Nat. Protoc.* 1 (6): 3088–3093.

20 Nejatishahidein, N., Kim, M., Jung, S.Y. et al. (2022). Scale-up issues for commercial depth filters in bioprocessing. *Biotechnol. Bioeng.* 119 (4): 1105–1114.

21 Ouranidis, A., Davidopoulou, C., Tashi, R.K., and Kachrimanis, K. (2021). Pharma 4.0 continuous mRNA drug products manufacturing. *Pharmaceutics* 13 (9): 1371.

22 Grier, A.E., Burleigh, S., Sahni, J. et al. (2016). pEVL: a linear plasmid for generating mRNA IVT templates with extended encoded poly(A) sequences. *Mol. Ther. Nucleic Acids* 5 (4): e306.

23 Ohlson, J. (2020). Plasmid manufacture is the bottleneck of the genetic medicine revolution. *Drug Discov. Today* 25 (11): 1891–1893.

24 Hill, V. (2010). Production of closed linear DNA. WO2010086626A1. https://patents.google.com/patent/WO2010086626A1/en (accessed 28 August 2022).

25 Bishop, D.C., Caproni, L., Gowrishankar, K. et al. (2020). CAR T cell generation by piggyBac transposition from linear doggybone DNA vectors requires transposon DNA-flanking regions. *Mol. Ther. Methods Clin. Dev.* 17: 359–368.

26 Mucker, E.M., Brocato, R.L., Principe, L.M. et al. (2022). SARS-CoV-2 doggybone DNA vaccine produces cross-variant neutralizing antibodies and is protective in a COVID-19 animal model. *Vaccines (Basel)* 10 (7): 1104.

27 Scott, V.L., Patel, A., Villarreal, D.O. et al. (2015). Novel synthetic plasmid and doggybone DNA vaccines induce neutralizing antibodies and provide protection from lethal influenza challenge in mice. *Hum. Vaccin. Immunother.* 11 (8): 1972–1982.

28 Thornton, C.D., Fielding, S., Karbowniczek, K. et al. (2021). Safe and stable generation of induced pluripotent stem cells using doggybone DNA vectors. *Mol. Ther. Methods Clin. Dev.* 23: 348–358.

29 Barreira, M., Kerridge, C., Jorda, S. et al. (2022). Enzymatically amplified linear dbDNA as a rapid and scalable solution to industrial lentiviral vector manufacturing. *Gene Ther.* 30 (1–2): 122–131.

30 Beckert, B. and Masquida, B. (2011). Synthesis of RNA by in vitro transcription. *Methods Mol. Biol.* 703: 29–41.

31 Hommelsheim, C.M., Frantzeskakis, L., Huang, M., and Ülker, B. (2014). PCR amplification of repetitive DNA: a limitation to genome editing technologies and many other applications. *Sci. Rep.* 4 (1): 5052.

32 Daniel, S., Kis, Z., Kontoravdi, C., and Shah, N. (2022). Quality by design for enabling RNA platform production processes. *Trends Biotechnol.* 40 (10): 1213–1228.

33 Niazi, S.K. (2022). Making COVID-19 mRNA vaccines accessible: challenges resolved. *Expert Rev. Vaccines* 21 (9): 1163–1176.

34 Samnuan, K., Blakney, A.K., McKay, P.F., and Shattock, R.J. (2021). Design-of-experiments in vitro transcription yield optimization of self-amplifying RNA. http://biorxiv.org/lookup/doi/10.1101/2021.01.08.425833 (accessed 18 August 2022).

35 Tersteeg, S., Mrozowich, T., Henrickson, A. et al. (2022). Purification and characterization of inorganic pyrophosphatase for in vitro RNA transcription. *Biochem. Cell Biol.* 100 (5): 425–436.

36 Elich, J., Rabideau, A., Shamashkin, M. et al. (2020). Fed-batch in vitro transcription process. https://patentscope.wipo.int/search/en/detail.jsf?docId=WO2020185811 (accessed 18 August 2022).

37 Wu, M.Z., Asahara, H., Tzertzinis, G., and Roy, B. (2020). Synthesis of low immunogenicity RNA with high-temperature in vitro transcription. *RNA* 26 (3): 345–360.

38 Szabó, G.T., Mahiny, A.J., and Vlatkovic, I. (2022). COVID-19 mRNA vaccines: platforms and current developments. *Mol. Ther.* 30 (5): 1850–1868.

39 Kim, S.C., Sekhon, S.S., Shin, W.R. et al. (2021). Modifications of mRNA vaccine structural elements for improving mRNA stability and translation efficiency. *Mol. Cell Toxicol.* 18 (1): 1–8.

40 Charenton, C. and Graille, M. (2018). mRNA decapping: finding the right structures. *Philos. Trans. R. Soc. Lond. Ser. B Biol. Sci.* 373 (1762): 20180164.

41 Wadhwa, A., Aljabbari, A., Lokras, A. et al. (2020). Opportunities and challenges in the delivery of mRNA-based vaccines. *Pharmaceutics* 12 (2): E102.

42 Kang, D.D., Li, H., and Dong, Y. (2023). Advancements of in vitro transcribed mRNA (IVT mRNA) to enable translation into the clinics. *Adv. Drug Deliv. Rev.* 199: 114961.

43 Shanmugasundaram, M., Senthilvelan, A., and Kore, A.R. (2022). Recent advances in modified cap analogs: synthesis, biochemical properties, and mRNA based vaccines. *Chem. Rec.* 22 (8): e202200005.

44 Kwon, S., Kwon, M., Im, S. et al. (2022). mRNA vaccines: the most recent clinical applications of synthetic mRNA. *Arch. Pharm. Res.* 45 (4): 245–262.

45 Henderson, J.M., Ujita, A., Hill, E. et al. (2021). Cap 1 messenger RNA synthesis with co-transcriptional CleanCap® analog by in vitro transcription. *Curr. Protocol.* 1 (2): e39.

46 Sahin, U., Muik, A., Vogler, I. et al. (2021). BNT162b2 vaccine induces neutralizing antibodies and poly-specific T cells in humans. *Nature* 595 (7868): 572–577.

47 Fang, E., Liu, X., Li, M. et al. (2022). Advances in COVID-19 mRNA vaccine development. *Signal Transduct. Target. Ther.* 7 (1): 94.

48 Corbett, K.S., Edwards, D.K., Leist, S.R. et al. (2020). SARS-CoV-2 mRNA vaccine design enabled by prototype pathogen preparedness. *Nature* 586 (7830): 567–571.

49 Linares-Fernández, S., Lacroix, C., Exposito, J.Y., and Verrier, B. (2020). Tailoring mRNA vaccine to balance innate/adaptive immune response. *Trends Mol. Med.* 26 (3): 311–323.

50 Grinsted, J., Liddell, J., Bouleghlimat, E. et al. (2022). Purification of therapeutic & prophylactic mRNA by affinity chromatography. *Cell Gene Ther. Insights* 8 (2): 335–349.

51 Stöcher, M. and Berg, J. (2004). Removal of template DNA from cRNA preparations by combined oligo (dT) affinity chromatography and DNase I digestion. *Biotechniques* 36 (3): 480–482.

52 Chaplin, D.D. (2010). Overview of the immune response. *J. Allergy Clin. Immunol.* 125 (2 Suppl 2): S3–S23.

53 Sebastián-Serrano, Á., de Diego-García, L., di Lauro, C. et al. (2019). Nucleotides regulate the common molecular mechanisms that underlie neurodegenerative diseases; therapeutic implications. *Brain Res. Bull.* 151: 84–91.

54 Vultaggio-Poma, V., Falzoni, S., Salvi, G. et al. (2022). Signalling by extracellular nucleotides in health and disease. *Biochim. Biophys. Acta, Mol. Cell Res.* 1869 (5): 119237.

55 Webb, C., Khadke, S., Tandrup Schmidt, S. et al. (2019). The impact of solvent selection: strategies to guide the manufacturing of liposomes using microfluidics. *Pharmaceutics* 11 (12): 653.

56 Roces, C.B., Lou, G., Jain, N. et al. (2020). Manufacturing considerations for the development of lipid nanoparticles using microfluidics. *Pharmaceutics* 12 (11): E1095.

57 To, K.K.W. and Cho, W.C.S. (2021). An overview of rational design of mRNA-based therapeutics and vaccines. *Expert Opin. Drug Discov.* 16 (11): 1307–1317.

58 Rosa, S.S., Prazeres, D.M.F., Azevedo, A.M., and Marques, M.P.C. (2021). mRNA vaccines manufacturing: challenges and bottlenecks. *Vaccine* 39 (16): 2190–2200.

59 Read, M.L., Singh, S., Ahmed, Z. et al. (2005). A versatile reducible polycation-based system for efficient delivery of a broad range of nucleic acids. *Nucleic Acids Res.* 33 (9): e86.

60 Gantier, M.P. and Williams, B.R.G. (2007). The response of mammalian cells to double-stranded RNA. *Cytokine Growth Factor Rev.* 18 (5–6): 363–371.

61 Whitley, J., Zwolinski, C., Denis, C. et al. (2022). Development of mRNA manufacturing for vaccines and therapeutics: mRNA platform requirements and development of a scalable production process to support early phase clinical trials. *Transl. Res.* 242: 38–55.

62 Jacobson, E. (2022). Quality control in mRNA vaccine manufacturing—the critical path. https://www.biocompare.com/Editorial-Articles/592381-Quality-Control-in-mRNA-Vaccine-Manufacturing-The-Critical-Path/ (accessed 31 October 2023).

63 Baronti, L., Karlsson, H., Marušič, M., and Petzold, K. (2018). A guide to large-scale RNA sample preparation. *Anal. Bioanal. Chem.* 410 (14): 3239–3252.

64 Pascolo, S. (2017). Messenger mRNA: the inexpensive biopharmaceutical. *J. Multidiscip. Eng. Sci. Technol.* 4: 6937.

65 Akash, M.S.H. and Rehman, K. (2020). Column chromatography. In: *Essentials of Pharmaceutical Analysis* (ed. M.S.H. Akash and K. Rehman), 167–174. Singapore: Springer https://doi.org/10.1007/978-981-15-1547-7_13.

66 Karlsson, H., Baronti, L., and Petzold, K. (2020). A robust and versatile method for production and purification of large-scale RNA samples for structural biology. *RNA* 26 (8): 1023–1037.

67 Karikó, K., Muramatsu, H., Ludwig, J., and Weissman, D. (2011). Generating the optimal mRNA for therapy: HPLC purification eliminates immune activation and improves translation of nucleoside-modified, protein-encoding mRNA. *Nucleic Acids Res.* 39 (21): e142.

68 Fahr, S., Peña-Benavides, S.A., Thiel, L. et al. (2022). Mobile on demand COVID-19 vaccine production units for developing countries. *Ind. Eng. Chem. Res.* 61: 13191–13204.

69 Funkner A, Dorner S, Sewing S et al. (2016). A method for producing and purifying RNA, comprising at least one step of tangential flow filtration. https://patentscope.wipo.int/search/en/detail.jsf?docId=WO2016193206 (accessed 13 August 2022).

70 Bancel, S., Issa, W.J., Aunins, J.G., and Chakraborty, T. (2014). Manufacturing methods for production of RNA transcripts. WO2014152027A1. https://patents.google.com/patent/WO2014152027A1/en (accessed 17 August 2022).

71 Heartlein, M., Derosa, F., Dias, A., and Karve, S. (2014). Methods for purification of messenger RNA. WO2014152966A1. https://patents.google.com/patent/WO2014152966A1/en (accessed 2 November 2021).

72 Thakor, N. and Holcik, M. (2012). RNA affinity chromatography. In: *Affinity Chromatography* (ed. S. Magdeldin). InTech http://www.intechopen.com/books/affinity-chromatography/affinity-purification-and-identification-of-ires-trans-acting-factors (accessed 25 August 2022).

73 Bryant, S. and Manning, D.L. (2000). Isolation of mRNA by affinity chromatography. In: *The Nucleic Acid Protocols Handbook*, Springer Protocols Handbooks (ed. R. Rapley), 9–11. Totowa, NJ: Humana Press https://doi.org/10.1385/1-59259-038-1:9.

74 Easton, L.E., Shibata, Y., and Lukavsky, P.J. (2010). Rapid, nondenaturing RNA purification using weak anion-exchange fast performance liquid chromatography. *RNA* 16 (3): 647–653.

75 Issa, W.J., Barberio, J.L., Aunins, J.G., and Afeyan, N.B. (2020). Ion exchange purification of mRNA. US10590161B2. https://patents.google.com/patent/US10590161B2/en?q=iON+EXCHANGE+PURIFICATION+OF+MRNA&oq=iON+EXCHANGE+PURIFICATION+OF+MRNA (accessed 2 November 2021).

76 Issa, W.J., Aunins, J.G., and Bancel, S. (2014). Ribonucleic acid purification. WO2014152031A1. https://patents.google.com/patent/WO2014152031A1/un (accessed 2 November 2021).

77 Weissman, D., Pardi, N., Muramatsu, H., and Karikó, K. (2013). HPLC purification of in vitro transcribed long RNA. In: *Synthetic Messenger RNA and Cell Metabolism Modulation*, Methods in Molecular Biology, vol. 969 (ed. P.M. Rabinovich), 43–54. Totowa, NJ: Humana Press http://link.springer.com/10.1007/978-1-62703-260-5_3 (accessed 17 August 2022).

78 Gagnon, P., Goričar, B., Peršič, Š. et al. (2020). Two new capture options for improved purification of large mRNA. *Cell Gene Ther. Insights* 6 (7): 1035–1046.

79 Scorza, F.B., Wen, Y., Geall, A., and Porter, F. (2018). RNA purification methods. EP2970948B1. https://patents.google.com/patent/EP2970948B1/en (accessed 18 August 2022).

80 Baiersdörfer, M., Boros, G., Muramatsu, H. et al. (2019). A facile method for the removal of dsRNA contaminant from in vitro-transcribed mRNA. *Mol. Ther. Nucleic Acids* 15: 26–35.

81 Abysalh, J., Derosa, F., Vargas, J., and Smith, C.M. (2020). Methods for purification of messenger RNA. WO2020232371A1. https://patents.google.com/patent/WO2020232371A1/en (accessed 18 August 2022).

82 Davis, J., Debear, J., and Cheng, C. (2017). Polynucleotide purification with monolith columns. WO/2017/205477. https://patentscope.wipo.int/search/en/detail.jsf?docId=WO2017205477 (accessed 16 August 2022).

83 Chatterjee, A., Mirer, P.L., Zaldivar Santamaria, E. et al. (2010). RNA isolation from mammalian cells using porous polymer monoliths: an approach for high-throughput automation. *Anal. Chem.* 82 (11): 4344–4356.

84 Blakney, A.K., Ip, S., and Geall, A.J. (2021). An update on self-amplifying mRNA vaccine development. *Vaccines* 9 (2): 97.

85 Reichmuth, A.M., Oberli, M.A., Jaklenec, A. et al. (2016). mRNA vaccine delivery using lipid nanoparticles. *Ther. Deliv.* 7 (5): 319–334.

86 Vavilis, T., Stamoula, E., Ainatzoglou, A. et al. (2023). mRNA in the context of protein replacement therapy. *Pharmaceutics* 15 (1): 166.

87 Bessis, N., GarciaCozar, F.J., and Boissier, M.C. (2004). Immune responses to gene therapy vectors: influence on vector function and effector mechanisms. *Gene Ther.* 11 (Suppl 1): S10–S17.

88 Baum, C., Kustikova, O., Modlich, U. et al. (2006). Mutagenesis and oncogenesis by chromosomal insertion of gene transfer vectors. *Hum. Gene Ther.* 17 (3): 253–263.

89 Waehler, R., Russell, S.J., and Curiel, D.T. (2007). Engineering targeted viral vectors for gene therapy. *Nat. Rev. Genet.* 8 (8): 573–587.

90 Bouard, D., Alazard-Dany, D., and Cosset, F.L. (2009). Viral vectors: from virology to transgene expression. *Br. J. Pharmacol.* 157 (2): 153–165.

91 Xu, L., Wang, X., Liu, Y. et al. (2022). Lipid nanoparticles for drug delivery. *Adv. NanoBiomed. Res.* 2 (2): 2100109.

92 Li, W. and Szoka, F.C. (2007). Lipid-based nanoparticles for nucleic acid delivery. *Pharm. Res.* 24 (3): 438–449.

93 Schoenmaker, L., Witzigmann, D., Kulkarni, J.A. et al. (2021). mRNA-lipid nanoparticle COVID-19 vaccines: structure and stability. *Int. J. Pharm.* 601: 120586.

94 Cheng, X. and Lee, R.J. (2016). The role of helper lipids in lipid nanoparticles (LNPs) designed for oligonucleotide delivery. *Adv. Drug Deliv. Rev.* 99 (Pt A): 129–137.

95 Kaur, R., Bramwell, V.W., Kirby, D.J., and Perrie, Y. (2012). Pegylation of DDA:TDB liposomal adjuvants reduces the vaccine depot effect and alters the Th1/Th2 immune responses. *J. Control. Release* 158 (1): 72–77.

96 Mishra, S., Webster, P., and Davis, M.E. (2004). PEGylation significantly affects cellular uptake and intracellular trafficking of non-viral gene delivery particles. *Eur. J. Cell Biol.* 83 (3): 97–111.

97 Remaut, K., Lucas, B., Braeckmans, K. et al. (2007). Pegylation of liposomes favours the endosomal degradation of the delivered phosphodiester oligonucleotides. *J. Control. Release* 117 (2): 256–266.

98 Judge, A., McClintock, K., Phelps, J.R., and Maclachlan, I. (2006). Hypersensitivity and loss of disease site targeting caused by antibody responses to PEGylated liposomes. *Mol. Ther.* 13 (2): 328–337.

99 Alameh, M.G., Tombácz, I., Bettini, E. et al. (2021). Lipid nanoparticles enhance the efficacy of mRNA and protein subunit vaccines by inducing robust T follicular helper cell and humoral responses. *Immunity* 54 (12): 2877–2892.e7.

100 Xie, C., Yao, R., and Xia, X. (2023). The advances of adjuvants in mRNA vaccines. *NPJ Vaccines* 8 (1): 1–6.

101 Lee, J., Woodruff, M.C., Kim, E.H., and Nam, J.H. (2023). Knife's edge: balancing immunogenicity and reactogenicity in mRNA vaccines. *Exp. Mol. Med.* 55 (7): 1305–1313.

102 Vlatkovic, I. (2021). Non-immunotherapy application of LNP-mRNA: maximizing efficacy and safety. *Biomedicines* 9 (5): 530.

103 Nag, K., Sarker, M.E.H., Kumar, S. et al. (2022). DoE-derived continuous and robust process for manufacturing of pharmaceutical-grade wide-range LNPs for RNA-vaccine/drug delivery. *Sci. Rep.* 12 (1): 9394.

104 Jeffs, L.B., Palmer, L.R., Ambegia, E.G. et al. (2005). A scalable, extrusion-free method for efficient liposomal encapsulation of plasmid DNA. *Pharm. Res.* 22 (3): 362–372.

105 Stroock, A.D., Dertinger, S.K.W., Ajdari, A. et al. (2002). Chaotic mixer for microchannels. *Science* 295 (5555): 647–651.

106 Trotta, M., Debernardi, F., and Caputo, O. (2003). Preparation of solid lipid nanoparticles by a solvent emulsification–diffusion technique. *Int. J. Pharm.* 257 (1–2): 153–160.

107 Dingler, A. and Gohla, S. (2002). Production of solid lipid nanoparticles (SLN): scaling up feasibilities. *J. Microencapsul.* 19 (1): 11–16.

108 Das, S., Ng, W.K., and Tan, R.B.H. (2012). Are nanostructured lipid carriers (NLCs) better than solid lipid nanoparticles (SLNs): development, characterizations and comparative evaluations of clotrimazole-loaded SLNs and NLCs? *Eur. J. Pharm. Sci.* 47 (1): 139–151.

109 Public Citizen. (2021). How to make enough vaccine for the world in one year. https://www.citizen.org/article/how-to-make-enough-vaccine-for-the-world-in-one-year/ (accessed 25 August 2022).

110 Kumar, V., Srinivasan, V., and Kumara, S. (2022). Smart vaccine manufacturing using novel biotechnology platforms: a study during COVID-19. *J. Comput. Inf. Sci. Eng.* 22 (4): 040903.

111 Kis, Z., Kontoravdi, C., Shattock, R., and Shah, N. (2020). Resources, production scales and time required for producing RNA vaccines for the global pandemic demand. *Vaccines* 9 (1): 3.

112 Crommelin, D.J.A., Anchordoquy, T.J., Volkin, D.B. et al. (2021). Addressing the cold reality of mRNA vaccine stability. *J. Pharm. Sci.* 110 (3): 997–1001.

113 Arteta, M.Y., Kjellman, T., Bartesaghi, S. et al. (2018). Successful reprogramming of cellular protein production through mRNA delivered by functionalized lipid nanoparticles. *PNAS* 115 (15): E3351–E3360.

114 Zhang, M., Hussain, A., Yang, H. et al. (2023). mRNA-based modalities for infectious disease management. *Nano Res.* 16 (1): 672–691. https://doi.org/10.1007/s12274-022-4627-5.

115 Zhao, P., Hou, X., Yan, J. et al. (2020). Long-term storage of lipid-like nanoparticles for mRNA delivery. *Bioact. Mater.* 5 (2): 358–363.

116 Muramatsu, H., Lam, K., Bajusz, C. et al. (2022). Lyophilization provides long-term stability for a lipid nanoparticle-formulated, nucleoside-modified mRNA vaccine. *Mol. Ther.* 30 (5): 1941–1951.

117 Lee, H., Jiang, D., and Pardridge, W.M. (2020). Lyoprotectant optimization for the freeze-drying of receptor-targeted Trojan horse liposomes for plasmid DNA delivery. *Mol. Pharm.* 17 (6): 2165–2174.

118 USP-NF. (2022). Analytical procedures for mRNA vaccine quality (draft guidelines). https://www.uspnf.com/notices/analytical-procedures-mrna-vaccines-20220210 (accessed 19 August 2022).

119 Vlatkovic, I., Ludwig, J., Boros, G. et al. (2022). Ribozyme assays to quantify the capping efficiency of in vitro-transcribed mRNA. *Pharmaceutics* 14 (2): 328.

120 Rayaprolu, B., Carr, C., Joest, E. et al. (2023). Defining the required critical quality attributes (CQAs) and phase requirements for mRNA/LNP product development and manufacture. *BioPhorum* https://www.biophorum.com/

download/defining-the-required-critical-quality-attributes-cqas-and-phase-requirements-for-mrna-lnp-product-development-and-manufacture/ (accessed 4 January 2024).

121 Knezevic, I., Liu, M.A., Peden, K. et al. (2021). Development of mRNA vaccines: scientific and regulatory issues. *Vaccines* 9 (2): 81.

122 Liu, M.A., Zhou, T., Sheets, R.L. et al. (2022). WHO informal consultation on regulatory considerations for evaluation of the quality, safety and efficacy of RNA-based prophylactic vaccines for infectious diseases, 20-22 April 2021. *Emerg. Microbes Infect.* 11 (1): 384–391.

123 van de Berg, D., Kis, Z., Behmer, C.F. et al. (2021). Quality by design modelling to support rapid RNA vaccine production against emerging infectious diseases. *NPJ Vaccines* 6 (1): 65.

124 Rele, S. (2021). COVID-19 vaccine development during pandemic: gap analysis, opportunities, and impact on future emerging infectious disease development strategies. *Hum. Vaccin. Immunother.* 17 (4): 1122–1127.

125 Kis, Z., Kontoravdi, C., Dey, A.K. et al. (2020). Rapid development and deployment of high-volume vaccines for pandemic response. *J. Adv. Manuf. Process.* 2 (3): e10060.

126 Kis, Z., Tak, K., Ibrahim, D. et al. (2022). Pandemic-response adenoviral vector and RNA vaccine manufacturing. *NPJ Vaccines* 7 (1): 1–10.

127 Vuksanaj, K. (2022). Key insights into overcoming mRNA process challenges. GEN - Genetic Engineering and Biotechnology News. https://www.genengnews.com/sponsored/key-insights-into-overcoming-mrna-process-challenges/ (accessed 17 August 2022).

128 Vickers, J., Cramer, P., Eardley-Patel, R., and Excell, O. (2022). Overcoming engineering challenges to enable commercial scale mRNA vaccine manufacturing. *BioPharm. Int.* 35 (8): 36–41.

129 Geiger, J. and Treml, M. (2020). mRNA purification by tangential flow filtration. WO2020165158A1. https://patents.google.com/patent/WO2020165158A1/en (accessed 24 August 2022).

130 Schmidt, A., Helgers, H., Vetter, F.L. et al. (2021). Fast and flexible mRNA vaccine manufacturing as a solution to pandemic situations by adopting chemical engineering good practice—continuous autonomous operation in stainless steel equipment concepts. *Processes* 9 (11): 1874.

131 Helgers, H., Hengelbrock, A., Schmidt, A., and Strube, J. (2021). Digital twins for continuous mRNA production. *Processes* 9 (11): 1967.

132 Ghaemmaghamian, Z., Zarghami, R., Walker, G. et al. (2022). Stabilizing vaccines via drying: quality by design considerations. *Adv. Drug Deliv. Rev.* 187: 114313.

133 Fukuda, I.M., Pinto, C.F.F., dos S Moreira, C. et al. (2018). Design of experiments (DoE) applied to pharmaceutical and analytical quality by design (QbD). *Braz. J. Pharm. Sci.* 54 (spe): http://www.scielo.br/scielo.php?script=sci_arttext&pid=S1984-82502018000700405&lng=en&tlng=en (accessed 24 August 2022).

134 Politis, S.N., Colombo, P., Colombo, G., and Rekkas, D.M. (2017). Design of experiments (DoE) in pharmaceutical development. *Drug Dev. Ind. Pharm.* 43 (6): 889–901.

135 Fahr, S., Thiel, L., and Sengoba, C. (2021). *Mobile on-Demand (MOD) mRNA Vaccine Production: A Design and Optimal Location Study*, 15. Aachener Verfahrenstechnik, RWTH Aachen University https://web.fe.up.pt/~fgm/eurecha/scp_2020/eurecha2020_mainreport_1stprize.pdf (accessed 24 August 2022).

136 BioNTech. Modern manufacturing processes for the production of the COVID-19 vaccine. https://www.biontech.com/int/en/home/manufacturing-and-services/production-network.html (accessed 14 August 2022).

7

mRNA Vaccination for Induction of Immune Tolerance Against Autoimmune Disease

Mark C. Gissler[1†], Felix S.R. Picard[2†], Timoteo Marchini[1], Holger Winkels[2], and Dennis Wolf[1]

[1] *University of Freiburg, Faculty of Medicine and University Heart Center, Department of Cardiology and Angiology, Hugstetter Str. 55, 79106, Freiburg im Breisgau, Germany*
[2] *University of Cologne, Faculty of Medicine and University Hospital Cologne, Department of Cardiology, Kerpener Strasse 62, 50937 Cologne, Germany*

7.1 Role of Adaptive Immune Cells in Autoimmunity and Tolerance

7.1.1 Development of the Adaptive Immune System – Defining the Boundaries of Autoimmunity

The immune system is an intricate and complex network of immune mediators, cells, and tissues. It protects the human body against pathogens and diseases of various kinds and can be divided into two complex defense systems. A first and primitive line of defense is provided by mechanical and chemical barriers, such as the skin and mucosa. Commensal bacteria residing at these surfaces provide a biological barrier by competing with pathogenic bacteria for nutrients and habitat [1]. The innate immune response is a multicellular and protein-based system, which is activated by the recognition of pathogen-associated molecular patterns (PAMPs) or damage-associated molecular patterns (DAMPs) in response to infection or injury. The immune responses triggered are dependent on the respective PAMP- or DAMP-mediated activation of pattern recognition receptors (PRRs), such as Toll-like receptors (TLRs). Their structure and function are linked to the genetically encoded receptor sequences of the respective organism [1].

7.1.2 Diversity of Adaptive Immunity

Acquired or adaptive immunity is the immunological response against foreign structural proteins and other particles with a harmful potential called antigens. Concerning cellular immunity, peptides from such antigens are presented by

† Mark C. Gissler and Felix S.R. Picard contributed equally.

Trends in mRNA Vaccine Research, First Edition. Edited by Gabor Tamas Szabo and Norbert Pardi.

major histocompatibility complexes (MHCs) and recognized by T-cell receptors (TCRs), leading to the activation of antigen-specific T cells that specifically recognize the combination of MHC and peptide. Alternatively, as part of the humoral immune response, an antigen is recognized directly by a specific B-cell receptor (BCR) expressed on B cells. Recognition of the cognate antigen via the BCR in combination with sufficient costimulatory signals, such as CD40–CD40L interaction, induces an immunoglobulin switch and the formation of B-memory and antibody-producing plasma cells. While natural antibodies are genetically encoded, the coding DNA sequences for the expression of most antibodies and antigen-recognizing TCRs and BCRs are subject to V(D)J recombination (V for variable, D for diversifying, and J for joining) [1]. This enables the formation of an immense diversity of highly specific receptors, which enable the recognition of any potential antigen: The entire T-cell repertoire comprises $5–10 \times 10^9$ different T-cell clones [2], while the TCR repertoire covers approximately $1–2 \times 10^8$ unique TCR sequences in young adults [3]. Both T and B cells derive from common lymphoid progenitors (CLPs), which differentiate from hematopoietic stem cells in the bone marrow. CLPs migrate into the thymus, enter the T-cell lineage, and develop into naïve T cells, which eventually leave the thymus and enter the periphery. During development, the recombined TCR is tested for reactivity against endogenous antigens presented in MHCs in a process called positive selection. Only cells with a functional TCR will receive survival signals, others die. In the second step, remaining T cells will be selected not to recognize self-antigens. If T cells respond to a self-antigen with strong TCR signals, T cells will be eliminated. Otherwise, T cells would be self-reactive. Yet, three subsets of unconventional T cells require strong agonistic TCR signals: Forkhead Box P3 $(Foxp3)^+$ regulatory T (T_{reg}) cells, invariant natural killer T (iNKT) cells, and $TCR\alpha\beta^+$ $CD8\alpha\alpha^+$ intestinal intraepithelial lymphocytes (IELs) [4–6]. T_{regs} are immunosuppressive cells that are selected for some autoantigens. Hence, autoimmunity is prevented by a protective limb of autoimmunity [7]. Notably, T cells specific for autoantigens with pathogenic phenotypes drive local tissue dysfunction and destruction in autoimmunity. T_{regs} with the same specificity can neutralize this pathogenic response. The balance of autoimmunity and health is therefore kept in check by the ratio of immunosuppressive T_{regs} and pathogenic T-cell clones.

7.1.3 Antigen-Specific T Cells

The resulting conventional T cells can be divided into $CD4^+$ (MHCII-restricted) and $CD8^+$ (MHCI-restricted) cells [8, 9]. These can be classified not only by their CD4/CD8 coreceptor expression but also by their main TCR composition: Alpha–beta T cells (αβ T cells), which express a TCR consisting of an alpha chain and a beta chain (αβ), represent most T cells in the human immune system. They recognize peptide antigens presented on MHC molecules. This recognition allows αβ T cells to detect and respond to a wide range of foreign pathogens, including viruses, bacteria, parasites, and also self-antigens, i.e. peptides from endogenous proteins. αβ T cells are involved in both cell-mediated and humoral immune responses, coordinating the actions of other immune cells and secreting cytokines to regulate immunity. Another subset of T cells that develops in the thymus rearranges a different TCR consisting of TCR-γ and TCR-δ chains (γδ T cells). γδ T cells are conserved throughout evolution and across species. Unlike αβ T cells, γδ T cells are not MHC-restricted, and their antigen recognition does not rely on CD4 or CD8 coreceptor expression although γδ T cells in the mouse intestine express the CD8αα dimer and several human γδ T-cell subsets also express CD8 [10]. γδ T cells recognize a broader range of antigens [11], including both peptide and nonpeptide molecules. They are mainly found in epithelial tissues, such as the skin, intestines, and lungs, where they serve as a first line of defense against infections. γδ T cells exhibit rapid and innate-like immune responses, contributing to the early control of infections and tissue repair [12]. The functional differences between αβ T cells and γδ T cells are partly attributed to their distinct tissue distributions and TCR specificities. αβ T cells predominantly populate lymphoid tissues, such as the lymph nodes and spleen, and participate in adaptive immune responses. They undergo clonal expansion upon antigen recognition and can differentiate into various effector cell types, including cytotoxic T cells and helper T cells. In contrast, γδ T cells are enriched in nonlymphoid tissues, particularly at barrier surfaces, where they act as a frontline defense mechanism against pathogens. They exhibit innate-like features and can rapidly produce effector molecules, such as cytokines and chemokines, without prior antigen exposure.

7.1.4 T-cell Phenotypes and Functions

Antigen-specific $CD4^+$ and $CD8^+$ T cells exist as effector cells that either activate further immune cells or actively kill target cells through cytokine release and secretion of lytic proteins. Alternatively, they appear as effector memory cells (T_{EM}), tissue-resident memory cells (T_{RM}), or central memory cells (T_{CM}) in secondary lymphoid organs. These cells are immediately reactivated upon renewed antigen contact and provide a new reservoir of antigen-specific effector cells through rapid proliferation [13].

7.1.4.1 $CD4^+$ T Cells

$CD4^+$ T cells are a specialized type of T cells that orchestrate and steer the activity of other immune cells and act as T-helper (T_H) cells that can differentiate into several effector states. They are classified by lineage transcription factors and the respective set of cytokines they secrete to shape the microenvironment and to steer immune responses: T_H1 cells are proinflammatory cells, which depend on the expression of the transcription factor T-bet and secrete interferon gamma (IFN-γ), and tumor necrosis factor alpha (TNF-α) [14]. They are important mediators of immune responses against cancer cells and intracellular pathogens such as viruses. Type 2 $CD4^+$ T-helper (T_H2) cells express the transcription factor Gata3 and secrete interleukin-4 (IL-4), IL-5, IL-10, and IL-13 [15]. They are involved in the activation of B cells and antibody production and are relevant for the defense of extracellular parasites and allergic responses. T_H9 cells are characterized by interferon regulating factor 4 (IRF4) expression, and IL-9 and IFN-γ production and engage in both allergic responses and anticancer defense [16]. T_H17 cells express the transcription factor RAR-related orphan receptor gamma2 (RORγT) and secrete IL-17 and IL-22 [15]. T_H17 cells initiate and maintain inflammatory reactions, particularly in the context of bacterial and fungal infections. Their proinflammatory potential makes T_H17 cells prone to mediate autoimmune diseases. T_{regs} are characterized by FoxP3 expression and are crucial for maintaining immune tolerance and preventing autoimmunity. They not only secrete the anti-inflammatory cytokine interleukin-10 (IL-10) and transforming growth factor beta (TGF-β) [3, 17] but also engage in other mechanisms to suppress activation of neighboring immune cells. A specialized subset of $CD4^+$ T cells, T follicular helper (T_{FH}) cells, is characterized by the expression of transcription factor BCL6 and the chemokine receptor CXCR5. T_{FH} cells secrete cytokines and express surface molecules important for B-cell maturation [18]. A small subset of naïve CD4 T cells expresses MHC class I-restricted T-cell-associated molecule (CRTAM), a surface marker commonly expressed by $CD8^+$ T cells and iNKT cells. $CRTAM^+$ $CD4^+$ T cells have the potential to differentiate into $CD4^+$ cytotoxic T lymphocytes (CTLs), which secrete classical T_H1 cytokines like IFN-γ and TNF-α, but also bear cytolytic potential by granzyme and perforin secretion [19].

7.1.4.2 $CD8^+$ T Cells

$CD8^+$ T cells are CTLs. They can kill other cells based on strong IFN-γ production and release of perforins and granzymes. Different effector types of $CD8^+$ T cells can be distinguished: proinflammatory IL-17-producing $CD8^+$ cells with a weak cytotoxic potential (T_C17) have been described in inflammatory diseases and autoimmunity in mice and humans [20, 21]. In addition, proinflammatory IL-9-secreting $CD8^+$ T cells, termed T_C9 [22] and IL-22-producing, proinflammatory T_C22 cells have been identified in atopic dermatitis [23, 24]. In analogy to $CD4^+$ T_{regs}, $CD8^+$ T_{regs} exert anti-inflammatory actions [25]. The plasticity and variable roles of $CD4^+$ and $CD8^+$ effector T-cell subtypes have been the subject of immunological research in recent decades.

7.1.5 Role of B Cells and Autoantibodies

7.1.5.1 Development of B Cells

Like T-cell progenitors, B-cell progenitors develop from hematopoietic stem cells in the bone marrow in adult humans, while the mesenchymal tissues of the yolk sac and fetal liver are primary sources of B cells in fetuses and newborns. However, unlike T-cell development, which is largely restricted to embryonic and neonatal life, B-cell progenitors and B cells form throughout the entire lifespan [26]. Deletion of self-reactive clones of B cells is an important part of the development of the antibody repertoire. Like T cells, each B-cell clone expresses a unique, antigen-specific membrane-bound version of the antibody produced and secreted by the cell, called the BCR. Unlike the MHC-restricted TCR, the BCR binds proteins, nucleic acids, carbohydrates, and lipid sequences (antigenic determinants) independently of their association with MHC proteins. Therefore, B cells can be activated by cell-bound and soluble antigens [27]. Clones of developing B cells that fail to successfully remodel their BCR or whose BCR is not stimulated within 1–3 days after export to the primary lymphoid organs (lymph nodes and spleen) die. Death of the newly developed B cells also occurs when antigenic stimulation occurs without immediate T_H cell-provided signals, e.g. ligation of CD40L with CD40 on the B-cell surface. Chronic stimulation of B cells by soluble antigens, such as serum antigens, from their earliest stages of development onwards induces anergy. Anergic B cells do not proliferate and mature into antibody-secreting cells upon antigenic restimulation and T-cell help. Anergic B cells, which are potentially autoreactive and thus might pose a threat, will leave the bone marrow and home into secondary lymphoid organs, where they are eliminated in two ways: (i) they remain in the periarteriolar zones and thus do not compete with nonanergic B cells for space and signals in the follicles and germinal centers, where further expansion and maturation occurs; or (ii) they are killed by activated T cells. Lysis of anergic B cells by T cells depends on the Fas/Fas ligand pathway. Adoptive transfer studies have shown that the elimination of these anergic B cells requires a functional Fas on the B cell and a functional Fas ligand on the T cell. Additional signals by other members of the TNF family are required, such as CD40–CD40L interactions. Stimulation of CD40 on anergic B cells induces expression of Fas, which induces cell death upon engagement of Fas ligand expressed on the T-cell surface. Interestingly, the same sequence of events is required for B-cell proliferation and maturation in normal B cells after acute antigen stimulation. Thus, the activation state of the B cell (chronic or acute) determines the functional outcome (death or expansion and maturation) of the T/B-cell interaction [28].

7.1.5.2 Somatic Hypermutations in B Cells – Refining High-Affinity Antibodies

Mature B cells, unlike mature T cells, can undergo somatic mutation of their BCR after antigen stimulation. This feature allows affinity maturation of the response in germinal centers to produce antibodies with higher affinity, but also poses a new risk for the development of autoantibodies and immunologic escape. Somatic mutations of the BCR are regulated by a complex process known as somatic hypermutation (SHM), which occurs during the maturation of B cells in the germinal centers of secondary lymphoid organs. SHM is a mechanism that introduces point mutations into the variable regions of the BCR genes, specifically in the genes encoding the immunoglobulin heavy and light chains. These mutations lead to the generation of BCR variants with diverse antigen-binding specificities, allowing the immune system to produce antibodies with increased affinity for the target antigen. B cells stimulated by antigen in the context of complement (e.g. on the surface of a bacterium) or complement on the surface of a specialized antigen-presenting cell (APC) (follicular dendritic cell, FDC) are not subject to apoptosis. Stimulation of germinal center B cells (centrocytes) by antigen in the absence of complement or CD23 stimulation results in deletion of these clones. This type of clonal deletion of mature B cells is independent of the Fas system. Complement or FDC stimulation of B cells induces expression of antiapoptotic molecules such as Bcl-2, and deletion of B cells that do not receive signals from both the BCR and the costimulator occurs via a pathway analog to the "neglect" pathway of thymocytes.

7.1.5.3 Noncanonical Functions of B Cells

B cells do not only exist as classical antibody producers, but more recent studies identified an IL-10-producing subtype with immunoregulatory and suppressive capabilities (B_{reg}) similar to classical immune regulators of the $CD4^+$ lineage [29, 30].

7.1.6 Autoimmune Diseases – Break of Tolerance Against Self-antigens

Immunological tolerance describes highly regulated mechanisms to prevent an immune response against a particular antigen. The unresponsiveness of the immune system to self-antigens (self-tolerance) is ensured through central and peripheral tolerance mechanisms. Central tolerance of newly developing T cells with high-affinity self-reactive TCR clones is mediated in the thymus through clonal deletion (elimination of potentially dangerous cells) or clonal diversion, the reprogramming of such cells into T_{reg} cells [31]. As these processes alone do not suffice to control self-reactivity in all circumstances, further mechanisms exist to prevent autoreactive T cells outside of the thymus from inflicting harmful immune responses against self-antigens. Peripheral tolerance mechanisms include maintenance of a functionally unresponsive state of self-reactive T cells in the absence of costimulation (termed "anergy") and homeostatic control through checkpoint proteins such as cytotoxic T-lymphocyte antigen 4 (CTLA-4) [32, 33]. The break of tolerance against self-antigens results in autoimmune diseases. The exact mechanisms behind the loss of immune tolerance in autoimmune diseases are not fully understood, but genetic predisposition, environmental factors, and dysregulation of the immune system are believed to be contributing factors. Interferences with a plethora of factors that maintain tolerance in an experimental setting may induce autoimmune diseases.

Besides T cells, antibodies are essential components of the immune system and provide protection against foreign invaders such as bacteria and viruses. In autoimmune diseases, the immune system recognizes self-antigens, which results in the production of autoantibodies which leads to a misguided attack of healthy tissue [34]. A breakdown of immune tolerance is the basis for generation of autoantibodies against self-antigens and can induce and/or contribute to autoimmune diseases. Once autoantibodies are produced, they can cause direct damage to cells or tissues through various mechanisms. Among those mechanisms is activation of the complement system, which consists of a series of proteins that amplify the immune response. The activation of the complement system can lead to inflammation and cell destruction. Autoantibodies can further initiate the process of antibody-dependent cellular cytotoxicity (ADCC) and recruit effector cells such as natural killer (NK) cells and macrophages, which bind with their Fc receptor antibodies and induce lysis of cells coated with autoantibodies [35]. In some cases, autoantibodies produced against specific target proteins may cross-react with other tissues, leading to a broader autoimmune response. These phenomena induce chronic inflammation and tissue damage in various organs and systems and lead to a myriad of autoimmune diseases such as rheumatoid arthritis, systemic lupus erythematosus (SLE), multiple sclerosis (MS), and type 1 diabetes (T1DM). The function of autoantibodies is exemplified by SLE. SLE is characterized by an autoimmune response that affects multiple tissue sites throughout the body including the skin, kidneys, blood cells, brain, heart, and lung. SLE is a prototypic autoimmune disorder that shows the occurrence and involvement of autoantibodies. Prominent autoantibodies in SLE are antinuclear antibodies (ANAs) [36]. ANAs are the most prevalent autoantibodies in lupus. They target various components found in the cell nucleus, including DNA, RNA, and proteins. ANAs are a hallmark of SLE and are detected in most lupus patients. They are also present in other autoimmune diseases, but their presence, along with other clinical symptoms, helps in diagnosing SLE. Anti-dsDNA antibodies are strongly associated with active lupus and are considered specific markers for the disease. Anti-dsDNA antibodies can form immune complexes that deposit in the kidneys, leading to lupus nephritis, a severe complication of SLE [37].

7.1.7 Immunomodulation of Autoimmune Diseases

Modulation of autoimmune diseases aims to suppress or modify the abnormal immune responses that contribute to the development and progression of autoimmune conditions. During the past decades, several different approaches have been developed and refined to dampen the activity of the immune system. Immunosuppressive drugs such as corticosteroids (prednisone and dexamethasone) are commonly used as a first-line immunosuppressive therapy. They exert their function by both inhibiting the production of proinflammatory cytokines like IL-1, IL-6, and TNF-α and reducing immune cell activation and migration [38]. Methotrexate (MTX), a cytostatic initially developed as chemotherapeutic agent, has been successfully in use as a second line immunosuppressant in several arthritis subtypes [39] and Morbus Crohn and MS [40]. Biologic therapies target specific components of the immune system involved in autoimmune diseases. Examples include monoclonal antibodies that block proinflammatory cytokines, such as TNF-α, interleukin-6 (IL-6), or interleukin-17 (IL-17). One of the biggest blockbuster drugs in rheumatoid arthritis has been Adilimumab/Humira, a fully human antibody against TNF-α [41]. Other biologics aim to inhibit specific immune cells, such as pathogenic B cells or T cells, or to promote the function of T_{regs} to suppress aberrant immune responses. For instance, T_{regs} can be expanded by T_{reg}-promoting cytokines such as IL-2 [42] or by an adoptive transfer of *ex vivo* expanded T_{regs} *in vivo*, which has been first tested in patients with T1DM [43, 44]. However, such therapies have to be regarded with caution: a low-dose IL-2 therapy in addition to polyclonal T_{reg} therapy did not only induce proliferation of immunosuppressive T_{regs} but also expansion of cytotoxic NK cells and CD8 T cells, which can have detrimental effects in the context of diabetes [43]. Cell-based therapies, such as hematopoietic stem cell transplantation (HSCT) or mesenchymal stem cell (MSC) therapy, are being explored as potential treatments for autoimmune diseases. HSCT involves the transplantation of hematopoietic stem cells, which can repopulate the immune system and potentially reset immune tolerance. MSCs have immunomodulatory properties and can suppress immune responses, making them attractive for cell-based therapies. Likewise, live-long target-unspecific immunosuppression that is at the risk of targeting beneficial immune function in host defense does not represent a causal treatment.

7.1.7.1 Tolerogenic Vaccination to Dampen MHC-II-Dependent Autoimmunity

Autoimmunity is the result of an aberrant response against specific autoantigens or self-antigens. Current therapies against autoimmunity aim at lowering overall reactivity of the immune system, which grounds on the lack of any other specific therapies. Immune-activating vaccination that is designed to protect against bacterial and viral infection certainly represents the most successful intervention of medical history [45]. The centerpiece of the concept of *immunomodulatory* or *tolerogenic* vaccination is to induce a preferable immune phenotype that is either protecting from *de novo* disease or attenuating established autoimmune diseases. Immunosuppressive T_{regs} are the best-described target cells for this concept; expanding the pool of T_{regs} holds great promise to enhance the natural counterpart of pathogenic autoreactive T cells. Preclinical approaches employing immunization primarily target at T cells, while the role of vaccination-induced antibodies that serve as biomarkers of disease activity has been less well understood. Tolerogenic vaccination has been demonstrated in mouse models of diabetes, MS, and atherosclerosis [46]. Most of these concepts have remained at a preclinical level. We will introduce and comment on tolerogenic vaccination in two autoimmune models, MS and atherosclerosis, in the following sections.

7.2 Atherosclerosis – An Unprecedented Autoimmune Disease

7.2.1 Autoimmune Component of Atherosclerosis

Atherosclerosis is a chronic inflammatory disease of medium- to large-size arteries that is characterized by the development of vessel occluding plaques [47, 48]. The clinical complications of atherogenesis arise from formation of arterial thrombi, vessel occlusion, and subsequent tissue ischemia. Myocardial infarction (MI) and ischemic stroke represent the leading causes of death worldwide [48, 49]. Evidence from experimental and clinical studies has identified the accumulation of low-density lipoprotein cholesterol (LDL-C) in the subintimal space of arteries triggered by cardiovascular risk factors, such as hyperglyceridemia and hypertension, as the major culprit of atherosclerosis [50]. The main protein component of the LDL-C particle is Apolipoprotein B 100 (ApoB-100), which contains the binding site for the hepatic LDL receptor (LDL-R) [51]. Within the vessel wall, LDL/ApoB-100 is subject to an oxidative modification [52] and subsequently taken up by monocyte-derived macrophages, which turn into "foam cells" that characterize and drive atherosclerotic disease progression by secretion of proinflammatory cytokines and matrix metalloproteinases (MMPs) that ultimately promote destabilization and rupture of the plaque [53–55]. Peptides from ApoB act as autoantigens and initiate an autoimmune response that comprises autoreactive T cells and B-cell-derived immunoglobulins binding epitopes of LDL/ApoB [48, 56]. The adaptive autoimmune response against LDL/ApoB is highly heterogeneous. For instance, the presence of autoantibodies in atherosclerosis can affect the vascular endothelium, smooth muscle cells, and foam cells. Yet, not all autoantibodies in atherosclerosis exert proinflammatory functions. A natural IgM antibody called E06, which is germline encoded, has been shown to bind the phosphocholine headgroup of oxidized phospholipid, prevent oxidized LDL (oxLDL) uptake by macrophages [57, 58], and reduce atherosclerosis in mouse models [59]. Recently, another protective antibody targeting a novel antigen in the atherosclerotic plaque, the mitochondrial dehydrogenase ALDH4A1, has been identified [60].

7.2.1.1 Role of Antigen-Specific T-Helper Cells in Atherosclerosis

T cells represent the largest leukocyte population in human atherosclerotic plaques with $CD4^+$ T-helper cells accounting for the majority of all lesional T cells [61, 62]. Antigen-specific helper T cells in the murine atherosclerotic plaque show distinct lineage commitment mainly comprising proatherogenic T_H1, antiatherogenic T_{reg}, and T_H17 phenotypes (as discussed in [63]). T_H1 cells express the transcription factor T bet, secrete the proinflammatory cytokine IFN-γ, and exacerbate atherosclerosis. T-regulatory (T_{reg}) cells express the transcription factor FoxP3 and IL-2 receptor (CD25), produce the anti-inflammatory cytokine IL-10 and TGF-β, and limit atherosclerosis by promoting self-tolerance [64]. T_H17 cells express the transcription factor RORγT, produce IL-17, and have been observed to show both pro- and anti-atherosclerotic properties in experimental models [65]. ApoB-specific T-helper cells in the plaque and lymph nodes show partially overlapping commitment to the latter that describe T_H phenotypes with T_H1-like or T_{reg}-like cells depending on concomitant cytokine/transcription factor expression of T-bet/IFN-γ or FoxP3/IL-10, respectively, as highlighted by recent insights from scRNA-seq [63]. Notably, T-cell lineage commitment of ApoB-reactive T-helper cells in atherogenesis is not necessarily permanent and can change in the course of atherogenesis. Initially, these cells have been found to exhibit an overall anti-inflammatory T_{reg} phenotype. However, this initial protective phenotype is gradually lost and replaced by a proinflammatory T_H1-/T_H17-like phenotype with only a residual T_{reg} transcriptome [66]. Hypothetically, it should be the aim of any tolerogenic vaccination approach to (i) maintain the T_{reg} phenotype over time or (ii) generate *de novo* IL-10-expressing T_{regs} or IL-10-expressing non-T_{regs} [63, 67].

7.2.1.2 B Cells and Autoantibodies in Atherosclerosis

Functional heterogeneity can also be found in the B-cell compartment: Protective B_1 cells produce IgM antibodies that cross-react with specific (neo-) epitopes that emerge during oxidation of LDL and prevent oxLDL uptake by macrophages and mostly protect from atherosclerosis without requiring participation of T cells. On the other hand, conventional B_2 cells secrete IgG antibodies that enhance vascular inflammation and promote atherosclerosis [63, 68] albeit the role of vaccination-induced antibodies is controversial (see Section 7.2.4). We and others have shown that antibodies recognizing LDL and ApoB correlate with cardiovascular outcomes and risk factors in humans [68, 69]. These observations underline the need to precisely delineate cellular targets for atheroprotective vaccination to selectively strengthen the anti-inflammatory portions of the immune system.

7.2.2 Established Autoantigens in Atherosclerosis

7.2.2.1 LDL-C and ApoB

Atherosclerosis is a lipid-associated disease driven by chronic inflammation. Since the adaptive immune component of atherosclerosis was discovered in 1986 by Hansson and colleagues, a handful of autoantigens have been identified in preclinical studies [70]. The most studied target autoantigens are LDL and oxLDL and its core protein ApoB [71]. LDL-cholesterol levels in humans correlate with increased coronary heart disease risk and adverse clinical outcomes [50]. Surprisingly, Palinski et al. 1995 first reported that immunization of LDL-R-deficient rabbits with homologous malondialdehyde-modified LDL reduces atherogenesis [72]. In line, further preclinical studies in rodent models including atherosclerotic-prone *Ldlr*$^{-/-}$ and *Apoe*$^{-/-}$ mice established that vaccination with either native or oxLDL ameliorates atherogenesis [73–77]. Mechanistically, atheroprotection has been proposed to be mediated by an anti-inflammatory T-cell response that comprises induction and proliferation of antigen-specific T cells, anti-inflammatory cytokine production [78], and a humoral antibody-driven response initiated by B cells [71]. Notably, the main immunogenic part of the LDL particle is its core protein ApoB. Consequently, vaccination with ApoB-100 peptides alone suffices to protect from atherosclerosis [79]. Up to date, nine distinct ApoB peptide epitopes have been validated to limit *de novo* atherosclerosis in preclinical studies: p3, p6, p18, p101, p102, p103, p210, p265, and p295 [66, 78–81]. Whereas atheroprotection after immunization of *Apoe*$^{-/-}$ mice with peptides p3, p6, p18, p101, p102, and p103 was mediated by an expansion of IL-10-producing T_{regs} and relevant antibody titers to these peptides, vaccination of p210, which has no biologically relevant binding affinity to the murine MHC-II allele I-A^b, does not confer atheroprotection by presentation in MHC-II complexes to induce T_{regs} but through alternative anti-inflammatory pathways as detailed below. An overview of experimental studies investigating immunization against LDL-related antigens in mice is provided in [71]. Upon vaccination with these ApoB peptides, a number of anti-inflammatory effects can be observed (previously reviewed in [63]). In summary, induction of ApoB-specific CD4$^+$ T cells and consecutively increased secretion of IL-10 by T_{reg} cells in the atherosclerotic aorta and spleen have been established as the main atherogenesis limiting mechanism [63]. In line, immunization with ApoB peptides fails to confer atheroprotection in atherosclerotic-prone *Apoe*$^{-/-}$ mice if T_{reg} cells are depleted [82]. Further, T_{reg}-independent IL-10 secretion by T_R1 cells [78, 83], immunosuppression by specific $CD8^+$ T-cell subsets [84, 85], and inhibition of T_H1 immunity [63] may contribute to atheroprotection.

7.2.2.2 Heat-Shock Proteins

Heat-shock proteins (HSPs) are constitutively expressed molecular chaperones that play a vital role in the cellular stress response. Intracellularly, HSPs protect proteins from denaturation or loss of function by facilitating protein (re-) folding [86]. Notably, extracellularly expressed HSPs can elicit immune responses as humans develop immune responses to modified autologous and/or bacterial HSPs [87]. As HSPs are rather large proteins, they may give rise to a plethora of potential epitopes with both pro- and anti-inflammatory properties [88]. Heat-shock protein 60 (HSP60) has been identified as a ubiquitous self-antigen expressed on the surface of endothelial cells (ECs) in response to traditional atherosclerotic risk factors [88]. In patients, antibodies against human HSP60 are associated with the presence and severity of coronary artery disease [89]. Detection of HSP60-specific IFN-γ-producing T_{eff} cells in early human atherosclerotic lesions has underlined the existence of HSP-related autoimmunity as a potential mediator of atherosclerosis [71, 90]. Notably, human HSP60 shares a molecular mimicry with chlamydial and mycobacterial HSP65 [91]. Induction of oral tolerance to HSP60 and HSP60 peptides in *Ldlr*$^{-/-}$ mice or some HSP65 peptides in *Apoe*$^{-/-}$ mice results in an increase in the number of T_{reg} cells and a significant decrease in plaque size [92, 93]. Whether the immunological activity against human HSPs causally evolves from human autoantigens or is rather a result of molecular mimicry with bacterial HSP is currently unclear [63].

7.2.2.3 Beta-2-Glycoprotein I

Beta-2-glycoprotein I (β2GPI) is a soluble protein circulating in blood that is implicated in the regulation of the complement system and of hemostasis. β2GPI is the antigenic target of pathogenic autoantibodies found in patients with antiphospholipid syndrome (APS) [94]. George et al. reported that β2GPI is abundantly expressed in the subendothelial regions and the intimal–medial border of human atherosclerotic plaques and colocalized with $CD4^+$ T cells [95]. *In vitro*, β2GPI binds to oxLDL and forms covalently bound oxLDL/β2GPI complexes [96], which associate with disease severity and an increased risk of adverse outcomes in patients with acute coronary syndromes [97]. Whether vaccination using β2GPI protects from experimental atherosclerosis *in vivo* is controversial [63].

7.2.2.4 Virus-Derived Antigens

Several viruses including herpes simplex virus, Epstein–Barr virus (EBV), Varicella Zoster virus (VZV), and Influenza virus have been detected in the vasculature [98, 99] and implicated with the pathogenesis of atherosclerosis [98]. Clinical observations have suggested that viral infections with VZV and Influenza increase the risk for atherosclerotic sequelae including MI and stroke [100]. In a meta-analysis of clinical trials, influenza vaccination was associated with a lower risk of major adverse cardiovascular events with the greatest treatment effect in high-risk patients with clinically relevant atherosclerosis [101]. Similarly, SARS-CoV-2 infection increased the risk of major adverse cardiovascular events and long-term cardiovascular outcomes while full and even partial vaccination against COVID-19 was associated with a lower risk of MACE after SARS-CoV-2 infection according to recent observational data [102, 103]. Notably, such associations might not exclusively derive from antigen-specific immune mechanisms but could at least partially be explained by broad systemic inflammatory effects secondary to local tissue injury and activation of thrombotic pathways [63, 104].

7.2.3 Mechanism of Tolerogenic Peptide Vaccination in Atherosclerosis

Several animal studies have reported that vaccination with either native, oxLDL, or peptides from ApoB induces an atheroprotective response [63, 71]. Vaccination with ApoB peptides was shown to generate antigen-specific T cells (recognizing the cognate antigen/peptide used for immunization), boost T-cell proliferation, and induce cytokine secretion [78]. ApoB-specific $CD4^+$ T cells have been found in the spleen and in the peritoneal cavity. Induction of IL-10-secreting T_{regs} in the atherosclerotic aorta and spleen has been proposed as the main mechanism [79, 105–107]. Pre-existing ApoB-specific T_{regs} or IL-10-secreting non-T_{regs} (T_R1 cells) selectively expand after vaccination with ApoB, either at the site of injection or in draining lymph nodes. Furthermore, cytokines secreted by ApoB-specific T cells may circulate and act on atherosclerotic plaques in a remote fashion (Figure 7.1). It has been proposed that ApoB-specific T cells migrate into the plaque and modulate plaque inflammation and architecture by direct and indirect interactions with stromal and other immune cells [104]. IL-10 seems to be the major propagator of this anti-inflammatory response, although the vast source of IL-10 in the plaque is produced by macrophages [108]. IL-10 is the counter-enzyme blocking pathogenic T_H1-immunity and differentiation of macrophages into the proinflammatory M1-like phenotype.

Classically, vaccination against infectious agents needs to be capable of inducing high-affinity B-cell-derived IgGs that bind to immunodominant epitopes and neutralize the antigen. In addition, vaccination-induced IgGs are biomarkers of vaccination efficacy and antigen-specific T cells support rapid recall responses.

Of note, the generation of neutralizing IgG antibodies requires a proinflammatory response with T_H1-polarized $CD4^+$ T cells, which fundamentally differs from an immunomodulatory immunization that aims to induce a protective response with immunosuppressive T_{regs}. Whether and how antibodies support this response is currently unknown.

7.2.4 Alternative Immunomodulation Against Cardiovascular Disease (CVD) Autoimmunity

7.2.4.1 DNA and mRNA Vaccination

Recombinant proteins, synthesized peptides, attenuated pathogens, and other more complex forms of vaccines (e.g. multivalent peptides displayed on liposomes or other nanoparticles) represent the most common form of antigens for immunomodulation

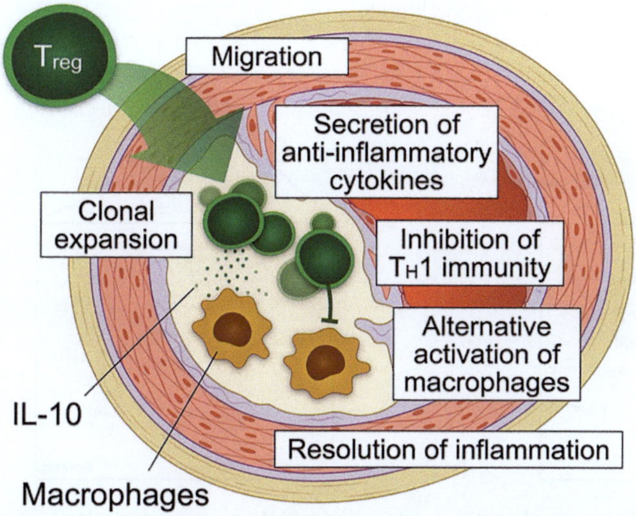

Figure 7.1 Function of T_{regs} induced by tolerogenic vaccination against ApoB peptides. Antigen-specific T cells induced by vaccination differentiate into IL-10-secreting regulatory T (T_{reg}) cells or IL-10-secreting non-T_{reg} (T_R1) in draining lymph nodes. LDL/ApoB-specific T cells then migrate into atherosclerotic plaques and redistribute to naturally draining lymph nodes (e.g. cervical and mediastinal lymph nodes in atherosclerotic animals). IL-10 suppresses cellular proliferation and activation of effector T cells in the plaque. In addition, T_{reg} cells inhibit pathogenic T_H1 pathways, induce less inflammatory alternative-activation pathways in macrophages, and support resolution of inflammation. These effects attenuate atherosclerotic lesion progression. Source: Dennis Wolf.

to elicit a specific immune response. More recently, peptides or entire proteins were delivered by a method referred to as DNA vaccination. There, naked DNA or DNA packed into plasmids that encodes for the antigen is therapeutically applied. DNA-guided expression of vaccines/antigens has been described in animal models of autoimmunity, including experimental autoimmune encephalomyelitis (EAE) and rheumatoid arthritis [109–111]. In the setting of atherosclerosis, vascular endothelial growth factor 2 (VEGF2) was expressed by an orally available DNA vaccine that induced cellular immunity against VEGF2-expressing cells. VEGF2 is known to be expressed by stressed endothelium. Interestingly, this resulted in the generation of $CD8^+$ cytotoxic T cells, which neutralized VEGF2-expressing ECs and therefore protected from atherosclerosis [112]. While this strategy was designed to induce broad and cell-unspecific expression of VEGF-2, mRNA vaccines that contain the messenger RNA (mRNA) coding for an antigen have been reported to be more cell specific and to achieve expression of the desired transcript directly in dendritic cells (DCs) in the spleen [113, 114]. Cell type-specific delivery of DNA that allows for transduction *in vivo* remains an experimental challenge, especially since several viral delivery systems would induce systemic infection-like inflammation [115]. mRNA vaccines have recently emerged as highly effective vaccines against SARS-CoV2. mRNA-based vaccination promises low-cost manufacturing, high safety, fast development, and high potency [116, 117].

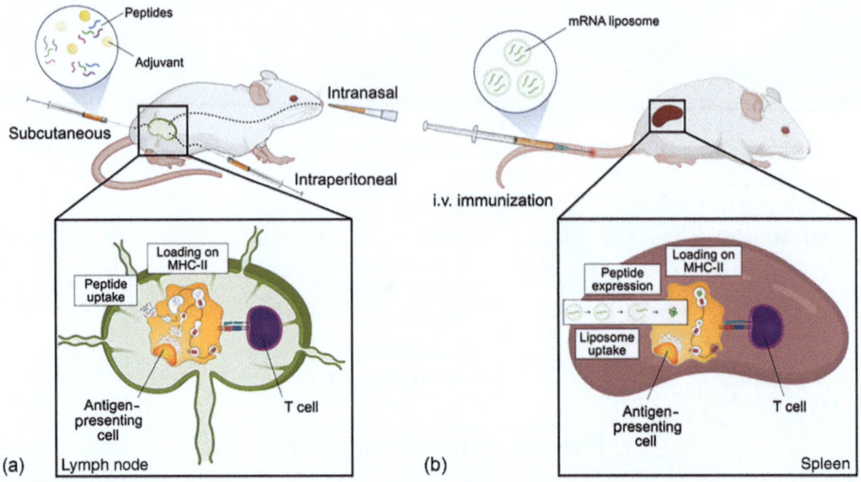

Figure 7.2 Mechanistic differences of peptide/protein and mRNA vaccination in mice. (a) For peptide/protein vaccination, the autoantigen (or peptide thereof) must be combined with an adjuvant (mostly CFA or IFA). The emulsion of adjuvant, oil, and protein is often injected subcutaneously or into the peritoneal cavity [118]. Intranasal application has been reported too [105]. From local injection sites, antigens are transported to locally draining lymph nodes, taken up by antigen-presenting cells (APCs), processed in the endosomes, and peptides from the antigen are presented to T cells. (b) mRNA-based vaccination in the mouse has been tested by intravenous injection [113]. Liposomes are transported to secondary lymphoid organs such as the spleen and locally draining lymph nodes, taken up, and the mRNA is released. mRNA-coding proteins are processed, and peptides thereof are presented on MHC-II. Source: Dennis Wolf.

It is important to note that the aim of antiviral immunity usually is the generation of T_H1 immunity with proinflammatory T-helper cells and high titers of IgG antibodies. Unlike, mRNA-based expression of peptides in a noninflammatory, tolerogenic setting bears the potential to induce immunosuppressive T_H responses with tolerogenic T_{regs} [113]. mRNA vaccines against LDL/ApoB have not yet been described. The principle challenge of DNA and mRNA vaccines to express peptides or entire autoantigens specifically in DCs to induce antigen presentation seems to have been circumvented by a nanoparticle-formulated 1-methylpseudouridine-modified messenger RNA (m1Ψ mRNA) that induced a strong T_{reg} response and prevented EAE in mice [113] (Figure 7.2).

7.2.4.2 Immunotherapy with Immunoglobulins

IgG antibodies against LDL and ApoB can be detected in healthy mice and humans. These partially correlate with clinical atherosclerosis. IgG antibody titers can be therapeutically induced by vaccination with LDL, ApoB, or ApoB peptides [67, 68, 72–74, 76, 78, 106, 119, 120]. It has been proven that IgG-antibody titers are highly effective in quantifying vaccination efficacy, whether these have a biological function, however, is highly controversial. This is exemplified by the fact that vaccination with peptides from the inner, nonhydrated core of LDL particles can be generated *in vivo*. These, however, are not likely to bind the cognate antigen. Both, pro- and anti-atherogenic, roles of passive vaccination with ApoB-induced IgG antibodies have been reported [121–124], while most IgM antibodies seem to be antiatherogenic (summarized in [68]). Existing evidence suggests that T-cell immunity works partially independent of humoral traits of autoimmunity.

7.2.4.3 TCR/CAR T-cell Immunotherapy

T cellular immunity can be mimicked by *ex vivo* constructed T cells expressing a chimeric antigen receptor (CAR T cells) or a transgenic TCR. Single-chain variable fragments (scFv) from antibodies that recognize a unique antigen in cancer cells are often used as CARs. For instance, $CD8^+$ cytotoxic T cells expressing a CAR with specificity toward a cancer antigen can neutralize cancer cells. Likewise, T cells can be constructed to express a TCR recognizing specific antigens, for instance, tumor antigens [125] or cardiac fibroblasts in mice [126], the latter strategy protecting from cardiac fibrosis. Notably, expression of recombinant CAR or TCR can be instructed by mRNA *in vitro* or *in vivo*.

7.3 The Autoimmune Component of MS

7.3.1 Pathophysiology of MS

MS is a neurodegenerative disease affecting the central nervous system (CNS), which is characterized by an autoimmune-driven inflammatory response targeting myelin [127, 128]. Autoreactive T and B cells infiltrate the CNS and secrete proinflammatory cytokines, such as IL-1β, INF-γ, and TNF-α, which promote inflammation, oligodendrocyte dysfunction, and apoptosis. Key autoantibodies and T cells are directed against myelin oligodendrocyte glycoprotein (MOG), the main autoantigen in MS. MOG is a protein found in the myelin sheath. MOG-specific autoantibodies bind and inactivate MOG and promote dysfunction of myelin. MOG autoantibodies are more common in certain subtypes of MS, such as in pediatric cases and those with atypical clinical presentations. The exact mechanisms by which autoantibodies contribute to demyelination and neurodegeneration in MS are still under investigation. The loss of myelin disrupts nerve signal transmission and leads to the formation of sclerotic plaques, characteristic of MS lesions [129]. As the disease progresses, axonal damage and neuronal loss occur, leading to a permanent neurological impairment. Additionally, MS involves the activation of microglia and astrocytes, which exacerbate inflammation and contribute to the neurodegenerative processes. Although the exact etiology of MS remains elusive, genetic susceptibility, environmental factors, and dysregulated immune responses have important roles in the development and progression of MS.

7.3.2 Role of Antigen-Specific Immunity in MS

The center of EAE and MS is an adaptive immune response with T_H1 and T_H17 cytokine-producing T cells that migrate into the CNS and accumulate. In the CNS,

T cells recognize their cognate antigen MOG presented by APCs (macrophages, microglia, DCs, and astrocytes). The main effector cell of this response is macrophages that are instructed by T cells. Myelin is phagocytosed by macrophages. The inflammatory response is further aggravated by antibodies, complement activation, and direct cytotoxic effects of T cells [130, 131]. Notably, anti-inflammatory T cells and their cytokines, mostly IL-10 and T_{regs}, have the ability to resolve this inflammatory response. Whether damaged axons with impaired functionality can regenerate ad integrum depends on the degree of destruction and the context [132]. T_H17 cells seem to be among the first to infiltrate the CNS [133]; IL-17 has a central role in mobilizing innate immune cells to the CNS and initiating IL-1β production [134]. T_{regs} counteract pathogenic immunity by suppressing T_H1 and T_H17 cells. Expansion of antigen-specific T_{regs} has therefore been promoted as an aim of tolerogenic vaccination. In addition to antigen-specific T_{regs}, T_{regs} cells can also act as nonspecific bystander cells [135]. Likewise, immunosuppression is supported by IL-10-expressing non-T_{regs} (T_R1 cells) [136].

7.3.3 Mimicking MS by EAE Model

Rodents do not spontaneously develop MS. The gold standard and most used model is EAE. EAE causes a strong autoimmune response against MOG that results in (i) central nervous inflammation, (ii) demyelination, (iii) axonal loss, and (iv) gliosis and therefore resembles key features of human disease [137]. The main difference between MS and EAE is that EAE requires an external activation of MOG-specific autoimmunity, usually by immunization against the cognate antigens together with immune-activating adjuvants [138, 139]. The choice of adjuvants (IFA versus CFA) seems to determine the degree of EAE [140].

7.3.4 Vaccination Approaches to Prevent EAE

Vaccination is one of the most effective and cost-efficient preventive therapies. Misguided information has led to the concern that vaccination against infectious agents contributes to MS incidence and may deteriorate the health of MS patients, but this has been largely debunked [141–143]. On the contrary, MS patients are at a higher risk of succumbing to vaccine-preventable infections. It is important that this vulnerable population receives protection against infectious agents. Vaccination strategies have not only been used to protect MS patients from infections but also to target pathomechanisms of MS [144]. Today, there are no clinically available vaccines against MS. Several strategies have been examined in EAE mice including TCR peptide vaccination and altered peptide ligand (APL) vaccination [145]. Pathogenic, MOG-reactive T cells have a limited number of variable TCR regions. Peptide sequences of these TCRs have been shown to successfully prevent EAE by boosting TCR-specific T_{regs} [146], a cell population that decreases in time in MS. MS patients show a greater diversity of their antigen-specific TCR repertoire, thus complicating the clinical implementation of a TCR-peptide-based approach. Of note, a trivalent TCR-peptide vaccine targeting three CDR2 regions prevalent on MS-specific T cells has been applied to 27 MS patients every four weeks for 48 weeks. At the end of the trial, MS subjects had similar or augmented Foxp3 expression among peptide-restimulated PBMCs, which also secreted more IL-10, thus demonstrating that this approach might boost immunoregulatory networks in the control of MS [147]. Oral immunization is known to induce tolerogenic antigen-specific immune responses. Mucosal immunization with EAE-related peptides such as MBP and PLP successfully suppressed EAE in rodent models [148–151]. However, a phase three clinical trial tested oral tolerance induction in MS patients and failed to detect any beneficial effects in comparison to placebo controls [151]. This was attributed to a high variance in the placebo control group but might be further attributed to the heterogeneity of the immune response in MS patients. Other experimental approaches for vaccines against MS included vaccination against axonal growth inhibitors associated with myelin, transfer of antigen pulsed, tolerogenic DCs, and vaccination against proinflammatory cytokines [144]. Yet, these strategies all bear significant side effects and might impair host immunity. Thus, novel strategies targeting the immune response in MS with high specificity and broad applicability are needed.

7.3.4.1 mRNA-Based Tolerogenic Vaccination Against EAE

MS is a chronic inflammatory disease driven by several autoantigens. Recent studies successfully established nanoparticulate delivery of nucleoside-modified autoantigen-encoding mRNA into lymphoid $CD11c^+$ APCs as a feasible therapeutic strategy for antigen-specific tolerization without systemic immune suppression [113]. While Kranz et al. previously developed RNA-lipoplexes (RNA-LPX) that are taken up by splenic DCs via macropinocytosis and after activation of Toll-like receptor 7 (TLR7) potently trigger antigen-specific immunity with strong effector and memory T-cell responses [114], Krienke et al. employed a nonimmunogenic lipoplex formulation to deliver an mRNA-based vaccine (Figure 7.2) that contained 1-methylpseudouridine (m1Ψ) in place of uridin, which results in a higher translational capacity while lowering activation of innate immune cells due to lack of TLR7 stimulation [113, 152, 153].

For proof of concept, the authors of this study tested whether m1Ψ mRNA vaccination-triggered antigen presentation in the absence of inflammation and costimulation could ameliorate autoimmunity in EAE mouse models of MS [113]. While autoreactive T cells drive EAE after immunization with the MOG peptide MOG_{35-55}, treatment with MOG m1Ψ mRNA reduced T-cell-driven inflammation, induced development of T_{reg} cell populations, and protected from EAE in mice. Notably, MOG-specific CTLA-4^+, $ICOS^+$, and IL-10^+ $Foxp3^+$ T_{reg} cells from m1Ψ mRNA-immunized mice were not only capable of suppressing antigen-specific autoreactive T_{eff} cells but also exerted effective bystander immunosuppression in models of EAE triggered by a different peptide ($PLP_{139-151}$) or a mixture of the autoantigens MOG_{35-55}, $PLP_{139-151}$, $PLP_{178-191}$, MBP_{84-104}, and $MOBP_{15-36}$. Importantly, m1Ψ mRNA administration did neither impair the capability of DCs to mount functional immune responses nor induce antigen-specific autoantibodies [113] (Figure 7.3). The landmark study of Krienke et al. demonstrates for the first

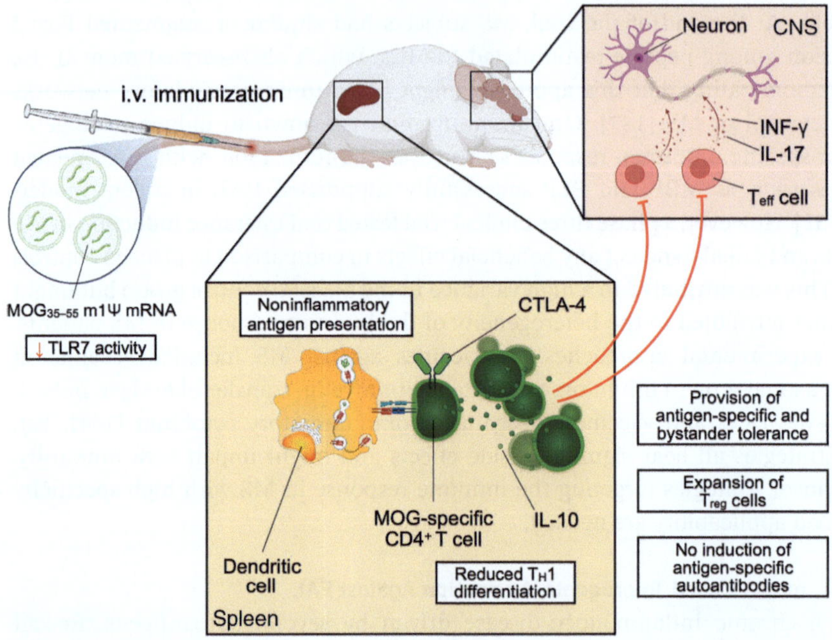

Figure 7.3 Tolerogenic mRNA vaccination against experimental autoimmune encephalitis (EAE) in mice. Following intravenous injection, nonimmunogenic lipid nanoparticles containing MOG_{35-55} 1-methylpseudouridine (m1Ψ) mRNA are specifically taken up by splenic dendritic cells, which present the translated peptide in an MHC-II dependent fashion to $CD4^+$ T cells. Immunization with MOG m1Ψ mRNA protects mice from EAE through reduced T-cell-driven inflammation and higher numbers of protective T_{reg} cells that mediated antigen-specific and bystander suppression. Notably, 1Ψ mRNA administration did not induce antigen-specific autoantibodies. Source: Dennis Wolf.

time that a specific mRNA-guided expression of antigenic peptides can induce peptide-specific T cells. This represents an important advantage over existing immunization strategies, in particular in comparison with peptide immunization (see Section 7.4.2). Notably, the lack of a proinflammatory adjuvant in nonimmunogenic m1Ψ mRNA lipoplex formulations results in the generation of a merely immunosuppressive and beneficial cellular response that does not require IgG antibodies. However, future studies are still required to evaluate the specificity of m1Ψ mRNA-induced immunoregulatory effects and whether repeat immunization is safe and effective in established disease [154] and in disease models more relevant to human disease, e.g. EAE induced by spinal cord homogenates [155].

7.4 Framework and Rationale for Future mRNA-Based Peptide Vaccination Strategies in Autoimmune Diseases

A large body of evidence has identified T-cell-driven inflammation as crucial in the pathophysiology of autoimmune diseases and their clinical complications [156].

Table 7.1 Conceptual aims of mRNA-based tolerogenic immunization in autoimmune diseases.

Autoantigen	– Antigenic peptide (cave: MHC-II matching necessary) – Entire antigen or fragment containing immunodominant epitopes (no need for MHC-II matching)
Target cells	– Expression selectively in dendritic cells (DCs) or – Cells licensed for antigen presentation (e.g. plasmacytoid DCs and tissue macrophages)
Mode of expression	– No inflammatory response after mRNA uptake/expression (measurable by IL-2, IL-12, and TNFα)
Result of T-cell stimulation	– Predominant generation of T_{regs} or IL-10-expressing T cells – No measurable IL-17, IFN-γ expression in T cells – Proof and monitoring of the expansion of antigen-specific T cells by Tetramer or ELISPOT [104]
Antibodies	– No generation of IgG antibodies or – Proof that IgG antibodies are not capable of accessing/binding to antigens *in vivo*
Efficacy	– Immunization needs to be effective in established diseases and in prevention of *de novo* diseases – Clinical biomarkers for disease activity necessary – Protective T-cell response needs to be sustained over long periods

The ideal treatment for such diseases would specifically target autoreactive cells without the need for broad and potentially harmful immunosuppressive therapy. The modification of the adaptive immune response using vaccines containing specific antigen(s) relevant for T-cell modulation has been identified as a feasible disease ameliorating strategy in preclinical studies of autoinflammatory diseases such as atherosclerosis and EAE [71, 157]. Induction of a specific, protective immune response against well-defined, disease-relevant antigens bears the potential of a targeted anti-inflammatory therapy without hampering host defense. Several prerequisites and aims of a successful tolerogenic immunization against autoimmune diseases using mRNA can be derived from previous studies and are summarized in Table 7.1.

7.4.1 Evidence for mRNA Vaccination to Induce Tolerance in Animal Models

Autoimmune diseases result from a breach of immunological self-tolerance and subsequent proinflammatory activity of autoreactive T cells. Current treatment options for systemic immune suppression come at the cost of potentially severe side effects such as an increased risk of infections. To date, vaccination has mostly been employed to elicit both cellular and humoral immune responses against infectious pathogens or cancer cells [158]. Former mRNA vaccines have been capable of inducing strong T-helper 1 (T_H1) responses via the activation of TLRs and have been boosted in their response by accompanying immunostimulatory, proinflammatory adjuvants [159]. Novel liposomal formulations of m1Ψ mRNA allow for antigen presentation by lymphoid tissue-resident $CD11c^+$ APCs [114] in a noninflammatory context and thereby induction of antigen-specific tolerance by (1) a nonimmunogenic lipoplex formulation intentionally purified to remove any residual immunostimulatory molecules and (2) the incorporation of m1Ψ instead of uracil, which allows for strongly reduced inflammatory properties [113].

7.4.2 Limitations of Traditional Peptide Vaccination

Traditionally, vaccines consist of live, attenuated, or inactivated pathogens, such as bacteria and viruses. This strategy has known limitations, such as uncontrollable immune responses even in the case of attenuated pathogens, potential cross-reaction of the pathogen with endogenous proteins, and the requirement to produce pathogens *in vitro*. It has been suggested to circumvent these limitations by using more specific vaccines consisting of immunodominant peptides that can be synthesized. This is exemplified by cancer vaccines that consist of certain highly specific immunodominant peptides that allow cytotoxic $CD8^+$ T cells to detect and destroy target cancer cells. In general, immunodominant peptides represent the smallest region of a protein that can elicit an immune response. In principle, the two arms of T-cell immunity, $CD8^+$ cytotoxic and $CD4^+$ T-helper cells, respond to peptides presented in an MHC-I- ($CD8^+$) and MHC-II- ($CD4^+$) dependent context. Here, we will focus on MHC-II-dependent peptides in the setting of autoimmunity. Loading of MHC-II with peptides can occur via a peptide-exchange mechanism, where an existing peptide loaded on MHC-II can be replaced by an alternative peptide antigen [160, 161]. Antigens are also taken up by micropinocytosis or via receptor-mediated events (BCR or Fc-receptor-mediated uptake of immune complexes). In the endosome, the protein antigen is processed by several proteases, mostly by cathepsins. Several peptide vaccines are currently in development, mostly for infectious pathogens and cancer treatment [162]. It is important to highlight that tolerogenic vaccination is distinguishable from the latter forms of vaccination by the lack of proinflammatory adjuvants and the desired immunosuppressive mechanism.

Mostly synthetic peptides are described in the literature. Limitations of synthetic peptides include weak immunogenicity and the lack of post-translational modifications that may occur in the naïve protein. Peptides also need to resist uptake and processing in the endosome of the APC. Peptide-based approaches require a limited set of immunogenic peptides that are highly dependent on the host's human leukocyte antigen (HLA) type or MHC-II alleles in the mouse, i.e. IA^b in C57BL/6 mice. Because the binding of a specific peptide to MHC/HLA differs across individuals and genetic backgrounds, peptides need to be selected for each

MHC-II allelic combination, making the unselective and broad use of certain single peptides in a population highly ineffective. One way to circumvent the latter limitation is the *in silico* and *in vitro* screening of a large number of peptides for MHC-II peptide binding affinities and function. This strategy has recently been described for ApoB self-peptides [66]. Peptides binding to MHC-II are on average 13 amino acids in length. Because the termini of class II peptides do not interact with MHC-II, peptides may be considerably longer. It has been shown that peptide's amino acid residues 1, 4, 6, and 9 interact with MHC-II, while others may be more important for interaction with the TCR [163]. Another limitation is that artificially selected peptides do not necessarily present naturally presented and processed peptides. Natural peptide and protein folding are also not represented by synthetic peptides. The requirement for additional adjuvants is likely the most important limitation of peptide vaccination since any type of adjuvant can skew the immune response (see below). Vaccination is performed by prime and repetitive booster injections, often in the peritoneal cavity, which is known to induce inflammation, skin irritation, and fibrosis over time. Emulsion droplets of oily adjuvants and proteins/peptides remain in the peritoneal cavity over weeks, which represents a major unwanted effect (Figure 7.4). Overall, these limitations may outweigh the potential advantages of peptide-based vaccination. Recently, mRNA has emerged as a highly efficient method to produce peptides and larger proteins in target cells, allowing natural antigen processing and induction of activating immune responses against CoV-SARS2 [117, 164, 165]. Notably, mRNA may work without classic adjuvants. Recently, it has been shown that mRNA is capable of inducing peptide expression targeted in DCs without additional inflammatory or TLR-stimulus (see Section 7.3.4.1). Several issues remain to be solved to develop an immunization-based therapy against human atherosclerotic cardiovascular disease (CVD).

7.4.3 Challenges of Future Vaccination Strategies

7.4.3.1 Antigen Targets and MHC Variability

In contrast to C57BL/6 mice used in experimental studies, which only express one single variant of MHC-II, humans express a multitude of MHC-II variants with eight different class II allotypes, which results in a total of approximately 10 000 different HLA allelic forms that all have different affinities to potential peptides and thus present a significant challenge for peptide vaccination: MHC-II alleles (and thereby their suitable antigenic peptide candidates) would need to be identified by sequencing for each prospective patient before vaccination [66]. The use of multitarget vaccines that combine several antigenic epitopes could increase the efficacy of antiatherosclerotic immunization strategies. However, each peptide may bind to different MHC-II alleles with distinct affinities, and the degree of binding affinity might influence resulting T-cell phenotypes [166]. mRNA vaccines recently emerged as a promising alternative to conventional protein vaccination because of their capacity for rapid development, potential for low cost, and high potency manufacture [116]. Krienke et al. reported the systemic delivery of nanoparticle-formulated m1Ψ mRNA for antigen presentation in the absence of costimulatory signals, which induced a strong T_{reg} response and ameliorated disease in mouse models of MS [113].

This concept holds great promise to develop further tolerogenic vaccination strategies. In particular, it needs to be tested whether entire antigens, such as the whole sequence of MOG or ApoB or its immunodominant fragments can be expressed specifically in DCs without affecting DC homeostasis (Table 7.1). Such strategy would bypass the need to select for naturally presented peptides. There have been no studies on mRNA vaccines against LDL/ApoB yet.

7.4.3.2 Clinically Applicable Adjuvants and Routes of Administration

Immunologic adjuvants modulate (i.e. enhancement of strength and/or duration) the antigen-specific immune response within an organism when given in combination with specific antigens. Frequently used vaccination adjuvants in mouse models are complete Freund's adjuvant (CFA) that consists of heat-inactivated mycobacterium tuberculosis in nonmetabolizable paraffin oil and mannide monooleate and incomplete Freund's adjuvant (IFA) that does not contain mycobacteria. ApoB-peptide vaccination with CFA–IFA as subcutaneous prime followed by 4× intraperitoneal boost injections, respectively, conferred atheroprotection in *Apoe*$^{-/-}$ mice after 13 weeks of western diet [78] while subcutaneous vaccination with CFA as prime and single boost injection exacerbated murine atherosclerosis after five weeks of western diet using the same antigen [167]. Modern clinically used adjuvants make use of aluminum compounds (alum) or cholera toxin B (CTB) subunit while CFA and IFA are obsolete now due to toxicity or safety

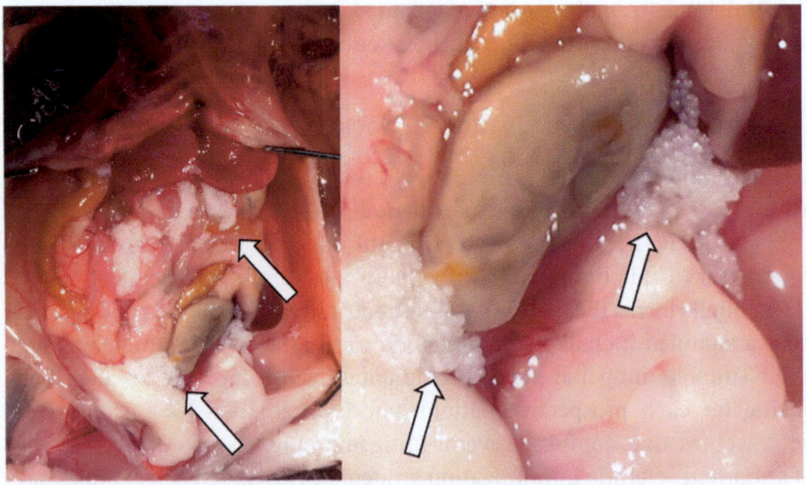

Figure 7.4 Lipid-emulsion droplets after intraperitoneal booster injection with incomplete Freund's adjuvant (IFA). Most tolerogenic vaccination protocols in the mouse have been established with combinations of complete Freund's adjuvant (CFA) or IFA. Often, booster injections of IFA and autoantigens (peptides/proteins) are injected in the peritoneal cavity, where emulsion droplets can remain for weeks and induce chronic inflammation (white arrows). It is also important that repetitive intraperitoneal injections are known to induce severe fibrotic changes in the peritoneum and mesenteries. Source: Dennis Wolf.

concerns [168]. Importantly, adjuvants alone may have the ability to modulate atherosclerosis, as shown for IFA and alum which may induce an atheroprotective immune response even in the absence of a specific antigen [169]. Recent evidence suggests that squalene-based adjuvants such as MF59 and Addavax are promising candidate adjuvants for developing a clinically effective atherosclerosis vaccine [107]. Notably, adjuvant-free, subcutaneous immunization with ApoB peptides in principle is possible and has been shown to significantly reduce atherosclerosis in *Apoe*$^{-/-}$ mice [170]. With regard to the root of antigen delivery, booster injections in mice are often made into the peritoneal cavity, which is not practical in humans and bears unwanted side effects (Figure 7.4). Alternative routes of administration for antigen delivery include oral, nasal, intravenous, and sub- or intracutaneous application [63] or mRNA-guided expression.

7.4.3.3 Effectiveness and Safety of Peptide Vaccination

Previous studies on LDL/ApoB vaccination in mice to dampen atherosclerosis have been primarily carried out in a preventative setting, where high efficacy in preventing *de novo* atherosclerosis has been demonstrated. However, whether tolerance mediating vaccination has the potential to dampen or even reverse established atherosclerotic disease is yet unknown. Notably, atherosclerosis typically develops over years and decades before symptoms arise. Autopsy studies have found signs of coronary atherosclerosis in 78% of patients <35 years old who died from noncardiac trauma [171]. Therefore, from a clinical perspective, the development of a vaccine with the potential to treat patients who already have developed atherosclerosis is highly desirable. Further, given the constantly transforming phenotype of ApoB-specific T cells during atherogenesis, a vaccine should be capable of either reversing the phenotype of late-stage T_H1-primed and proinflammatory T cells back to an anti-inflammatory T_{reg}-like phenotype or generating new, more stable, immunosuppressive T_{regs}. Induction of proinflammatory or unstable anti-inflammatory ApoB-specific T cells could potentially lead to adverse destabilization of existing atherosclerosis.

7.4.3.4 Requirement of Clinical Biomarkers

It remains questionable whether tolerogenic vaccination has the ability to reverse established disease or only to prevent *de novo* autoimmune diseases. In fact, most studies (using peptide, DNA or mRNA vaccination) have tested preventive settings in tolerogenic vaccination and vaccination may not work in mid- or end-stage disease when protective autoimmunity has already vanished [66, 104]. It is therefore important to define clinical tools and workflows to define and treat individuals at a specific high risk for autoimmune diseases. We propose the following workflow: Healthy individuals carry a specific risk for autoimmune diseases based on genetics, acquired lifestyle or environmental risk factors, and other chronic-inflammatory diseases (1). In a high-risk scenario, novel biomarkers that allow screening for levels and polarization of the antigen-specific immune response need to be established and validated. In principle, cellular biomarkers, i.e. tetramer- or ELISPOT-identified autoantigen-specific cells, antibodies, traditional protein or

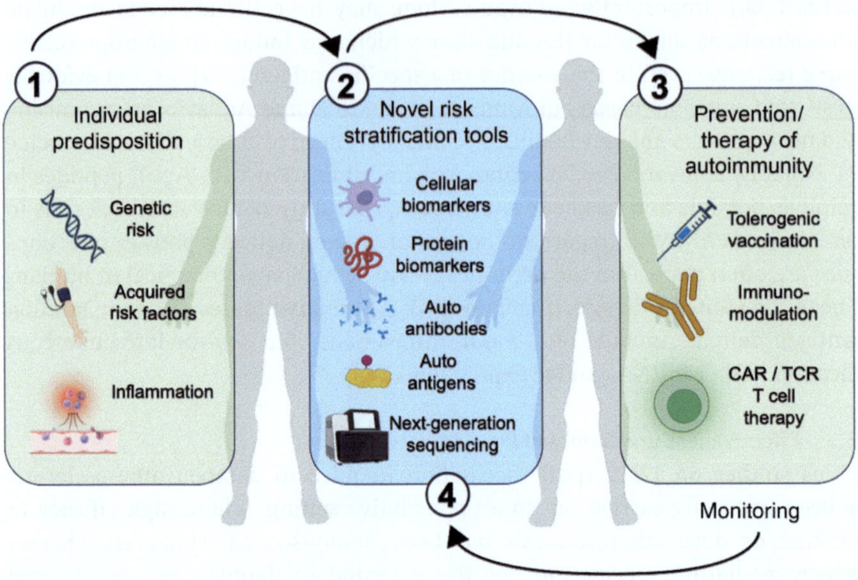

Figure 7.5 Proposed workflow of future mRNA tolerogenic vaccination in patients. Healthy individuals carry a specific risk for autoimmune diseases based on genetics, acquired lifestyle or environmental risk factors, and other chronic-inflammatory diseases (1). In a high-risk scenario, novel biomarkers testing the existence or polarization of the antigen-specific immune response need to be tested. In principle, cellular biomarkers, i.e. tetramer-identified autoantigen-specific cells, antibodies, traditional protein or lipid biomarkers, or transcriptional signatures, could be developed and validated for risk prediction (2). If a high-risk scenario is confirmed and biomarkers are indicative of future autoimmune diseases, specific preventive treatments are initiated. mRNA vaccination, as well as other biological-based immunomodulation, is possible (3). Therapeutic efficacy is monitored by a set of biomarkers tailored to detect the targets of immunomodulation (4). Source: Dennis Wolf.

lipid biomarkers, or transcriptional signatures, could be developed and validated for risk prediction (2). If a high-risk scenario is confirmed and biomarkers are indicative of future autoimmune diseases, specific, preventive treatments are initiated. mRNA vaccination, as well as other biological-based immunomodulation, is possible (3). Therapeutic efficacy is monitored by a set of biomarkers tailored to detect the targets of immunomodulation (4) (Figure 7.5). In atherosclerosis, immune-specific tools for risk stratification could involve quantification of antibodies against LDL/ApoB or ApoB-specific T cells by restimulation assays or tetramers [104, 119].

7.4.4 Outlook: Chances of mRNA-Based Approaches in Future Clinical Immunomodulation in Allergy

mRNA-based approaches represent a versatile technology with a great potential for future clinical immunomodulation in humans. Recent studies have demonstrated an optimized, partial cell-type specific *in vivo* delivery of mRNA with sustained protein expression. In autoimmune diseases, mRNA-based protein vaccines hold the promise to induce an antigen-specific immune tolerance that efficiently limits inflammation and improves disease-specific outcomes in mice [113]. It is important to note that mRNA-based therapies are *per se* not confined to autoimmunity. This is exemplified by recent reports that have induced immune tolerance by mRNA in allergic diseases. In allergies, the immune system recognizes otherwise harmless non-self-antigens, such as proteins from peanuts, pollen, or bee venom [172]. On the contrary, autoimmunity is strictly confined to endogenously expressed self-proteins. However, allergy and autoimmunity share some important homologies: for instance, both pathologies are maintained by the inability of the immune system to mount effective tolerogenic responses that prevent its overactivation against antigens/allergens. Likewise, peptides from allergens are presented in APC/MHC-II-dependent context. Besides other important cellular and humoral mechanisms, allergens are recognized by allergen-specific T_H2 cells that produce the T_H2 signature cytokines IL-4, IL-5, IL-9, and IL-13. T_H2-associated cytokines mediate subsequent infiltration and activation of eosinophils and boost antibody isotype switching to IgE. Allergen cross-linking of IgE bound to adjacent high-affinity receptor (FcεRI) on mast cells and basophils triggers the release of histamine and other mediators including prostaglandin D2 and leukotrienes [173]. Further, allergen–IgE complexes facilitate T_H2 development via binding to surface low-affinity receptor for IgE (FcεRII) on B cells [174, 175]. It was first established in 1911 that allergen-specific immunotherapy (ASI), a form of vaccination with allergens, can effectively ameliorate disease-specific symptoms. In ASI, allergens are repeatedly injected subcutaneously in increasing doses or given by an oral route [176]. ASI is usually performed over three years with gradually increasing antigen doses and causes effective desensitization, but no long-lasting tolerance over a greater lifespan. Key mechanisms of ASI include a reduction of allergen-specific T_H2 cells and the induction of immunosuppressive T_{regs} and B-regulatory cells (B_{regs}), a subtype of IL-10-expressing B cells, which promote an anti-inflammatory environment that limits IgE production and induces the generation of allergen-specific IgG subclasses such as IgG4 [177]. Allergen-specific IgG competes with IgE for allergen, which effectively results in inhibition of allergen–IgE–complex mediated activation of mast cells and basophils as well as IgE-facilitated T_H2 development [178, 179]. In addition, regulatory innate lymphoid cells (ILC_{reg}) and regulatory natural killer cells (NK_{reg}) have been implicated in suppressing allergen-specific inflammation via IL-10 production ([180], Figure 7.6).

However, ASI has important limitations: First, exposure to cognate allergens is at the risk of inducing potentially life-threatening allergies – a risk that may be addressable by using recombinant hypoallergenic variants of the antigen or by using alternative adjuvants [181, 182]. Second, ASI is usually not capable of inducing long-term immune tolerance. Third, the duration of ASI remains highly variable and depends on the allergen, routes, and doses. These limitations have sparked the idea that mRNA-guided delivery of allergens may be superior to conventional protein-based approaches. While initial evidence on naked mRNA vaccination suggested that immunization with mRNA preferentially induces a T_H2-biased T-helper cell polarization, which would have had the ability to drive allergies [183],

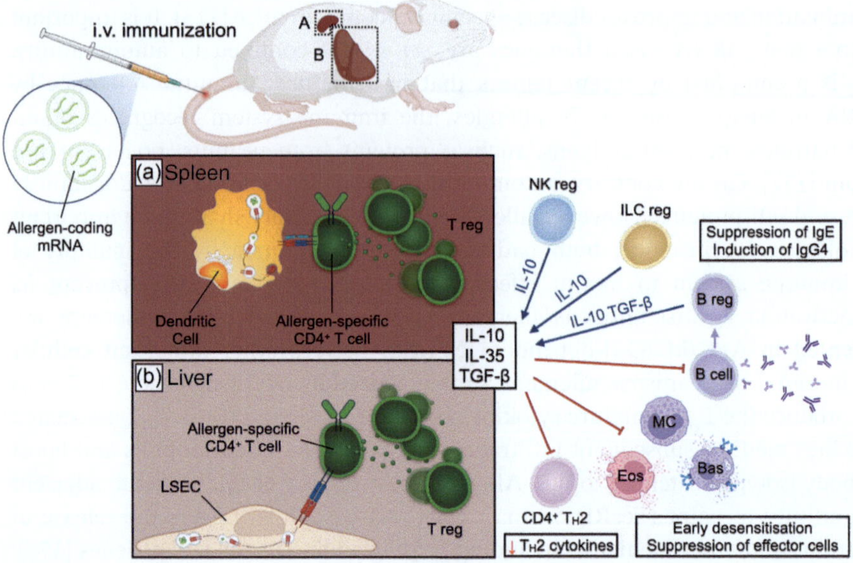

Figure 7.6 Proposed regulation of allergic immune responses by tolerogenic mRNA vaccination. Allergen-specific CD4$^+$ T_{regs} may be induced in the spleen (a) or liver (b) by intravenous immunization with allergen-coding mRNA. Allergen-specific T_{regs} cells express the anti-inflammatory cytokines IL-10, TGF-β, and IL-35 that suppress T_H2 cells, eosinophils (Eos), and basophils (Bas), while promoting the generation of allergen-specific B-regulatory (B_{reg}) cells. This suppressive environment limits the production of IgE and promotes the generation of IgG4 by B cells. Additionally, regulatory natural killer (NK) cells (NK_{reg}) and regulatory innate lymphoid cells (ILC_{reg}) help establish and maintain allergen-specific tolerance. After [177]. Source: Dennis Wolf.

other reports have shown that mRNA vaccines, depending on context and type of mRNA delivery, can induce proinflammatory, immune-activating T_H1 responses [184] or anti-inflammatory, immune-suppressive T_{regs} [173]. Notably, prophylactic mRNA vaccination against allergy in mice is capable of conferring robust and long-term T memory responses, arguing for the potential for long-lasting effects of mRNA immunotherapy [185].

Efficient tolerance induction requires the expansion and activation of allergen-specific T_{regs} that can suppress allergen-specific T_H2 responses [186] as previously shown for noninflammatory m1Ψ mRNA [113]. Recently, it has been shown that a liver-targeting immune-tolerogenic mRNA lipid nanoparticle platform (LNP) may allow to treat peanut-induced anaphylaxis by single- and multiple-epitope nucleotide sequence delivery. The authors employed an mRNA strand comprising nucleotide sequences encoding for nonallergenic MHC-II binding T-cell epitopes that were identified in "Ara h2," the dominant peanut protein allergen. Codon-optimized mRNA was used for microfluidics synthesis of LNPs with an ionizable cationic lipid and a lipid-anchored mannose ligand for targeting liver sinusoidal ECs. Prophylactic administration of nondecorated (mAra h2#4/LNP) or decorated (mAra h2#4/LNP-Man) LNP delivering mAra h2#4 was performed at 0 and 7 days in female C3H/HeJ mice, followed by sensitization through oral administration of 100 mg/kg crude peanut extract (CPE) and 0.5 mg/kg cholera toxin at 14, 21, and 28 days before peritoneal challenge with CPE on day 35 to induce anaphylaxis. Therapy with mRNA/LNP *in vivo* alleviated physical manifestations of anaphylaxis and led to a suppression of mast cell release, T_H2-mediated cytokine production, and IgE synthesis. Further, treatment with mAra h2#4/LNP or mAra h2#4/LNP-Man significantly expanded the splenic pool of IL-10-producing $CD25^+FoxP3^+T$ cells assessed at seven days after i.v. injection [187].

Collectively, mRNA-based approaches remain readily adaptable to any protein antigen feasible while being cost effective at the same time allowing for a wide and specific delivery and presentation of single or combined epitopes to induce tolerance against allergy and autoimmune diseases [154].

List of Abbreviations

ApoB-100	Apolipoprotein B 100
BCR	B-cell receptor
CFA	Complete Freund's adjuvant
CLP	Common lymphoid progenitor
CRTAM	Class 1-restricted T-cell-associated molecule
CTB	Cholera toxin B subunit
CTLs	Cytotoxic T lymphocytes
CVD	Cardiovascular disease
FDC	Follicular dendritic cell
IFA	Incomplete Freund's adjuvant
IFN-γ	Interferon gamma
iNKT	Invariant natural killer T cell
IRF4	Interferon regulating factor 4
LDL-C	Low-density lipoprotein cholesterol
LDL-R	LDL receptor
MHC	Major histocompatibility complex
MI	Myocardial infarction
MMPs	Matrix metalloproteinases
MS	Multiple sclerosis
oxLDL	Oxidized low-density lipoprotein particle
RORγT	RAR-related orphan receptor gamma
SHM	Somatic hypermutation
SLE	Systemic lupus erythematosus
T_C22	IL-22-secreting $CD8^+$ T cell
T_C9	IL-9-secreting $CD8^+$ T cell

T_{CM}	Central memory T cell
TCR	T-cell receptor
T_{EM}	Effector memory T cell
TGF-β	Transforming growth factor beta
TNF-α	Tumor necrosis factor alpha
T_{reg}	Regulatory T cell
T_{RM}	Tissue-resident memory T cell

Acknowledgements

Mark C. Gissler was funded by the IMM-PACT-Program for Clinician Scientists, Department of Medicine II, Medical Center – University of Freiburg and Faculty of Medicine, University of Freiburg, funded by the Deutsche Forschungsgemeinschaft (DFG, German Research Foundation) – 413517907. Dennis Wolf is a member of SFB1425, funded by the Deutsche Forschungsgemeinschaft (DFG, German Research Foundation). Figures were generated with schematics from Biorender.com.

Conflict of Interest

The authors declare no conflict of interest.

References

1 Janeway, C.A. and Murphy, K. (2018). *Immunologie*. Heidelberg: Springer Berlin Heidelberg.

2 Watkins, T.S. and Miles, J.J. (2021). The human T-cell receptor repertoire in health and disease and potential for omics integration. *Immunol. Cell Biol.* 99 (2): 135–145.

3 Qi, Q., Liu, Y., Cheng, Y. et al. (2014). Diversity and clonal selection in the human T-cell repertoire. *Proc. Natl. Acad. Sci. U. S. A.* 111 (36): 13139–13144.

4 Hsieh, A.C., Liu, Y., Edlind, M.P. et al. (2012). The translational landscape of mTOR signalling steers cancer initiation and metastasis. *Nature* 485 (7396): 55–61.

5 Kronenberg, M. and Gapin, L. (2002). The unconventional lifestyle of NKT cells. *Nat. Rev. Immunol.* 2 (8): 557–568.

6 Lambolez, F., Kronenberg, M., and Cheroutre, H. (2007). Thymic differentiation of $TCR\alpha\beta^+$ $CD8\alpha\alpha^+$ IELs. *Immunol. Rev.* 215 (1): 178–188.

7 Ley, K. (2016). 2015 Russell Ross memorial lecture in vascular biology: protective autoimmunity in atherosclerosis. *Arterioscler. Thromb. Vasc. Biol.* 36 (3): 429–438.

8 Vignali, D.A., Collison, L.W., and Workman, C.J. (2008). How regulatory T cells work. *Nat. Rev. Immunol.* 8 (7): 523–532.

9 Germain, R.N. (2002). T-cell development and the CD4-CD8 lineage decision. *Nat. Rev. Immunol.* 2 (5): 309–322.

10 Föhse, L., Reinhardt, A., Oberdörfer, L. et al. (2013). Differential postselection proliferation dynamics of αβ T cells, Foxp3 + regulatory T cells, and invariant NKT cells monitored by genetic pulse labeling. *J. Immunol.* 191 (5): 2384–2392.

11 Mallick-Wood, C.A., Pao, W., Cheng, A.M. et al. (1996). Disruption of epithelial gamma delta T cell repertoires by mutation of the Syk tyrosine kinase. *Proc. Natl. Acad. Sci. U. S. A.* 93 (18): 9704–9709.

12 Bonneville, M., O'Brien, R.L., and Born, W.K. (2010). γδ T cell effector functions: a blend of innate programming and acquired plasticity. *Nat. Rev. Immunol.* 10 (7): 467–478.

13 Sallusto, F., Geginat, J., and Lanzavecchia, A. (2004). Central memory and effector memory T cell subsets: function, generation, and maintenance. *Annu. Rev. Immunol.* 22 (1): 745–763.

14 Mahnke, J., Schumacher, V., Ahrens, S. et al. (2016). Interferon regulatory factor 4 controls TH1 cell effector function and metabolism. *Sci. Rep.* 6 (1): 35521.

15 Nakayamada, S., Takahashi, H., Kanno, Y., and O'Shea, J.J. (2012). Helper T cell diversity and plasticity. *Curr. Opin. Immunol.* 24 (3): 297–302.

16 Kaplan, M.H. (2013). Th9 cells: differentiation and disease. *Immunol. Rev.* 252 (1): 104–115.

17 Sakaguchi, S., Yamaguchi, T., Nomura, T., and Ono, M. (2008). Regulatory T cells and immune tolerance. *Cell* 133 (5): 775–787.

18 Crotty, S. (2019). T follicular helper cell biology: a decade of discovery and diseases. *Immunity* 50 (5): 1132–1148.

19 Takeuchi, A. and Saito, T. (2017). CD4 CTL, a cytotoxic subset of CD4(+) T cells, their differentiation and function. *Front. Immunol.* 8: 194.

20 Huber, M., Heink, S., Grothe, H. et al. (2009). Th17-like developmental process leads to CD8+ Tc17 cells with reduced cytotoxic activity. *Eur. J. Immunol.* 39 (7): 1716–1725.

21 Srenathan, U., Steel, K., and Taams, L.S. (2016). IL-17+ CD8+ T cells: differentiation, phenotype and role in inflammatory disease. *Immunol. Lett.* 178: 20–26.

22 Visekruna, A., Ritter, J., Scholz, T. et al. (2013). Tc9 cells, a new subset of $CD8^+$ T cells, support Th2-mediated airway inflammation. *Eur. J. Immunol.* 43 (3): 606–618.

23 Liu, Y., Yang, B., Ma, J. et al. (2011). Interleukin-21 induces the differentiation of human Tc22 cells via phosphorylation of signal transducers and activators of transcription. *Immunology* 132 (4): 540–548.

24 de Jesús-Gil, C., Sans-de San Nicolàs, L., García-Jiménez, I. et al. (2021). Human CLA(+) memory T cell and cytokines in psoriasis. *Front. Med.* 8: 731911.

25 Churlaud, G., Pitoiset, F., Jebbawi, F. et al. (2015). Human and mouse CD8+CD25+FOXP3+ regulatory T cells at steady state and during interleukin-2 therapy. *Front. Immunol.* 6 (MAR): 171.

26 Ramírez, J., Lukin, K., and Hagman, J. (2010). From hematopoietic progenitors to B cells: mechanisms of lineage restriction and commitment. *Curr. Opin. Immunol.* 22 (2): 177–184.

27 Pelanda, R. and Torres, R.M. (2012). Central B-cell tolerance: where selection begins. *Cold Spring Harb. Perspect. Biol.* 4 (4): a007146.

28 Rathmell, J.C., Townsend, S.E., Xu, J.C. et al. (1996). Expansion or elimination of B cells in vivo: dual roles for CD40- and Fas (CD95)-ligands modulated by the B cell antigen receptor. *Cell* 87 (2): 319–329.

29 Mauri, C. and Bosma, A. (2012). Immune regulatory function of B Cells. *Annu. Rev. Immunol.* 30 (1): 221–241.

30 Catalán, D., Mansilla, M.A., Ferrier, A. et al. (2021). Immunosuppressive mechanisms of regulatory B cells. *Front. Immunol.* 12: 611795.

31 Xing, Y. and Hogquist, K.A. (2012). T-cell tolerance: central and peripheral. *Cold Spring Harb. Perspect. Biol.* 4 (6): a006957.

32 Mackay, I.R. (2001). Tolerance and autoimmunity. *West. J. Med.* 174 (2): 118–123.

33 Fife, B.T. and Bluestone, J.A. (2008). Control of peripheral T-cell tolerance and autoimmunity via the CTLA-4 and PD-1 pathways. *Immunol. Rev.* 224: 166–182.

34 Xiao, Z.X., Miller, J.S., and Zheng, S.G. (2021). An updated advance of autoantibodies in autoimmune diseases. *Autoimmun. Rev.* 20 (2): 102743.

35 Narvekar, A., Pardeshi, A., Jain, R., and Dandekar, P. (2022). ADCC enhancement: a conundrum or a boon to mAb therapy? *Biologicals* 79: 10–18.

36 Pisetsky, D.S. and Lipsky, P.E. (2020). New insights into the role of antinuclear antibodies in systemic lupus erythematosus. *Nat. Rev. Rheumatol.* 16 (10): 565–579.

37 Rekvig, O.P. (2019). The dsDNA, anti-dsDNA antibody, and lupus nephritis: what we agree on, what must be done, and what the best strategy forward could be. *Front. Immunol.* 10: 1104.

38 Madamsetty, V.S., Mohammadinejad, R., Uzieliene, I. et al. (2022). Dexamethasone: insights into pharmacological aspects, therapeutic mechanisms, and delivery systems. *ACS Biomater. Sci. Eng.* 8 (5): 1763–1790.

39 Keystone, E., Heijde, D.V.D., Mason, D. et al. (2008). Certolizumab pegol plus methotrexate is significantly more effective than placebo plus methotrexate in active rheumatoid arthritis: findings of a fifty-two-week, phase III, multicenter, randomized, double-blind, placebo-controlled, parallel-group study. *Arthritis Rheum.* 58 (11): 3319–3329.

40 Gray, O., McDonnell, G.V., and Forbes, R.B. (2004). Methotrexate for multiple sclerosis. *Cochrane Database Syst. Rev.* 2004 (10): CD003208.

41 Bain, B. and Brazil, M. (2003). Adalimumab. *Nat. Rev. Drug Discov.* 2 (9): 693–694.

42 La Cava, A. (2008). Tregs are regulated by cytokines: implications for autoimmunity. *Autoimmun. Rev.* 8 (1): 83–87.

43 Dong, S., Hiam-Galvez, K.J., Mowery, C.T. et al. (2021). The effect of low-dose IL-2 and Treg adoptive cell therapy in patients with type 1 diabetes. *JCI Insight* 6 (18): e147474.

44 Bluestone, J.A., Buckner, J.H., Fitch, M. et al. (2015). Type 1 diabetes immunotherapy using polyclonal regulatory T cells. *Sci. Transl. Med.* 7 (315): 315ra189.

45 Greenwood, B. (2014). The contribution of vaccination to global health: past, present and future. *Philos. Trans. R. Soc. Lond. Ser. B Biol. Sci.* 369 (1645): 20130433.

46 Moorman, C.D., Sohn, S.J., and Phee, H. (2021). Emerging therapeutics for immune tolerance: tolerogenic vaccines, T cell therapy, and IL-2 therapy. *Front. Immunol.* 12: 657768.

47 Gissler, M.C., Stachon, P., Wolf, D., and Marchini, T. (2022). The role of tumor necrosis factor associated factors (TRAFs) in vascular inflammation and atherosclerosis. *Front. Cardiovasc. Med.* 9: 826630.

48 Wolf, D. and Ley, K. (2019). Immunity and inflammation in atherosclerosis. *Circ. Res.* 124 (2): 315–327.

49 Kruk, M.E., Gage, A.D., Joseph, N.T. et al. (2018). Mortality due to low-quality health systems in the universal health coverage era: a systematic analysis of amenable deaths in 137 countries. *Lancet* 392 (10160): 2203–2212.

50 Colantonio, L.D., Bittner, V., Reynolds, K. et al. (2016). Association of serum lipids and coronary heart disease in contemporary observational studies. *Circulation* 133 (3): 256–264.

51 Glass, C.K. and Witztum, J.L. (2001). Atherosclerosis. the road ahead. *Cell* 104 (4): 503–516.

52 de Winther, M.P., van Dijk, K.W., Havekes, L.M., and Hofker, M.H. (2000). Macrophage scavenger receptor class A: a multifunctional receptor in atherosclerosis. *Arterioscler. Thromb. Vasc. Biol.* 20 (2): 290–297.

53 Ketelhuth, D.F. and Hansson, G.K. (2016). Adaptive response of T and B cells in atherosclerosis. *Circ. Res.* 118 (4): 668–678.

54 Mitra, S., Goyal, T., and Mehta, J.L. (2011). Oxidized LDL, LOX-1 and atherosclerosis. *Cardiovasc. Drugs Ther.* 25 (5): 419–429.

55 Halvorsen, B., Otterdal, K., Dahl, T.B. et al. (2008). Atherosclerotic plaque stability–what determines the fate of a plaque? *Prog. Cardiovasc. Dis.* 51 (3): 183–194.

56 Stemme, S., Faber, B., Holm, J. et al. (1995). T lymphocytes from human atherosclerotic plaques recognize oxidized low density lipoprotein. *Proc. Natl. Acad. Sci. U. S. A.* 92 (9): 3893–3897.

57 Chang, M.K., Binder, C.J., Miller, Y.I. et al. (2004). Apoptotic cells with oxidation-specific epitopes are immunogenic and proinflammatory. *J. Exp. Med.* 200 (11): 1359–1370.

58 Shaw, P.X., Horkko, S., Chang, M.K. et al. (2000). Natural antibodies with the T15 idiotype may act in atherosclerosis, apoptotic clearance, and protective immunity. *J. Clin. Invest.* 105 (12): 1731–1740.

59 Que, X., Hung, M.Y., Yeang, C. et al. (2018). Oxidized phospholipids are proinflammatory and proatherogenic in hypercholesterolaemic mice. *Nature* 558 (7709): 301–306.

60 Lorenzo, C., Delgado, P., Busse, C.E. et al. (2021). ALDH4A1 is an atherosclerosis auto-antigen targeted by protective antibodies. *Nature* 589 (7841): 287–292.

61 Winkels, H., Ehinger, E., Vassallo, M. et al. (2018). Atlas of the immune cell repertoire in mouse atherosclerosis defined by single-cell RNA-sequencing and mass cytometry. *Circ. Res.* 122 (12): 1675–1688.

62 Fernandez, D.M., Rahman, A.H., Fernandez, N.F. et al. (2019). Single-cell immune landscape of human atherosclerotic plaques. *Nat. Med.* 25 (10): 1576–1588.

63 Marchini, T., Abogunloko, T., and Wolf, D. (2021). Modulating autoimmunity against LDL: development of a vaccine against atherosclerosis. *Hamostaseologie* 41 (6): 447–457.

64 Meng, X., Yang, J., Dong, M. et al. (2016). Regulatory T cells in cardiovascular diseases. *Nat. Rev. Cardiol.* 13 (3): 167–179.

65 Saigusa, R., Winkels, H., and Ley, K. (2020). T cell subsets and functions in atherosclerosis. *Nat. Rev. Cardiol.* 17 (7): 387–401.

66 Wolf, D., Gerhardt, T., Winkels, H. et al. (2020). Pathogenic autoimmunity in atherosclerosis evolves from initially protective apolipoprotein B(100)-reactive CD4(+) T-regulatory cells. *Circulation* 142 (13): 1279–1293.

67 Wolf, D., Gerhardt, T., and Ley, K. (2017). *Vaccination to Prevent Cardiovascular Disease*, Cardiac and Vascular Biology, 29–52. Springer International Publishing.

68 Tsiantoulas, D., Diehl, C.J., Witztum, J.L., and Binder, C.J. (2014). B cells and humoral immunity in atherosclerosis. *Circ. Res.* 114 (11): 1743–1756.

69 Marchini, T., Malchow, S., Caceres, L. et al. (2022). Circulating autoantibodies recognizing immunodominant epitopes from human apolipoprotein B associate with cardiometabolic risk factors, but not with atherosclerotic disease. *Front. Cardiovasc. Med.* 9: 826729.

70 Jonasson, L., Holm, J., Skalli, O. et al. (1986). Regional accumulations of T cells, macrophages, and smooth muscle cells in the human atherosclerotic plaque. *Arteriosclerosis* 6 (2): 131–138.

71 Nettersheim, F.S., De Vore, L., and Winkels, H. (2020). Vaccination in atherosclerosis. *Cells* 9 (12): 2560.

72 Palinski, W., Miller, E., and Witztum, J.L. (1995). Immunization of low density lipoprotein (LDL) receptor-deficient rabbits with homologous malondialdehyde-modified LDL reduces atherogenesis. *Proc. Natl. Acad. Sci. U. S. A.* 92 (3): 821–825.

73 Freigang, S., Horkko, S., Miller, E. et al. (1998). Immunization of LDL receptor-deficient mice with homologous malondialdehyde-modified and native LDL reduces progression of atherosclerosis by mechanisms other than induction of high titers of antibodies to oxidative neoepitopes. *Arterioscler. Thromb. Vasc. Biol.* 18 (12): 1972–1982.

74 Ameli, S., Hultgardh-Nilsson, A., Regnstrom, J. et al. (1996). Effect of immunization with homologous LDL and oxidized LDL on early atherosclerosis in hypercholesterolemic rabbits. *Arterioscler. Thromb. Vasc. Biol.* 16 (8): 1074–1079.

75 George, J., Afek, A., Gilburd, B. et al. (1998). Hyperimmunization of apo-E-deficient mice with homologous malondialdehyde low-density lipoprotein suppresses early atherogenesis. *Atherosclerosis* 138 (1): 147–152.

76 Zhou, X., Caligiuri, G., Hamsten, A. et al. (2001). LDL immunization induces T-cell-dependent antibody formation and protection against atherosclerosis. *Arterioscler. Thromb. Vasc. Biol.* 21 (1): 108–114.

77 Chyu, K.Y., Reyes, O.S., Zhao, X. et al. (2004). Timing affects the efficacy of LDL immunization on atherosclerotic lesions in apo E (-/-) mice. *Atherosclerosis* 176 (1): 27–35.

78 Tse, K., Gonen, A., Sidney, J. et al. (2013). Atheroprotective vaccination with MHC-II restricted peptides from ApoB-100. *Front. Immunol.* 4: 493.

79 Hermansson, A., Johansson, D.K., Ketelhuth, D.F. et al. (2011). Immunotherapy with tolerogenic apolipoprotein B-100-loaded dendritic cells attenuates atherosclerosis in hypercholesterolemic mice. *Circulation* 123 (10): 1083–1091.

80 Gisterå, A., Hermansson, A., Strodthoff, D. et al. (2017). Vaccination against T-cell epitopes of native ApoB100 reduces vascular inflammation and disease in a humanized mouse model of atherosclerosis. *J. Intern. Med.* 281 (4): 383–397.

81 Kimura, T., Kobiyama, K., Winkels, H. et al. (2018). Regulatory CD4(+) T cells recognize major histocompatibility complex class II molecule-restricted peptide epitopes of apolipoprotein B. *Circulation* 138 (11): 1130–1143.

82 Wigren, M., Kolbus, D., Duner, P. et al. (2011). Evidence for a role of regulatory T cells in mediating the atheroprotective effect of apolipoprotein B peptide vaccine. *J. Intern. Med.* 269 (5): 546–556.

83 Wigren, M., Bengtsson, D., Duner, P. et al. (2009). Atheroprotective effects of Alum are associated with capture of oxidized LDL antigens and activation of regulatory T cells. *Circ. Res.* 104 (12): e62–e70.

84 Chyu, K.Y., Zhao, X., Dimayuga, P.C. et al. (2012). CD8+ T cells mediate the athero-protective effect of immunization with an ApoB-100 peptide. *PLoS One* 7 (2): e30780.

85 Zhou, J., Dimayuga, P.C., Zhao, X. et al. (2014). CD8(+)CD25(+) T cells reduce atherosclerosis in apoE(-/-) mice. *Biochem. Biophys. Res. Commun.* 443 (3): 864–870.

86 Young, J.C., Agashe, V.R., Siegers, K., and Hartl, F.U. (2004). Pathways of chaperone-mediated protein folding in the cytosol. *Nat. Rev. Mol. Cell Biol.* 5 (10): 781–791.

87 Kilic, A. and Mandal, K. (2012). Heat shock proteins: pathogenic role in atherosclerosis and potential therapeutic implications. *Autoimmun. Dis.* 2012: 502813.

88 Wick, C. (2016). Tolerization against atherosclerosis using heat shock protein 60. *Cell Stress Chaperones* 21 (2): 201–211.

89 Zhu, J., Quyyumi, A.A., Rott, D. et al. (2001). Antibodies to human heat-shock protein 60 are associated with the presence and severity of coronary artery disease: evidence for an autoimmune component of atherogenesis. *Circulation* 103 (8): 1071–1075.

90 Almanzar, G., Öllinger, R., Leuenberger, J. et al. (2012). Autoreactive HSP60 epitope-specific T-cells in early human atherosclerotic lesions. *J. Autoimmun.* 39 (4): 441–450.

91 Kimura, T., Tse, K., Sette, A., and Ley, K. (2015). Vaccination to modulate atherosclerosis. *Autoimmunity* 48 (3): 152–160.

92 van Puijvelde, G.H., van Es, T., van Wanrooij, E.J. et al. (2007). Induction of oral tolerance to HSP60 or an HSP60-peptide activates T cell regulation and reduces atherosclerosis. *Arterioscler. Thromb. Vasc. Biol.* 27 (12): 2677–2683.

93 Grundtman, C., Jakic, B., Buszko, M. et al. (2015). Mycobacterial heat shock protein 65 (mbHSP65)-induced atherosclerosis: preventive oral tolerization and definition of atheroprotective and atherogenic mbHSP65 peptides. *Atherosclerosis* 242 (1): 303–310.

94 McDonnell, T., Wincup, C., Buchholz, I. et al. (2020). The role of beta-2-glycoprotein I in health and disease associating structure with function: more than just APS. *Blood Rev.* 39: 100610.

95 George, J., Harats, D., Gilburd, B. et al. (1999). Immunolocalization of beta2-glycoprotein I (apolipoprotein H) to human atherosclerotic plaques: potential implications for lesion progression. *Circulation* 99 (17): 2227–2230.

96 Kobayashi, K., Matsuura, E., Liu, Q. et al. (2001). A specific ligand for beta(2)-glycoprotein I mediates autoantibody-dependent uptake of oxidized low density lipoprotein by macrophages. *J. Lipid Res.* 42 (5): 697–709.

97 Greco, T.P., Conti-Kelly, A.M., Anthony, J.R. et al. (2010). Oxidized-LDL/beta(2)-glycoprotein I complexes are associated with disease severity and increased risk for adverse outcomes in patients with acute coronary syndromes. *Am. J. Clin. Pathol.* 133 (5): 737–743.

98 Gopal, R., Marinelli, M.A., and Alcorn, J.F. (2020). Immune mechanisms in cardiovascular diseases associated with viral infection. *Front. Immunol.* 11: 570681.

99 Ibrahim, A.I., Obeid, M.T., Jouma, M.J. et al. (2005). Detection of herpes simplex virus, cytomegalovirus and Epstein-Barr virus DNA in atherosclerotic plaques and in unaffected bypass grafts. *J. Clin. Virol.* 32 (1): 29–32.

100 Shah, P.K. (2019). Inflammation, infection and atherosclerosis. *Trends Cardiovasc. Med.* 29 (8): 468–472.

101 Udell, J.A., Zawi, R., Bhatt, D.L. et al. (2013). Association between influenza vaccination and cardiovascular outcomes in high-risk patients: a meta-analysis. *JAMA* 310 (16): 1711–1720.

102 Jiang, J., Chan, L., Kauffman, J. et al. (2023). Impact of vaccination on major adverse cardiovascular events in patients with COVID-19 infection. *J. Am. Coll. Cardiol.* 81 (9): 928–930.

103 Xie, Y., Xu, E., Bowe, B., and Al-Aly, Z. (2022). Long-term cardiovascular outcomes of COVID-19. *Nat. Med.* 28 (3): 583–590.

104 Marchini, T., Hansen, S., and Wolf, D. (2021). ApoB-specific CD4(+) T cells in mouse and human atherosclerosis. *Cells* 10 (2): 446.

105 Klingenberg, R., Lebens, M., Hermansson, A. et al. (2010). Intranasal immunization with an apolipoprotein B-100 fusion protein induces antigen-specific regulatory T cells and reduces atherosclerosis. *Arterioscler. Thromb. Vasc. Biol.* 30 (5): 946–952.

106 Kimura, T., Tse, K., McArdle, S. et al. (2017). Atheroprotective vaccination with MHC-II-restricted ApoB peptides induces peritoneal IL-10-producing CD4 T cells. *Am. J. Physiol. Heart Circ. Physiol.* 312 (4): H781–H790.

107 Kobiyama, K., Vassallo, M., Mitzi, J. et al. (2018). A clinically applicable adjuvant for an atherosclerosis vaccine in mice. *Eur. J. Immunol.* 48 (9): 1580–1587.

108 Orecchioni, M., Wolf, D., Suryawanshi, V. et al. (2022). Deleting interleukin-10 from myeloid cells exacerbates atherosclerosis in Apoe(-/-) mice. *Cell. Mol. Life Sci.* 80 (1): 10.

109 Walczak, A., Szymanska, B., and Selmaj, K. (2004). Differential prevention of experimental autoimmune encephalomyelitis with antigen-specific DNA vaccination. *Clin. Neurol. Neurosurg.* 106 (3): 241–245.

110 Kutzler, M.A. and Weiner, D.B. (2008). DNA vaccines: ready for prime time? *Nat. Rev. Genet.* 9 (10): 776–788.

111 Shen, Y., Chen, J., Zhang, X. et al. (2007). Human TNF-alpha gene vaccination prevents collagen-induced arthritis in mice. *Int. Immunopharmacol.* 7 (9): 1140–1149.

112 Hauer, A.D., van Puijvelde, G.H., Peterse, N. et al. (2007). Vaccination against VEGFR2 attenuates initiation and progression of atherosclerosis. *Arterioscler. Thromb. Vasc. Biol.* 27 (9): 2050–2057.

113 Krienke, C., Kolb, L., Diken, E. et al. (2021). A noninflammatory mRNA vaccine for treatment of experimental autoimmune encephalomyelitis. *Science* 371 (6525): 145–153.

114 Kranz, L.M., Diken, M., Haas, H. et al. (2016). Systemic RNA delivery to dendritic cells exploits antiviral defence for cancer immunotherapy. *Nature* 534 (7607): 396–401.

115 Parks, R.J. and Gussoni, E. (2018). Building immune tolerance through DNA vaccination. *Proc. Natl. Acad. Sci. U. S. A.* 115 (39): 9652–9654.

116 Pardi, N., Hogan, M.J., Porter, F.W., and Weissman, D. (2018). mRNA vaccines - a new era in vaccinology. *Nat. Rev. Drug Discov.* 17 (4): 261–279.

117 Szabo, G.T., Mahiny, A.J., and Vlatkovic, I. (2022). COVID-19 mRNA vaccines: platforms and current developments. *Mol. Ther.* 30 (5): 1850–1868.

118 Greenfield, E.A. (2019). Routes of antigen injection in mice and rats. *Cold Spring Harb. Protoc.* 2019 (6): https://doi.org/10.1101/pdb.prot100230.

119 Kimura, T., Kobiyama, K., Winkels, H. et al. (2018). Regulatory CD4(+) T cells recognize MHC-II-restricted peptide epitopes of apolipoprotein B. *Circulation* 138 (11): 1130–1143.

120 Gistera, A., Klement, M.L., Polyzos, K.A. et al. (2018). LDL-reactive T cells regulate plasma cholesterol levels and development of atherosclerosis in humanized hypercholesterolemic mice. *Circulation* 38 (22): 2513–2526.

121 Xu, Q., Dietrich, H., Steiner, H.J. et al. (1992). Induction of arteriosclerosis in normocholesterolemic rabbits by immunization with heat shock protein 65. *Arterioscler. Thromb.* 12 (7): 789–799.

122 Tay, C., Liu, Y.H., Kanellakis, P. et al. (2018). Follicular B cells promote atherosclerosis via T cell-mediated differentiation into plasma cells and secreting pathogenic immunoglobulin G. *Arterioscler. Thromb. Vasc. Biol.* 38 (5): e71–e84.

123 Schiopu, A., Bengtsson, J., Soderberg, I. et al. (2004). Recombinant human antibodies against aldehyde-modified apolipoprotein B-100 peptide sequences inhibit atherosclerosis. *Circulation* 110 (14): 2047–2052.

124 Schiopu, A., Frendeus, B., Jansson, B. et al. (2007). Recombinant antibodies to an oxidized low-density lipoprotein epitope induce rapid regression of atherosclerosis in apobec-1(-/-)/low-density lipoprotein receptor(-/-) mice. *J. Am. Coll. Cardiol.* 50 (24): 2313–2318.

125 Mullard, A. (2017). FDA approves first CAR T therapy. *Nat. Rev. Drug Discov.* 16 (10): 669.

126 Aghajanian, H., Kimura, T., Rurik, J.G. et al. (2019). Targeting cardiac fibrosis with engineered T cells. *Nature* 573 (7774): 430–433.

127 McGinley, M.P., Goldschmidt, C.H., and Rae-Grant, A.D. (2021). Diagnosis and treatment of multiple sclerosis: a review. *JAMA* 325 (8): 765–779.

128 Filippi, M., Bar-Or, A., Piehl, F. et al. (2018). Multiple sclerosis. *Nat. Rev. Dis. Primers* 4 (1): 43.

129 Dulamea, A.O. (2017). Role of oligodendrocyte dysfunction in demyelination, remyelination and neurodegeneration in multiple sclerosis. *Adv. Exp. Med. Biol.* 958: 91–127.

130 Hemmer, B., Nessler, S., Zhou, D. et al. (2006). Immunopathogenesis and immunotherapy of multiple sclerosis. *Nat. Clin. Pract. Neurol.* 2 (4): 201–211.

131 Fletcher, J.M., Lalor, S.J., Sweeney, C.M. et al. (2010). T cells in multiple sclerosis and experimental autoimmune encephalomyelitis. *Clin. Exp. Immunol.* 162 (1): 1–11.

132 Piaton, G., Williams, A., Seilhean, D., and Lubetzki, C. (2009). Remyelination in multiple sclerosis. *Prog. Brain Res.* 175: 453–464.

133 Reboldi, A., Coisne, C., Baumjohann, D. et al. (2009). C-C chemokine receptor 6-regulated entry of TH-17 cells into the CNS through the choroid plexus is required for the initiation of EAE. *Nat. Immunol.* 10 (5): 514–523.

134 McGinley, A.M., Sutton, C.E., Edwards, S.C. et al. (2020). Interleukin-17A serves a priming role in autoimmunity by recruiting IL-1beta-producing myeloid cells that promote pathogenic T cells. *Immunity* 52 (2): 342–356 e6.

135 Thornton, A.M. and Shevach, E.M. (2000). Suppressor effector function of CD4+CD25+ immunoregulatory T cells is antigen nonspecific. *J. Immunol.* 164 (1): 183–190.

136 Clemente-Casares, X., Blanco, J., Ambalavanan, P. et al. (2016). Expanding antigen-specific regulatory networks to treat autoimmunity. *Nature* 530 (7591): 434–440.

137 Constantinescu, C.S., Farooqi, N., O'Brien, K., and Gran, B. (2011). Experimental autoimmune encephalomyelitis (EAE) as a model for multiple sclerosis (MS). *Br. J. Pharmacol.* 164 (4): 1079–1106.

138 Robinson, A.P., Harp, C.T., Noronha, A., and Miller, S.D. (2014). The experimental autoimmune encephalomyelitis (EAE) model of MS: utility for understanding disease pathophysiology and treatment. *Handb. Clin. Neurol.* 122: 173–189.

139 Libbey, J.E. and Fujinami, R.S. (2011). Experimental autoimmune encephalomyelitis as a testing paradigm for adjuvants and vaccines. *Vaccine* 29 (17): 3356–3362.

140 Kap, Y.S., Smith, P., Jagessar, S.A. et al. (2008). Fast progression of recombinant human myelin/oligodendrocyte glycoprotein (MOG)-induced experimental autoimmune encephalomyelitis in marmosets is associated with the activation of MOG34-56-specific cytotoxic T cells. *J. Immunol.* 180 (3): 1326–1337.

141 Mailand, M.T. and Frederiksen, J.L. (2017). Vaccines and multiple sclerosis: a systematic review. *J. Neurol.* 264 (6): 1035–1050.

142 Otero-Romero, S., Lebrun-Frenay, C., Reyes, S. et al. (2023). European Committee for Treatment and Research in Multiple Sclerosis and European Academy of Neurology consensus on vaccination in people with multiple sclerosis: improving immunization strategies in the era of highly active immunotherapeutic drugs. *Eur. J. Neurol.* 30 (8): 2144–2176.

143 Reyes, S., Ramsay, M., Ladhani, S. et al. (2020). Protecting people with multiple sclerosis through vaccination. *Pract. Neurol.* 20 (6): 435–445.

144 Correale, J., Farez, M., and Gilmore, W. (2008). Vaccines for multiple sclerosis: progress to date. *CNS Drugs* 22 (3): 175–198.

145 Badawi, A.H. and Siahaan, T.J. (2012). Immune modulating peptides for the treatment and suppression of multiple sclerosis. *Clin. Immunol.* 144 (2): 127–138.

146 Mattes, P.M. and Mattes, W.B. (1992). Alpha-naphthyl butyrate carboxylesterase activity in human and rat nasal tissue. *Toxicol. Appl. Pharmacol.* 114 (1): 71–76.

147 Vandenbark, A.A., Culbertson, N.E., Bartholomew, R.M. et al. (2008). Therapeutic vaccination with a trivalent T-cell receptor (TCR) peptide vaccine restores deficient FoxP3 expression and TCR recognition in subjects with multiple sclerosis. *Immunology* 123 (1): 66–78.

148 Higgins, P.J. and Weiner, H.L. (1988). Suppression of experimental autoimmune encephalomyelitis by oral administration of myelin basic protein and its fragments. *J. Immunol.* 140 (2): 440–445.

149 Javed, N.H., Gienapp, I.E., Cox, K.L., and Whitacre, C.C. (1995). Exquisite peptide specificity of oral tolerance in experimental autoimmune encephalomyelitis. *J. Immunol.* 155 (3): 1599–1605.

150 Karpus, W.J., Kennedy, K.J., Smith, W.S., and Miller, S.D. (1996). Inhibition of relapsing experimental autoimmune encephalomyelitis in SJL mice by feeding the immunodominant PLP139-151 peptide. *J. Neurosci. Res.* 45 (4): 410–423.

151 al-Sabbagh, A., Miller, A., Santos, L.M., and Weiner, H.L. (1994). Antigen-driven tissue-specific suppression following oral tolerance: orally administered myelin basic protein suppresses proteolipid protein-induced experimental autoimmune encephalomyelitis in the SJL mouse. *Eur. J. Immunol.* 24 (9): 2104–2109.

152 Karikó, K., Muramatsu, H., Welsh, F.A. et al. (2008). Incorporation of pseudouridine into mRNA yields superior nonimmunogenic vector with increased translational capacity and biological stability. *Mol. Ther.* 16 (11): 1833–1840.

153 Karikó, K., Buckstein, M., Ni, H., and Weissman, D. (2005). Suppression of RNA recognition by Toll-like receptors: the impact of nucleoside modification and the evolutionary origin of RNA. *Immunity* 23 (2): 165–175.

154 Wardell, C.M. and Levings, M.K. (2021). mRNA vaccines take on immune tolerance. *Nat. Biotechnol.* 39 (4): 419–421.

155 Furlan, R. (2021). A tolerizing mRNA vaccine against autoimmunity? *Mol. Ther.* 29 (3): 896–897.

156 Khan, U. and Ghazanfar, H. (2018). T lymphocytes and autoimmunity. *Int. Rev. Cell Mol. Biol.* 341: 125–168.

157 Pfeil, J., Simonetti, M., Lauer, U. et al. (2021). Prevention of EAE by tolerogenic vaccination with PEGylated antigenic peptides. *Ther. Adv. Chronic Dis.* 12: 20406223211037830.

158 Pascolo, S. (2004). Messenger RNA-based vaccines. *Expert. Opin. Biol. Ther.* 4 (8): 1285–1294.

159 Verbeke, R., Hogan, M.J., Loré, K., and Pardi, N. (2022). Innate immune mechanisms of mRNA vaccines. *Immunity* 55 (11): 1993–2005.

160 Falk, K., Lau, J.M., Santambrogio, L. et al. (2002). Ligand exchange of major histocompatibility complex class II proteins is triggered by H-bond donor groups of small molecules. *J. Biol. Chem.* 277 (4): 2709–2715.

161 Abualrous, E.T., Stolzenberg, S., Sticht, J. et al. (2023). MHC-II dynamics are maintained in HLA-DR allotypes to ensure catalyzed peptide exchange. *Nat. Chem. Biol.* 19 (10): 1196–1204.

162 Purcell, A.W., McCluskey, J., and Rossjohn, J. (2007). More than one reason to rethink the use of peptides in vaccine design. *Nat. Rev. Drug Discov.* 6 (5): 404–414.

163 Rammensee, H.G. (1995). Chemistry of peptides associated with MHC class I and class II molecules. *Curr. Opin. Immunol.* 7 (1): 85–96.

164 Geall, A.J., Mandl, C.W., and Ulmer, J.B. (2013). RNA: the new revolution in nucleic acid vaccines. *Semin. Immunol.* 25 (2): 152–159.

165 Sahin, U., Kariko, K., and Tureci, O. (2014). mRNA-based therapeutics–developing a new class of drugs. *Nat. Rev. Drug Discov.* 13 (10): 759–780.

166 Han, A., Glanville, J., Hansmann, L., and Davis, M.M. (2014). Linking T-cell receptor sequence to functional phenotype at the single-cell level. *Nat. Biotechnol.* 32 (7): 684–692.

167 Shaw, M.K., Tse, K.Y., Zhao, X. et al. (2017). T-cells specific for a self-peptide of ApoB-100 exacerbate aortic atheroma in murine atherosclerosis. *Front. Immunol.* 8: 95.

168 Brunner, R., Jensen-Jarolim, E., and Pali-Scholl, I. (2010). The ABC of clinical and experimental adjuvants–a brief overview. *Immunol. Lett.* 128 (1): 29–35.

169 Khallou-Laschet, J., Tupin, E., Caligiuri, G. et al. (2006). Atheroprotective effect of adjuvants in apolipoprotein E knockout mice. *Atherosclerosis* 184 (2): 330–341.

170 Herbin, O., Ait-Oufella, H., Yu, W. et al. (2012). Regulatory T-cell response to apolipoprotein B100-derived peptides reduces the development and progression of atherosclerosis in mice. *Arterioscler. Thromb. Vasc. Biol.* 32 (3): 605–612.

171 Joseph, A., Ackerman, D., Talley, J.D. et al. (1993). Manifestations of coronary atherosclerosis in young trauma victims–an autopsy study. *J. Am. Coll. Cardiol.* 22 (2): 459–467.

172 Platts-Mills, T.A. (2015). The allergy epidemics: 1870-2010. *J. Allergy Clin. Immunol.* 136 (1): 3–13.

173 Stone, K.D., Prussin, C., and Metcalfe, D.D. (2010). IgE, mast cells, basophils, and eosinophils. *J. Allergy Clin. Immunol.* 125 (2 Suppl 2): S73–S80.

174 van der Heijden, F.L., Joost van Neerven, R.J., van Katwijk, M. et al. (1993). Serum-IgE-facilitated allergen presentation in atopic disease. *J. Immunol.* 150 (8 Pt 1): 3643–3650.

175 Wachholz, P.A., Soni, N.K., Till, S.J., and Durham, S.R. (2003). Inhibition of allergen-IgE binding to B cells by IgG antibodies after grass pollen immunotherapy. *J. Allergy Clin. Immunol.* 112 (5): 915–922.

176 Durham, S.R. and Shamji, M.H. (2023). Allergen immunotherapy: past, present and future. *Nat. Rev. Immunol.* 23 (5): 317–328.

177 Kucuksezer, U.C., Ozdemir, C., Cevhertas, L. et al. (2020). Mechanisms of allergen-specific immunotherapy and allergen tolerance. *Allergol. Int.* 69 (4): 549–560.

178 Würtzen, P.A., Lund, G., Lund, K. et al. (2008). A double-blind placebo-controlled birch allergy vaccination study II: correlation between inhibition of IgE binding, histamine release and facilitated allergen presentation. *Clin. Exp. Allergy* 38 (8): 1290–1301.

179 Shamji, M.H., Valenta, R., Jardetzky, T. et al. (2021). The role of allergen-specific IgE, IgG and IgA in allergic disease. *Allergy* 76 (12): 3627–3641.

180 Deniz, G., Erten, G., Kücüksezer, U.C. et al. (2008). Regulatory NK cells suppress antigen-specific T cell responses. *J. Immunol.* 180 (2): 850–857.

181 Pauli, G., Larsen, T.H., Rak, S. et al. (2008). Efficacy of recombinant birch pollen vaccine for the treatment of birch-allergic rhinoconjunctivitis. *J. Allergy Clin. Immunol.* 122 (5): 951–960.

182 Niederberger, V., Horak, F., Vrtala, S. et al. (2004). Vaccination with genetically engineered allergens prevents progression of allergic disease. *Proc. Natl. Acad. Sci. U. S. A.* 101 Suppl 2 (Suppl 2): 14677–14682.

183 Carralot, J.P., Probst, J., Hoerr, I. et al. (2004). Polarization of immunity induced by direct injection of naked sequence-stabilized mRNA vaccines. *Cell. Mol. Life Sci.* 61 (18): 2418–2424.

184 Roesler, E., Weiss, R., Weinberger, E.E. et al. (2009). Immunize and disappear-safety-optimized mRNA vaccination with a panel of 29 allergens. *J. Allergy Clin. Immunol.* 124 (5): 1070-7.e1–1070-7.e11.

185 Hattinger, E., Scheiblhofer, S., Roesler, E. et al. (2015). Prophylactic mRNA vaccination against allergy confers long-term memory responses and persistent protection in mice. *J Immunol Res* 2015: 797421.

186 Abdel-Gadir, A., Massoud, A.H., and Chatila, T.A. (2018). Antigen-specific Treg cells in immunological tolerance: implications for allergic diseases. *F1000Res.* 7: 38.

187 Xu, X., Wang, X., Liao, Y.P. et al. (2023). Use of a liver-targeting immune-tolerogenic mRNA lipid nanoparticle platform to treat peanut-induced anaphylaxis by single- and multiple-epitope nucleotide sequence delivery. *ACS Nano* 17 (5): 4942–4957.

Part II

Recent Progress in Vaccine Research and Development

8

Design and Development of mRNA Vaccines to Combat the COVID-19 Pandemic

Istvan Tombacz

University of Pennsylvania, Perelman School of Medicine, Department of Medicine, 1 uCity Square, 25 N 38th Street, Philadelphia, PA 19104, USA

8.1 Introduction

Severe acute respiratory coronavirus 2 (SARS-CoV-2) has spread across the globe since its discovery in China at the end of 2019, causing the global pandemic of coronavirus disease 2019. As of today, there have been close to 700 million registered cases and 7 million registered deaths associated with it worldwide [1], with serious socioeconomic consequences. After the outbreak, academia and the biotech industry worked at breakneck pace to develop safe, effective, and affordable vaccines to mitigate the spread of the virus and prevent severe health events. Since then, multiple vaccines employing different modalities have been approved throughout the world [2, 3].

Messenger RNA has emerged as a possible and promising vaccine platform in the last two decades. It offers lower costs, easier and faster design, and manufacturing because of its relatively simple properties as a material and its synthetic production process. Multiple preclinical and clinical studies have demonstrated the utility and efficacy of this modality [4, 5]. At the outbreak of the COVID-19 pandemic, two biotechnology companies, which had already been working on applications for the mRNA platform, immediately started working on vaccines against SARS-CoV-2. Moderna Inc. produced a GMP-quality mRNA vaccine candidate (mRNA-1273) for human trials in only 42 days after receiving the nucleotide sequence of SARS-CoV-2, demonstrating the superiority of this platform regarding ease of design and manufacture. Both Moderna and Pfizer/BioNTech started phase III clinical trials in July 2020, and both vaccine candidates (mRNA-1273 and BNT162b2, respectively) showed over 90% efficacy within a six-month follow-up [6–9]. Both vaccines received emergency approval in multiple countries over the world shortly after, and full approval later, allowing hundreds of millions of people to be immunized against SARS-CoV-2, which contributed to significantly reduced morbidity and mortality from COVID-19. This success is both a blessing and a curse for future mRNA vaccines. It is certain that the increased interest will lead to many more applications in the future (mainly infectious diseases and cancer) now that the mRNA platform

Trends in mRNA Vaccine Research, First Edition. Edited by Gabor Tamas Szabo and Norbert Pardi.

has proved itself, but unprecedented quickness of development and deployment of a previously unknown vaccine type has garnered worrying levels of distrust and skepticism among the general populace.

In this chapter, we review the development of the two approved mRNA-based SARS-CoV-2 vaccines from Moderna and Pfizer/BioNTech, focusing on design, preclinical and clinical data, challenges, and current and future directions.

8.2 SARS-CoV-2 Vaccine Design

The genome sequence data of SARS-CoV-2 was first deposited into GenBank in January 2020. Analysis of the sequence began immediately all over the world. Knowledge gained from previous outbreaks of coronaviruses (SARS-CoV-1 and MERS-CoV) was pivotal in identifying promising antigens as vaccine targets. Coronaviruses employ a surface glycoprotein, Spike (S), to enter target cells; this S protein also gives them a distinctive halo or corona in electron microscopy images. Immune response against Spike can generate neutralizing antibodies, preventing viral entry, thus practically all SARS-CoV-2 vaccines use Spike as an antigen. The S protein contains two subunits. S1 includes the receptor-binding domain (RBD) and other neutralizing epitopes, while S2 is responsible for viral fusion with the host cell membrane [10]. Previous experience gained from MERS-CoV resulted in a modified version of Spike carrying two proline substitutions in S2 (K986P and V987P), which stabilize S in a prefusion state to induce higher levels of neutralizing antibodies compared to wild-type (WT) Spike [11]. Both Moderna's and Pfizer/BioNTech's vaccine employ this S-2P variant, but BioNTech also tested a shorter sequence containing the RBD only. Multiple other companies have started clinical trials utilizing various strategies involving mRNA (Table 8.1) [12, 13]. Some vaccines utilize a modification where the furin cleavage site between S1 and S2 is mutated, so that no cleavage occurs. The contribution of this modification to vaccine efficacy has not been elucidated.

mRNA vaccines fall into two categories. Self-amplifying mRNA is based on alphaviruses, carrying an antigen-coding sequence along with viral genome replication protein-coding sequences. On the other hand, nonreplicating mRNA encodes only the antigen and can be unmodified or contain modified nucleosides [4, 14]. Both Moderna's and Pfizer/BioNTech's vaccine utilize nonreplicating, nucleoside-modified mRNA (containing 1-methyl-pseudouridine instead of uridine), encapsulated in lipid nanoparticles (LNPs) [15]. Moderna committed to this approach only, while BioNTech initiated a phase I trial (NCT04380701) with four candidates. BNT162a1 and BNT162b1 encoded only the RBD on either unmodified or nucleoside-modified mRNA, respectively [16, 17]. BNT162b2, the eventual commercial vaccine, utilizes nucleoside-modified mRNA encoding full S-2P [6]. Finally, BNT162c2 was a self-amplifying mRNA of S-2P. In this trial, BNT162b2 induced similar levels of antibody responses but lower frequency and intensity of adverse effects as BNT162b1, thus phase II/III trials were initiated with the former [18]. No data have been released regarding BNT162a1 and BNT162c2.

Table 8.1 mRNA-based vaccines currently or previously in development.

Name	Developer	Type	Clinical phase	Antigen	Dose (μg) and route of administration
BNT162b2[a)]		nr-nm	I/II/III/IV	S2-P, codon-optimized	30; im
BNT162b1	Pfizer/BioNTech	nr-nm	I/II/III	RBD, secreted	1–100; im
BNT162b3		nr-nm	I/II	RBD trans-membrane	nd; im
mRNA-1273[a)]	Moderna/NIAID/BARDA	nr-nm	III	S2-P	100; im
TAK-919	Takeda/Moderna	nr-nm	I/II	S2-P	100; im
ChulaCov19	Chulalongkorn University	nr-nm	II	WT Spike	10–50; im
CVnCoV	CureVac	nr-um	II/III	S2-P	12; im
BNT162a1	Pfizer/BioNTech	nr-um	I	RBD, secreted	nd; im
MRT5500 (VAW00001)	Translate Bio/Sanofi	nr-um	I/II	S2-P, furin cleavage modified	15–135; im
ARCoV	AMS/Walvax/Suzhou	nr-um	II/III	RBD	15; im
PTX-COVID19B	Providence Therapeutics	nr-um	I/II	WT Spike	16–100; im
DS5670	Daiichi Sankyo	nr-um	I/II	Not disclosed	10–100; im
SW-0123	Stemirna Therapeutics/Shanghai East Hospital	nr-um	I/II/III	WT Spike	10–100; im
EG-COVID	eyeGENE	nr-um	I/II	WT Spike	100, 200; im
BNT162c2	Pfizer/BioNTech	sa	I	S2-P	nd; im
LNP-nCoVsaRNA	Imperial College London	sa	I/II	S2-P	0.1–10; im
LNP-nCOVsaRNA-02	ICL/MRC/UVRI/LSHTM/Uganda Research Unit	sa	I	S2-P	5; route not disclosed, possibly im

(Continued)

Table 8.1 (Continued)

Name	Developer	Type	Clinical phase	Antigen	Dose (μg) and route of administration
EXG5003	Elixirgen Therapeutics	sa	I/II	RBD	nd; id
ARCT 021[a]	Arcturus Therapeutics/Duke-NUS Medical School	sa	I/II/III	S2-P	5, 7.5; im
CoV2 SAM LNP	GSK	sa	I	WT Spike	1, im
HDT301 (repRNA-CoV2S; HGCO19)	SENAI Cimatec/HDT/Gennova/Quratis	sa	I	WT Spike	1–25; im
VLPCOV-01	VLP Therapeutics Japan	sa	I	RBD trans-membrane	0.3–3; im
SAM-SARS-CoV-2	Gritstone	sa	I	S2-P, furin cleavage modified	10; im

Type: nr-nm: nonreplicating, nucleoside-modified; nr-um: nonreplicating, unmodified; sa: self-amplifying. Dose and route of administration: nd: not disclosed; im: intramuscular; id: intradermal.

a) Multiple booster candidates against variants are available or in development.

mRNA-1273 and BNT162b2 received Emergency Use Authorization in the United States by the Food and Drug Administration (FDA) and in Europe by the European Medicines Agency (EMA) at the turn of 2020/2021. BNT162b2 was fully approved in the United States on August 23, 2021, and mRNA-1273 received full approval on January 31, 2022. To date, these are the only two vaccines against COVID-19 utilizing mRNA that received approval from any agency.

8.3 Development of SARS-CoV-2 mRNA Vaccines

8.3.1 mRNA-1273 – Moderna

In a joint effort with the Vaccine Research Center on the National Institute of Health, Moderna developed and produced a GMP-grade batch of their nucleoside-modified mRNA vaccine candidate, mRNA-1273, 43 days after receiving the genome sequence of SARS-CoV-2. Preclinical evaluation in mice and phase I clinical trials were begun in parallel [19, 20]. They reported induction of Th1-biased S-specific $CD4^+$ T cells (advantageous for antiviral immunity as opposed to possible Th2-related vaccine-enhanced disease [21]), $CD8^+$ T cells, and strong neutralizing antibody responses. Sterilizing protection was achieved with a single immunization of 1 μg mRNA–LNP [19]. In nonhuman primates, two immunizations of 10 or 100 μg elicited dose-dependent S-specific $CD4^+$ T cell responses, T follicular helper cell and neutralizing antibody responses [20]. However, $CD8^+$ T cells were not abundantly present in blood. A very high level of protection from viral replication in the bronchoalveolar lavage fluid and nasal swabs was observed after two immunizations with a 100-μg dose.

Phase I clinical trial started with 45 healthy individuals aged 18–55 in March 2021 [22]. The immunization regimen consisted of two intramuscular injections of 25, 100, or 250 μg of the vaccine two weeks apart. Adverse events were dose dependent and significantly stronger after the second dose. S-specific IgG titers and virus neutralization assays indicated robust, dose-dependent humoral responses, which were boosted after the second immunization. The trial was later expanded with 40 people in two additional groups, aged 56–70 and 71+ years [23]. The vaccine induced mild and moderate adverse events in these groups, and neutralizing antibody levels were similar to the 18–55-year-old group. S-specific $CD4^+$ T cell responses were strong and Th1-biased, while $CD8^+$ T cell responses were low and variable, like in nonhuman primates. While $CD8^+$ T cell levels were lower than in Pfizer's/BioNTech's trial, an independent study using a different detection method (activation-induced marker expression versus intracellular cytokine staining in the trial) found similar, good $CD8^+$ T cell responses with both vaccines [24].

An observer-blinded phase III clinical trial was started based on this safety and immunogenicity data, involving 30 420 people, aged 18–65 years, receiving two injections of placebo or 100 μg of the vaccine four weeks apart [7]. Local adverse events after the second dose were mild to moderate, while systemic adverse events were reported as moderate to severe. Efficacy at preventing COVID-19 was reported to be 94.1%, with complete protection from severe illness during a median follow-up of 64 days. Efficacy remained high after a six-month follow-up (90+% against contracting COVID-19 and 95+% against severe illness). Vaccine-induced neutralizing antibody titers against multiple SARS-CoV-2 variants decreased gradually over 180 days to roughly 20% of peak levels, according to recent studies [25, 26]. Immune responses will be followed for two years to evaluate long-term durability. Emergency use authorization for individuals aged 18 and older was granted in the United States on December 18, 2020, and in the EU on January 6, 2021 based on these clinical trial data. The vaccine received full authorization in the United States on January 31, 2022. As of the end of September 2022, over 550 million doses (counted individually) have been administered worldwide [27].

8.3.2 BNT162b2 – Pfizer/BioNTech

Development of BNT162b2 started practically the same time as Moderna's mRNA-1273, utilizing the same strategy of nucleoside-modified mRNA encoding S-2P, encapsulated in LNP [6, 18, 28–31]. In preclinical studies, BNT162b2 induced strong cellular and humoral immune responses in mice immunized with 0.2–5 μg mRNA. In rhesus macaques, 30 or 100 μg doses prompted similarly high and robust protective immune responses [31].

BNT162b1 and BNT162b2 were evaluated in a phase I clinical trial for safety starting at the end of April 2020. A total of 195 individuals, aged 18–55 and 65–85, were enrolled, separated into 13 groups of 15 people, 3 of which received placebo and 12 received vaccine. Groups were defined by age of participants, vaccine candidate, and dosage (10, 20, and 30 μg). One group received a single dose of 100 μg BNT162b1, while all other groups received two doses 21 days apart. BNT162b2 was associated with a lower incidence and severity of systemic reactions than BNT162b1, especially in older adults. The two vaccine candidates elicited similar, dose-dependent neutralizing titers in both age groups, comparable to convalescent sera, with small differences between dose groups [18]. Based on these phase I data obtained in the United States and previous interim data of BNT162b1 from Germany and the United States, BNT162b2 was selected to be advanced to phase II/III.

Phase III evaluation of BNT162b2 is still ongoing in a multinational observer-blinded study (NCT04368728). Originally, 43 548 volunteers, 16 years or older, were assigned 1:1 to placebo or vaccine groups. Two doses of 30 μg of BNT162b2 were administered 21 days apart. Adverse reactions were mild to moderate and self-limiting. Serious (grade 4) adverse events occurred at similar, low frequencies in both the vaccine and the placebo group (0.6% and 0.5%, respectively). During a median follow-up of two months, 8 cases of COVID-19 (onset at least seven days after the second dose) occurred in the vaccine group, and 162 cases were found in the placebo group, resulting in an efficacy of 95%.

In a follow-up evaluation six months after vaccination, overall efficacy remained high, 91.3%, among people without evidence of previous SARS-CoV-2 infection and 83.7% between 4 and 7.5 months after the second dose [9]. In total, 2264 participants aged 12–15 were included in this study. The vaccine continued to be safe, and efficacy against severe COVID-19 was measured to be 96.7%, with at least one dose of BNT162b2 received.

Based on these safety, immunogenicity, and efficacy data, Pfizer/BioNTech's vaccine has received approval in over 100 countries. It received emergency use authorization for individuals aged 16 and older in the United States on December 11, 2020, and in the EU on December 21, 2020. Full approval was granted in the United States on August 23, 2021, and in the EU on October 10, 2022. As of the end of September 2022, over 1.5 billion doses (counted individually) have been administered [27].

8.4 Other SARS-CoV-2 mRNA Vaccines Developments

8.4.1 CVnCoV – CureVac

CureVac opted for a slightly different strategy than Moderna and Pfizer/BioNTech. Instead of using modified nucleosides, CureVac's vaccine, CVnCoV, is unmodified but sequence-engineered to be GC-rich [32]. The mRNA encodes S-2P, like the former two. In preclinical studies, the vaccine-induced strong $CD4^+$ and $CD8^+$ T cell and neutralizing antibody responses in mice after two immunizations with 2 μg mRNA–LNP [33]. While significantly lower neutralizing antibody responses were observed in Syrian golden hamsters after two doses of 10 μg, the vaccine still elicited high levels of protection from viral replication in the lungs. In nonhuman primates, two doses of 8 μg vaccine induced robust cellular and humoral immune responses and high levels of protection from viral replication [34].

Phase I evaluation of CVnCoV started in June 2020 (NCT04449276). Two immunizations of a range of vaccine doses (2, 4, 6, 8, 12, 16, and 20 μg) were evaluated in 250 healthy individuals [35]. Dose-dependent adverse events were observed. Although the safety profile of the vaccine was generally acceptable, app. 35% of people in the 12 μg group (which was selected later for phase II/III trials, as higher doses were lesser tolerated) experienced severe adverse events after the second shot. Notably, this is a higher percentage than in the case of Moderna's and Pfizer/BioNTech's higher dose, nucleoside-modified vaccines [6, 7]. Dose-dependent antigen-specific antibody responses were measured, but significant variability was observed in the 12 μg group.

A phase II/III clinical trial (NCT04652102) was started with 39 680 participants from ten countries split 1:1 into vaccine and placebo groups [36]. Two immunizations with 12 μg vaccine were administered 28 days apart. Primary vaccine efficacy was calculated to be 48.2%, efficacy against severe COVID-19 was 70.7%, both significantly lower than in the case of Moderna's and Pfizer/BioNTech's vaccines. Adverse events, mostly systemic, were common in the vaccine group (27% versus 3% in the placebo group). Based on these data, CureVac withdrew its application for emergency approval.

The reason for the less-than-favorable efficacy of CVnCoV has been a point of debate [37]. CureVac stipulated that the low efficacy was caused by then-circulating newer variants of concern (VOC), as their phase III trial took place later than Moderna's and Pfizer/BioNTech's but used the same S-2P sequence of the original Wuhan strain, making direct comparison difficult. The trial scientists sequenced the virus in 124 participants who got sick and found 13 different variants. Only 1 of the infected people had a SARS-CoV-2 whose Spike matched the mRNA used in the vaccine. In total, 41% of these cases and 91% of the 44 cases in Europe were caused by the Alpha strain. However, other trials at the time found that the Beta strain has the biggest impact on the vaccines' ability to protect against the disease, and Moderna's and Pfizer/BioNTech's vaccines work well against Alpha. It has been proposed that the low efficacy of CVnCoV may not only be attributed to different viral strains. It has been pointed out that in their phase I study, neutralizing antibody levels induced by the vaccine were lower than in people who became infected naturally, suggesting that the vaccine is simply not immunogenic enough in people. A number of explanations have been offered for lower immunogenicity [37]. First, unmodified mRNA can induce interferon production, which can decrease protein translation and block T helper cell generation, in turn, impeding the production of antibodies by B cells. It may also be responsible for the higher frequency of adverse effects. Second, it has been suggested that the dose used may have been too low. CureVac's dose of 12 μg is significantly lower than Moderna's 100 μg or Pfizer/BioNTech's 30 μg. Third, mRNA vaccines use LNPs to protect and deliver the mRNA payload. It has been shown that ionizable lipids used for LNP formulations act as adjuvants [38, 39]. All three previously mentioned mRNA vaccines use different ionizable lipids, which may be responsible for differences in safety, immunogenicity, and efficacy.

8.4.2 Additional mRNA-based SARS-CoV-2 Vaccines Evaluated in Clinical Trials

The Academy of Military Medical Sciences (Beijing), Walvax Biotechnology, and Suzhou Abogen Biosciences are developing a Spike RBD-encoding modified mRNA–LNP vaccine (ARCoV). In mice, 2 and 10 μg prime-boost immunizations induced strong neutralizing antibody responses, $CD4^+$ and $CD8^+$ T cell responses, and protection from SARS-CoV-2 infection [40]. Two immunizations with 100 and 1000 μg in cynomolgus macaques induced potent neutralizing antibody responses. A phase III clinical trial with app. 28 000 participants is underway (NCT04847102). An updated version of the vaccine was also developed in response to the Omicron strain.

Sanofi/Translate Bio tested an unmodified mRNA–LNP vaccine encoding S-2P/GSAS (MRT5500) [41]. This is a modified version in which the furin cleavage site is mutated (RRAR to GSAS at position 682–685). Preclinical studies in mice and nonhuman primates were promising, and a phase I/II trial was started in March 2021 [42]. Positive interim data at the end of September 2021 confirmed the capabilities of Sanofi's platform, according to the company. Despite this, Sanofi decided to not initiate a phase III trial with this vaccine candidate, focusing on its recombinant protein-based vaccine in collaboration with GlaxoSmithKline instead [43]. Among the reasons, Sanofi cited the wide availability of existing mRNA-based SARS-CoV-2 and the difficulties of starting a placebo-controlled clinical trial in countries with high vaccination rates.

The Imperial College of London evaluated a SARS-CoV-2 vaccine based on self-amplifying mRNA–LNP (LNP-nCoVsaRNA). Two immunizations with a very low dose of 10 ng S-2P encoding saRNA induced robust cellular and humoral immune responses in mice [44]. A phase I/II clinical trial was started, however, the vaccine failed to induce seroconversion in a significant percentage of participants. Thus, development was halted. A phase I trial (NCT04934111) is currently underway with a redesigned saRNA backbone (LNP-nCoVsaRNA-02).

Arcturus and Duke-NUS Medical School is developing a WT S-encoding self-amplifying mRNA vaccine (ARCT-021). Strong cellular and humoral responses were induced in mice using a single immunization of 2 μg [45]. In addition, protective immune responses were induced in B-cell depleted but not in $CD8^+$ T-cell-depleted mice [46]. In monkeys, two immunizations with 5 μg or a single immunization with 20 μg induced high levels of protection from viral replication. ARCT-021 was entered into a phase I/II clinical trial. Immunization regimes included a single dose of 5 or 7.5 μg, two doses of 5 μg, or placebo. The vaccine was well-tolerated but induced low neutralizing antibody responses despite good $CD4^+$ and $CD8^+$ T-cell responses. Further evaluation is ongoing. Arcturus is also investigating modified antigen-encoding sequences for boosting against VOC Alpha, Beta, Gamma, Delta, and Omicron (ARCT-154 and -165) [47].

There are multiple other RNA-based COVID-19 vaccine candidates in various stages of development and clinical trials (Table 8.1) [12, 13].

8.5 Booster Immunizations and Variants of Concern

Initial efficacy data of both the Moderna and the Pfizer/BioNTech vaccine was excellent; however, later follow-up studies found increasing frequencies of breakthrough infections attributed to waning immune responses and emerging VOC due to the rapid evolution of SARS-CoV-2 [48–50]. Major variant Alpha (B.1.1.7) was first documented in September 2020 in the United Kingdom, Beta (B.1.351) in May 2020 in South Africa, Gamma (P.1) in November 2020 in Brazil, Delta (B.1.617.2) in October 2020 in India, and Omicron (B.1.1.529) in November 2021 in multiple countries. Among the earlier variants, Beta was the most resistant to antibodies raised by the vaccines or previous infections, and Delta showed modest resistance to neutralization and an extremely high rate of transmission [26, 51]. To combat the decreased efficacy of their vaccines, both companies initiated studies to evaluate the usefulness of booster vaccinations with either the original vaccines based on the WT Spike sequence or modified sequences reflecting VOCs.

Following promising results in mice [52], Moderna launched a clinical trial to examine booster immunizations with WT and variant Spike sequences. The vaccines were found to be safe and well tolerated. All boosters increased neutralization titers against the WT D614G strain and tested VOCs, including Beta, Gamma, and Delta. Moderna received emergency approval from the FDA for a single booster shot of the original mRNA-1273 on October 20, 2021, and from the EU on October 25, 2021. As the mRNA-1273 booster showed equally good results against VOCs as variant vaccine boosters, and since most variants had been overcome by Delta at that point, deploying a variant vaccine booster was unnecessary. With the emergence of Omicron, this strategy was reevaluated, as Omicron carries 30 mutations in the Spike protein, more than any previous VOCs, resulting in drastically higher transmissibility and high immune evasion capability. Moderna opted to roll out bivalent vaccines containing the original sequence and mRNA encoding Spike of Omicron [53]. Authorization from the FDA for the bivalent booster against Omicron BA.4/BA.5 (mRNA-1273.222) was received on August 31, 2022, based on data from trials of a booster against BA.1 (mRNA-1273.214), accepting it as relevant and supportive of BA.4/BA.5 booster safety and immunogenicity. The EU approved the BA.1 booster on September 6, 2022 and is evaluating the BA.4/BA.5 booster for approval. As the Omicron variant continued to evolve, a monovalent vaccine against the XBB.1.5 strain was developed (Spikevax 2023–2024), and the FDA approved the updated vaccine in September 2023. The approvals and authorizations for the bivalent vaccine were revoked.

BioNTech followed a similar path regarding booster immunizations. The ongoing clinical trial (NCT04368728) was expanded to include a third immunization with BNT162b2 or BNT162b2SA, a variant encoding the Spike of the Beta strain (SA as in South Africa). While results with the latter were not published, in a serum neutralization assay, the booster shot with the original vaccine produced fivefold to sevenfold higher neutralization geometric mean titers against the WT virus one month after the third dose compared to titers one month after the second dose [54]. Interestingly, titers against the Beta variant increased even more, 15–20 times, mitigating the decrease in efficacy of the original prime-boost regimen against Beta. Israel approved a third dose of BNT162b2 for people above the age of 60 who received the second dose at least five months prior on July 30, 2021, and a study was published in September of the same year examining patient records to evaluate the efficacy of the additional dose [55]. At least 12 days after the booster dose, the number of confirmed infections dropped 11-fold compared to the nonboosted group, while the rate of severe illness was lower by a factor of 19.5. A third dose of BNT162b2 as a single booster shot was granted emergency use approval in the United States on September 22, 2021, and in the EU on October 4, 2021. Similarly to Moderna, BioNTech also produced and deployed bivalent boosters against the now dominant Omicron strain. They were approved simultaneously with the Moderna boosters, on August 31, 2022 by the FDA (for BA.4/BA.5 boost), and on September 6, 2022 by the EMA (for BA.1 boost). BioNTech also developed a monovalent vaccine against the XBB.1.5 strain (Comirnaty 2023–2024), and the FDA authorization was amended in September 2023. The authorization for the bivalent vaccine was revoked.

8.6 Future Directions

The mRNA–LNP platform has been at the forefront of biomedical research for some time now, especially in the fields of cancer and infectious disease vaccines, and protein replacement therapy. The COVID-19 pandemic has allowed this vaccine modality to prove itself by vastly reducing the morbidity and mortality of this disease. Advantages of the platform were demonstrated, as the mRNA-based vaccines were the first to be designed, manufactured, and deployed, and also presented the highest efficacy compared to traditional inactivated virus vaccines and even to vaccines based on adenoviruses, which platform is a newcomer to the vaccine field, just like mRNA–LNP. With a convincing entry like this, we can expect mRNA-based vaccines against other pathogens to be developed, most probably in the near future.

One area where the mRNA vaccines fall behind other modalities is storage conditions. Originally, the Moderna vaccine needed to be kept at −20 °C and the Pfizer/BioNTech vaccine at −70 °C up to a couple of days before administration. This caused logistical problems, especially in developing countries, where the cold chain was difficult to maintain according to guidelines (in addition to the issue of limited availability and developed countries reserving almost all of the available production capacity). These guidelines were later adjusted. Currently, the Moderna vaccine can be kept at 2–8 °C for up to a month and the Pfizer/BioNTech vaccine up to 10 weeks, while the shelf life of the inactivated virus SARS-CoV-2 vaccine from Sinopharm (VeroCell) is 24 months at 2–8 °C. Similarly, all or most inactivated virus vaccines are stable for a considerable time at this temperature. Thus, one of the possible directions for improvement is developing new lipids capable of remaining stable for longer periods of time or even withstanding lyophilization [56].

Although the SARS-CoV-2 mRNA vaccines were generally well tolerated, adverse event prevalence and severity were higher than in the case of other vaccines [57, 58]. While fatigue, fever, and headaches were not uncommon, these were not a serious issue. There were more concerning cases, however, for example, a number of people – mostly adolescents – who developed myocarditis and needed to be hospitalized [59–61]. Adverse events might be attributed to the encoded antigen, or the lipid the mRNA is formulated with [62]. The mechanism of action of these mRNA vaccines needs to be investigated in detail to shed light on this problem and to avoid similar occurrences in the future [39]. Developing new lipids may also help in this regard.

As SARS-CoV-2 cannot be expected to be eradicated in the near future, it is possible that the vaccines will become seasonal, to be taken at least by people in risk groups, similarly to influenza shots. Both Moderna and Pfizer/BioNTech are already working on combination vaccines against influenza and SARS-CoV-2 (and Respiratory Syncytial Virus, in the case of Moderna) [63, 64]. Current CDC guidelines (as of October 2023) recommend everyone five years and older to get one dose of the updated 2023–2024 vaccines. Moderately or severely immunocompromised people may get additional doses.

References

1 Worldometer. (2023). COVID Live - Coronavirus Statistics. https://www.worldometers.info/coronavirus/#countries (accessed 9 October 2023).

2 Krammer, F. (2020). SARS-CoV-2 vaccines in development. *Nature* 586 (7830): 516–527.

3 Wouters, O.J., Shadlen, K.C., Salcher-Konrad, M. et al. (2021). Challenges in ensuring global access to COVID-19 vaccines: production, affordability, allocation, and deployment. *Lancet* 397 (10278): 1023–1034.

4 Pardi, N., Hogan, M.J., Porter, F.W., and Weissman, D. (2018). mRNA vaccines — a new era in vaccinology. *Nat. Rev. Drug Discov.* 17 (4): 261–279.

5 Pardi, N., Hogan, M.J., and Weissman, D. (2020). Recent advances in mRNA vaccine technology. *Curr. Opin. Immunol.* 65: 14–20.

6 Polack, F.P., Thomas, S.J., Kitchin, N. et al. (2020). Safety and efficacy of the BNT162b2 mRNA Covid-19 vaccine. *N. Engl. J. Med.* 383 (27): 2603–2615.

7 Baden, L.R., El Sahly, H.M., Essink, B. et al. (2021). Efficacy and safety of the mRNA-1273 SARS-CoV-2 vaccine. *N. Engl. J. Med.* 384 (5): 403–416.

8 Dagan, N., Barda, N., Kepten, E. et al. (2021). BNT162b2 mRNA Covid-19 vaccine in a nationwide mass vaccination setting. *N. Engl. J. Med.* 384 (15): 1412–1423.

9 Thomas, S.J., Moreira, E.D., Kitchin, N. et al. (2021). Safety and efficacy of the BNT162b2 mRNA Covid-19 vaccine through 6 months. *N. Engl. J. Med.* 385 (19): 1761–1773.

10 Dai, L. and Gao, G.F. (2021). Viral targets for vaccines against COVID-19. *Nat. Rev. Immunol.* 21 (2): 73–82.

11 Pallesen, J., Wang, N., Corbett, K.S. et al. (2017). Immunogenicity and structures of a rationally designed prefusion MERS-CoV spike antigen. *Proc. Natl. Acad. Sci. U. S. A.* 114 (35): E7348–E7357.

12 Hogan, M.J. and Pardi, N. (2022). mRNA vaccines in the COVID-19 pandemic and beyond. *Annu. Rev. Med.* 73 (1): 17–39.

13 Szabó, G.T., Mahiny, A.J., and Vlatkovic, I. (2022). COVID-19 mRNA vaccines: platforms and current developments. *Mol. Ther.* 30 (5): 1850–1868.

14 Ghattas, M., Dwivedi, G., Lavertu, M., and Alameh, M.G. (2021). Vaccine technologies and platforms for infectious diseases: current progress, challenges, and opportunities. *Vaccines* 9 (12): 1490.

15 Alameh, M.G., Weissman, D., and Pardi, N. (2020). Messenger RNA-based vaccines against infectious diseases. *Curr. Top. Microbiol. Immunol.* 440: 111–145.

16 Mulligan, M.J., Lyke, K.E., Kitchin, N. et al. (2020). Phase I/II study of COVID-19 RNA vaccine BNT162b1 in adults. *Nature* 586 (7830): 589–593.

17 Sahin, U., Muik, A., Derhovanessian, E. et al. (2020). COVID-19 vaccine BNT162b1 elicits human antibody and TH1 T cell responses. *Nature* 586 (7830): 594–599.

18 Walsh, E.E., Frenck, R.W., Falsey, A.R. et al. (2020). Safety and immunogenicity of two RNA-based Covid-19 vaccine candidates. *N. Engl. J. Med.* 383 (25): 2439–2450.

19 Corbett, K.S., Edwards, D.K., Leist, S.R. et al. (2020). SARS-CoV-2 mRNA vaccine design enabled by prototype pathogen preparedness. *Nature* 586 (7830): 567–571.

20 Corbett, K.S., Flynn, B., Foulds, K.E. et al. (2020). Evaluation of the mRNA-1273 vaccine against SARS-CoV-2 in nonhuman primates. *N. Engl. J. Med.* 383 (16): 1544–1555.

21 Lee, W.S., Wheatley, A.K., Kent, S.J., and DeKosky, B.J. (2020). Antibody-dependent enhancement and SARS-CoV-2 vaccines and therapies. *Nat. Microbiol.* 5 (10): 1185–1191.

22 Jackson, L.A., Anderson, E.J., Rouphael, N.G. et al. (2020). An mRNA vaccine against SARS-CoV-2 — preliminary report. *N. Engl. J. Med.* 383 (20): 1920–1931.

23 Anderson, E.J., Rouphael, N.G., Widge, A.T. et al. (2020). Safety and immunogenicity of SARS-CoV-2 mRNA-1273 vaccine in older adults. *N. Engl. J. Med.* 383 (25): 2427–2438.

24 Tarke, A., Sidney, J., Methot, N. et al. (2021). Impact of SARS-CoV-2 variants on the total CD4+ and CD8+ T cell reactivity in infected or vaccinated individuals. *Cell Rep. Med.* 2 (7): 100355.

25 Doria-Rose, N., Suthar, M.S., Makowski, M. et al. (2021). Antibody persistence through 6 months after the second dose of mRNA-1273 vaccine for Covid-19. *N. Engl. J. Med.* 384 (23): 2259–2261.

26 Pegu, A., O'Connell, S.E., Schmidt, S.D. et al. (2021). Durability of mRNA-1273 vaccine–induced antibodies against SARS-CoV-2 variants. *Science* 373 (6561): 1372–1377.

27 Our World in Data. (2022). COVID-19 vaccine doses administered by manufacturer. https://ourworldindata.org/grapher/covid-vaccine-doses-by-manufacturer (accessed 10 November 2022).

28 Liu, Y., Liu, J., Xia, H. et al. (2021). Neutralizing activity of BNT162b2-elicited serum. *N. Engl. J. Med.* 384 (15): 1466–1468.

29 Muik, A., Wallisch, A.K., Sänger, B. et al. (2021). Neutralization of SARS-CoV-2 lineage B.1.1.7 pseudovirus by BNT162b2 vaccine–elicited human sera. *Science* 371 (6534): 1152–1153.

30 Sahin, U., Muik, A., Vogler, I. et al. (2021). BNT162b2 vaccine induces neutralizing antibodies and poly-specific T cells in humans. *Nature* 595 (7868): 572–577.

31 Vogel, A.B., Kanevsky, I., Che, Y. et al. (2021). BNT162b vaccines protect rhesus macaques from SARS-CoV-2. *Nature* 592 (7853): 283–289.

32 Thess, A., Grund, S., Mui, B.L. et al. (2015). Sequence-engineered mRNA without chemical nucleoside modifications enables an effective protein therapy in large animals. *Mol. Ther.* 23 (9): 1456–1464.

33 Rauch, S., Roth, N., Schwendt, K. et al. (2021). mRNA-based SARS-CoV-2 vaccine candidate CVnCoV induces high levels of virus-neutralising antibodies and mediates protection in rodents. *NPJ Vaccines* 6 (1): 1–9.

34 Rauch, S., Gooch, K., Hall, Y. et al. (2020). mRNA vaccine CVnCoV protects non-human primates from SARS-CoV-2 challenge infection. bioRxiv. p. 2020.12.23.424138. https://www.biorxiv.org/content/10.1101/2020.12.23.424138v1 (accessed 11 November 2022).

35 Kremsner, P.G., Mann, P., Kroidl, A. et al. (2021). Safety and immunogenicity of an mRNA-lipid nanoparticle vaccine candidate against SARS-CoV-2. *Wien. Klin. Wochenschr.* 133 (17): 931–941.

36 Kremsner, P.G., Ahuad Guerrero, R.A., Arana-Arri, E. et al. (2022). Efficacy and safety of the CVnCoV SARS-CoV-2 mRNA vaccine candidate in ten countries in Europe and Latin America (HERALD): a randomised, observer-blinded, placebo-controlled, phase 2b/3 trial. *Lancet Infect. Dis.* 22 (3): 329–340.

37 Cohen, J. (2021). What went wrong with CureVac's highly anticipated new mRNA vaccine for COVID-19? https://www.science.org/content/article/what-went-wrong-curevac-s-highly-anticipated-new-mrna-vaccine-covid-19 (accessed 18 November 2022).

38 Alameh, M.G., Tombácz, I., Bettini, E. et al. (2021). Lipid nanoparticles enhance the efficacy of mRNA and protein subunit vaccines by inducing robust T follicular helper cell and humoral responses. *Immunity* 54 (12): 2877–2892.e7.

39 Verbeke, R., Hogan, M.J., Loré, K., and Pardi, N. (2022). Innate immune mechanisms of mRNA vaccines. *Immunity* 55 (11): 1993–2005.

40 Zhang, N.N., Li, X.F., Deng, Y.Q. et al. (2020). A thermostable mRNA vaccine against COVID-19. *Cell* 182 (5): 1271–1283.e16.

41 Kalnin, K.V., Plitnik, T., Kishko, M. et al. (2021). Immunogenicity and efficacy of mRNA COVID-19 vaccine MRT5500 in preclinical animal models. *NPJ Vaccines* 6 (1): 1–12.

42 Sanofi. (2021). Sanofi and Translate Bio initiate Phase 1/2 clinical trial of mRNA COVID-19 vaccine candidate. https://www.sanofi.com/en/media-room/press-releases/2021/2021-03-12-06-00-00-2191846 (accessed 11 November 2022).

43 Sanofi. (2021). Sanofi to focus its COVID-19 development efforts on the recombinant vaccine candidate. https://www.sanofi.com/en/media-room/press-releases/2021/2021-09-28-16-44-47-2304800 (accessed 11 November 2022).

44 McKay, P.F., Hu, K., Blakney, A.K. et al. (2020). Self-amplifying RNA SARS-CoV-2 lipid nanoparticle vaccine candidate induces high neutralizing antibody titers in mice. *Nat. Commun.* 11 (1): 3523.

45 de Alwis, R., Gan, E.S., Chen, S. et al. (2021). A single dose of self-transcribing and replicating RNA-based SARS-CoV-2 vaccine produces protective adaptive immunity in mice. *Mol. Ther.* 29 (6): 1970–1983.

46 Arcturus Therapeutics, Inc. (2020). Arcturus therapeutics received approval from Singapore health sciences authority to proceed with phase 2 study of ARCT-021 (LUNAR-COV19) vaccine candidate and provides new and updated clinical and preclinical data. https://ir.arcturusrx.com/news-releases/news-release-details/arcturus-therapeutics-received-approval-singapore-health (accessed 11 November 2022).

47 Arcturus Therapeutics, Inc. (2022). Arcturus therapeutics reports new data demonstrating neutralizing antibody immune response to the SARS-CoV-2 omicron variant from ARCT-154 and ARCT-165 booster clinical trial. https://ir.arcturusrx.com/news-releases/news-release-details/arcturus-therapeutics-reports-new-data-demonstrating (accessed 22 November 2022).

48 Puranik, A., Lenehan, P.J., Silvert, E. et al. (2021). Comparison of two highly-effective mRNA vaccines for COVID-19 during periods of Alpha and Delta variant prevalence. medRxiv. p. 2021.08.06.21261707. https://www.medrxiv.org/content/10.1101/2021.08.06.21261707v3 (accessed 14 November 2022).

49 Goldberg Y, Mandel M, Bar-On YM, et al. (2021). Waning immunity of the BNT162b2 vaccine: a nationwide study from Israel. medRxiv.

p. 2021.08.24.21262423. https://www.medrxiv.org/content/10.1101/2021.08.24.21262423v1 (accessed 14 November 2021).

50 Pouwels, K.B., Pritchard, E., Matthews, P.C. et al. (2021). Effect of Delta variant on viral burden and vaccine effectiveness against new SARS-CoV-2 infections in the UK. *Nat. Med.* 27 (12): 2127–2135.

51 Planas, D., Veyer, D., Baidaliuk, A. et al. (2021). Reduced sensitivity of SARS-CoV-2 variant Delta to antibody neutralization. *Nature* 596 (7871): 276–280.

52 Wu, K., Choi, A., Koch, M. et al. (2021). Variant SARS-CoV-2 mRNA vaccines confer broad neutralization as primary or booster series in mice. *Vaccine* 39 (51): 7394–7400.

53 Chalkias, S., Harper, C., Vrbicky, K. et al. (2022). A bivalent omicron-containing booster vaccine against Covid-19. *N. Engl. J. Med.* 387 (14): 1279–1291.

54 Falsey, A.R., Frenck, R.W., Walsh, E.E. et al. (2021). SARS-CoV-2 neutralization with BNT162b2 vaccine dose 3. *N. Engl. J. Med.* 385 (17): 1627–1629.

55 Bar-On, Y.M., Goldberg, Y., Mandel, M. et al. (2021). Protection of BNT162b2 vaccine booster against Covid-19 in Israel. *N. Engl. J. Med.* 385 (15): 1393–1400.

56 Muramatsu, H., Lam, K., Bajusz, C. et al. (2022). Lyophilization provides long-term stability for a lipid nanoparticle-formulated, nucleoside-modified mRNA vaccine. *Mol. Ther. J. Am. Soc. Gene Ther.* 30 (5): 1941–1951.

57 Kouhpayeh, H. and Ansari, H. (2022). Adverse events following COVID-19 vaccination: a systematic review and meta-analysis. *Int. Immunopharmacol.* 109: 108906.

58 Guo, W., Deguise, J., Tian, Y. et al. (2022). Profiling COVID-19 vaccine adverse events by statistical and ontological analysis of VAERS case reports. *Front. Pharmacol.* 13. https://www.frontiersin.org/articles/10.3389/fphar.2022.870599 (accessed 14 November 2022).

59 Krug, A., Stevenson, J., and Høeg, T.B. (2022). BNT162b2 vaccine-associated myo/pericarditis in adolescents: a stratified risk-benefit analysis. *Eur. J. Clin. Investig.* 52 (5): e13759.

60 Li, X., Lai, F.T.T., Chua, G.T. et al. (2022). Myocarditis following COVID-19 BNT162b2 vaccination among adolescents in Hong Kong. *JAMA Pediatr.* 176 (6): 612–614.

61 Montgomery, J., Ryan, M., Engler, R. et al. (2021). Myocarditis following immunization with mRNA COVID-19 vaccines in members of the US military. *JAMA Cardiol.* 6 (10): 1202–1206.

62 Trougakos, I.P., Terpos, E., Alexopoulos, H. et al. (2022). Adverse effects of COVID-19 mRNA vaccines: the spike hypothesis. *Trends Mol. Med.* 28 (7): 542–554.

63 Moderna. (2022). Moderna announces first participants dosed in phase 3 study of seasonal influenza vaccine candidate (mRNA-1010). https://investors.modernatx.com/news/news-details/2022/Moderna-Announces-First-Participants-Dosed-in-Phase-3-Study-of-Seasonal-Influenza-Vaccine-Candidate-mRNA-1010/default.aspx (accessed 14 November 2022).

64 Pfizer. (2022). Pfizer and BioNTech initiate phase 1 study of single dose mRNA-based combination vaccine candidate for influenza and COVID-19. https://www.pfizer.com/news/announcements/pfizer-and-biontech-initiate-phase-1-study-single-dose-mrna-based-combination (accessed 14 November 2022).

9

mRNA Vaccines for HIV-1

Paolo Lusso

National Institute of Allergy and Infectious Diseases, Laboratory of Immunoregulation, Building 10, Room 6A11, 10 Center drive, Bethesda, MD 20892, USA

9.1 Introduction

9.1.1 A Long and Winding Road: 40 Years and Counting

More than four decades have passed since June 5, 1981, the day when the Centers for Disease Control (CDC)'s Morbidity and Mortality Weekly Report (MMWR) bulletin reported "five cases of *Pneumocystis carinii* pneumonia (PCP) among previously healthy young men in Los Angeles" [1], which heralded the recognition of a new disease, later defined as the acquired immunodeficiency syndrome (AIDS). Yet, an effective vaccine against its causative agent, human immunodeficiency type 1 (HIV-1), is not in sight yet on the horizon. Immediately after its discovery, HIV-1 started to appear as a very challenging foe. First, being a retrovirus, it has the ability to stably integrate its own genome into the host chromosomal DNA and become latent, thereby establishing a lifelong persistent infection that remains essentially ineradicable, at least for today's technology. Second, it became rapidly evident that HIV-1 has a preferential tropism for immune cells, especially $CD4^+$ T lymphocytes that represent the concertmasters of adaptive immune responses, thereby directly striking the immune system at the core of its command center. Third, the outer envelope (Env) of HIV-1, which is the sole target of protective neutralizing antibodies, shows a remarkable degree of antigenic variability, thereby continuously escaping immune control. If these obstacles were not sufficient, the deepening knowledge of the biochemical and structural features of the HIV-1 Env over the past three decades has progressively unraveled an extraordinary armamentarium of immune-evasion tactics that has no precedents in virology [2]. Most notable are the protected configuration of conserved neutralization epitopes, due to the extensive glycan shield that covers almost the entire exposed surface of Env, and the intrinsic flexibility of the trimeric Env structure, which leads to a peculiar conformational masking of critical sites. For all these reasons, science has faced an unprecedented challenge to develop an effective vaccine against HIV-1. And the quest is still on.

Trends in mRNA Vaccine Research, First Edition. Edited by Gabor Tamas Szabo and Norbert Pardi.

9.1.2 A Very High Bar: Failure of Traditional Approaches

If we do not have an HIV-1 vaccine yet, after more than four decades, it has not been for the lack of trying. A variety of traditional approaches have been tested in preclinical models and, in selected cases, in clinical trials, but they have almost invariably failed. The only vaccine that has shown limited efficacy in a human trial – a prime-boost protocol conducted in a large volunteer cohort in Thailand (RV144) – was able to reduce the risk of infection by a mere ~30% and only transiently [3]. Furthermore, subsequent attempts to replicate this result with analogous protocols in South Africa have failed [4]. Many comprehensive reviews on the wide array of efforts toward the development of an HIV-1 vaccine in the pre-mRNA (messenger RNA) era have been published [5–7].

The main reason why conventional vaccine approaches have been ineffective against HIV-1 is that the bar to achieve protection is extremely high. Protection, in the case of HIV-1, equals "sterilizing" immunity, i.e. prevention of even a single successful infection event within the organism. The reason for this high bar is that for HIV-1, unlike most other infectious agents, prevention of the acute illness that accompanies primary infection is of no relevance to protection. The real disease caused by HIV-1 is a progressive immunodeficiency that develops over the course of several years of chronic infection. Once the virus gets its foot in the door and integrates its genome into the host DNA, the clock starts. And the disease will almost invariably progress unless effective antiretroviral treatment is started and continued indefinitely with strict adherence. Thus, the only way to protect against HIV-1 disease would be to lock the virus completely out of the body from square one: that is "sterilizing" immunity.

9.1.3 A New Era: An HIV-1 Vaccine Is Feasible

A series of breakthrough discoveries in protein structure and antibody cloning technologies over the past 15 years has opened a new era, providing the long-awaited proof-of-principle that a protective HIV-1 vaccine is effectively feasible. Pioneering observations on the sterilizing effects of neutralizing human monoclonal antibodies were reported as early as 1999, with passive immunoprophylaxis studies conducted in nonhuman primates [8–10]. However, the antibodies utilized initially had limited potency and breadth. Starting from the late 2000s, however, several groups started to apply improved technologies for the efficient cloning and expansion of individual B cells as well as for the direct cloning of antibody genes from sorted B cells, which led to the isolation of a growing panel of broadly neutralizing antibodies (bNAbs) from chronically HIV-1-infected patients [5–7, 11]. Potent bNAbs were then utilized in passive infusion studies to confer protection from hybrid simian–human immunodeficiency virus (SHIV) in macaque models [12–14]. The simultaneous recognition that the human immune system has the ability, albeit in a limited proportion of individuals, to produce bNAbs against vulnerable sites in the HIV-1 Env and that such bNAbs mediate complete protection from relevant virus challenge in suitable preclinical models has provided conclusive evidence that an HIV-1 vaccine is feasible.

All of this happened before the arrival of mRNA on the stage of vaccine development. This chapter is focused on the prolific effects that have stemmed from the encounter between the HIV-1 vaccine field and mRNA technology. Although the application of mRNA to HIV-1 vaccines is still at an early stage of development, it has already provided some important proof-of-principle of its exceptional versatility and potential efficacy.

9.2 Strategies for HIV-1 Vaccine Design

There is wide consensus in the field that in order to confer protection from the majority of circulating HIV-1 strains, which predominantly fall in the tier-2 category of neutralization sensitivity, a vaccine must be able to induce bNAbs, although other protective mechanisms are likely to be involved, if not necessary. The isolation, over the past decade, of a growing collection of bNAbs from HIV-infected individuals and the extraordinary progress made in the structural definition of the HIV-1 Env trimer have been major propulsors of HIV-1 vaccine research, which has seen a dramatic acceleration in recent years. The main strategies for the development of bNAb-inducing HIV-1 vaccines are described in several recent reviews [6, 7, 11, 15]. This chapter provides only the general concepts of HIV-1 vaccine design being focalized on the most recent approaches that use mRNA as a platform for vaccine delivery (Section 9.4).

9.2.1 Main Strategies

Four main strategies, nonmutually exclusive, are currently being pursued in the development of HIV-1 vaccines:

9.2.1.1 Lineage-Based Vaccines

A detailed reconstruction of the lineage evolution of several bNAbs has been obtained by high-throughput sequencing of immunoglobulin genes within the individuals who originated these antibodies [16–18]. The genealogic tree of the bNAbs can then serve as a roadmap for vaccine design. First, by computational methods, the putative germline antibody precursor, also termed unmutated common ancestor (UCA), as well as ancestral intermediate forms, are inferred. The next step is to identify HIV-1 Envs, derived either from the same donor over the course of bNAb evolution or from unrelated individuals, which bind with sufficient affinity to the UCA and the intermediate forms. Often, specific modifications of the Envs are required to increase their binding affinity for the UCAs, such as targeted deglycosylations or variable-loop shortening. This is the case for the 426c Env, a clade-C Env consensus sequence derived from a single donor, which acquires increasing affinity for the VRC01-class UCA antibodies (targeting the CD4-binding site) upon deletion of one (N276) or, even better, three (N276, N460, and N463) *N*-glycans that surround the CD4-binding site [19]. After the most effective Envs are defined, a sequential immunization protocol is designed, starting from priming with a UCA-engaging Env, followed by booster immunizations with Envs that progressively recapitulate the entire history of the bNAb lineage evolution. By shepherding specific B cells through all the sequential steps of such evolution, the aim of this approach is to confer selective advantage at each passage to B cells expressing antibodies that carry the improbable mutations required for progressive affinity maturation toward the final, high-affinity, mature bNAb.

9.2.1.2 Mutation-Guided Vaccines

A variation of the B-cell shepherding approach, mutation-guided strategies aim to identify critical improbable mutations that occur during bNAb evolution and use them to inform the structure-based rational design of Env immunogens, even totally unrelated to the Envs detected in the patients who originated the bNAb, that could specifically select for such mutations [20, 21]. The resulting mutation-guided Env forms will then be sequentially utilized for immunization as done in the lineage-based approaches.

9.2.1.3 Structure-Based Vaccines

Structure-based immunogen design is based on the precise definition of the atomic structure of the antigenic supersites of vulnerability targeted by bNAbs [7, 15, 22]. The structural definition of antigenic supersites is typically obtained by crystallization or cryo-electron microscopy (cryoEM) of bNAbs in complex with soluble HIV-1 Env trimers such as SOSIP trimers. The closer the trimer conformation is to that adopted by native, unbound Env trimers on the virion surface, the more relevant the structure will be for vaccine purposes. The trimer itself that is employed for structural analysis may represent a suitable immunogen, provided that it binds with sufficient affinity to the desired bNAbs. However, further structural analysis coupled with *in silico* modeling is commonly used to refine the template for final immunogen design. Aims of this refinement process include structural stabilization of the antigenic supersites (e.g. by the introduction of neo-disulfide bonds or cavity-filling mutations), optimization of the bNAb interface (e.g. by structure-guided mutagenesis), enhancement of epitope accessibility (e.g. by targeted deglycosylation or other mutagenesis), and masking or elimination of off-target epitopes or regions that may distract the immune system focusing on the desired target regions (e.g. by removal of the variable loops or glycan shielding of the trimer base).

9.2.1.4 Epitope-Based Vaccines

Targeting of specific epitopes within antigenic supersites of HIV-1 vulnerability can also be achieved by alternative approaches, including the more traditional peptide-mediated immunization. In this case, it is the composition of the individual epitope, rather than the conformation of the entire supersite, that guides immunogen design [15, 23]. The epitope can be presented in the context of a compatible scaffold, both to increase its size and to facilitate the native folding of the antigenic site, or conjugated to an appropriate carrier. This approach allows for the simultaneous use of epitope sequences from multiple HIV-1 strains that reflect the antigenic diversity among circulating viral populations. Typically, the initial epitope-specific priming is followed by boosting with increasingly complex immunogens such as soluble trimers.

9.2.1.5 Combination Strategies

Although an HIV-1 vaccine approach may be primarily inspired by one of the strategies outlined above, a combination of different strategies is often utilized to design complex vaccine protocols in an attempt to overcome the limitations of each individual approach. Thus, germline-targeting Env immunogens are generally utilized during the priming phase regardless of the subsequent choice of boosting regimens. Likewise, structure-guided Env modifications are commonly included in most approaches, as they can help to overcome the immune-evasion tactics of the HIV-1 Env trimer. It is increasingly clear that a single immunogen or a simple immunization protocol is unlikely to overcome the formidable challenge of recruiting rare bNAb precursors and shepherd them through a very demanding affinity-maturation path. But within the last decade the HIV-1 vaccine field has seen a remarkable progress, which has raised realistic hopes for the imminent development of at least a partially effective vaccine. And mRNA is likely to play an important part in this endeavor.

9.3 mRNA-Based HIV-1 Vaccines

9.3.1 Why mRNA?

Until a few years ago, the efficient delivery of mRNA to a living organism to induce the *in vivo* expression of therapeutic proteins or vaccines would have been considered a "mission impossible." However, a series of technological breakthroughs over the last two decades have made mRNA one of the most promising current technologies for nucleic acid-based therapies and vaccines. One of the most salient properties of mRNA is its utilization of the host cellular machinery for protein manufacturing. Hence, the body becomes the factory of the vaccine or therapeutic protein. This feature carries some fundamental benefits for proteins that require particular posttranslational modifications, such as native N-linked glycosylation, because industrial production in continuous cell lines can never yield proteins with the desired characteristics. In addition, endogenous protein expression directed by mRNA within the host cells allows for the production of membrane-embedded glycoproteins, which adopt a native antigenic configuration analogous to that of virion-associated glycoproteins. Although endogenous *in vivo* production can also be achieved using other delivery platforms, such as DNA or viral vectors, mRNA offers a series of important advantages, as summarized in Table 9.1 [and reviewed in [24]]. First and foremost, safety: mRNA is a simple and homogeneous substance, nearly identical to a physiological molecule, devoid of infectivity or ability to integrate into the host chromosomes and cause DNA mutagenesis, and has a finite *in vivo* persistence. Although mRNA possesses inherent immune-stimulating activities, this property can be significantly reduced

Table 9.1 Major advantages related to the use of mRNA for HIV-1 vaccine delivery.

	Advantage	Features	Keys to success
1	Safety	• Simple and homogeneous substance • Nearly identical to a physiological molecule • Lack of infectivity • Lack of ability to integrate into host chromosomes and cause DNA mutagenesis • Finite *in vivo* persistence	Nucleotide modification
2	Versatility	• Universally applicable to any pathological process or agent	Uses code of life
3	Rapidity of development	• Requires only the availability of specific genetic sequences • Single production line to manufacture any new mRNA product	Single biological product (only sequence varies)
4	Efficiency	• Both delivery and expression markedly more efficient than with DNA-based therapies or vaccines	LNP encapsulation; codon optimization
5	Lack of immunogenicity	• No anti-vector immunity elicited even after multiple administrations	Physiological molecule; lipid encapsulation
6	Low cost	• Scalable manufacturing at contained costs after the initial investment in the production facility	High efficiency of *in vitro* translation

by nucleotide modification. Second, versatility: as every physiological process requires the expression of genetic information, mRNA can be applied to virtually any pathological process or agent as long as the relevant genetic sequences are known. Third, rapidness of development: the design and production of mRNA require only the input of specific genetic sequences, with a single production line being suitable for manufacturing any number of mRNA products. This is the reason why mRNA therapies and vaccines can be deployed almost in "real time." Fourth, efficiency: both the delivery and the expression of mRNA are orders of magnitude more efficient than with DNA-based therapies or vaccines. This is because mRNA needs to cross only a single bio-membrane, the cytoplasmic membrane, and is directly translated to protein by ribosomes without the need for the synthesis of intermediate messenger molecules. Moreover, codon optimization strategies and other modifications have substantially improved the translation efficiency of exogenous mRNA in mammalian cells. Fifth, lack of immunogenicity: since mRNA is typically encapsulated into a lipidic envelope, no anti-vector immunity develops even after multiple administrations. Sixth, low cost: apart from the initial investment to establish a dedicated production facility, scalable manufacturing of mRNA can subsequently be achieved with relatively contained costs due to the efficiency of high-throughput *in vitro* transcription.

Due to the favorable features listed above, in 2020 mRNA technology has swiftly emerged as the cornerstone technology in the fight against COVID-19, the most devastating pandemic to have plagued the world in over a century. If one had asked people in the street "what is mRNA?" during the early days of the pandemic, in the spring of 2020, hardly anybody would have even heard of it. Before 2015, even scientists would have generally been skeptical that RNA transcripts could safely and efficiently be transduced into living cells *in vivo* and direct the endogenous production of therapeutic proteins or vaccines. But it happened. Thanks to the vision and extraordinary work of a group of pioneers who pursued what appeared to be an impossible dream. In fact, when the first cases of an unknown severe pulmonary infection first emerged in the city of Wuhan, China, at the end of 2019 [25], the mRNA technology was already well established and was being developed as a vaccine delivery system against one of the severe acute respiratory syndrome coronavirus-2 (SARS-CoV-2)'s first-grade cousins, Middle East respiratory syndrome coronavirus (MERS-CoV) [26]. Owing to the exceptional versatility of the mRNA platform, the transfer of the new pathogen sequences, the vaccine design and production, and the clinical experimentation all happened within the span of a few months [27]. The rest is in the history books. The field of mRNA vaccines in the pre-COVID-19 era has been comprehensively reviewed by Pardi et al. [24].

9.3.2 Key Technological Breakthroughs

At its inception, the mRNA field faced extraordinary challenges to evolve toward clinical applicability, mainly due to difficulties related to RNA stabilization, delivery and reactogenicity. After the original discovery of mRNA in 1961 [28], it took more than 25 years to establish the concept that *in vitro*-transcribed mRNA could be delivered to living cells and effectively inform protein expression both *in vitro* [29] and *in vivo* [30]. Two years later, the first evidence of a therapeutic effect of exogenously injected mRNA was reported [31]. However, a series of major hurdles had to be overcome. When Drew Weissman and Katalin Karikò, in the early 2000s' set out to develop an mRNA vaccine against HIV-1, they swiftly realized that the potent inflammatory response triggered by the inoculation of exogenous mRNA would have created a major obstacle. Their elegant solution, reported in 2005, was the replacement of the innate-stimulating uridine with pseudouridine, a breakthrough that opened the doors of the clinical realm [32]. The importance of mRNA purity was also recognized, especially the removal of contaminating double-stranded mRNA, which is a potent inducer of innate immune responses [33]. Subsequent work pioneered the application to mRNA of lipid-encapsulation techniques originally developed for silencing-RNA (siRNA) delivery [34]. Thus, mRNA would be efficiently transferred through the cellular membrane for endogenous translation into proteins and, at the same time, protected from degradation by ubiquitous RNases.

9.3.3 Main Platforms for mRNA-Based HIV-1 Vaccines

Over the past 15 years, two main types of mRNA vaccine platforms for HIV-1 have been designed and tested in preclinical models: mRNA-transduced dendritic cells (DCs) and direct *in vivo* mRNA delivery. A list of mRNA-based HIV-1 vaccines evaluated or under evaluation in nonhuman primate models or in clinical trials is presented in Table 9.2.

Table 9.2 mRNA vaccines evaluated against HIV-1 or SHIV in clinical trials and nonhuman primate models.

mRNA and delivery system	Clinical trial or NHP model	Main outcomes	References
Autologous DCs transfected with HIV-1 Gag, Vpr, Rev, Nef + CD40L	Clinical trial in ART-suppressed infected subjects (AGS-004)	HIV-specific proliferative cellular responses	Routy et al. [35]
Autologous DCs transfected with HIV-1 Gag	Clinical trial in ART-suppressed infected subjects	HIV-1-specific interferon (IFN)-γ responses; increase in *ex vivo* CD8-mediated HIV-suppressive activity	Van Gulck et al. [36]
Autologous DCs transfected with HIV-1 Gag and Nef	Clinical trial in ART-uninfected volunteers (PARC002)	No significant $CD4^+$ or $CD8^+$ T-cell responses	Gandhi et al. [37]
Autologous DCs transfected with HIV-1 Gag	Cynomolgus macaques	Gag-specific $CD4^+$ and $CD8^+$ T cells that produced IFN-γ, TNF-α, MIP-1β and/or IL-2	Romain et al. [38]
Naked mRNA expressing HIVACAT T-cell immunogen + TLR4, CD40 ligand and CD70	Clinical trials in ART-suppressed infected subjects (iHIVARNA)	No significant immunogenicity	Leal et al. [39]; de Jong et al. [40]
LNP-formulated mRNA expressing a clade-C HIV-1 Env	Rhesus macaques	HIV-1 specific, polyfunctional $CD4^+$ T cell responses, neutralizing antibody responses	Pardi et al. [41, 42]
Cationic nanoemulsion-formulated SAM (VEEV) expressing a clade-C HIV-1 Env gp140	Rhesus macaques	Potent Th1 cellular immune responses neutralizing antibodies	Bogers et al. [43]
PLX nanoparticle-formulated SAM (VEEV) expressing a stabilized HIV-1 Env trimer (ConSOSL.UFO)	Rhesus macaques	High Env-specific IgG responses	Aldon et al. [44]
LNP-coformulated multiclade *env* + *gag* mRNA (VLP-forming)	Rhesus macaques	Robust anti-Env Th1 and TFH responses, low-titer broadly neutralizing antibodies, protection from heterologous tier-2 challenge	Zhang et al. [45]
LNP-formulated mRNA expressing a gp120-derived core (eOD-GT8 60mer)	Clinical trial (IAVI G003)	Activation and expansion of VRC01-like UCA-expressing B cells (preliminary data)	Schief et al. study in progress
LNP-formulated mRNA expressing membrane-bound HIV-1 Env trimers	Clinical trial (HVTN 302)	Robust anti-Env antibody responses (preliminary data)	Schief et al. study in progress

9.3.3.1 mRNA-Transduced Dendritic Cells

Initial attempts to design an HIV-1 mRNA vaccine were inspired by cancer immunotherapy, where the *in vivo* delivery of *ex vivo*-transduced autologous DCs was being explored to present tumor-specific antigens to the immune system [46]. This technology was first validated *in vitro* using HIV-1 antigens [47] and then evaluated in both preclinical and clinical studies. One of the earliest clinical protocols, AGS-004, enrolled 10 infected adults under antiretroviral therapy (ART) who were inoculated monthly with autologous monocyte-derived DCs electroporated with mRNA encoding CD40 ligand, an immunostimulatory molecule, and four HIV-1 proteins: Gag, Vpr, Rev, and Nef. The recipients developed HIV antigen-specific proliferative cellular responses, especially by $CD8^+$ T cells, without major adverse events [35]. Similar protocols were tested in subsequent studies yielding mixed results. Van Gulck et al. showed a significant vaccine-induced increase in the magnitude and breadth of HIV-1-specific interferon (IFN)-γ responses, particularly to Gag, in HIV-1-infected patients under ART treatment, as well as an increase in CD8-mediated HIV-suppressive activity tested *ex vivo* [36]. Different results were instead obtained by Gandhi et al. in uninfected healthy volunteers, in whom inoculation of autologous DCs expressing HIV-1 Gag and Nef failed to induce significant $CD4^+$ or $CD8^+$ T-cell responses [37]. Whether this lack of response was a consequence of the immunologically naïve status of the healthy volunteers enrolled in this study remains to be ascertained. In contrast, immunization of uninfected cynomolgus macaques with autologous CD34-derived DCs transduced with HIV-1 Gag was reported to induce virus-specific cell-mediated immune responses: the animals developed Gag-specific $CD4^+$ and $CD8^+$ T cells that produced IFN-γ, tumor necrosis factor (TNF)-α, macrophage inflammatory protein (MIP)-1β, and/or interleukin (IL)-2. The number of polyfunctional $CD8^+$ T cells increased with repeated booster injections [38].

In summary, despite their potential effectiveness, DC-mediated vaccine approaches have major limitations for widespread use related to their high cost, the need for an *ad personam* manufacturing process, and the difficulties in vaccine standardization. While their use in oncology may be justified by the relative rarity and life-threatening nature of certain forms of cancers, especially those for which effective treatments are lacking, large-scale use of DC-mediated approaches for vaccination campaigns in the general population would be inconceivable.

9.3.3.2 Direct *In Vivo* mRNA Delivery

The direct *in vivo* delivery of mRNA offers several advantages over DC-mediated vaccine approaches because it is widely applicable without the need for personalized production, it is scalable, it can be accurately standardized, and it has more contained costs. Two main platforms for the parenteral delivery of mRNA vaccines against HIV-1 have been explored: non-replicating mRNA and self-amplifying mRNA (SAM). The first platform simply delivers a defined amount of *in vitro*-transcribed mRNA that is translated to protein *in vivo* over a limited time period and is eventually degraded by cellular processes. The second utilizes the RNA replication mechanism of a virus, typically an alphavirus such as Venezuelan equine encephalitis virus (VEEV), to multiply *in vivo* the delivered mRNA. The most important advantage of SAM is the net quantitative increase in the amount of mRNA available *in vivo*, which allows for the administration of smaller vaccine doses, results in augmented protein production, and mimics the increasing antigenic load that occurs during natural infection; moreover, protein expression continues over a prolonged period of time compared to non-replicating mRNA. The main downsides of SAM are related to the use of components from a heterologous virus, which may create additional safety concerns, induce anti-vector immunity, and impose limitations on the size of deliverable mRNA.

Major efforts have been made over the past decade to develop increasingly efficient methods for the direct *in vivo* delivery of mRNA. Even injection of naked mRNA was initially considered after it was shown to result in detectable protein expression *in vivo* [30]; however, the inherent instability of unprotected RNA made its clinical development very challenging. A naked mRNA vaccine for the therapeutic immunization of HIV-infected individuals, named iHIVARNA, was nevertheless developed and evaluated in Phase-I and Phase-II clinical trials [39, 40]. The vaccine, which encompassed mRNAs expressing an HIV immunogen (HIVACAT T-cell immunogen or HTI, a polypeptide generated by joining 16 fragments of 10–70 amino acids each, encoding immunodominant epitopes from HIV-1 Gag, Pol, Vif, and Nef identified in long-term non-progressors or virus controllers) along with three mRNAs expressing immunostimulatory molecules (TLR4, CD40 ligand, and CD70; also known as TriMix), was administered to ART-suppressed HIV-infected individuals by intranodal injection. As largely predictable, the results of the trials failed to show sufficient immunogenicity to justify the continuation of these studies.

A variety of methods have been devised to protect and stabilize mRNA for its efficient *in vivo* delivery. One of the earliest to be explored was based on the ability of bacteriophage MS2 to package mRNA inside virus-like particles (VLPs). When tested in mice, MS2-packaged HIV-1 *gag* mRNA was found to elicit Gag-specific antibody responses [48]. However, most of the mRNA delivery systems were based on encapsulation by cationic lipids. Using *gag* mRNA complexed with a cationic lipid (1,2-dioleoyl-3trimethylammonium-propane/1,2-dioleoyl-*sn*-glycero-3-phosphoethanolamine, or DOTAP/DOPE), Pollard et al. reported the elicitation of robust Gag-specific functional T-cell responses and humoral responses in mice [49]. Specific immune responses were similarly induced using *gag* mRNA delivered by self-assembling cationic nanomicelles based on polyethyleneiminestearic acid (PSA) copolymer [50]. An original approach was the use of *env (gp120)* mRNA complexed with cationic cyclodextrin-polyethylenimine 2k (CP 2k), which has the unique property of reversibly opening the tight junctions between mucosal cells, thereby facilitating mRNA transfer through the mucosal epithelial barrier and enhancing its paracellular delivery. Using this method, Li et al. were able to induce both systemic and mucosal anti-HIV immune responses by intranasal delivery in mice, with a balanced production of Th1, Th2, and Th17 cytokines [51]. A self-adjuvanted system based on mRNA complexing with polycationic peptide protamine has also been developed. Using this system, Gebre et al. evaluated in mice the early immunologic responses to a clade-C HIV-1 Env gp140 mRNA vaccine in comparison to DNA, protein, and rhesus adenovirus 52 (RhAd52) vaccines expressing the same Env. Envelope-specific antibodies were detected as early as day 5 following mRNA vaccination, while they were delayed until days 7–14 following DNA, protein, or RhAd52 vaccination. No cellular immune responses were detected within the short time frame of this study [52].

9.3.3.3 The Rise of the LNPs

A key advance for the *in vivo* delivery of mRNA that rapidly gained widespread attention was the development of lipid nanoparticles (LNPs) [53], liposome-like protective bubbles formed by a mixture of different lipids including an ionizable cationic lipid, which offer significant advantages in terms of both efficiency and stability. LNP-formulated mRNA encoding influenza hemagglutinin delivered by either the intramuscular or the intradermal route was reported to efficiently target and activate antigen-presenting cells in macaques, resulting in upregulation of type-I interferon-inducible genes and priming of antigen-specific $CD4^+$ T cells in the draining lymph nodes [54]. Importantly, LNP formulations were shown to possess an intrinsic adjuvant activity that promotes a robust induction of T-follicular helper (TFH) cell responses, which in turn facilitate durable antibody responses. The intrinsic adjuvanticity of LNPs depends on the ionizable lipid component and was shown to be superior to that of a widely used adjuvant, MF59 [55]. Several studies over the past few years have investigated whether an LNP-delivered mRNA vaccine for HIV-1 is immunogenic at levels at least comparable to those of traditional vaccines. Using nucleoside-modified, purified mRNA encapsulated into lipid nanoparticles (mRNA–LNPs), Pardi et al. documented the induction of polyfunctional, antigen-specific, $CD4^+$ T cell responses and autologous neutralizing antibody responses against HIV-1 Env by intradermal vaccination of mice and nonhuman primates. They provided evidence that even a single dose of membrane-bound *env (gp160)* mRNA induces higher levels of TFH cells in draining lymph nodes compared to homologous protein trimers adjuvanted with double-stranded RNA. Multiple mRNA immunizations induced strong antigen-specific TFH cell responses and high numbers of specific germinal center (GC) B cells and plasma cells, which were associated with long-lived and high-affinity neutralizing antibodies. $CD8^+$ T-cell responses were also induced [41]. The same authors subsequently tested the same intradermal LNP platform in rabbits with nucleoside-modified mRNA expressing a clade C transmitted/founder (T/F) HIV-1 Env (1086C). Rabbits were immunized with 50 μg of mRNA at weeks 0, 6, 18, and 30, and started to develop tier-1A heterologous neutralizing antibodies and classic antibody-dependent cellular cytotoxicity (ADCC) after the second immunization. The same study also included a complete longitudinal analysis of the six macaques described in the previous report [55], which had been immunized with 50 μg of mRNA at weeks 0, 4, 20, 32, and 48. Tier-1A heterologous neutralization started to appear in all animals after the second immunization, while tier-1B heterologous neutralization was detected in 5 of 6 animals but at lower titer and only after completion of all five immunizations (week 50); two macaques also developed neutralizing antibodies against the autologous virus, which is classified as tier-2, but autologous tier-2 neutralization is of questionable relevance to protective immunity because it only targets isolate-specific epitopes, most often corresponding to glycan holes. ADCC activity was also detected [42]. Together, the two studies by Pardi and colleagues demonstrated that an LNP-delivered Env-expressing mRNA vaccine is highly immunogenic and has the potential to elicit robust virus-specific cellular immune responses, especially TFH, and neutralizing antibodies. The study design, with the use of a single non-UCA-engaging Env strain, was not expected to induce broad spectrum tier-2 neutralization, but the mRNA/LNP platform was shown to be as effective, if not superior, to traditional adjuvanted-protein vaccines. A similar conclusion was subsequently reached by Melzi et al., who evaluated the efficiency of mRNA/LNP-mediated expression of optimized membrane-bound HIV-1 Env trimers in transgenic mice expressing the germline B-cell receptor of a V2-glycan-targeted bNAb, PCT64 [56]. Although a direct comparison with mRNA-expressed soluble trimers was not performed, mRNA-expressed membrane-bound Env trimers were shown to induce efficient activation and GC recruitment of specific B cells, both of which were more pronounced than with adjuvanted protein immunization and led to the accumulation of rare mutations associated with the initial steps of bNAb PCT64 maturation.

9.3.3.4 Self-Amplifying mRNA

Vaccine approaches based on SAM platforms have also been explored. A pre-clinical study was conducted in nonhuman primates using SAM formulated with a cationic nanoemulsion delivery system and expressing a clade-C HIV-1 Env gp140 (TV1). The SAM was based on an alphavirus genome containing the genes encoding the alphavirus RNA replication machinery but lacking the genes encoding the viral structural proteins required to make an infectious alphavirus particle. The SAM vaccine (50 μg/dose) was tested in a group of six rhesus macaques and compared with three other groups immunized with pre-formed viral replicon particles (VRPs), recombinant gp140 protein mixed with MF59 adjuvant, or a sham VRP/SAM control, respectively. Three immunizations were performed, at weeks 0, 4, and 12, followed by two protein boosters with adjuvanted gp140 protein in all experimental groups. Neutralizing antibodies against a tier-1A heterologous strain were induced in all groups, although they were higher in the SAM group and the adjuvanted-gp140 group, while neutralization of the autologous virus and two tier-1 simian-human immunodeficiency viruses (SHIVs) (1157pEL-p and SF162p4) appeared only late and remained at low titers. The SAM vaccine induced potent Th1 cellular immune responses, which were markedly higher than in animals immunized with pre-formed VRPs or with adjuvanted proteins; IL-4 production was also detected in response to viral antigens, but it was slightly higher in the adjuvanted-protein group than in the SAM group [43]. This study provided the first evidence in a suitable preclinical model that HIV-1 vaccination with SAM is safe and immunogenic, eliciting both humoral and cellular immune responses.

Another study with SAM was conducted in mice immunized with a mosaic T-cell antigen, termed tHIVconsvX. The vaccine induced broadly specific, polyfunctional $CD8^+$ and $CD4^+$ T cells, which remained detectable at a relatively high frequency over a period of at least 22 weeks postimmunization [57]. More recently, Aldon et al. evaluated in mice the relative immunogenicity of two alternative SAM platforms expressing a stabilized HIV-1 Env trimer (ConSOSL.UFO). They showed that a VEEV-based SAM delivered via a polyplex (PLX) nanoparticle formulation induced stronger humoral immune responses than a Semliki Forest virus (SFV)-delivered SAM. Moreover, they observed that membrane-bound Env elicited a humoral response more rapidly than the homologous soluble trimer. In larger animals, including guinea pigs, rabbits, and macaques, a dose as low as 5 μg of PLX-formulated SAM was found to induce high Env-specific immunoglobulin G (IgG) responses [44]. These studies confirmed that the SAM platform allows to reduce the mRNA dose without compromising the efficacy of immunization.

9.4 Recent Advances in HIV-1 mRNA Vaccine Design

9.4.1 The Medium Is Not the Message

Despite the encouraging proof-of-principle that mRNA could perform as well as, or even better than other vaccine platforms against HIV-1 in preclinical models, as discussed above, simple immunization schemes based on single mRNA-encoded HIV-1 immunogens cannot be expected to elicit the production of bNAbs or other forms of protective immunity. Thus, although mRNA has proven to be an excellent vehicle endowed with a series of specific advantages for an HIV-1 vaccine, the vehicle alone cannot solve the formidable challenges that are inherent to eliciting broad-spectrum HIV-1 neutralization and protection. The medium is not the message. Or rather, in this case, the messenger is not the message. To elicit bNAbs, complex and accurately designed and timed vaccine protocols must be devised for initially stimulating and expanding rare breeds of B-cell precursors and, subsequently, for pushing their maturation through a very narrow path until they acquire high-affinity binding for a few tightly protected sites of vulnerability on the HIV-1 Env trimer.

Three decades of research have proven that in order to offer any hope of protection, an HIV-1 vaccine requires a complex design encompassing diverse and accurately selected or engineered Env immunogens, along with an appropriately timed sequence of immunizations. Critical elements for the development of an effective HIV-1 vaccine are summarized in Table 9.3. Over the past five years, a limited number of innovative mRNA vaccine approaches for HIV-1 have been designed, which have the potential to elicit broad-spectrum neutralization and protective immunity. Studies in preclinical models have further corroborated the power of mRNA technology when applied to optimized vaccine protocols.

9.4.2 Specific Approaches

This section illustrates a few selected approaches that have recently been developed and evaluated in preclinical models, yielding promising results.

Table 9.3 Key elements for the development of an effective HIV-1 vaccine.

	Element	Objectives	Strategies
1	Native antigenicity	Present the HIV-1 Env trimer with the conformation and antigenic profile displayed by native virus	Endogenous expression (e.g. mRNA); production of Gag-containing VLPs
2	Exclusion of non-neutralizing or off-target epitopes	Avoid immune system stimulation with distracting immunodominant epitopes	Use of membrane-anchored Env; trimer stabilization
3	Optimal GC stimulation	Expand GCs, increase number of Env-specific GC B cells, accumulate improbable mutations	Production of VLPs; dose-escalation priming, multiple booster immunizations
4	UCA bNAb engagement	Recruit UCA-expressing B cells; initiate bNAb lineage evolution	Use of GL-targeting Envs
5	bNAb maturation	Preferentially expand/affinity mature B cells containing bNAb-lineage specific mutations	Multiple booster immunizations with multiclade heterologous tier-2 Envs

Abbreviations used: VLP, virus-like particles; UCA, unmutated common ancestor; GC, germinal center.

9.4.2.1 A VLP-Forming *env-gag* mRNA Platform

The extraordinary versatility of mRNA as an expression system offers the opportunity to design complex vaccine protocols with the inclusion of diverse elements that may favor the recruitment and expansion of bNAbs, along with other protective immune responses. Zhang et al. [45] took full advantage of such versatility to develop an HIV-1 vaccine platform that combines a set of unique features: (i) utilization of mRNA-encoded Env immunogens; (ii) use of membrane-anchored (either full-length or minimally truncated) HIV-1 Env; (iii) production of VLPs *in vivo* by co-formulation of *env* with *gag* mRNA; (iv) priming with Envs that engage germline bNAb precursors; (v) intensive boosting with rationally selected heterologous tier-2 Envs. Thus, this vaccine utilized a combination of both lineage-based and structure-based strategies.

After validation of the VLP-forming platform in mice, the *env-gag* mRNA vaccine was tested in a complex immunization-challenge study in rhesus macaques. The animals were sequentially vaccinated with mRNA encoding four different Envs derived from three HIV-1 clades (i.e. WITO-Δ276 and WITO wild-type, T/F clade B; BG505, T/F clade A; and DU422, clade C), each co-formulated with SIVmac239 *gag* mRNA. The choice of SIV Gag was justified by the use of a hybrid SHIV virus for the final challenge, which contains HIV-1 Env and SIV Gag. The initial priming was performed with WITO-Δ276, which is deglycosylated at amino acid 276 in gp120 to facilitate recognition of the CD4-binding site by putative macaque UCAs; moreover, WITO naturally engages the UCA of human bNAb CH01. After three immunizations with WITO (autologous phase), the animals received multiple booster immunizations with mixed heterologous Envs (heterologous phase) for a total of 10 sequential immunizations over a period of 58 weeks. In one study subgroup, the final boosts in each phase were performed with adjuvanted homologous proteins (SOSIP trimers). The vaccine was well tolerated in spite of the multiple immunizations with high mRNA doses (up to 400 μg per dose). Both autologous and heterologous trimer-binding antibodies were rapidly induced as were autologous neutralizing antibodies, which became more durable after the booster immunizations. Strikingly, after the third heterologous immunization, heterologous tier-2 neutralizing antibodies started to appear in all animals, with the eventual development of broadly tier-2 neutralizing antibodies that were effective against 11 out of 12 HIV-1 strains included in a reference global panel. However, the neutralization titers remained low (reciprocal half-maximal inhibitory concentrations [IC_{50}] titers, 10–125). The vaccine also elicited robust polyfunctional virus-specific $CD4^+$ T-cell responses mainly directed against HIV-1 Env, with significant activation of TFH cells, a key subpopulation for GC functionality and generation of neutralizing antibody responses. Most importantly, vaccinated animals showed a significantly reduced risk of mucosal infection with a difficult-to-neutralize heterologous tier-2 SHIV strain (AD8), inoculated intrarectally at low weekly doses for 13 weeks. No differences in neutralizing antibody titers and protection were seen between animals which received a final protein boost and those which received almost exclusively mRNA.

Analysis of protection correlates identified an association with the presence of antibodies to the CD4-binding site, as evaluated by immunoassays using an engineered gp120 outer-domain probe (eOD-GT8) designed to engage VRC01-lineage UCAs [58]. Nevertheless, the vaccine elicited a wide range of antibodies against other Env regions, as well as ADCC-mediating antibodies. The authors concluded that protection was presumably due to a combination of immunological responses, with a major role played by Env-specific antibodies, some of which had broadly neutralizing activity. Importantly, the results of this study have recently been confirmed in a second macaque study that used a similar VLP-forming *env-gag* mRNA vaccine platform but enrolled a higher number of animals (P. Zhang et al. unpublished data).

The results obtained with the VLP-forming *env-gag* mRNA vaccine platform were encouraging. One of the merits of this platform is the fact that it is a complete vaccine protocol, not just restricted to the priming and early boosting phases, and that it was followed by live virus challenge to test its efficacy. Besides employing mRNA, which allows for the endogenous expression of Env glycoproteins decorated with its own native N-linked glycosylation, the presumable reasons for the success of this vaccine included the predominant use of membrane-anchored gp160, which adopts a *bona fide* native antigenic configuration without exposure of distractive immunodominant epitopes, and especially the *in vivo* production of VLPs, which are believed to be better immunogens than subunit vaccines because they closely mimic native viral particles in terms of size, shape, mobility and antigenic configuration. Remarkably, mRNA-mediated co-expression of Env and Gag was shown to yield VLPs with high numbers of Env spikes displayed on their surface, markedly higher than in native HIV-1 virions. Finally, this protocol combined a lineage-based approach, which promoted the early engagement of germline bNAb precursors, with repeated boosting with heterologous tier-2 Envs selected for optimal engagement of mature bNAbs. Based on the favorable preclinical results, a Phase-I clinical trial modeled after the *env-gag* mRNA platform has been designed (HIV Vaccine Trials Network (HVTN) 310) and is expected to be launched in 2025.

9.4.2.2 Self-Assembling Nanoparticles

An alternative approach to Env-Gag co-formulation for the production of multivalent HIV-1 Env immunogens using mRNA is the generation of self-assembling nanoparticles, as recently reported by Mu et al. [59]. Specific strategies for Env stabilization were initially validated using LNP-encapsulated gp160 mRNA from the clade-C Env CH848 using knock-in mice carrying the UCA of bNAb DH270 (which targets the V3-glycan supersite). After three immunizations, the mice developed high titers of autologous neutralizing antibodies, and their B cells acquired key DH270-lineage mutations. The selected stabilized Env bearing additional mutations was then fused at its C-terminus with the *Helicobacter pylori* ferritin gene through a linker to produce a single-chain hybrid protein capable of trimerizing and self-assembling into ferritin nanoparticles (termed CH848 10.17DT SOSIP trimer-ferritin NP). Knock-in mice were immunized with LNP-encapsulated mRNA encoding such hybrid protein. After three immunizations, the mice developed robust GC responses, high titers of autologous neutralizing antibodies and improbable mutations that are essential for the maturation of bNAb DH270. Analysis of a total of 397 DH270-related heavy- and light-chain pairs after six sequential immunizations showed a high frequency of improbable mutations, with three cloned mAbs capable of neutralizing the majority of 17 heterologous HIV-1 isolates that were previously shown to be neutralized by the first intermediate ancestor antibody in the DH270 ancestry lineage (DH270 IA4). In most cases, however, neutralization was relatively modest, with IC_{50} greater than 1 μg/ml. This study nevertheless provided evidence that an mRNA vaccine expressing self-assembling nanoparticles can drive a bNAb precursor through the first critical step of the affinity maturation path. Despite the limitations of studies performed in knock-in mice, which possess high numbers of GL-antibody precursor B cells, these results identified self-assembling nanoparticles as a promising strategy for application to different immunogens and immunization schemes. More recently, through mutation-based design of booster mRNA immunogens, Wiehe et al. were able to elicit affinity-matured antibodies bearing key improbable mutations, which acquired some degree of neutralization breadth [60]. To validate this vaccine concept in humans, a clinical trial (HVTN 307) was recently launched, which employs protein nanoparticles displaying the DH270gl-engaging V3G CH848 Pr-NP1 for priming and mRNA encoding a glycan-repaired form of the same Env for boosting (B. Haynes, personal communication).

9.4.2.3 Engineered Germline-Engaging gp120 Cores

Another strategy that has recently been evaluated using mRNA as a vehicle is the use of the germline-targeting engineered core protein eOD-GT8. This immunogen was originally designed by Schief and colleagues to prime human B cells expressing germline precursors of VRC01-class bNAbs [58]. After validating a self-assembling nanoparticle-forming version of the immunogen (eOD-GT8 60mer) as a protein vaccine both in preclinical models and in a Phase-I clinical trial [61], eOD-GT8 60mer has recently been tested in mice in a SAM form, encapsulated in DOTAP-based LNPs, based on an alphavirus replicon [62]. In contrast to nonreplicating mRNA, whose expression was low and short-lived, SAM induced robust protein expression after a single intramuscular injection, which lasted for up to 30 days. Following immunization of mice, eOD-GT8 60-mer-encoding replicons elicited high titers of gp120-specific antibodies and higher levels of antigen-specific GC B cells compared with protein immunization. Likewise, immunization of knock-in mice expressing human inferred VRC01 UCA heavy chains induced efficient priming of B cells and somatic hypermutations consistent with VRC01-class antibody development. Although restricted to the early priming phase of vaccination, this concept represents a promising first step for the efficient recruitment of germline precursors for a specific bNAb class (VRC01) and is currently being evaluated in a Phase-I clinical trial using non-replicating LNP-encapsulated mRNA [63]. More recently, first-boost immunization strategies following priming with *eOD-GT8* mRNA were evaluated in VRC01-UCA knock-in mouse models [64, 65]. Boosting with a gp120 core-based nanoparticle immunogen derived from a CXCR4-tropic HIV-1 molecular clone, HXB2, and lacking the key N276 glycan (core-g28v2 60mer) resulted in an increased frequency of B-cell clones bearing VRC01-lineage mutations and capable of neutralizing selected heterologous pseudoviruses, albeit only when lacking the N276 glycan [64, 65]. It remains unclear whether these early intermediate VRC01-like antibodies have the capability of progressing toward the final bNAb maturation stages.

9.5 The Future

The amazing journey of mRNA from an unlikely concept to a life-saving vaccine implemented on a worldwide scale has raised high hopes that this extraordinary technology might be applied to resolve many of the challenges of modern medicine, including the development of an HIV-1 vaccine. But will mRNA be a universal solution to "deliver us from evil?". The simple answer is no. mRNA is a wonderful tool but not a solution. However, mRNA can offer fundamental help on the way to finding better solutions for many medical challenges, especially those that pose a very high bar. Its safety, rapid implementation, versatility, efficiency, lack of immunogenicity, and relatively low cost make mRNA an ideal platform for vaccine development [66]. This is especially true in the case of an HIV-1 vaccine where presentation of the Env in its native antigenic conformation, as can be achieved through endogenous production by host cells, could be a key factor for success. In fact, besides a growing number of preclinical studies, a few clinical trials for mRNA-based HIV-1 vaccines have recently been initiated or are in the planning to be launched soon. The future has started.

9.5.1 Room for Improvement

The initial attempts to produce mRNA vaccines against HIV-1 have recently been reviewed [67, 68]. Although mRNA-based vaccines have already demonstrated signs of increased efficacy relative to traditional vaccine platforms, further improvement is unquestionably needed. The elicitation of broad-spectrum neutralizing antibodies, active against multiple heterologous tier-2 viral strains, remains the gold standard for HIV-1 vaccine efficacy, yet it has rarely been achieved and only at very low titers. The durability of neutralizing antibody responses is also an issue, as is their isotype, since IgG is less prone than immunoglobulin A (IgA) to concentrate at mucosal surfaces where viral transmission occurs. Moreover, despite the ability of LNP-encapsulated mRNA to elicit strong polyfunctional $CD4^+$ T-cell responses, including TFH cells, an area of potential improvement is the limited elicitation of specific $CD8^+$ T-cell responses.

The following is a list of possible improvements of current mRNA platforms that might be used to optimize the delivery of HIV-1 mRNA vaccines and enhance specific protective responses.

9.5.1.1 Mucosal Delivery and Other Alternative Routes

With rare exceptions, transmission of HIV-1 occurs by the mucosal route, and it is at mucosal surfaces, especially the genital and rectal mucosae, that the protective mechanisms should be primarily effective. Thus, induction of IgA and tissue-resident memory (TRM) $CD8^+$ T cells at these locations is desirable, but intramuscular immunization elicits them inefficiently. An ideal alternative might be the direct mucosal delivery of mRNA, which should elicit strong local responses and favor the production of secretory IgA and TRM $CD8^+$ T cells. Although there are many physical obstacles that may reduce the efficiency of mRNA delivery at mucosal surfaces, the interest in this approach is increasing [69]. Another option is intradermal delivery, which was shown to be effective for mRNA [54] and superior to the intramuscular route for a modified vaccinia Ankara (MVA) vaccine to induce protection from vaginal SHIV challenge in female macaques [70].

A variety of other routes of mRNA administration may also be explored, besides the classic intramuscular route, to increase vaccine efficacy and facilitate specific organ targeting by mRNA. Intravenous delivery is unlikely to offer advantages since the mRNA will be rapidly cleared from the circulation and concentrated in the liver and, to some extent, in the kidneys and lungs. Subcutaneous and intradermal inoculations have been tested in various studies and may offer some advantages compared to the intramuscular route. In the case of HIV-1, an attractive possibility is intranodal inoculation, as utilized in an early clinical trial with naked mRNA [39], which might significantly enhance the efficiency of antigen presentation and GL activation.

9.5.1.2 Slow Delivery

An approach that has received considerable attention in the HIV-1 vaccine field is slow delivery [71], with special emphasis on the priming phase, where the administration of multiple escalating doses over a period of two weeks was shown to be particularly effective in inducing strong and durable GC responses presumably by increasing long-term antigen retention in these structures [72]. Can these concepts be applied to mRNA vaccines? Besides repeated injections, which are impractical, there are several other potential approaches to utilize slow-delivery systems, including subcutaneous osmotic pumps and silica encapsulation platforms. A major question regards the long-term stability of mRNA at a temperature close to 37 °C, as required for slow delivery. Conversely, one of the major benefits of slow-delivery approaches would be to mimic the sustained antigenic exposure that occurs in chronically HIV-1-infected individuals who eventually succeed, over a long period of time, in developing bNAbs.

9.5.1.3 Env-Gag VLP Optimization

Although a VLP-forming *env-gag* mRNA vaccine platform has shown promising results in mice and nonhuman primates [45], as further confirmed by preliminary studies conducted in germline VRC01-knock-in mice (L. Stamatatos et al. unpublished observations), there is undoubtedly room for further optimization. First, the protocol utilized in the first study was long and cumbersome, and therefore difficult to implement in a human trial. Second, the broad-spectrum neutralization elicited was low in titer and did not reach levels that are considered to be protective *in vivo*. Third, the protective effect was only partial, with a small number of animals remaining fully protected after 13 sequential low-dose virus inoculations. Fourth, the duration of the protective effect was not evaluated. One aspect of this approach that can be improved, among others, is the quality of the VLPs because Gag, in the absence of the viral protease, remains uncleaved and generates only immature VLPs. Thus, efforts have been made to include the viral protease in the form of a full-length or truncated *gagpol* mRNA transcript. Preliminary results, obtained both *in vitro* and *in vivo*, indicate that the addition of *gagpol* mRNA yields mature VLPs that contain fully processed Gag and are more effective than immature VLPs in eliciting robust priming responses, broad-spectrum neutralizing antibodies and protection (P. Zhang et al. unpublished observations). The mechanism underlying the increased efficacy of mature vs. immature VLPs may be related to increased Env mobility that promotes Env clustering on the VLP surface.

9.5.1.4 Multiple-Array Antigen Presentation

It is well established that the immune system responds more efficiently to an ordered array of protein antigens displayed on a solid or semi-solid surface [73]. HIV-1, like most viruses, presents multiple copies of its Env spike on the virion surface, although they are typically sparse, which may help to explain the relatively low immunogenicity of Env during natural infection. However, there is an increasing choice of platforms in the field that generate pre-formed or self-assembling nanoparticles or other types of multiple-array antigen platforms, which can stimulate specific immune responses with high efficiency [22, 59]. Besides presenting the antigen in multiple, well-ordered sets, these immunogens are also of larger size than individual subunit proteins, which is another beneficial feature. One of the concerns with these approaches is that the Env antigenic configuration may be altered by expression as a fusion protein, for example, with ferritin or other scaffolds, or by chemical conjugation to a solid support.

9.5.1.5 Supplemental Adjuvants

Although LNP-encapsulated mRNA is a self-adjuvanted vaccine, owing to its inherent ability to activate innate immune sensors, the immune responses it elicits are heavily biased toward T-helper type 1 (Th1) and TFH responses [45, 55]. This may cause an unbalanced vaccine response, with very strong $CD4^+$ T-cell responses that promote the development of antibodies and relatively low antiviral effectors such as $CD8^+$ T cells. In addition, the durability of the protective immunity elicited by mRNA vaccines is not optimal and might be extended through the early recruitment of specific elements of the innate immune system. To expand the narrow selectivity of mRNA vaccine responses, it is conceivable to supplement an mRNA vaccine with additional adjuvants to stimulate a broader range of immune responses. For example, specific cytokines or Toll-like receptor activators could be co-delivered with the vaccine either as mRNA or as proteins. The induction of broader and more balanced vaccine responses might further increase the efficacy and durability of current mRNA vaccines.

9.5.1.6 Combination of mRNA with Other Platforms

Finally, mRNA should not be considered as an exclusive platform because its many virtues might be further enhanced by combining it with other delivery systems that may exert complementary and even synergistic effects. Combination platforms could be implemented by both sequential and simultaneous administration and during both the priming and the boosting phases. Examples of combinations include but are not limited to, mRNA priming followed by boosting with adjuvanted proteins (e.g. soluble trimers), pre-formed nanoparticles (e.g. self-assembling ferritin nanoparticles), or Env-expressing viral vectors (e.g. adenovirus or MVA). These regimens might help to modulate the dominant Th1/TFH responses induced by LNP/mRNA, broaden the immunological milieu, and induce a more balanced $CD4^+$ versus $CD8^+$ T-cell activation at the end of the immunization scheme. Alternatively, mRNA priming might be complemented by simultaneous co-priming with other platforms, especially viral vectors that could more effectively prime $CD8^+$ T-cell responses. Combination attempts of mRNA with other vaccine platforms are already being explored as a follow-up to ongoing or completed vaccine trials, as is the case of the planned extension of the HVTN 133 trial, which will evaluate whether mRNA encoding a transmembrane gp41 MPER can boost and affinity mature existing heterologous neutralizing bNAbs to greater breadth and potency (B. Haynes, personal communication). Without diminishing the importance of mRNA, creative combinations of delivery systems, supplemental adjuvants, and diverse vaccine platforms could in the long term achieve results that remain beyond the reach of each individual approach.

9.6 Concluding Remarks

The recent application of mRNA technology to HIV-1 vaccines has started to unravel the extraordinary potential of mRNA as a vehicle for vaccine delivery. While mRNA by itself will not be sufficient to solve the riddle of HIV-1 vaccine development, it possesses unique features that can greatly facilitate progress in this endeavor and, eventually, might tilt the balance in favor of cleverly designed protocols based on effective immunogens. The future of HIV-1 vaccines has started, and mRNA is destined to play an important role in this quest.

Acknowledgment

I am grateful to Drs. Barton F. Haynes and William R. Schief for sharing unpublished data. This work was supported by the Intramural Research Program of NIAID, NIH.

References

1 Centers for Disease Control (CDC) (1981). Pneumocystis pneumonia—Los Angeles. *MMWR Morb. Mortal Wkly. Rep.* 30: 250–252.

2 Wei, X., Decker, J.M., Wang, S. et al. (2003). Antibody neutralization and escape by HIV-1. *Nature* 422: 307–312.

3 Rerks-Ngarm, S., Pitisuttithum, P., Nitayaphan, S. et al. (2009). Vaccination with ALVAC and AIDSVAX to prevent HIV-1 infection in Thailand. *N. Engl. J. Med.* 361: 2209–2220.

4 Gray, G.E., Bekker, L.G., Laher, F. et al. (2021). Vaccine efficacy of ALVAC-HIV and bivalent subtype C gp120–MF59 in adults. *N. Engl. J. Med.* 384: 1089–1100.

5 Mascola, J.R. and Haynes, B.F. (2013). HIV-1 neutralizing antibodies: understanding nature's pathways. *Immunol. Rev.* 254: 225–244.

6 Burton, D.R. and Hangartner, L. (2016). Broadly neutralizing antibodies to HIV and their role in vaccine design. *Annu. Rev. Immunol.* 34: 635–659.

7 Kwong, P. and Mascola, J.P. (2018). HIV-1 vaccines based on antibody identification, B cell ontogeny and epitope structure. *Immunity* 48: 855–871.

8 Baba, T.W., Liska, V., Hofmann-Lehmann, R. et al. (2000). Human neutralizing monoclonal antibodies of the IgG1 subtype protect against mucosal simian-human immunodeficiency virus infection. *Nat. Med.* 6: 200–206.

9 Mascola, J.R., Lewis, M.G., Stiegler, G. et al. (1999). Protection of macaques against pathogenic simian/human immunodeficiency virus 89.6PD by passive transfer of neutralizing antibodies. *J. Virol.* 73: 4009–4018.

10 Mascola, J.R., Stiegler, G., Van Cott, T.C. et al. (2000). Protection of macaques against vaginal transmission of a pathogenic HIV-1/SIV chimeric virus by passive infusion of neutralizing antibodies. *Nat. Med.* 6: 207–210.

11 Haynes, B.F., Wiehe, K., Borrow, P. et al. (2022). Strategies for HIV-1 vaccines that induce broadly neutralizing antibodies. *Nat. Rev. Immunol.* 12: 1–17.

12 Moldt, B., Rakasz, E.G., Schultz, N. et al. (2012). Highly potent HIV-specific antibody neutralization in vitro translates into effective protection against mucosal SHIV challenge in vivo. *Proc. Natl. Acad. Sci. U. S. A.* 109 (46): 18921–18925.

13 Pegu, A., Yang, Z.Y., Boyington, J.C. et al. (2014). Neutralizing antibodies to HIV-1 envelope protect more effectively in vivo than those to the CD4 receptor. *Sci. Transl. Med.* 6: 243ra88.

14 Shingai, M., Donau, O.K., Plishka, R.J. et al. (2014). Passive transfer of modest titers of potent and broadly neutralizing anti-HIV monoclonal antibodies block SHIV infection in macaques. *J. Exp. Med.* 211: 2061–2074.

15 Kwong, P.D., Dekosky, B.J., and Ulmer, J.B. (2020). Antibody-guided structure-based vaccines. *Semin. Immunol.* 50: 101428.

16 Liao, H.X., Linch, R., Zhou, T. et al. (2013). Co-evolution of a broadly neutralizing HIV-1 antibody and founder virus. *Nature* 496: 469–476.

17 Doria-Rose, N.A., Schramm, C.A., Gorman, J. et al. (2014). Developmental pathway for potent V1V2-directed HIV-neutralizing antibodies. *Nature* 509: 55–62.

18 Bonsignori, M., Zhou, T., Sheng, Z. et al. (2016). Maturation pathway from germline to broad HIV-1 neutralizer of a CD4-mimic antibody. *Cell* 165: 449–463.

19 McGuire, A.T., Hoot, S., Dreyer, A.M. et al. (2013). Engineering HIV envelope protein to activate germline B cell receptors of broadly neutralizing anti-CD4 binding site antibodies. *J. Exp. Med.* 210: 655–663.

20 Steichen, J.M., Kulp, D.W., Tokatlian, T. et al. (2016). HIV vaccine design to target germline precursors of glycan-dependent broadly neutralizing antibodies. *Immunity* 45: 483–496.

21 Wiehe, K., Bradley, T., Meyerhoff, R.R. et al. (2018). Functional relevance of improbable antibody mutations for HIV broadly neutralizing antibody development. *Cell Host Microbe* 23: 759–765.e6.

22 Graham, B.S., Gilman, M.S.A., McLellan, J.S. et al. (2019). Structure-based vaccine antigen design. *Annu. Rev. Med.* 70: 91–104.

23 Xu, K., Acharya, P., Kong, R. et al. (2018). Epitope-based vaccine design yields fusion peptide-directed antibodies that neutralize diverse strains of HIV-1. *Nat. Med.* 24: 857–867.

24 Pardi, N., Hogan, M.J., Porter, W., and Weissman, D. (2018). mRNA vaccines a new era in vaccinology. *Nat. Rev. Drug Discov.* 17: 261–279.

25 Zhu, N., Zhang, D., Wang, W. et al. (2020). A novel coronavirus from patients with pneumonia in China, 2019. *N. Engl. J. Med.* 382: 727–733.

26 Corbett, K.S., Edwards, D.K., Leist, S.R. et al. (2020). SARS-CoV-2 mRNA vaccine design enabled by prototype pathogen preparedness. *Nature* 586: 567–571.

27 Jackson, L.A., Anderson, E.J., Rouphael, N.G. et al. (2020). An mRNA vaccine against SARS-CoV-2 - preliminary report. *N. Engl. J. Med.* 383: 1920–1931.

28 Brenner, S., Jacob, F., and Meselson, M. (1961). An unstable intermediate carrying information from genes to ribosomes for protein synthesis. *Nature* 190: 576–581.

29 Malone, R.W., Felgner, P.L., and Verma, I.M. (1989). Cationic liposome-mediated RNA transfection. *Proc. Natl. Acad. Sci. U. S. A.* 86: 6077–6081.

30 Wolff, J.A., Malone, R.W., Williams, P. et al. (1990). Direct gene transfer into mouse muscle in vivo. *Science* 247: 1465–1468.

31 Jirikowski, G.F., Sanna, P.P., Maciejewski-Lenoir, D., and Bloom, F.E. (1992). Reversal of diabetes insipidus in Brattleboro rats: intrahypothalamic injection of vasopressin mRNA. *Science* 255: 996–998.

32 Kariko, K., Buckstein, M., Ni, H., and Weissman, D. (2005). Suppression of RNA recognition by Toll-like receptors: the impact of nucleoside modification and the evolutionary origin of RNA. *Immunity* 23: 165–175.

33 Kariko, K., Muramatsu, H., Luwig, J., and Weissman, D. (2011). Generating the optimal mRNA for therapy: HPLC purification eliminates immune activation and improves translation of nucleoside-modified, protein-encoding mRNA. *Nucleic Acids Res.* 39: e142.

34 Allen, T.M. and Cullis, P.R. (2013). Liposomal drug delivery systems: from concept to clinical applications. *Adv. Drug Deliv. Rev.* 65: 1–148.

35 Routy, J.P., Boulassel, M.R., Yassine-Diab, B. et al. (2010). Immunologic activity and safety of autologous HIV RNA-electroporated dendritic cells in HIV-1 infected patients receiving antiretroviral therapy. *Clin. Immunol.* 134: 140–147.

36 Van Gulck, E., Vlieghe, E., Vekemans, M. et al. (2012). mRNA-based dendritic cell vaccination induces potent antiviral T-cell responses in HIV-1-infected patients. *AIDS* 26: F1–F12.

37 Gandhi, R.T., Kwon, D.S., Macklin, E.A. et al. (2016). Immunization of HIV-1-infected persons with autologous dendritic cells transfected with mRNA encoding HIV-1 Gag and Nef: results of a randomized, placebo-controlled clinical trial. *JAIDS* 71: 246–253.

38 Romain, G., Van Gulck, E., Epaulard, O. et al. (2012). CD34-derived dendritic cells transfected ex vivo with HIV-Gag mRNA induce polyfunctional T-cell responses in nonhuman primates. *Eur. J. Immunol.* 42: 2019–2030.

39 Leal, L., Guard, A.C., Moron-Lopez, S. et al. (2018). Phase I clinical trial of an intranodally administered mRNA-based therapeutic vaccine against HIV-1 infection. *AIDS* 32: 2533–2545.

40 de Jong, W., Aerts, J., Allard, S. et al. (2019). iHIVARNA phase IIa, a randomized, placebo-controlled, double-blinded trial to evaluate the safety and immunogenicity of iHIVARNA-01 in chronically HIV-infected patients under stable combined antiretroviral therapy. *Trials* 20: 361.

41 Pardi, N., Hogan, M.J., Naradikian, M.S. et al. (2018). Nucleoside-modified mRNA vaccines induce potent T follicular helper and germinal center B cell responses. *J. Exp. Med.* 215: 1571–1588.

42 Pardi, N., LaBranche, C.C., Ferrari, G. et al. (2019). Characterization of HIV-1 nucleoside-modified mRNA vaccines in rabbits and rhesus macaques. *Mol. Ther. Nucleic Acids* 15: 36–47.

43 Bogers, W.M., Oostermeijer, H., Mooij, P. et al. (2015). Potent immune responses in rhesus macaques induced by nonviral delivery of a self-amplifying RNA vaccine expressing HIV type 1 envelope with a cationic nanoemulsion. *J. Infect. Dis.* 211: 947–955.

44 Aldon, Y., McKay, P.F., Moreno Herrero, J. et al. (2021). Immunogenicity of stabilized HIV-1 Env trimers delivered by self-amplifying mRNA. *Mol. Ther. Nucleic Acids* 25: 483–493.

45 Zhang, P., Narayanan, E., Liu, Q. et al. (2021). A multiclade env–gag VLP mRNA vaccine elicits tier-2 HIV-1-neutralizing antibodies and reduces the risk of heterologous SHIV infection in macaques. *Nat. Med.* 27: 2234–2245.

46 Sullenger, B.A. and Gilboa, E. (2002). Emerging clinical applications of RNA. *Nature* 418: 252–258.

47 Weissman, D., Ni, H., Scales, D. et al. (2000). HIV Gag mRNA transfection of dendritic cells (DC) delivers encoded antigen to MHC class I and II molecules, causes DC maturation, and induces a potent human in vitro primary immune response. *J. Immunol.* 165: 4710–4717.

48 Sun, S., Li, W., Sun, Y. et al. (2011). A new RNA vaccine platform based on MS2 virus-like particles produced in *Saccharomyces cerevisiae*. *Biochem. Biophys. Res. Commun.* 407: 124–128.

49 Pollard, C., Rejman, J., De Haes, W. et al. (2013). Type I IFN counteracts the induction of antigen-specific immune responses by lipid-based delivery of mRNA vaccines. *Mol. Ther.* 21: 251–259.

50 Zhao, M., Li, M., Zhang, Z. et al. (2016). Induction of HIV-1 gag specific immune responses by cationic micelles mediated delivery of gag mRNA. *Drug Deliv.* 23: 2596–2607.

51 Li, M., Zhao, M., Fu, Y. et al. (2016). Enhanced intranasal delivery of mRNA vaccine by overcoming the nasal epithelial barrier via intra- and paracellular pathways. *J. Control. Release* 228: 9–19.

52 Gebre, M.S., Rauch, S., Roth, N. et al. (2022). mRNA vaccines induce rapid antibody responses in mice. *NPJ Vaccines* 7: 88.

53 Geall, A.J., Verma, A., Otten, G.R. et al. (2012). Nonviral delivery of self-amplifying RNA vaccines. *Proc. Natl. Acad. Sci. U. S. A.* 109: 14604–14609.

54 Liang, F., Lindgren, G., Lin, A. et al. (2017). Efficient targeting and activation of antigen-presenting cells in vivo after modified mRNA vaccine administration in rhesus macaques. *Mol. Ther.* 25: 2635–2647.

55 Alameh, M.G., Tombácz, I., Bettini, E. et al. (2021). Lipid nanoparticles enhance the efficacy of mRNA and protein subunit vaccines by inducing robust T follicular helper cell and humoral responses. *Immunity* 54: 2877–2892.e7.

56 Melzi, E., Willis, J.R., Ma, K.M. et al. (2022). Membrane-bound mRNA immunogens lower the threshold to activate HIV Env V2 apex-directed broadly neutralizing B cell precursors in humanized mice. *Immunity* 55: 1–19.

57 Moyo, N., Vogel, A.B., Buus, S. et al. (2018). Efficient induction of T cells against conserved HIV-1 regions by mosaic vaccines delivered as self-amplifying mRNA. *Mol. Ther. Methods Clin. Dev.* 12: 32–46.

58 Jardine, J., Julien, J.P., Menis, S. et al. (2013). Rational HIV immunogen design to target specific germline B cell receptors. *Science* 340: 711–716.

59 Mu, Z., Wiehe, K., Saunders, K.O. et al. (2022). mRNA-encoded HIV-1 Env trimer ferritin nanoparticles induce monoclonal antibodies that neutralize heterologous HIV-1 isolates in mice. *Cell Rep.* 38: 110514.

60 Wiehe, K., Saunders, K.O., Stalls, V. et al. (2024). Mutation-guided vaccine design: a process for developing boosting immunogens for HIV broadly neutralizing antibody induction. *Cell Host Microbe* 32: 1–17.

61 International AIDS Vaccine Initiative. (2022). A phase 1 trial to evaluate the safety and immunogenicity of eOD-GT8 60mer vaccine, adjuvanted. https://clinicaltrials.gov/ct2/show/study/NCT03547245?term=eod-gt8&cond=Hiv&draw=2&rank=1 (accessed 23 December 2023).

62 Melo, M., Porter, E., Zhang, Y. et al. (2019). Immunogenicity of RNA replicons encoding HIV Env immunogens designed for self-assembly into nanoparticles. *Mol. Ther.* 27: 2080–2090.

63 International AIDS Vaccine Initiative. (2023). A study to evaluate the safety and immunogenicity of eOD-GT8 60mer mRNA vaccine (mRNA-1644). https://clinicaltrials.gov/ct2/show/NCT05414786?term=mrna&cond=Hiv&draw=2&rank=3 (accessed 23 December 2023).

64 Cottrell, C.A., Hu, X., Lee, J.H. et al. (2024). Heterologous prime-boost vaccination drives early maturation of HIV broadly neutralizing antibody precursors in humanized mice. *Sci. Transl. Med.* 16: eadn0223.

65 Wang, X., Cottrell, C.A., Hu, X. et al. (2024). mRNA-LNP prime boost evolves precursors toward VRC01-like broadly neutralizing antibodies in preclinical humanized mouse models. *Sci. Immunol.* 9: eadn0622.

66 Lusso, P. (2023). The quest for an HIV-1 vaccine: will mRNA deliver us from evil? *Expert Rev. Vaccines* 22: 267–269.

67 Mu, Z., Haynes, B.F., and Cain, D.W. (2021). HIV mRNA vaccines — progress and future paths. *Vaccines* 9: 134.

68 Khalid, K., Padda, J., Khedr, A. et al. (2021). HIV and messenger RNA (mRNA) vaccine. *Cureus* 13: e16197.

69 Hameed, S.A., Paul, S., Dellosa, G.K.Y. et al. (2022). Towards the future exploration of mucosal mRNA vaccines against emerging viral diseases; lessons from existing next-generation mucosal vaccine strategies. *NPJ Vaccines* 7: 71.

70 Bollimpelli, V.S., Reddy, P.B.J., Gangadhara, S. et al. (2023). Intradermal but not intramuscular modified vaccinia Ankara immunizations protect against intravaginal tier2 simian-human immunodeficiency virus challenges in female macaques. *Nat. Commun.* 14: 4789.

71 Cirelli, K.M., Carnathan, D.G., Nogal, B. et al. (2019). Slow delivery immunization enhances HIV neutralizing antibody and germinal center responses via modulation of immunodominance. *Cell* 177: 1153–1171.

72 Tam, H.H., Melo, M.B., Kang, M. et al. (2016). Sustained antigen availability during germinal center initiation enhances antibody responses to vaccination. *Proc. Natl. Acad. Sci. U. S. A.* 113: E6639–E6648.

73 Chackerian, B., Durfee, M.R., and Schiller, J.T. (2008). Virus-like display of a neo-self antigen reverses B cell anergy in a B cell receptor transgenic mouse model. *J. Immunol.* 180: 5816–5825.

10

mRNA Vaccines Against Tick-borne Diseases

Gunjan Arora and Erol Fikrig

Yale University School of Medicine, Department of Internal Medicine, Section of Infectious Diseases, New Haven, CT 06520, USA

10.1 Introduction

The word vaccine comes from the Latin word *vacca* which means cow. The term was first used following Edward Jenner's seminal work with cowpox virus, which was used as a vaccine against smallpox [1]. Artificial active immunization or vaccination against infectious agents remains one of the most effective ways to prevent microbial diseases. Vaccination can generate immunity against most pathogens, and in many cases, it provides long-term protection. A vaccine's success depends on memory T-cell responses that are essential to generate cellular and humoral immunity. T-cells help B-cells produce neutralizing antibodies against a foreign antigen [2–7]. The selection of a target antigen is often one of the first challenges in designing a vaccine. In some cases, antibody-mediated protection is effective when the target is linked to pathogenesis [8–11]. In addition, pathogens use diverse evasion strategies, such as antigenic variation, to express a variety of antigens on the surface, which creates obstacles in target identification, especially in the case of intracellular pathogens [12–16]. Therefore, developing vaccines remains challenging for many vector-borne diseases.

10.2 Vector-borne Diseases

According to the World Health Organization, more than 17% of all infectious diseases are transmitted by vectors. Vector-borne diseases cause more than 700 000 deaths annually. Blood-feeding arthropods, such as mosquitoes, ticks, sandflies, tsetse flies, and fleas transmit diverse pathogens, including Dengue virus, West Nile virus, *Borrelia spirochetes*, Leishmania, Trypanosomes, and Plasmodium to humans and animals [17–22]. In North America, tick-borne infections are among the most common vector-borne illnesses, and Lyme borreliosis is the most frequently diagnosed tick-borne illness. Ticks also transmit at least 14 other

Trends in mRNA Vaccine Research, First Edition. Edited by Gabor Tamas Szabo and Norbert Pardi.

pathogens including relapsing fever causing *Borrelia* sp., Powassan virus, *Babesia*, and *Anaplasma* (Table 10.1). Control of mosquitoes and ticks remains challenging due to the large geographical spread of these vectors, cost, safety issues as well as the emergence of insecticide resistance. There is an urgent need to develop effective therapeutic strategies including drugs, vaccines, and insecticides to control and prevent arthropod-borne infections.

10.3 Tick-borne Diseases

Ticks are a distinct form of parasitic arachnid that are part of the mite superorder. There are over 700 hard ticks from the family *Ixodidae* and almost 190 soft ticks in the *Argasida* family [77]. There are four major stages in a tick's life cycle – egg, larva, nymph, and adult. To develop from one life stage to the next, ticks require a blood meal and, in the process, can transmit pathogens to a vertebrate host. Though the exact number of tick-borne diseases remains unknown, ticks can spread infections caused by bacteria, viruses, or parasites to humans or animals.

Ixodes scapularis is one of the major tick species that is widely distributed across the eastern United States [78]. *I. scapularis* nymphs and adults transmit the agents of Lyme disease, Babesiosis, Anaplasmosis, and Powassan disease, among other infections. Studies also suggest that in the past two decades, the geographic range of *I. scapularis* has also expanded [17, 79, 80]. According to the Centers for Disease Control and Prevention (CDC), there were over 50 000 tick-borne disease cases reported annually between 2016 and 2019. In addition, the number of reported tick-borne diseases doubled between 2004 and 2016 years. During this period, Lyme disease accounted for 82% of all tick-borne diseases in North America, but spotted fever Rickettsioses, Babesiosis, and Anaplasmosis/Ehrlichiosis cases also increased [78]. The infections are more commonly reported in the late spring and summer but can occur year round.

Ticks are also known carriers of Relapsing Fever causing Borrelia species which is mainly transmitted by argasid vectors also known as "soft ticks" of the genus Ornithodoros. Different ticks also transmit many viruses that can cause infection in humans, e.g. Powassan virus, louping ill virus (LIV), Central European encephalitis (CEE) virus, Greek goat encephalitis virus, Russian spring–summer encephalitis (RSSE), Omsk Hemorrhagic Fever, Crimean–Congo hemorrhagic fever virus (CCHFV), Alkhurma hemorrhagic fever (AHF) Kyasanur forest disease virus (KFDV).

10.4 Tick Saliva Antigens as Vaccine Candidates

The proteins secreted by salivary glands of infected ticks are deposited at the bite site along with the pathogens and help tick engorge on the host [81–83]. Tick saliva is a dynamic mixture of antigens whose composition may not be same all along

Table 10.1 List of tick-borne diseases.

No.	Disease	Pathogen	Tick genus	Reference
1.	Lyme	*Borrelia burgdorferi senso lato*	*Ixodes*	[17, 23–29]
2.	Human granulocytic anaplasmosis	*Anaplasma phagocytophilum*	*Ixodes*	[30–34]
3.	Ehrlichiosis	*Ehrlichia chaffeensis, Ehrlichia ewingii*, or *Ehrlichia muris eauclairensis*	*Amblyomma* and *Ixodes*	[35–38]
4.	Rocky mountain spotted fever	*Rickettsia species*	Dermacentor, *Amblyomma, Rhipicephalus*	[32, 39–42]
5.	Powassan virus	Powassan virus	*Ixodes* and *Dermacentor*	[43–48]
6.	Colorado tick fever or mountain tick fever	Colorado tick fever (CTF) virus	*Dermacentor*	[49–51]
7.	Bourbon virus	Bourbon virus genus Thogotovirus	*Amblyomma*	[52–55]
8.	Relapsing fever	Relapsing causing *Borrelia* sp. *Borrelia miyamotoi, Borrelia hermsii, Borrelia crocidurai, Borrelia hispanica*	*Ornithodoros*	[13, 56–58]
9.	Babesiosis	*Babesia microti, Babesia bovis, Babesia bigemina*	*Ixodes, Rhipicephalus*	[59, 60]
10.	Theileriosis	*Theileria equi* and *Theileria orientalis*	*Ixodes, Rhipicephalus*	[59–61]
11.	Jingmen tick virus (JMTV)	Jingmen tick virus (JMTV)	Amblyomma	[62–64]
12.	Tick-borne encephalitis	Tick-borne encephalitis virus complex, e.g. Central European encephalitis (CEE) virus and Russian spring–summer encephalitis (RSSE) virus	*Ixodes, Dermacentor, Ornithodoros*	[65–69]
13.	Heartland virus disease	Heartland virus of Family Bunyaviridae	*Amblyomma*	[55, 70–72]
14.	Crimean–Congo hemorrhagic fever (CCHF)	Crimean–Congo hemorrhagic fever orthonairovirus (CCHFV) belongs to the Jingmen virus group	*Rhipicephalus*	[73–75]
15.	Siberian tick typhus	*Rickettsia sibirica*	*Dermacentor* and *Haemaphysalis*	[76]

and is dependent on the type of tick species, life stage, feeding, among other factors [84–91]. Some antigens present in the saliva facilitate the pathogens survival at the entry point in the host [92–96]. Therefore, many studies have been devoted to identifying the tick sialome and functional characterization of individual salivary antigens. Their efforts are supported by results that show immunization with tick saliva is sufficient to elicit tick resistance. Recent efforts are focused on developing a cocktail of tick saliva components that can be used as a new multivalent vaccine against tick-borne diseases.

10.5 Vaccines Targeting Pathogens That Cause Tick-borne Diseases

Since Lyme disease is the most common tick-borne disease in North America and Eurasia, major efforts to make vaccines were focused on *Borrelia burgdorferi*. The first breakthrough to develop a Lyme vaccine was achieved when it was demonstrated that immunization with outer-surface protein A (OspA) prevented *B. burgdorferi* infection in mice and other animal models [97–101]. In human clinical trials, the vaccine was shown to be safe and effective. The vaccine showed 76% efficacy in preventing clinical Lyme disease and 100% in preventing asymptomatic infection [102]. Subsequently, the first OspA-based Lyme vaccine "LYMErix" was approved for humans in 1998. This vaccine was discontinued later citing insufficient consumer demand. Other OspA-based protein vaccines have been developed by other companies including Baxter Bioscience, and VLA15 (developed by Valneva Austria GmbH) [103, 104]. An OspA-based protein vaccine may again become available in the future. In addition, mRNA technology could be useful in developing new OspA-based vaccines against Lyme disease.

While there is no vaccine for humans, Merck has a vaccine for Lyme disease in dogs eight weeks of age or older called "Nobivac-Lyme" [105]. This vaccine is *B. burgdorferi* BACTERIN, which is a suspension of killed or attenuated bacteria. Other vaccines (LymeVax® Zoetis, and Recombitek® Lyme, Merial) and Merilym® 3, Merial and Virbagen Canis-B, Virbac) based on inactivated Bacterial suspensions are used against Lyme borreliosis in animals. There is currently an urgent need to develop new vaccines against Lyme disease and other tick-borne diseases.

10.6 mRNA Vaccines

Nucleic acid vaccines such as mRNA vaccines represent a pathbreaking approach to rapidly develop vaccines and overcome challenges with traditional vaccines (Figure 10.1). The first report on the successful use of *in vitro* transcribed (IVT) mRNA in animals was published in 1990 [106, 107]. The engineered mRNA allows mRNA to be more stable and better delivered overcoming traditional barriers to using mRNA as a vaccine. mRNA vaccines are noninfectious and therefore are considered safer than killed and live attenuated viruses. Further, the risk of adding

Vaccine platform	Advantages	Disadvantages
Protein vaccines	• Stable • Lower quantities required • Final product is used directly • No integration with the host genome • Many FDA approved vaccines	• Present for a limited time, boosting required • Production hassles: Soluble protein, correct modifications, and folding pattern required • Endotoxin contamination possible
DNA vaccines	• Stable expression • Can produce multiple mRNAs • Easy production • Protein is produced, folded, and post-translationally modified in the host cell • Approved (ZyCoV-D) for COVID-19 in India	• Must enter the nucleus, higher amounts required • Possibility of integration with the host genome • Endotoxin contamination
mRNA vaccines	• Flexibility of mRNA vaccine design, codon optimization, and production • Protein is produced, folded, and post-translationally modified in the host • Easy production • No integration with the host genome • Approved for COVID-19	• Unstable • Costly

Figure 10.1 Comparison of protein, DNA and mRNA vaccine platforms.

mutation in DNA-based vaccines is not present in the mRNA platform. Since mRNA stability can be regulated by modifications in the base and delivery methods, it is considered safer for *in vivo* delivery [106, 108, 109].

To increase the translation activity of mRNA modifications carrier molecules such as LNP, which also serves as an adjuvant are key. mRNA does not need any other viral vector for delivery and therefore, is not affected by anti-vector immunity which is a problem for adenovirus-based vaccines. Since mRNA can be generated by a chemical *in vitro* transcription reaction the production can be controlled and easily scaled up or down in no time. The breakthrough for the mRNA vaccine field came during the COVID-19 pandemic when the first two vaccines approved by the United States Food and Drug Administration (FDA) were mRNA-based vaccines that were shown to be over 90% efficacious in clinical trials [110–112]. This breaks the barrier for this new technology and preclinical data is now available for many other diseases for some promising vaccines human clinical trials are also underway. For tick-borne diseases, there are a few examples where mRNA vaccines have been tested using the genes of pathogen origin (and not the tick), such as mRNA vaccine encoding the Powassan virus (tick-transmitted) *prM* and *E* gene [113], and tick-borne encephalitis virus Capsid protein C [114]. Recently, we have developed an mRNA vaccine consisting of tick saliva antigens that can block blood feeding ability of ticks and causes tick rejection [115].

10.7 An mRNA Vaccine Against Ticks

After repeated exposure to ticks, animals develop acquired resistance to tick, bites a phenomenon that is described as "tick immunity." This was first observed in 1939 by Trager [116]. Acquired resistance to *I. scapularis* is mostly observed in animals such as guinea pigs, rabbits, and cows, as well as in humans. These host species are not essential in the natural life cycle of *I. scapularis.* People who gained immunity to tick bites show dermal hypersensitivity following the bite of *I. scapularis* [117]. Acquiring tick immunity in guinea pigs can also restrict the tick's ability to spread *B. burgdorferi* [118].

It has been shown that naturally acquired tick resistance is related to the host's ability to mount robust immune responses against tick salivary gland antigens that are secreted by a tick during bite and present in saliva and cement. Tick salivary proteins play an important role in blood feeding, and many of these proteins have functional properties that can influence host immune responses, inflammation, and coagulation. Immunization with tick saliva led to a substantial degree of tick rejection in two to three days, which indicates that salivary components play a direct role in tick immunity. In addition, immunization with tick salivary antigens such as sialostatin L2, provide diminished tick feeding and detachment. Immunization with a combination of two salivary proteins, tick lectin pathway inhibitor (TSLPI) and Salp14 provided modest rejection in tick attachment [119].

There are primarily three challenges in developing a vaccine that can mimic tick immunity. First is to identify the optimum number of antigens that can provide robust immunity, second is to determine the adjuvant or vaccine platform that can increase the host response against these antigens, and third is to develop a robust model system that closely resembles tick bite in humans and can be used to screen different combinations in time, cost-efficient manner. We have selected several candidate antigens that are involved in tick feeding or that were shown to be part of the tick sialome to develop a cocktail of 19 salivary antigens using the mRNA lipid nanoparticle (mRNA–LNP) platform. Most of these antigens are shown to be highly immunogenic and, in many cases, their functional effect was known. Lipid nanoparticles (LNPs; I9ISP) that encapsulated mRNAs encoding the selected 19 *I. scapularis* proteins with modified nucleosides were used. The advantage to use this platform is it ensures *in vivo* delivery and protects mRNA from degradation.

In the first experiments, it was assessed if I9ISP-LNP (lipid-nanoparticle–containing nucleoside-modified mRNAs encoding 19 *I. scapularis* salivary proteins) can affect the *I. scapularis* ability to feed on a host and thereby prevent *B. burgdorferi* infection [115]. The primary animal model used in this study was guinea pigs.

When 19ISP mRNA vaccine immunized guinea pigs were challenged with *I. scapularis* they developed erythema at the bite site shortly after ticks began to attach, which indicates early response by host immunity. Further, in 19ISP-vaccinated guinea pigs and not in control animal's, ticks detach much earlier. Engorgement weights of ticks collected from 19ISP vaccinated Guinea pigs were also decreased. More importantly, 19ISP immunization in the guinea pigs also decreases overall *B. burgdorferi* transmission. The early induction of local immune response in the skin within 12 h of tick attachment may have affected the tick's ability to feed on the animals. These results also suggest that 19ISP is a promising direction in which arthropod vaccines can be developed either to be used alone in the future or in conjunction with traditional pathogen-based vaccines for the prevention of tick-borne diseases.

10.8 Powassan Vaccine

Powassan virus is a tick-borne infection that has recently gained attention due to the increase in cases and severity of the disease [120]. Powassan virus is a flavivirus that derives its name from Powassan in Canada. The virus was first isolated in 1958 from the brain of a child who died of encephalitis [121]. In the United States, most incidences occur in the northeast and Great Lakes regions from late spring through the mid-fall season. Powassan virus infection can lead to severe or even fatal neuroinvasive diseases that include infection of the brain (encephalitis) or the membranes around the brain and spinal cord (meningitis).

The outcome of severe Powassan disease can be fatal for about 10% of people. About 50% of people who survive severe disease suffer from long-term neurological sequelae such as recurring headaches and memory problems [44, 47, 48, 120]. Based on geographical and host associations, two genetic lineages of the Powassan virus are evident in North America. Powassan virus lineage I strains are present in *Ixodes cookei* ticks and whereas lineage II strains are present in *I. scapularis*. The two lineages share a strong identity in the amino acid sequence level of envelope (E) proteins and further are also serologically and clinically similar [122]. Since there are no approved vaccines for the Powassan virus and the looming threat of the Powassan epidemic prompted VanBlargan et al. to design an mRNA vaccine against this virus [113]. The vaccine uses a LNP-encapsulated modified mRNA encoding the structural premembrane (prM) protein of the Powassan virus and E protein genes. This is based on their strategy against other viruses that indicates co-expression of prM, and E proteins leads to the secretion of subviral particles that mimic virions and are capable of eliciting neutralizing antibody response in the host. LNP-encapsulated Powassan vaccine that contains modified mRNAs that encode the prM-E of the Powassan virus can induce robust antibody response in mice [113]. More importantly, this vaccine protects against Powassan virus strains of both lineages. Other than protecting against the Powassan virus this vaccine also induced cross-neutralizing antibodies against other tick-borne flaviviruses and even protects mice against the Langat virus which is distantly related to the Powassan virus [113]. Overall, this study shows an example of the power of the mRNA vaccine in developing an efficacious vaccine indicating the vaccine leads to the induction of cross-neutralization antibody response against other tick-borne flaviviruses.

10.9 RNA Vaccine Against Crimean–Congo Hemorrhagic Fever Virus

A tick-borne RNA bunyavirus, CCHFV is listed as a high-priority pathogen for the development of antiviral countermeasures by the World Health Organization lists [123]. The main reservoir of this virus is *Hyalomma* genus ticks and cases are prevalent in parts of Europe, Africa, and Asia [124]. Following the bite of infected ticks, the infected individual shows febrile illness with symptoms including sudden fever, myalgia, diarrhea, nausea, and vomiting. The disease symptoms in the hemorrhagic phase include severe bruising and uncontrolled bleeding and among patients who are hospitalized the fatality rates can be up to 50% [125]. At present, there is no efficacious vaccine or therapeutic available against this disease. This tri-segmented RNA virus belongs to the *Nairoviridae family. The* small genomic segment of the virus encodes the nucleoprotein (NP), the medium encodes the glycoprotein precursor (GPC), and the large segment encodes the viral RNA-dependent RNA-polymerase. The two antigens GPC and NP are considered prime target for vaccine development and studies have been performed to evaluate the efficacy of either individual or dual antigens with varied results. NP and GPC can induce antibody and T-cell responses, and studies have shown that NP is more conserved among diverse CCHFV strains. Recently, CCHFV antigens NP or GPC efficacy was evaluated in a novel alphavirus-based replicon RNA (repRNA) vaccine platform [126]. The Replicon-based RNA vaccine platform is shown to be advantageous for its ability to stimulate host innate immunity as well as mimic viral infection. In a recent study, CCHFV specific vaccine is developed using the repRNAs platform. A low-dose repRNAs could elicit robust CCHFV-specific B- and CD8+ T-cell responses in only a single dose [126]. Further, this repRNA vaccine protects mice when challenged with another divergent CCHFV strain. Since this vaccine had two antigens, the study further shows the vaccine-related protection was mediated mostly through the NP antigen and the immune response to GPC antigen plays role in improving viral infection [126]. When the vaccine was given to immune-deficient mice it was clear that vaccine-induced humoral response protects mice from the disease. Overall results show this repRNA vaccine platform could be used to develop the CCHFV vaccine.

10.10 Conclusions

Vaccines are one of the most effective healthcare prevention measures that have been developed. In the eighteenth century, diseases such as smallpox, typhus, cholera, plague, yellow fever, and scarlet fever caused epidemics that killed millions of people throughout the world. In the next two centuries, widespread vaccination efforts led to the eradication of the smallpox virus while numerous lives were saved from infectious disease-related illnesses every year. Early vaccines were mostly attenuated or inactivated pathogens. Advances in vaccinology led to the development of subunit vaccines, e.g. toxoids or surface antigens. There are still many other diseases for which vaccine development remains challenging [127]. Another issue is the delivery of cost-effective vaccines in resource limited regions. For *Plasmodium* which cause malaria, and are transmitted by Anopheles mosquitoes, mosquitoes are being considered for vaccine delivery [128–130]. As an example, transgenic mosquitoes can deliver an anti-*Plasmodium falciparum* circumsporozoite protein

(PfCSP) single-chain antibody into a host's skin during a mosquito bite. Delivery of specific antibodies that bind to the circumsporozoite protein on the surface of the *Plasmodium sporoczoite* can reduce the infectivity of transgenic mosquitoes. Therefore, mosquito-specific expression of malaria vaccine candidates could be a unique strategy for block transmission of *Plasmodium*, however, much more research is required to evaluate the potential of such strategies in human field studies. Similarly, future attempts can be made to create genetically modified ticks that can deliver vaccines against tick-borne pathogens.

As the incidence of tick-borne diseases is on the rise, two kinds of vaccine development efforts are going in parallel. First approach focuses on pathogen-specific vaccine and second approach provide broad umbrella protection from tick bite and ability of ticks to transmit pathogens. This approach is based on the fact that tick saliva plays important role in blood feeding [83, 90, 91, 131–133] and in assisting pathogen transmission [18, 134, 135]. Advances in mRNA vaccine technology provide a major advance in new generation vaccines that target specific antigens expressed by pathogens or ticks. Initial results with mRNA LNP multiantigen vaccine are promising. Reductionist approaches will help in identifying minimum number of antigens required to recapitulate tick immunity [93, 119, 136]. Therefore, development of mRNA vaccines consisting of microbial or salivary antigens that play major role in feeding and transmission is key strategy to control multiple tick-transmitted diseases.

References

1 Doherty, M. and Robertson, M.J. (2004). Some early trends in immunology. *Trends Immunol.* 25: 623–631.

2 Messina, N.L., Zimmermann, P., and Curtis, N. (2019). The impact of vaccines on heterologous adaptive immunity. *Clin. Microbiol. Infect.* 25: 1484–1493.

3 Dorner, T. and Radbruch, A. (2007). Antibodies and B cell memory in viral immunity. *Immunity* 27: 384–392.

4 Seder, R.A. and Hill, A.V. (2000). Vaccines against intracellular infections requiring cellular immunity. *Nature* 406: 793–798.

5 Li, G., Teleki, C., and Wang, T. (2018). Memory T cells in flavivirus vaccination. *Vaccines (Basel)* 6: 73.

6 Blom, K., Cuapio, A., Sandberg, J.T. et al. (2018). Cell-mediated immune responses and immunopathogenesis of human tick-borne encephalitis virus-infection. *Front. Immunol.* 9: 2174.

7 Ohta, T., Yoshikawa, S., Tabakawa, Y. et al. (2017). Skin CD4(+) memory T cells play an essential role in acquired anti-tick immunity through interleukin-3-mediated basophil recruitment to tick-feeding sites. *Front. Immunol.* 8: 1348.

8 Poljak, A., Comstedt, P., Hanner, M. et al. (2012). Identification and characterization of *Borrelia* antigens as potential vaccine candidates against Lyme borreliosis. *Vaccine* 30: 4398–4406.

9 Ishii, N., Isogai, E., Isogai, H. et al. (1995). T cell response to *Borrelia garinii*, *Borrelia afzelii*, and *Borrelia japonica* in various congenic mouse strains. *Microbiol. Immunol.* 39: 929–935.

10 Barthold, S.W. (1993). Antigenic stability of *Borrelia burgdorferi* during chronic infections of immunocompetent mice. *Infect. Immun.* 61: 4955–4961.

11 Doritchamou, J., Teo, A., Morrison, R. et al. (2019). Functional antibodies against placental malaria parasites are variant dependent and differ by geographic region. *Infect. Immun.* 87: e00865-18.

12 Arora, G., Hart, G.T., Manzella-Lapeira, J. et al. (2018). NK cells inhibit *Plasmodium falciparum* growth in red blood cells via antibody-dependent cellular cytotoxicity. *elife* 7: e36806.

13 Arora, G., Lynn, G.E., Tang, X. et al. (2022). CD55 facilitates immune evasion by *Borrelia crocidurae*, an agent of relapsing fever. *MBio* 13: e0116122.

14 Dieng, M.M., Diawara, A., Manikandan, V. et al. (2020). Integrative genomic analysis reveals mechanisms of immune evasion in *P. falciparum* malaria. *Nat. Commun.* 11: 5093.

15 Ngono, A.E. and Shresta, S. (2018). Immune response to dengue and zika. *Annu. Rev. Immunol.* 36: 279–308.

16 Deitsch, K.W., Lukehart, S.A., and Stringer, J.R. (2009). Common strategies for antigenic variation by bacterial, fungal and protozoan pathogens. *Nat. Rev. Microbiol.* 7: 493–503.

17 Couret, J., Schofield, S., and Narasimhan, S. (2022). The environment, the tick, and the pathogen - It is an ensemble. *Front. Cell. Infect. Microbiol.* 12: 1049646.

18 Embers, M.E. and Narasimhan, S. (2013). Vaccination against Lyme disease: past, present, and future. *Front. Cell. Infect. Microbiol.* 3: 6.

19 Gratz, N.G. (1999). Emerging and resurging vector-borne diseases. *Annu. Rev. Entomol.* 44: 51–75.

20 Ribeiro, J.M. (1987). Role of saliva in blood-feeding by arthropods. *Annu. Rev. Entomol.* 32: 463–478.

21 Arora, G., Tang, X., Cui, Y. et al. (2024). mosGILT controls innate immunity and germ cell development in *Anopheles gambiae*. *BMC Genomics* 25: 42.

22 van Vuuren, M. and Penzhorn, B.L. (2015). Geographic range of vector-borne infections and their vectors: the role of African wildlife. *Rev. Sci. Tech.* 34: 139–149.

23 Rana, V.S., Kitsou, C., Dumler, J.S., and Pal, U. (2023). Immune evasion strategies of major tick-transmitted bacterial pathogens. *Trends Microbiol.* 31: 62–75.

24 Pal, U., Kitsou, C., Drecktrah, D. et al. (2021). Interactions between ticks and Lyme disease spirochetes. *Curr. Issues Mol. Biol.* 42: 113–144.

25 Eisen, L. (2020). Vector competence studies with hard ticks and *Borrelia burgdorferi sensu lato* spirochetes: a review. *Ticks Tick Borne Dis.* 11: 101359.

26 Hovius, J.W., van Dam, A.P., and Fikrig, E. (2007). Tick-host-pathogen interactions in Lyme borreliosis. *Trends Parasitol.* 23: 434–438.

27 Anguita, J., Hedrick, M.N., and Fikrig, E. (2003). Adaptation of *Borrelia burgdorferi* in the tick and the mammalian host. *FEMS Microbiol. Rev.* 27: 493–504.

28 Pal, U. and Fikrig, E. (2003). Adaptation of *Borrelia burgdorferi* in the vector and vertebrate host. *Microbes Infect.* 5: 659–666.

29 Gupta, A., Arora, G., Rosen, C.E. et al. (2020). A human secretome library screen reveals a role for peptidoglycan recognition protein 1 in Lyme borreliosis. *PLoS Pathog.* 16: e1009030.

30 Liu, L., Dai, J., Zhao, Y.O. et al. (2012). *Ixodes scapularis* JAK-STAT pathway regulates tick antimicrobial peptides, thereby controlling the agent of human granulocytic anaplasmosis. *J. Infect. Dis.* 206: 1233–1241.

31 Naimi, W.A., Green, R.S., Cockburn, C.L., and Carlyon, J.A. (2018). Differential susceptibility of male versus female laboratory mice to *Anaplasma phagocytophilum* infection. *Trop. Med. Infect. Dis.* 3: 78.

32 Rocha, S.C., Velasquez, C.V., Aquib, A. et al. (2022). Transmission cycle of tick-borne infections and co-infections, animal models and diseases. *Pathogens* 11: 1309.

33 Seidman, D., Ojogun, N., Walker, N.J. et al. (2014). *Anaplasma phagocytophilum* surface protein AipA mediates invasion of mammalian host cells. *Cell. Microbiol.* 16: 1133–1145.

34 Sukumaran, B., Narasimhan, S., Anderson, J.F. et al. (2006). An *Ixodes scapularis* protein required for survival of *Anaplasma phagocytophilum* in tick salivary glands. *J. Exp. Med.* 203: 1507–1517.

35 Hodzic, E., Fish, D., Maretzki, C.M. et al. (1998). Acquisition and transmission of the agent of human granulocytic ehrlichiosis by *Ixodes scapularis* ticks. *J. Clin. Microbiol.* 36: 3574–3578.

36 Hodzic, E., Ijdo, J.W., Feng, S. et al. (1998). Granulocytic ehrlichiosis in the laboratory mouse. *J. Infect. Dis.* 177: 737–745.

37 Daniels, T.J., Falco, R.C., Schwartz, I. et al. (1997). Deer ticks (*Ixodes scapularis*) and the agents of Lyme disease and human granulocytic ehrlichiosis in a New York City park. *Emerg. Infect. Dis.* 3: 353–355.

38 Des Vignes, F. and Fish, D. (1997). Transmission of the agent of human granulocytic ehrlichiosis by host-seeking *Ixodus scapularis* (Acari: *Ixodidae*) in southern New York state. *J. Med. Entomol.* 34: 379–382.

39 Voss, O.H., Cobb, J., Gaytan, H. et al. (2022). Pathogenic, but Not Nonpathogenic, *Rickettsia* spp. evade inflammasome-dependent IL-1 responses to establish an intracytosolic replication niche. *MBio* 13: e0291821.

40 Noguchi, H. (1926). Cultivation of *Rickettsia*-like microorganisms from the Rocky Mountain spotted fever tick, *Dermacentor andersoni*. *J. Exp. Med.* 43: 515–532.

41 Heinze, D.M., Carmical, J.R., Aronson, J.F. et al. (2014). Murine cutaneous responses to the Rocky Mountain spotted fever vector, *Dermacentor andersoni*, feeding. *Front. Microbiol.* 5: 198.

42 Burgdorfer, W. (1969). Ecology of tick vectors of American spotted fever. *Bull. World Health Organ.* 40: 375–381.

43 Feder, H.M., Telford, S., Goethert, H.K., and Wormser, G.P. (2021). Powassan virus encephalitis following brief attachment of Connecticut deer ticks. *Clin. Infect. Dis.* 73: e2350–e2354.

44 Campbell, O. and Krause, P.J. (2020). The emergence of human Powassan virus infection in North America. *Ticks Tick Borne Dis.* 11: 101540.

45 Koester, T.M., Timothy, P., Meece, J.K. et al. (2020). Suspected neuro-invasive Powassan virus infection in a pediatric patient. *Clin. Med. Res.* 18: 95–98.

46 Kemenesi, G. and Banyai, K. (2019). Tick-borne flaviviruses, with a focus on Powassan virus. *Clin. Microbiol. Rev.* 32: e00106-17.

47 Hermance, M.E. and Thangamani, S. (2017). Powassan virus: an emerging arbovirus of public health concern in North America. *Vector Borne Zoonotic Dis.* 17: 453–462.

48 Ebel, G.D. (2010). Update on Powassan virus: emergence of a North American tick-borne flavivirus. *Annu. Rev. Entomol.* 55: 95–110.

49 Padgett, K.A., Kjemtrup, A., Novak, M. et al. (2022). Colorado tick fever virus in the far west: forgotten, but not gone. *Vector Borne Zoonotic Dis.* 22: 443–448.

50 Kadkhoda, K., Semus, M., Jelic, T., and Walkty, A. (2018). Case report: a case of Colorado tick fever acquired in Southwestern Saskatchewan. *Am. J. Trop. Med. Hyg.* 98: 891–893.

51 Burgdorfer, W. (1977). Tick-borne diseases in the United States: Rocky Mountain spotted fever and Colorado tick fever. A review. *Acta Trop.* 34: 103–126.

52 Savage, H.M., Burkhalter, K.L., Godsey, M.S. Jr. et al. (2017). Bourbon virus in field-collected ticks, Missouri, USA. *Emerg. Infect. Dis.* 23: 2017–2022.

53 Lambert, A.J., Velez, J.O., Brault, A.C. et al. (2015). Molecular, serological and in vitro culture-based characterization of Bourbon virus, a newly described human pathogen of the genus Thogotovirus. *J. Clin. Virol.* 73: 127–132.

54 Kosoy, O.I., Lambert, A.J., Hawkinson, D.J. et al. (2015). Novel Thogotovirus associated with febrile illness and death, United States, 2014. *Emerg. Infect. Dis.* 21: 760–764.

55 Savage, H.M., Godsey, M.S. Jr., Panella, N.A. et al. (2018). Surveillance for tick-borne viruses near the location of a fatal human case of bourbon virus (family Orthomyxoviridae: genus thogotovirus) in Eastern Kansas, 2015. *J. Med. Entomol.* 55: 701–705.

56 Lopez, J., Hovius, J.W., and Bergstrom, S. (2021). Pathogenesis of relapsing fever. *Curr. Issues Mol. Biol.* 42: 519–550.

57 Cutler, S.J. (2015). Relapsing fever Borreliae: a global review. *Clin. Lab. Med.* 35: 847–865.

58 Dworkin, M.S., Schwan, T.G., Anderson, D.E. Jr., and Borchardt, S.M. (2008). Tick-borne relapsing fever. *Infect. Dis. Clin. North Am.* 22: 449–468, viii.

59 Almazan, C., Scimeca, R.C., Reichard, M.V., and Mosqueda, J. (2022). Babesiosis and theileriosis in North America. *Pathogens* 11: 168.

60 Scoles, G.A., Lohmeyer, K.H., Ueti, M.W. et al. (2021). Stray Mexico origin cattle captured crossing into Southern Texas carry *Babesia bovis* and other tick-borne pathogens. *Ticks Tick Borne Dis.* 12: 101708.

61 Telionis, A., Lahmers, K., Todd, M. et al. (2022). Distribution of *Theileria orientalis* in Virginia Market Cattle, 2018-2020. *Pathogens* 11: 1353.

62 Zhang, Y., Li, Z., Pang, Z. et al. (2022). Identification of Jingmen tick virus (JMTV) in *Amblyomma testudinarium* from Fujian Province, southeastern China. *Parasit. Vectors* 15: 339.

63 Pang, Z., Jin, Y., Pan, M. et al. (2022). Geographical distribution and phylogenetic analysis of Jingmen tick virus in China. *iScience* 25: 105007.

64 Guo, J.J., Lin, X.D., Chen, Y.M. et al. (2020). Diversity and circulation of Jingmen tick virus in ticks and mammals. *Virus Evol.* 6: veaa051.

65 Phipps, L.P. and Johnson, N. (2022). Tick-borne encephalitis virus. *J. Med. Microbiol.* 71: https://doi.org/10.1099/jmm.0.001492.

66 Kaiser, R. (2008). Tick-borne encephalitis. *Infect. Dis. Clin. North Am.* 22: 561–575, x.

67 Gustafson, R. (1994). Epidemiological studies of Lyme borreliosis and tick-borne encephalitis. *Scand. J. Infect. Dis. Suppl.* 92: 1–63.

68 Kozuch, O., Labuda, M., Lysy, J. et al. (1990). Longitudinal study of natural foci of Central European encephalitis virus in West Slovakia. *Acta Virol.* 34: 537–544.

69 Work, T.H. (1963). Tick-borne viruses. A review of an arthropod-borne virus problem of growing importance in the tropics. *Bull. World Health Organ.* 29: 59–74.

70 Aziati, I.D., Jnr, D.M., Antia, A. et al. (2023). Prevalence of Bourbon and Heartland viruses in field collected ticks at an environmental field station in St. Louis County, Missouri, USA. *Ticks Tick Borne Dis.* 14: 102080.

71 Savage, H.M., Godscy, M.S. Jr., Tatman, J. et al. (2018). Surveillance for Heartland and Bourbon viruses in Eastern Kansas, June 2016. *J. Med. Entomol.* 55: 1613–1616.

72 Savage, H.M., Godsey, M.S. Jr., Panella, N.A. et al. (2016). Surveillance for Heartland virus (Bunyaviridae: Phlebovirus) in Missouri during 2013: first detection of virus in adults of *Amblyomma americanum* (Acari: *Ixodidae*). *J. Med. Entomol.* 53: 607–612.

73 Mhamadi, M., Badji, A., Dieng, I. et al. (2022). Crimean-Congo hemorrhagic fever virus survey in humans, ticks, and livestock in agnam (Northeastern Senegal) from February 2021 to March 2022. *Trop. Med. Infect. Dis.* 7: 324.

74 Emmerich, P., Jakupi, X., von Possel, R. et al. (2018). Viral metagenomics, genetic and evolutionary characteristics of Crimean-Congo hemorrhagic fever orthonairovirus in humans, Kosovo. *Infect. Genet. Evol.* 65: 6–11.

75 Mhamadi, M., Badji, A., Dieng, I. et al. (2022). Multiple genotypes of Crimean-Congo hemorrhagic fever virus detected in ticks during a one health survey in Agnam, Northeastern Senegal. *Emerg. Microbes Infect.* 11: 2711–2714.

76 Parola, P., Paddock, C.D., and Raoult, D. (2005). Tick-borne rickettsioses around the world: emerging diseases challenging old concepts. *Clin. Microbiol. Rev.* 18: 719–756.

77 Beati, L. and Klompen, H. (2019). Phylogeography of ticks (Acari: *Ixodida*). *Annu. Rev. Entomol.* 64: 379–397.

78 Rosenberg, R., Lindsey, N., Fischer, M. et al. (2018). Vital Signs: Trends in Reported Vectorborne Disease Cases — United States and Territories, 2004–2016. *Morb. Mortal. Wkly Rep.* 67: 496–501.

79 Eisen, R.J. and Eisen, L. (2018). The blacklegged tick, *Ixodes scapularis*: an increasing public health concern. *Trends Parasitol.* 34: 295–309.

80 Eisen, R.J., Eisen, L., and Beard, C.B. (2016). County-scale distribution of *Ixodes scapularis* and *Ixodes pacificus* (Acari: *Ixodidae*) in the continental United States. *J. Med. Entomol.* 53: 349–386.

81 Wikel, S. (2013). Ticks and tick-borne pathogens at the cutaneous interface: host defenses, tick countermeasures, and a suitable environment for pathogen establishment. *Front. Microbiol.* 4: 337.

82 Kazimirova, M. and Stibraniova, I. (2013). Tick salivary compounds: their role in modulation of host defences and pathogen transmission. *Front. Cell. Infect. Microbiol.* 3: 43.

83 Ribeiro, J.M. and Francischetti, I.M. (2003). Role of arthropod saliva in blood feeding: sialome and post-sialome perspectives. *Annu. Rev. Entomol.* 48: 73–88.

84 Perner, J., Kropackova, S., Kopacek, P., and Ribeiro, J.M.C. (2018). Sialome diversity of ticks revealed by RNAseq of single tick salivary glands. *PLoS Negl. Trop. Dis.* 12: e0006410.

85 Kim, T.K., Tirloni, L., Pinto, A.F. et al. (2016). *Ixodes scapularis* tick saliva proteins sequentially secreted every 24 h during blood feeding. *PLoS Negl. Trop. Dis.* 10: e0004323.

86 Francischetti, I.M., Sa-Nunes, A., Mans, B.J. et al. (2009). The role of saliva in tick feeding. *Front. Biosci. (Landmark Ed.)* 14: 2051–2088.

87 Mulenga, A., Sugimoto, C., and Onuma, M. (2000). Issues in tick vaccine development: identification and characterization of potential candidate vaccine antigens. *Microbes Infect.* 2: 1353–1361.

88 Nuttall, P.A. (2019). Wonders of tick saliva. *Ticks Tick Borne Dis.* 10: 470–481.

89 Kim, T.K., Tirloni, L., Pinto, A.F.M. et al. (2020). Time-resolved proteomic profile of *Amblyomma americanum* tick saliva during feeding. *PLoS Negl. Trop. Dis.* 14: e0007758.

90 Lynn, G.E., Cerny, J., Kurokawa, C. et al. (2022). Immunization of guinea pigs with cement extract induces resistance against *Ixodes scapularis* ticks. *Ticks Tick Borne Dis.* 13: 102017.

91 Cerny, J., Lynn, G., DePonte, K. et al. (2020). Fractionation of tick saliva reveals proteins associated with the development of acquired resistance to *Ixodes scapularis*. *Vaccine* 38: 8121–8129.

92 Ramamoorthi, N., Narasimhan, S., Pal, U. et al. (2005). The Lyme disease agent exploits a tick protein to infect the mammalian host. *Nature* 436: 573–577.

93 Narasimhan, S., Kurokawa, C., DeBlasio, M. et al. (2021). Acquired tick resistance: the trail is hot. *Parasite Immunol.* 43: e12808.

94 Tang, X., Arora, G., Matias, J. et al. (2022). A tick C1q protein alters infectivity of the Lyme disease agent by modulating interferon gamma. *Cell Rep.* 41: 111673.

95 Cao, Y., Rosen, C., Arora, G. et al. (2020). An *Ixodes scapularis* protein disulfide isomerase contributes to *Borrelia burgdorferi* colonization of the vector. *Infect. Immun.* 88: e00426-20.

96 Arora, G., Sajid, A., Chuang, Y.M. et al. (2021). Immunomodulation by mosquito salivary protein AgSAP contributes to early host infection by *Plasmodium. MBio* 12: e0309121.

97 Fikrig, E., Barthold, S.W., Kantor, F.S., and Flavell, R.A. (1990). Protection of mice against the Lyme disease agent by immunizing with recombinant OspA. *Science* 250: 553–556.

98 Schaible, U.E., Kramer, M.D., Eichmann, K. et al. (1990). Monoclonal antibodies specific for the outer surface protein A (OspA) of *Borrelia burgdorferi* prevent Lyme borreliosis in severe combined immunodeficiency (scid) mice. *Proc. Natl. Acad. Sci. U. S. A.* 87: 3768–3772.

99 Gomes-Solecki, M. (2014). Blocking pathogen transmission at the source: reservoir targeted OspA-based vaccines against *Borrelia burgdorferi. Front. Cell. Infect. Microbiol.* 4: 136.

100 Fikrig, E., Barthold, S.W., Kantor, F.S., and Flavell, R.A. (1992). Long-term protection of mice from Lyme disease by vaccination with OspA. *Infect. Immun.* 60: 773–777.

101 Fikrig, E., Barthold, S.W., Kantor, F.S., and Flavell, R.A. (1991). Protection of mice from Lyme borreliosis by oral vaccination with Escherichia coli expressing OspA. *J. Infect. Dis.* 164: 1224–1227.

102 Steere, A.C., Sikand, V.K., Meurice, F. et al. (1998). Vaccination against Lyme disease with recombinant *Borrelia burgdorferi* outer-surface lipoprotein A with adjuvant. Lyme Disease Vaccine Study Group. *N. Engl. J. Med.* 339: 209–215.

103 Carpenter, A., Waltenburg, M.A., Hall, A. et al. (2022). Vaccine preventable zoonotic diseases: challenges and opportunities for public health progress. *Vaccines (Basel)* 10: 993.

104 Wressnigg, N., Pollabauer, E.M., Aichinger, G. et al. (2013). Safety and immunogenicity of a novel multivalent OspA vaccine against Lyme borreliosis in healthy adults: a double-blind, randomised, dose-escalation phase 1/2 trial. *Lancet Infect. Dis.* 13: 680–689.

105 Dantas-Torres, F. and Otranto, D. (2016). Best practices for preventing vector-borne diseases in dogs and humans. *Trends Parasitol.* 32: 43–55.

106 Pardi, N., Hogan, M.J., Porter, F.W., and Weissman, D. (2018). mRNA vaccines - a new era in vaccinology. *Nat. Rev. Drug Discov.* 17: 261–279.

107 Wolff, J.A., Malone, R.W., Williams, P. et al. (1990). Direct gene transfer into mouse muscle in vivo. *Science* 247: 1465–1468.

108 Jung, H.N., Lee, S.Y., Lee, S. et al. (2022). Lipid nanoparticles for delivery of RNA therapeutics: current status and the role of in vivo imaging. *Theranostics* 12: 7509–7531.

109 Pardi, N., Tuyishime, S., Muramatsu, H. et al. (2015). Expression kinetics of nucleoside-modified mRNA delivered in lipid nanoparticles to mice by various routes. *J. Control. Release* 217: 345–351.

110 Cai, C., Peng, Y., Shen, E. et al. (2021). A comprehensive analysis of the efficacy and safety of COVID-19 vaccines. *Mol. Ther.* 29: 2794–2805.

111 Deplanque, D. and Launay, O. (2021). Efficacy of COVID-19 vaccines: from clinical trials to real life. *Therapie* 76: 277–283.

112 Baden, L.R., El Sahly, H.M., Essink, B. et al. (2021). Efficacy and safety of the mRNA-1273 SARS-CoV-2 vaccine. *N. Engl. J. Med.* 384: 403–416.

113 VanBlargan, L.A., Himansu, S., Foreman, B.M. et al. (2018). An mRNA vaccine protects mice against multiple tick-transmitted flavivirus infections. *Cell Rep.* 25: 3382–3392 e3383.

114 Aberle, J.H., Aberle, S.W., Kofler, R.M., and Mandl, C.W. (2005). Humoral and cellular immune response to RNA immunization with flavivirus replicons derived from tick-borne encephalitis virus. *J. Virol.* 79: 15107–15113.

115 Sajid, A., Matias, J., Arora, G. et al. (2021). mRNA vaccination induces tick resistance and prevents transmission of the Lyme disease agent. *Sci. Transl. Med.* 13: eabj9827.

116 Trager, W. (1939). Acquired immunity to ticks. *J. Parasitol.* 25: 57–81.

117 Burke, G., Wikel, S.K., Spielman, A. et al. (2005). Hypersensitivity to ticks and Lyme disease risk. *Emerg. Infect. Dis.* 11: 36–41.

118 Nazario, S., Das, S., de Silva, A.M. et al. (1998). Prevention of *Borrelia burgdorferi* transmission in guinea pigs by tick immunity. *Am. J. Trop. Med. Hyg.* 58: 780–785.

119 Matias, J., Kurokawa, C., Sajid, A. et al. (2021). Tick immunity using mRNA, DNA and protein-based Salp14 delivery strategies. *Vaccine* 39: 7661–7668.

120 Anonymous. Centers for Disease Control and Prevention, National Center for Emerging and Zoonotic Infectious Diseases (NCEZID), Division of Vector-Borne Diseases (DVBD). https://www.cdc.gov/powassan/index.html (accessed 11 January 2024).

121 Mc, L.D. and Donohue, W.L. (1959). Powassan virus: isolation of virus from a fatal case of encephalitis. *Can. Med. Assoc. J.* 80: 708–711.

122 Ebel, G.D., Spielman, A., and Telford, S.R. (2001). Phylogeny of North American Powassan virus. *J. Gen. Virol.* 82: 1657–1665.

123 Dai, S., Deng, F., Wang, H., and Ning, Y. (2021). Crimean-Congo hemorrhagic fever virus: current advances and future prospects of antiviral strategies. *Viruses* 13: 1195.

124 Portillo, A., Palomar, A.M., Santibanez, P., and Oteo, J.A. (2021). Epidemiological aspects of Crimean-Congo hemorrhagic fever in Western Europe: what about the future? *Microorganisms* 9: 649.

125 Niazi, A.U., Jawad, M.J., Amirnajad, A. et al. (2019). Crimean-Congo hemorrhagic fever, Herat Province, Afghanistan, 2017. *Emerg. Infect. Dis.* 25: 1596–1598.

126 Leventhal, S.S., Meade-White, K., Rao, D. et al. (2022). Replicating RNA vaccination elicits an unexpected immune response that efficiently protects mice against lethal Crimean-Congo hemorrhagic fever virus challenge. *EBioMedicine.* 82: 104188.

127 Arora, G., Chuang, Y.M., Sinnis, P. et al. (2023). Malaria: influence of Anopheles mosquito saliva on Plasmodium infection. *Trends Immunol.* 44: 256–265.

128 Sumitani, M., Kasashima, K., Yamamoto, D.S. et al. (2013). Reduction of malaria transmission by transgenic mosquitoes expressing an antisporozoite antibody in their salivary glands. *Insect Mol. Biol.* 22: 41–51.

129 Yamamoto, D.S., Sumitani, M., Nagumo, H. et al. (2012). Induction of antisporozoite antibodies by biting of transgenic *Anopheles stephensi* delivering malarial antigen via blood feeding. *Insect Mol. Biol.* 21: 223–233.

130 Matsuoka, H., Ikezawa, T., and Hirai, M. (2010). Production of a transgenic mosquito expressing circumsporozoite protein, a malarial protein, in the salivary gland of *Anopheles stephensi* (Diptera: *Culicidae*). *Acta Med. Okayama* 64: 233–241.

131 Narasimhan, S., Kurokawa, C., Diktas, H. et al. (2020). *Ixodes scapularis* saliva components that elicit responses associated with acquired tick-resistance. *Ticks Tick Borne Dis.* 11: 101369.

132 Kotal, J., Langhansova, H., Lieskovska, J. et al. (2015). Modulation of host immunity by tick saliva. *J. Proteome* 128: 58–68.

133 Hovius, J.W., Levi, M., and Fikrig, E. (2008). Salivating for knowledge: potential pharmacological agents in tick saliva. *PLoS Med.* 5: e43.

134 Simo, L., Kazimirova, M., Richardson, J., and Bonnet, S.I. (2017). The essential role of tick salivary glands and saliva in tick feeding and pathogen transmission. *Front. Cell. Infect. Microbiol.* 7: 281.

135 Nuttall, P.A. and Labuda, M. (2004). Tick-host interactions: saliva-activated transmission. *Parasitology* 129 (Suppl): S177–S189.

136 Murfin, K.E. and Fikrig, E. (2017). Tick bioactive molecules as novel therapeutics: beyond vaccine targets. *Front. Cell. Infect. Microbiol.* 7: 222.

11

mRNA Vaccines for Malaria and Other Parasitic Pathogens

Leroy Versteeg[1,2,3] *and Jeroen Pollet*[1,2]

[1] *Baylor College of Medicine, Section of Tropical Medicine, Department of Pediatrics, 1 Baylor Plaza, Houston, TX 77030, USA*
[2] *Texas Children's Hospital Center for Vaccine Development, 1102 Bates Ave, Suite 560, Houston, TX 77030, USA*
[3] *Wageningen University & Research, Cell Biology and Immunology Group, Department of Cell Biology and Immunology, De Elst 1, 6708 WD Wageningen, The Netherlands*

11.1 The Global Burden of Parasitic Pathogens

Parasitic infections are a major cause of morbidity and mortality rates in poverty-stricken regions of the (sub)tropics. Malaria is among the most studied parasite-induced diseases and is responsible for more than 400 000 deaths annually; however, many other lesser-known, and thus oftentimes neglected, diseases caused by protozoa and helminths are responsible for high morbidity rates among the *bottom-billion*, living in poverty worldwide (Table 11.1). Those living in underdeveloped rural areas, as well as the urban slums of predominantly low- and middle-income countries (LMICs), are among the most affected, due to the lack of access to clean drinking water, decent sanitation, adequate housing, and healthcare services. The burden of disease in these communities slows down economic development, perpetuating the cycle of poverty-associated disease burden.

The World Health Organization (WHO), together with multiple international aid organizations, have committed remarkable efforts to prevent, control, and even eliminate certain parasitic diseases [2]. For malaria and other mosquito-borne diseases, new strategies to improve vector control include increasing the delivery of insecticide-treated nets, improving chemical formulations for indoor spraying, and new interventions that target outdoor-biting mosquitoes. For helminthic diseases, there have been large programs of mass drug administration targeting multiple parasite infections simultaneously, combined with community-level transmission control measures. Despite some clear successes, the toll of parasitic diseases remains unacceptably high. While vector elimination and recurrent mass drug administration are often effective in achieving temporary control over parasitic diseases, they typically fail to prevent diseases from returning to communities in the long term, as they do not prevent reinfection [3–5]. For other parasitic diseases such

Trends in mRNA Vaccine Research, First Edition. Edited by Gabor Tamas Szabo and Norbert Pardi.

Table 11.1 Prevalence of the most common parasitic infections globally.

Disease	Prevalence[a)]	Affected regions[a)]	Clinical trials and vaccines approved[b)]
Global numbers on parasitic infections			
Protozoan diseases			
Plasmodium (malaria)	163–203 million	>100 countries in the tropics and subtropics	206 clinical trials completed, 2 approved (RTS, S [Mosquirix™], R21/Matrix-M)
Toxoplasmosis	40 million in the United States[c)]	Worldwide	No clinical trials completed
American trypanosomiasis (Chagas disease)	6–7 million	South and Central America	No clinical trials completed
Leishmaniasis (Kala-azar)	4–6 million	>90 countries in the tropics and subtropics	14 clinical trials completed, no vaccines approved
African trypanosomiasis (sleeping sickness)	2000–7000	36 countries in Sub-Sahara Africa	No clinical trials completed
Amoebiasis	500 million	Worldwide	No clinical trials completed
Intestinal helminth diseases			
Ascariasis (roundworm)	394–511 million	Worldwide	No clinical trials completed
Hookworm	159–187 million	Worldwide	Nine clinical trials completed, no vaccines approved
Trichuriasis (whipworm)	316–413 million	Worldwide	No clinical trials completed
Other helminth diseases			
Schistosomiasis (snail fever)	117–166 million	>70 countries in Africa, Asia, and South America	10 clinical trials completed, no vaccines approved
Lymphatic filariasis (elephantiasis)	59–96 million	49 countries in Africa, Asia, and South America	No clinical trials completed

Table 11.1 (Continued)

Disease	Prevalence[a)]	Affected regions[a)]	Clinical trials and vaccines approved[b)]
Strongyloidiasis (threadworm)	30–100 million[c)]	Tropics and subtropics	No clinical trials completed
Cysticercosis (taeniasis)	4–6 million	Worldwide	No clinical trials completed
Onchocerciasis (river blindness)	17–21 million	31 African countries in the tropics	No clinical trials completed

a) Data was obtained from the 2019 Global Burden of Disease, Institute for Health Metrics and Evaluation, University of Washington.
b) Sources: clinicaltrials.gov, trialsearch.who.int
c) Source: CDC.gov

as Chagas disease, leishmaniasis, and toxoplasmosis, the available antiparasitic drugs have severe side effects and they offer low protection to prevent the chronic disease, making mass drug administration risky and ineffective. Overall, there is an urgent need for low-cost, long-lasting, easy-to-administer solutions to mitigate the burden of tropical parasitic infection in underserved populations.

11.2 Challenges of Vaccine Development Against Parasitic Pathogens

Vaccines are a potentially lucrative therapeutic modality in addressing parasitic diseases; however, progress in developing vaccines for such pathogens has been slow and only a handful have been tested in clinical trials. Despite many decades of research, only a few vaccine candidates against parasitic infections have been picked up by pharmaceutical companies and tested in clinical trials (Table 11.1).

A major barrier to progress in development of vaccines for parasitic pathogens is the absence of an economic incentive, which limits the interest of multinational organizations in taking a lead in clinical development. However, the absence of financial incentives is not the sole reason why there are currently no vaccines available. Developing vaccines to effectively prevent or control parasitic diseases is extremely difficult from a technical perspective relative to development of vaccines targeting viral and bacterial pathogens [6, 7].

Traditional vaccine platforms like inactivated vaccines or live-attenuated vaccines have proven very successful against infectious diseases, such as smallpox, measles, diphtheria, and tetanus [8–11]. These types of vaccines induce predominantly a robust humoral response and are generally capable of neutralizing viruses and bacteria. However, establishing vaccine-induced protection against parasites presents additional challenges.

Parasites are much more complex organisms than viruses or bacteria. Viruses typically only have a few dozen genes, while some parasites have more than 5000 genes that can comprise complex multigene families [12]. These genes can selectively be expressed depending on the parasitic life stage or based on the host they reside in Ref. [13]. Furthermore, parasites have learned to adapt to their hosts' immune defenses and can have longer host interactions, causing chronic infections. To evade the host's natural immunity, parasites typically have multifaceted life cycles, with different forms and stages inside and outside the host. Many have vast repertoires of polymorphic proteins, which overwhelm the hosts' immune system with epitopes, thus reducing the effectiveness of parasite clearance. Also, parasites cover their surface with proteins expressing antigenic variation, preventing the antibodies secreted by the hosts' humoral immune response from recognizing the parasitic pathogens for opsonization. The protozoan *Trypanosoma cruzi*, for example, is coated by polymorphic surface mucins on its plasma membrane, enabling immune invasion and persistent infection [14]. Similarly, the surface of *Trypanosoma brucei* parasites is covered by variant surface glycoproteins, which help to elude the immune response and prevent lytic factors present in plasma from binding to the parasite [15]. Furthermore, various parasites secrete immune-modulating proteins, which can downregulate different parts of the immune system.

While most vaccines against viruses or bacteria rely primarily on the induction of single-antigen neutralizing and opsonizing antibodies, antibody-based protection does not work well against many eukaryotic parasites. Some parasites such as plasmodium or trypanosomes reside at least partially intracellularly. They have different ways of entering the cells, which makes neutralization of the cell entry hard to target. Furthermore, protection based on neutralizing antibodies is naturally not very long lived due to the loss of memory B-cell responses [16]. Other studies revealed that malaria might induce changes to dendritic cells, which decreases their capacity to support memory B-cell survival [17]. With the limitation of humoral immunity, the most effective way to target parasite-infected cells is by potent $CD8^+$ T-cell responses [11]. Effective vaccine formulations against parasitic infection therefore typically rely on a strong Th1-skewed immune response.

Parasites can escape natural immunity by modulating immune responses. People typically do not develop long-lasting natural immunity and are typically subject to reinfection. Consequently, vaccine-induced immunity will have to either outperform the natural immune response or restore the function of the natural immunity during infection. One strategy may be to block immune signals or include proteins to mimic signals absent during infection to reinstate immunity and accelerate clearance of the parasite [7]; however, the cost and difficulty of coformulating different antigens limit the feasibility of this approach currently.

Preclinical investigations are often limited for many parasitic diseases, as there are no suitable animal models that recapitulate the human condition. Several candidate vaccines that demonstrate excellent protection in preclinical studies ultimately fail to protect in later clinical studies [18]. For instance, in the realm of malaria, despite over 40 vaccine candidates undergoing examination – based on whole inactivated sporozoites or subunit antigens – in more than 200 clinical trials, nearly all have fallen short in delivering substantial protection [7]. Even RTS,S/AS01 (Mosquirix™, GlaxoSmithKline [GSK]), the first approved malaria vaccine, was found to provide only modest protection against both mild and severe malaria, especially in infants [19, 20]. Better results are achieved using the second WHO-approved malaria vaccine R21/Matrix-M [21], which showed protection up to 77% in children aged 5–17 months in a phase 2b study in Burkina Faso [22]. Although the vaccine exhibits much better efficacy, it still fails to break the infection circle as it does not hinder the transmission of gametocytes from infected humans to mosquitoes.

11.3 mRNA Technology to Accelerate the Development of Advanced Next-Generation Vaccines

Parasites are complex organisms that have been thriving in human hosts since the beginning of time. To date, not many effective vaccine solutions against parasites have been developed, debatably due to limitations of the current vaccine technologies. The mRNA vaccine platform has hallmark features that resolve certain technological limitations, which may accelerate the development of more advanced vaccine solutions against parasitic infections.

- *mRNA vaccine antigens are highly immunogenic*
- mRNA-based vaccines have the capacity to stimulate strong humoral (antibody) and cellular (T-cell) immunity, specifically directed toward the vaccine antigens [23]. Based on a side-by-side immunogenicity study of mRNA COVID-19 vaccines [20], RNA vaccines induced the highest levels of humoral and cellular responses followed by adenovirus vaccines and then by inactivated vaccines [24, 25]. Other studies demonstrated the superior cellular immune response elicited by mRNA compared to recombinant protein vaccines [26]. The immunogenicity of mRNA vaccine candidates can be regulated, for example, using various nucleoside modifications [27] as well as delivery methods. Typically, no supplementary adjuvants are required, but certain immunostimulants can be included with RNA formulations, to steer toward a desired immune response [28]. There are even mRNA-based adjuvants available that stimulate dendritic cells into increased activation of $CD4^+$ and $CD8^+$ T-cell responses [29]. Further technology improvements are ongoing to make the mRNA platform more efficient. Nucleoside modifications, specific untranslated regions (UTRs), and improved coding sequences can lead to enhanced immunogenicity. Many other groups are exploring the use of self-amplifying RNA or circular RNA to lower the required mRNA doses [30].
- *mRNA vaccine development and production are comparatively simple, scalable, and rapid.*
- A main feature of the mRNA platform is its standardized production process, allowing for the rapid development of newly identified vaccine candidates in only a few weeks. The value of increased development timelines is obvious for emerging diseases and has been demonstrated during the COVID-19 pandemic. However, this shorter development time may also be a key advantage in producing and testing large numbers of vaccine candidates for parasitic diseases. Many new

tools and assays have become available to search for new vaccine epitopes, such as *in silico* epitope prediction [31–33] and immunopeptidomic screening using mass spectrometry [34, 35]. As a result, the list of potential new target candidates is long and growing. Using mRNA vaccine technology, newly identified candidates can more easily be made and evaluated in parallel, increasing the chance of finding effective targets. RNA delivery, to a certain extent, has also been standardized, with most researchers using similar formulations of well-characterized lipid nanoparticles (LNPs). Therefore, any selected candidate can readily be scaled up for clinical trials as small-scale lab protocols will closely mimic those used in good manufacturing practice (GMP) production facilities.

- *mRNA formulation allows for complex multivalent vaccine combinations*
- The mRNA platform allows for the less complicated production of multivalent vaccines, either as monocistronic sequence repetitions in the same construct or as coformulated individual sequences [36, 37]. This is another key advantage over subunit vaccines for which protein chimeras often produce low yields, coformulations can be unstable, and individual antigens require independent production [38]. Complex mRNA vaccine may therefore more easily combine multiple antigen targets that are essential for parasite development at different stages of its life cycle with antigen targets that are involved, for example, in the downregulation of the host immune system.
- The potential of multivalent mRNA vaccines in combating multiple genes within multicellular organisms was recently demonstrated by Lyme disease researchers [39]. Sajid et al. conducted experiments on Guinea pigs, administering a multivalent mRNA vaccine targeting 19 salivary proteins found in black-legged ticks to prevent them from transmitting Lyme infection. Vaccination triggered robust immunity against 10 saliva antigens, prompting early skin redness upon tick attachment. This reaction led to hindered tick feeding and rapid tick detachment before ticks could pass on *Borrelia burgdorferi* (Lyme disease agent) infection.
- *mRNA vaccines have an excellent widespread safety record*
- *In vitro* transcribed mRNA is noninfectious and after translation, it can be naturally degraded by the transfected cell. Furthermore, there is no risk for insertional mutagenesis as there may be for DNA-based vaccines [29]. An extensive worldwide safety profile has been established for mRNA vaccines in a short time frame during the coronavirus pandemic (2020–2022). The COVID mRNA vaccines have been administered to hundreds of million people and have generally been proven safe. Also, regulatory agencies are now familiar with the technology and many unfounded reservations by the public about using mRNA vaccines may be by now partially removed.

11.4 Accessibility, Manufacturing Capacity, and Logistics of mRNA for Low- and Mid-Income Countries

Successful implementation of a vaccine solution in an LMIC setting requires local large-scale GMP-manufacturing sites that can procure vaccines at a low per-dose cost to ensure broad accessibility. Although multiple initiatives have been started, at this point no such facility is in operation for mRNA products.

At the beginning of COVID-19 vaccination programs, COVID-19 mRNA vaccines were barely administered in LMICs. Their governments were outpriced by the wealthy nations, resulting in a major gap in the supply chain of these coveted mRNA vaccines [40]. Despite generous research funding and an enormous scale of production [41, 42], the first-generation COVID-19 mRNA vaccines were sold to governments at prices between $14 and $25 per dose and later versions were sold for over $100 per dose, which far exceeded the prices of the vaccines made with other technologies ($2–$5/dose) [40, 42]. Contributions through COVAX, the international organization meant to facilitate global vaccine distribution for COVID-19, have been limited and virtually no mRNA vaccines were sent to poorer countries [43]. Consequently, the hefty price tag of the COVID-19 mRNA vaccines may cause many to think that mRNA technology is not within reach of LMICs. However, this may be misleading as the cost was believed to be inflated by high demand and short supply by only two manufacturers. In contrast, multiple studies estimate that the total cost of production of mRNA vaccines is not prohibitive and in the same range as that of most other vaccines [40, 44–46]. Raw supplies are mostly available, the production technology is straightforward, and establishing a manufacturing facility is not more expensive compared to other current good manufacturing practice (cGMP) facilities [44].

Manufacturing capacity for mRNA vaccines is however rapidly expanding, as multiple biotech institutes have made significant investments to attain the capability to develop and manufacture cGMP-grade mRNA vaccines [47]. BioNTech, another pioneer in mRNA technology, recently initiated the construction of Africa's first mRNA Vaccine Factory in the capital of Rwanda and aims to start mRNA vaccine output in 2025 [48]. It will be used in support of their malaria project, funded by the WHO and the kENUP Foundation. Additionally, the WHO has initiated a global mRNA technology transfer program intending to support LMICs to design and develop next-generation mRNA vaccines and scale-up production to increase global access [49, 50]. The initial focus of the WHO mRNA technology transfer hub (Table 11.2) was to produce vaccines against COVID-19, but the capacity-building initiative will allow for the facilities to master the technology and prepare for large-scale manufacturing and distribution of any new mRNA vaccine in the future. Intense close collaboration with local governments, regulators, and centers for disease control should ensure swift regulatory alignment and policy transfer, and distribution to get new vaccines from the manufacturing facilities to the local communities.

These new mRNA facilities have the potential to prepare the LMICs for both new epidemics and ancient diseases such as those caused by parasites. Manufacturers of mRNA vaccines for parasitic diseases may eventually become profitable due to the standardized process, which allows switching between the production of different mRNA vaccines and therapeutics with minimal changes to the production line. In due course, even a one-dollar-per-dose manufacturing cost may become realistic, and these vaccines could be sold for 3–4 times the production value. Furthermore,

Table 11.2 Recipients of mRNA technology from the WHO mRNA technology transfer hub [50].[a)]

Country	mRNA technology recipient
Argentina	Sinergium Biotech
Bangladesh	Incepta Vaccine Ltd
Brazil	Bio-Manguinhos
Egypt	BioGeneric Pharma S.A.E
India	BiologicalE (Bio E)
Indonesia	Biofarma
Kenya	BioVAx
Nigeria	Biovaccines Nigeria Limited
Pakistan	National Institute of Health
Senegal	Institut Pasteur de Dakar
Serbia	Institut Torlak
South Africa	Biovac, Afrigen[a)]
Tunisia	Institut Pasteur de Tunis
Ukraine	Darnitsa
Viet Nam	Polyvac

a) Afrigen (South Africa) is the central institute of the WHO mRNA hub.

the developers could potentially sell the vaccines in bulk to other countries to reduce their capital expenditure in establishing or expanding their fill-and-finish facility [44].

Despite all ongoing initiatives to increase capacity building, at this time, under the current regulations, whether (generic) mRNA vaccines can be made affordable for the needs of LMICs may largely depend on the willingness of the leading manufacturers and suppliers of formulation components to share certain key intellectual property (IP) rights. The involved patents include nucleoside modifications, cap structures, poly(A) tail sequences, and lipids applied in the formulation [51, 52]. The coding region of an mRNA vaccine is usually not patentable because the sequence of the translated protein is part of the public domain. For the duration of the COVID-19 pandemic, Moderna, one of the key mRNA vaccine technology patent holders, communicated an openness to licensing for its COVID-19 vaccine technology without claiming infringement [44]. Specific agreements made through collaboration around mRNA vaccine IP would potentially benefit nonprofit humanitarian vaccine development projects. Furthermore, the IP landscape for mRNA applications seems to be still open for debate and certain creative solutions may become available in this research-intensive field [53]. Regardless, in our opinion, all people should have equal access to healthcare innovations, independent of their place of birth or residence.

After manufacturing or acquiring an mRNA vaccine, organizers must also consider the logistical challenges of how to effectively distribute doses to the public. If the vaccines need to be kept at arctic temperatures, then this may be prohibitively challenging in most resource-poor countries. In general, the current generation of COVID-19 mRNA vaccines guarantees stability for 30 days at 2–8 °C and for 6 months at −20 °C. However, for long-term stability, storage at −80 °C is recommended [54]. Lyophilization may offer a possible solution to overcome the long-term storage-related limitations of mRNA–LNP vaccines. Recent data indicate that with the addition of 5–10% low-cost sugars to the vaccine formulation, mRNA-LNP vaccines can be lyophilized without an impact on their physicochemical properties [55]. The stability of the lyophilized material does not significantly change for at least 6 months after storage at 4 °C. A study published in Molecular Therapy evaluated a reconstituted lyophilized mRNA influenza virus vaccine in mice and found no decrease in immunogenicity [56]. More information will come from a recently completed phase 3 clinical study, comparing the safety and tolerability of lyophilized BNT162b2 presented in single-dose vials to that of frozen-liquid BNT162b2 in multidose vials and determining whether the immune response is noninferior [57].

11.5 Published Data on mRNA Vaccines Against Parasitic Pathogens

At this time, the publicly available literature on mRNA vaccines for parasitic infections is still limited to a dozen manuscripts (Table 11.3); however, as the mRNA platform rapidly matures and projects receive funding, we expect to see much more data over the next five years. Hopefully, this will further result in more successful clinical data. Below, we summarize some of the pioneering publications in the field of mRNA vaccines for malaria, toxoplasmosis, Chagas disease, and leishmaniasis.

11.5.1 Malaria

In 1998, Tsuji et al. reported the first use of an RNA-based vaccine candidate against malaria, using a recombinant alpha-RNA virus that expressed a cytotoxic T-cell epitope of *Plasmodium yoelii* circumsporozoite protein (CSP) [58]. Peptide-specific $CD8^+$ T-cell responses were confirmed before a challenge with *P. yoelii* sporozoites, two weeks after immunization. The immunized mice had an approximate decrease of 80% in hepatic parasite rRNA levels compared to naive controls. A few years later, Anderson et al. published the first results on an *in vitro* transcribed self-amplifying RNA vaccine, which was coding for part of the *Plasmodium falciparum* antigen Pf332 [59]. The study reported a modest humoral immune response in mice and found that the mode of delivery of the RNA (naked RNA versus RNA encapsulated in viral particles) impacted the antibody subclasses. It would take over 15 years before the next RNA-based malaria vaccine paper was published.

Table 11.3 List of published research evaluating mRNA vaccines for parasitic diseases.

RNA vaccine	Vaccine target	Dose regimen	Efficacy	Ref
		Malaria		
Self-amplifying Sindbis virus RNA	*P. yoelii* CSP peptide epitope	10^7–10^8 PFU (mice)	Significant reduction in plasmodium RNA measured in liver	[58]
Self-amplifying Semliki Forest virus RNA	Pf332	10^6 PFU (mice)	N/A	[59]
Self-amplifying alpha virus RNA	PMIF	15 μg (mice)	Improved control over first infection, 100% protection to reinfection	[60]
Nucleoside-modified mRNA construct	PfGARP-A	50 μg (monkeys)	Significant, 3.5-fold reduction in blood parasitemia	[61]
Nucleoside-modified and unmodified mRNA construct	PfCSP	10 μg (mice)	Up to 88% sterile protection, measured by blood-stage parasite detection using microscopy	[62]
Nucleoside-modified mRNA construct	PfCSP, Pfs25	0.1–30 μg (mice)	>90% reduction in liver stage burden, four immunizations for full protection	[63]
Nucleoside-modified mRNA construct + NKT cell agonists	RPL6	1–30 μg (mice)	Sterile protection with a single dose of vaccine	[64]
		Toxoplasmosis		
Modified dendrimer nanoparticles, containing RNA replicons	AMA1, GRA6, ROP2A, ROP18, SAG1, SAG2A	40 μg (mice)	100% survival after challenge, no clinical indications of disease	[65]
Nucleoside-modified mRNA construct	TG_200	100 μg (mice)	Survival vaccinated mice after the challenge was significantly increased	[66]

Table 11.3 (Continued)

RNA vaccine	Vaccine target	Dose regimen	Efficacy	Ref
		Leishmaniasis		
Self-amplifying alpha virus RNA	PpSP15-LmSTI1	0.5–2 μg in BHK-12 cells	N/A	[67, 68]
Alphavirus RNA replicon, heterologous vaccine strategy	LEISH-F2	10 μg RNA followed by 5 μg recombinant protein (mice)	Significant reduction in parasite burden in the liver	[69]
		Chagas disease		
Nucleoside-modified mRNA construct	Tc24	10 μg (mice)	N/A	[70]

The table excludes manuscripts that discuss the potential of mRNA vaccines based on *in silico* analysis without experimental data.

In 2018, Baeza Garcia et al. presented results of a unique RNA vaccine that targeted one of the immune-modulating antigens secreted by plasmodium [60]. PMIF is a plasmodium ortholog of the cytokine macrophage migration inhibitory factor (MIF), which can evoke a receptor-dependent inflammatory response. This inflammation interferes with the differentiation of plasmodium-specific CD4 T effector cells into long-lived memory precursors. The study demonstrated that mice immunized with PMIF encoded by an RNA replicon induced a strong antigen-specific cellular and humoral immune response. The vaccine-induced PMIF antibodies were found to block the pro-inflammatory action of PMIF, without inhibiting the function of host MIF. In a challenge study infecting BALB/C mice with *Plasmodium berghei*, the authors showed that vaccinated mice had improved control of liver and blood-stage infection and even complete protection from reinfection. Further research has been ongoing in a collaboration between Yale University and GSK, and preparations are being made for a clinical trial [71]. The PMIF mRNA vaccine could synergize with other malaria mRNA vaccines and the approach could also be adapted for vaccines against other parasitic protozoan and helminthic parasites that are known to secrete MIF orthologs.

Raj et al. published about an mRNA vaccine candidate expressing *P. falciparum* glutamic-acid-rich protein (PfGARP) [61]. This parasite antigen is expressed on the surface of erythrocytes that are infected by early-to-late-trophozoite-stage parasites, and it is uniquely recognized by plasma derived from a specific group of children who appear less susceptible to *P. falciparum*. *In vitro* data was used to demonstrate that antibodies against PfGARP can kill trophozoite-infected erythrocytes by inducing programmed cell death in the parasites, and preclinical data of vaccinated non-human primates with PfGARP mRNA showed partial protection against a challenge with *P. falciparum*. To induce full protection, PfGARP mRNA may be coformulated with mRNA vaccines that target parasite invasion of hepatocytes or erythrocytes.

To improve the efficacy of the approved protein-based vaccine RTS,S (Mosquirix™), Mallorey et al. published the optimization of an mRNA vaccine alternative that targets parts of the CSP [62]. The mRNA vaccine induced strong humoral and cellular responses that offered full protection in mice challenged with *P. berghei* PfCSP-transgenic parasite strains. Further research led by Hayashi et al. pursued a combined vaccine strategy to halt malaria transmission, focusing on Pfs25 and PfCSP [63]. Notably, their findings showcased the exceptional immunogenicity of Pfs25 mRNA–LNPs, eliciting robust antibody responses and significant transmission-blocking activity even at low vaccine doses of 1 μg mRNA. Coadministration of Pfs25 and PfCSP mRNA–LNPs did not diminish antibody responses or functional efficacy, hinting at the practicality of leveraging the mRNA–LNP platform for combining multiple vaccines.

Lastly, Ganley et al. [64] explored using an adjuvanted mRNA vaccine to specifically drive the immune response toward generating liver tissue-resident memory T cells (T_{rm} cells) targeting the large ribosomal subunit protein L6 (RPL6) of *P. berghei*, given the essential role of T_{rm} cells in managing liver-stage infections. The researchers observed that a conventional lipoplex mRNA vaccine failed to stimulate substantial T_{rm} cell production or provide protection against *P. berghei* in mice. However, when they incorporated a modified version of an natural killer T (NKT) cell agonist (α-galactosylceramide) into the liposome formulation, a significant increase in T_{rm} cell generation was noted, resulting in effective protection. While NKT cell agonists exhibit promise for human applications, further investigation is necessary to ensure the safety and efficacy of this approach during translation.

Starting in 2023, BioNTech has commenced a first-in-human Phase I study of the first candidate from its malaria vaccine program (NCT05581641). They intend to assess two vaccine candidates (BNT165 and BNT165b1) featuring certain parts of CSP as previously optimized in their preclinical research program [72].

11.5.2 Toxoplasmosis

Characteristic of most protozoans, *Toxoplasma gondii* has a complex life cycle with different life stages. Latent parasites that surround themselves in a cyst can escape the host's immune response. A protective immune response against *T. gondii* infection requires a Th-1 biased response with activation of NK cells and $CD4^+$ and $CD8^+$ T cells that secrete high levels of interferon gamma (IFN-γ) [73]. These cytokines promote the expression of inducible nitric oxide synthase (iNOS) and reactive oxygen species (ROS), which hinder the replication of *T. gondii*. Certain *T. gondii*-specific antibodies that target extracellular parasites may further assist in protection [74].

Chahal et al. developed a single immunization approach using a multivalent mRNA vaccine that achieved protective immunity against lethal doses of different infectious diseases [65]. Modified dendrimer nanoparticles were developed, in which mRNA replicons were encapsulated, encoding for six different replicons antigens from *T. gondii*; apical membrane antigen 1 (AMA1), dense granule protein 6 (GRA6), rhoptry protein 2A (ROP2A), rhoptry protein 18 (ROP18), surface antigen 1 (SAG1), and surface antigen 2A (SAG2A). These antigens were selected for their conserved properties between multiple strains and their expression in multiple stages in the life cycle of *T. gondii*. The mRNA replicons were based on the genome of the Venezuelan equine encephalitis virus (VEEV) to support the self-amplification of the mRNA [75]. Mice vaccinated with multivalent mRNA were challenged with a lethal dose of wild-type PRU-delta HXGPRT *T. gondii* tachyzoites after 32 days. Twelve days after the challenge, all control mice received mRNA encoding an irrelevant antigen, succumbed to the challenge. However, all mice that had received mRNA containing the six different replicons lived for six months (when the study was terminated) without clinical symptoms from the challenge, indicating the effectiveness of this multivalent vaccine.

Zhang et al. identified a novel *T. gondii* antigen, named TG_200, using bioinformatic screening analysis, and utilized its sequence to develop a TG_200 mRNA–LNP vaccine [66]. Though the authors only present data for high-dose vaccination, administering three intramuscular doses of 100 μg RNA elicited a robust immune response, in terms of both humoral and cellular immunity. Vaccination induced specific proliferation of immune cells targeting *T. gondii* and stimulated the production of cytotoxic T lymphocytes (CTLs). Vaccinated mice displayed significantly improved survival after a subsequent *T. gondii* challenge (challenged with 102 tachyzoites of the RH strain) compared to the control group.

11.5.3 Leishmaniasis

Savar et al. investigated the use of a fusion antigen in a self-amplifying mRNA vaccine construct against leishmaniasis [67]. The fusion protein PpSP15-LmSTI1 consists of the SP-15 salivary protein from the sandfly *Phlebotomus papatasi*, and the stress-inducible protein 1 from *Leishmania major*, both of which have shown promising results as vaccine targets [68]. When RNA replicons containing the antigen sequence with the RNA genome of Semliki Forest virus (SFV) were used to transfect BHK-12 cells, robust expression levels of the RNA were measured by reverse transcriptase (RT)-qPCR. In a follow-up manuscript, Savar et al. tested different fusion forms of PpSP15-LmSTI1 and showed successful protein translation *in vitro* [68]. To note, *in vivo* immunogenicity and challenge studies using *Leishmania* parasites have yet to be done to fully evaluate the efficacy of the PpSP15-LmSTI1 SAM vaccine construct.

In another study, the potential of a heterologous mRNA–subunit vaccine strategy was demonstrated by Duthie et al. [69] An alphavirus RNA replicon encoding for the LEISH-F2 sequence was created and administered to mice followed by a booster with recombinant LEISH-F2 protein in glucopyranosyl lipid A in a stable oil-in-water emulsion (second-generation lipid adjuvant – stable emulsion [SLA-SE]) at day 21. Potent antigen-specific Th1 responses were measured through IFN-γ secretion by CD4 and CD8 T cells as well as a robust IFN-γ /tumor necrosis factor alpha (TNF-α) polyfunctional CD4 T cells response and F2-specific immunoglobulin G (IgG) titers. A challenge with *Leishmania donovani* showed that this heterologous vaccination strategy significantly reduced parasite burden in the liver compared to naïve mice or mice that received two vaccinations with F2-RNA or with recombinant protein. These results were linked with improved antigen-specific Th1 responses. Interestingly, when the draining lymph nodes were assessed after vaccination, a more pronounced adjustment of the T cell-to-B cell ratio was observed in the case of F2-RNA vaccinations. These findings highlight that antigen presentation by the different vaccine platforms has an impact on immune response, and the eventual protection against a challenge with pathogens.

11.5.4 Chagas Disease

Poveda et al. evaluated and compared the immunogenicity of *T. cruzi* antigens through mRNA vaccines, employing both homologous and heterologous prime/boost approaches [70]. The results revealed a consistent immunogenicity profile for Tc24-specific vaccines in a C57BL/6 mouse model, akin to earlier studies with protein-alone vaccines in Balb/C mice [76]. Because their intent is to deliver the vaccine during or after an acute infection, the therapeutic vaccine must not induce a strong inflammatory response, since that could aggravate cardiac disease [77, 78]. Instead, the group aims to induce a balanced Th1/Th2/Th17 immune response, with significantly high numbers of antigen-specific $CD8^+$ T cells, which can eliminate *T. cruzi*-infected cells and reduce parasite burden and cardiac tissue pathology [79, 80]. Notably, the authors showcased enhanced immunogenicity with the heterologous mRNA/protein vaccine, leading to significantly increased levels of activated $CD4^+$ and $CD8^+$ T cells, augmented cytokine-producing $CD4^+$ and $CD8^+$ T cells, and a balanced Th1/Th2/Th17 cytokine profile. A crucial observation was the significant induction of polyfunctional $CD8^+$ T cells, simultaneously producing various cytokines, particularly under the heterologous vaccination strategy. Polyfunctional T-cell responses, known for their association with effective *T. cruzi* infection control, make them a desirable attribute for a T-cell-based vaccine.

Multiple other groups have proposed the development of an mRNA vaccine against Chagas disease [31, 76]. Michel-Todó et al. performed an *in silico* analysis of the proteome of *T. cruzi* to identify important $CD4^+$, $CD8^+$, and B-cell epitopes [31]. Criteria for the epitopes were conserved protein sequences between parasitic strains, low identity to the human and human microbiome proteome, and high projected coverage of the human leukocyte antigen (HLA)'s alleles prevalent in the Latin American populations. This screening resulted in the selection of 2 $CD4^+$ T-cell epitopes, 18 $CD8^+$ T-cell epitopes, and 10 B-cell epitopes that in total originate from 25 different *T. cruzi* antigens. An epitope-based vaccine was proposed using all the epitopes separated by linker sequences. mRNA was chosen as the preferred vaccine platform to ease and costs of development. A second suggestion for a

T. cruzi mRNA vaccine was made by Maldonado et al. [77]. This group suggests an mRNA-based vaccine that encodes a chimeric antigen comprised of three *T. cruzi* antigens: Cruzipain (GP57/61, or Cz), Tc52 (N-terminal domain only), and shed acute-phase antigen (SAPA). These antigens are thought to be well conserved, present in all parasitic life stages, highly immunogenic, located on the cell surface of *T. cruzi*, and essential for its survival.

11.5.5 Helminths

At present, no research papers on mRNA vaccines against helminthic diseases have been published. The application has however been suggested and discussed by us and others in multiple review papers [67, 81–84]. Multiple partially effective vaccine antigens have already been studied and even tested in the clinic [81] and are ideally suited for testing as multivalent mRNA vaccines to protect against helminths.

11.6 Conclusions and Prospects

Parasitic infections cause a tremendous burden of disease in LMICs all over the world, particularly among those living in poverty. Vaccines have been the most successful measure against viral and bacterial infections but they yet must prove their effectiveness against parasites. While the lack of economic incentives may have been holding back the involvement of commercial pharmaceutical companies, there also may have been a technical gap preventing the development of vaccine solutions against these more complex organisms.

The success of mRNA COVID-19 vaccines has led to greater acceptance of mRNA as a safe and effective vaccine platform. This vaccine revolution has not gone unnoticed in the field of parasitology. Multiple groups have started mRNA vaccine research programs to learn, evaluate, and experiment with the new vaccine platform. Vaccine development using the mRNA platform has a potentially faster development process, which will accelerate screening of new candidates. Similarly, the recent emergence of mRNA vaccine production facilities will more easily accommodate GMP production for clinical doses for future trials.

The number of people suffering from parasitic infections might well exceed the number of dollars that can be made available by governments in LMICs. It is however a general misconception that mRNA vaccines are more expensive to produce than other vaccine platforms. IP rights are probably the sole limitation of a rapid technology transfer to LMICs. The equipment and biological supplies are globally available, so the cost of establishing a manufacturing facility can be affordable even for LMICs. Setting up large-scale mRNA production facilities in LMICs may even offer them an investment opportunity to take care of local humanitarian needs while boosting the economy. Self-sufficiency in producing mRNA products can indeed bring many rewards in the future, including the production of novel antiparasitic vaccines, managing future pandemics, and converting traditional vaccines into lower-cost and more effective multivalent mRNA vaccines. In this

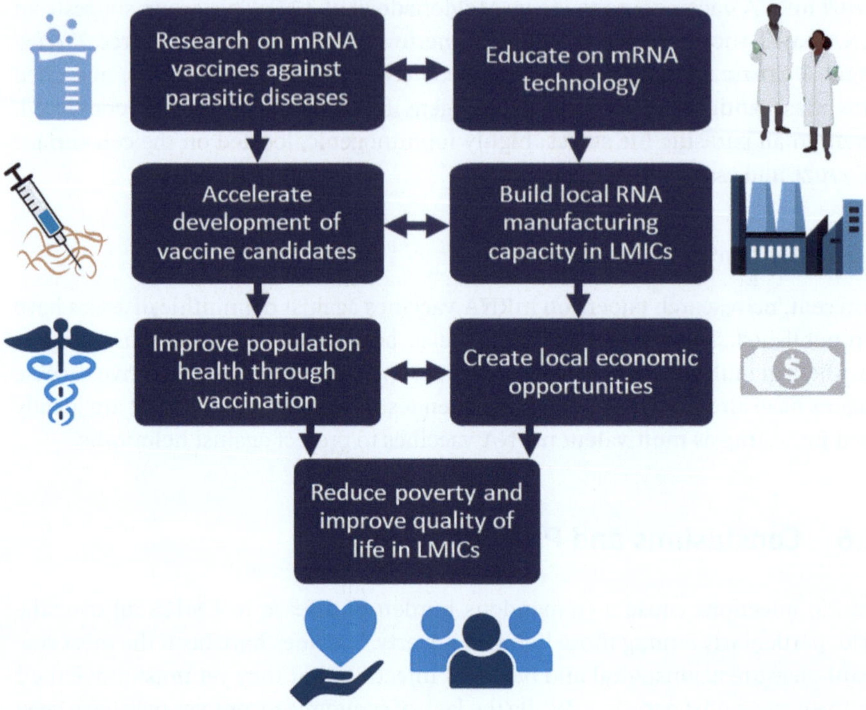

Figure 11.1 Schematic illustration of the possible health and economic opportunities of mRNA vaccines for communities in LMICs.

way, mRNA vaccines may offer both improved health and economic prospects to improve the quality of life in LMICs (Figure 11.1).

The groundwork for broader adoption of mRNA vaccine technology has been laid and has resulted in the publication of exciting early-stage research data, the appointment of mRNA technology hubs in LMICs by the WHO, and the construction of the GMP mRNA vaccine manufacturing facilities including the first of such facilities in Africa. We are further hopeful that mRNA technology will mature over the next years and that the platform will help accelerate the search for vaccine solutions against parasitic diseases.

References

1 RePORTER. https://reporter.nih.gov/search/exmbW_-yDkmGG53_RWc3WA/projects/charts (accessed 1 October 2022).

2 World Health Organization. (1987). Prevention and control of intestinal parasitic infections: WHO Technical Report Series N°749. https://www.who.int/publications-detail-redirect/WHO-TRS-749 (accessed 2 October 2022).

3 White, N.J., Day, N.P.J., Ashley, E.A. et al. (2022). Have we really failed to roll back malaria? *Lancet* 399: 799–800.

4 Bartsch, S.M. et al. (2016). Modeling the Economic and Epidemiologic Impact of Hookworm Vaccine and Mass Drug Administration (MDA) in Brazil, a high transmission setting. *Vaccine* 34: 2197–2206.

5 Kura, K. et al. (2020). The impact of mass drug administration on *Schistosoma haematobium* infection: what is required to achieve morbidity control and elimination? *Parasit. Vectors* 13: 554.

6 Sacks, D.L. (2014). Vaccines against tropical parasitic diseases: a persisting answer to a persisting problem. *Nat. Immunol.* 15: 403–405.

7 Wykes, M.N. (2013). Why haven't we made an efficacious vaccine for malaria? *EMBO Rep.* 14: 661.

8 Dhillon, S. and Pace, D. (2017). Meningococcal Quadrivalent Tetanus Toxoid Conjugate Vaccine (MenACWY-TT; Nimenrix®): a review. *Drugs* 77: 1881–1896.

9 Song, J.-Y. et al. (2021). Safety, tolerability, and immunogenicity of V114, a 15-valent pneumococcal conjugate vaccine, followed by sequential PPSV23 vaccination in healthy adults aged ≥50 years: a randomized phase III trial (PNEU-PATH). *Vaccine* 39: 6422–6436.

10 Halperin, S.A. et al. (2003). A phase I study of the safety and immunogenicity of recombinant hepatitis B surface antigen co-administered with an immunostimulatory phosphorothioate oligonucleotide adjuvant. *Vaccine* 21: 2461–2467.

11 Zhang, C., Maruggi, G., Shan, H., and Li, J. (2019). Advances in mRNA vaccines for infectious diseases. *Front. Immunol.* 10.

12 Herreros-Cabello, A., Callejas-Hernández, F., Gironès, N., and Fresno, M. (2020). *Trypanosoma cruzi* genome: organization, multi-gene families, transcription, and biological implications. *Genes* 11: 1196.

13 Versteeg, L. et al. (2021). Location and expression kinetics of Tc24 in different life stages of *Trypanosoma cruzi*. *PLoS Negl. Trop. Dis.* 15: e0009689.

14 Buscaglia, C.A., Campo, V.A., Frasch, A.C.C., and Di Noia, J.M. (2006). *Trypanosoma cruzi* surface mucins: host-dependent coat diversity. *Nat. Rev. Microbiol.* 4: 229–236.

15 Burri, C., Chappuis, F., and Brun, R. (2014). 45 - Human African trypanosomiasis. In: *Manson's Tropical Infectious Diseases, 23*e (ed. J. Farrar et al.), 606–621.e4. W.B. Saunders https://doi.org/10.1016/B978-0-7020-5101-2.00046-7.

16 Weiss, G.E. et al. (2010). The *Plasmodium falciparum*-specific human memory B cell compartment expands gradually with repeated malaria infections. *PLoS Pathog.* 6: e1000912.

17 Osii, R.S., Otto, T.D., Garside, P. et al. (2020). The impact of malaria parasites on dendritic cell–T cell interaction. *Front. Immunol.* 11: 1597.

18 Schwartz, L., Brown, G.V., Genton, B., and Moorthy, V.S. (2012). A review of malaria vaccine clinical projects based on the WHO rainbow table. *Malar. J.* 11: 11.

19 Laurens, M.B. (2019). RTS,S/AS01 vaccine (Mosquirix^{TM}): an overview. *Hum. Vaccin. Immunother.* 16: 480–489.

20 Duffy, P.E. and Patrick Gorres, J. (2020). Malaria vaccines since 2000: progress, priorities, products. *NPJ Vaccines* 5: 1–9.

21 Datoo, M.S. et al. (2022). Efficacy and immunogenicity of R21/Matrix-M vaccine against clinical malaria after 2 years' follow-up in children in Burkina Faso: a phase 1/2b randomised controlled trial. *Lancet Infect. Dis.* 22: 1728–1736.

22 Gsell, P.-S. et al. (2023). Key considerations for the development of novel mRNA candidate vaccines in LMICs: a WHO/MPP mRNA Technology Transfer Programme meeting report. *Vaccine* 41: 7307–7312.

23 Salleh, M.Z., Norazmi, M.N., and Deris, Z.Z. (2022). Immunogenicity mechanism of mRNA vaccines and their limitations in promoting adaptive protection against SARS-CoV-2. *PeerJ* 10: e13083.

24 Lim, W.W., Mak, L., Leung, G.M. et al. (2021). Comparative immunogenicity of mRNA and inactivated vaccines against COVID-19. *Lancet Microbe* 2: e423.

25 Ben Ahmed, M. et al. (2022). Humoral and cellular immunogenicity of six different vaccines against SARS-CoV-2 in adults: a comparative study in Tunisia (North Africa). *Vaccines* 10: 1189.

26 Wu, Y., Zhang, H., Meng, L. et al. (2022). Comparison of immune responses elicited by SARS-CoV-2 mRNA and recombinant protein vaccine candidates. *Front. Immunol.* 13: 906457.

27 Edwards, D.K., Jasny, E., Yoon, H. et al. (2017). Adjuvant effects of a sequence-engineered mRNA vaccine: translational profiling demonstrates similar human and murine innate response. *J. Transl. Med.* 15: 1. https://translational-medicine.biomedcentral.com/articles/10.1186/s12967-016-1111-6 (accessed 2 October 2022).

28 Yang, J. et al. (2019). Hybrid nanovaccine for the co-delivery of the mRNA antigen and adjuvant. *Nanoscale* 11: 21782–21789.

29 Pardi, N., Hogan, M.J., Porter, F.W., and Weissman, D. (2018). mRNA vaccines — a new era in vaccinology. *Nat. Rev. Drug Discov.* 17: 261–279.

30 Lundstrom, K. (2021). Self-replicating RNA viruses for vaccine development against infectious diseases and cancer. *Vaccines* 9: 1187.

31 Michel-Todó, L. et al. (2019). In silico design of an epitope-based vaccine ensemble for Chagas disease. *Front. Immunol.* 10: 2698.

32 Ajibola, O. et al. (2021). In silico characterisation of putative *Plasmodium falciparum* vaccine candidates in African malaria populations. *Sci. Rep.* 11: 16215.

33 Zawawi, A. et al. (2020). In silico design of a T-cell epitope vaccine candidate for parasitic helminth infection. *PLoS Pathog.* 16: e1008243.

34 Becker, J.P. and Riemer, A.B. (2022). The importance of being presented: target validation by immunopeptidomics for epitope-specific immunotherapies. *Front. Immunol.* 13: 883989.

35 Leddy, O.K., White, F.M., and Bryson, B.D. (2021). Leveraging immunopeptidomics to study and combat infectious disease. *mSystems* 6: e0031021.

36 Chivukula, S. et al. (2021). Development of multivalent mRNA vaccine candidates for seasonal or pandemic influenza. *NPJ Vaccines* 6: 1–15.

37 Peng, L. et al. (2022). Multiplexed LNP-mRNA vaccination against pathogenic coronavirus species. *Cell Rep.* 40: 111160.

38 Mueller, C., Altenburger, U., and Mohl, S. (2018). Challenges for the pharmaceutical technical development of protein coformulations. *J. Pharm. Pharmacol.* 70: 666–674.

39 Sajid, A. et al. (2021). mRNA vaccination induces tick resistance and prevents transmission of the Lyme disease agent. *Sci. Transl. Med.* 13: eabj9827.

40 Light, D.W. and Lexchin, J. (2021). The costs of coronavirus vaccines and their pricing. *J. R. Soc. Med.* 114: 502–504.

41 Wouters, O.J. et al. (2021). Challenges in ensuring global access to COVID-19 vaccines: production, affordability, allocation, and deployment. *Lancet* 397: 1023–1034.

42 Dyer, O. (2021). Covid-19: countries are learning what others paid for vaccines. *BMJ* 372: n281.

43 World Health Organization. COVAX. https://www.who.int/initiatives/act-accelerator/covax (accessed 30 September 2022).

44 Niazi, S.K. (2022). Making COVID-19 mRNA vaccines accessible: challenges resolved. *Expert Rev. Vaccines* 21: 1163–1176.

45 Prabhala, A. and Alsalhani, A. (2022). Developing countries can make the mRNA vaccines they need. *Nat. Hum. Behav.* 6: 167.

46 Rosa, S.S., Prazeres, D.M.F., Azevedo, A.M., and Marques, M.P.C. (2021). mRNA vaccines manufacturing: challenges and bottlenecks. *Vaccine* 39: 2190–2200.

47 VaccinesWork. (2022). Hunting the 'perfect protein' for malaria mRNA vaccine. https://www.gavi.org/vaccineswork/hunting-perfect-protein-malaria-mrna vaccine (accessed 21 June 2022).

48 kENUP. https://www.kenup.eu/ (accessed 30 September 2022).

49 Pan American Health Organization. (2022). For vaccine equity: producers work together to advance mRNA technology in Latin America - PAHO/WHO. https://www.paho.org/en/stories/vaccine-equity-producers-work-together-advance-mrna-technology-latin-america (accessed 30 September 2022).

50 World Health Organization. Recipients of mRNA technology from the WHO mRNA technology transfer hub. https://www.who.int/initiatives/the-mrna-vaccine-technology-transfer-hub/recipients-of-mrna-technology-from-the-who-mrna-technology-transfer-hub (accessed 30 September 2022).

51 Lyu, M. et al. (2023). The global patent landscape of mRNA for diagnosis and therapy. *Nat. Biotechnol.* 41: 1193–1199.

52 Gaviria, M. and Kilic, B. (2021). A network analysis of COVID-19 mRNA vaccine patents. *Nat. Biotechnol.* 39: 546–548.

53 Martin, C. and Lowery, D. (2020). mRNA vaccines: intellectual property landscape. *Nat. Rev. Drug Discov.* 19: 578.

54 Uddin, M.N. and Roni, M.A. (2021). Challenges of storage and stability of mRNA-based COVID-19 vaccines. *Vaccines* 9: 1033.

55 Ball, R.L., Bajaj, P., and Whitehead, K.A. (2016). Achieving long-term stability of lipid nanoparticles: examining the effect of pH, temperature, and lyophilization. *Int. J. Nanomedicine* 12: 305–315.

56 Muramatsu, H. et al. (2022). Lyophilization provides long-term stability for a lipid nanoparticle-formulated, nucleoside-modified mRNA vaccine. *Mol. Ther.* 30: 1941–1951.

57 BioNTech SE. (2022). A phase 3, randomized, observer-blind study to evaluate the safety, tolerability, and immunogenicity of multiple formulations of the vaccine candidate BNT162B2 against COVID 19 in healthy adults 18 through 55 years of age. https://clinicaltrials.gov/ct2/show/NCT04816669 (accessed 29 September 2022).

58 Tsuji, M. et al. (1998). Recombinant Sindbis viruses expressing a cytotoxic T-lymphocyte epitope of a malaria parasite or of influenza virus elicit protection against the corresponding pathogen in mice. *J. Virol.* 72: 6907–6910.

59 Andersson, C. et al. (2001). Comparative immunization study using RNA and DNA constructs encoding a part of the *Plasmodium falciparum* antigen Pf332. *Scand. J. Immunol.* 54: 117–124.

60 Baeza Garcia, A. et al. (2018). Neutralization of the Plasmodium- encoded MIF ortholog confers protective immunity against malaria infection. *Nat. Commun.* 9: 2714.

61 Raj, D.K. et al. (2020). Anti-PfGARP activates programmed cell death of parasites and reduces severe malaria. *Nature* 582: 104–108.

62 Mallory, K.L. et al. (2021). Messenger RNA expressing PfCSP induces functional, protective immune responses against malaria in mice. *NPJ Vaccines* 6: 1–12.

63 Hayashi, C.T.H. et al. (2022). mRNA-LNP expressing PfCSP and Pfs25 vaccine candidates targeting infection and transmission of *Plasmodium falciparum. NPJ Vaccines* 7: 1–14.

64 Ganley, M. et al. (2023). mRNA vaccine against malaria tailored for liver-resident memory T cells. *Nat. Immunol.* 24: 1487–1498.

65 Chahal, J.S. et al. (2016). Dendrimer-RNA nanoparticles generate protective immunity against lethal Ebola, H1N1 influenza, and *Toxoplasma gondii* challenges with a single dose. *Proc. Natl. Acad. Sci. U. S. A.* 113: E4133–E4142.

66 Zhang, Y. et al. (2023). Immunization with a novel mRNA vaccine, TGGT1_216200 mRNA-LNP, prolongs survival time in BALB/c mice against acute toxoplasmosis. *Front. Immunol.* 14: 1161507.

67 Savar, N.S. et al. (2021). Quantitative evaluation of PpSP15-LmSTI1 fusion gene expression following transfection with an alphavirus-derived self-amplifying mRNA and conventional DNA vaccine platforms. *Mol. Cell. Probes* 59: 101749.

68 Savar, N.S. et al. (2022). An alphavirus-derived self-amplifying mRNA encoding PpSP15-LmSTI1 fusion protein for the design of a vaccine against leishmaniasis. *Parasitol. Int.* 89: 102577.

69 Duthie, M.S. et al. (2018). Heterologous immunization with defined RNA and subunit vaccines enhances T cell responses that protect against *Leishmania donovani. Front. Immunol.* 9: 2420.

70 Poveda, C. et al. (2023). Heterologous mRNA-protein vaccination with Tc24 induces a robust cellular immune response against *Trypanosoma cruzi*, characterized by an increased level of polyfunctional CD8+ T-cells. *Curr. Res. Immunol.* 4: 100066.

71 Lowe, D. (2021). A malaria vaccine candidate. https://www.science.org/content/blog-post/malaria-vaccine-candidate (accessed 1 August 2022).

72 BioNTech. (2021). BioNTech provides update on plans to develop sustainable solutions to address infectious diseases on the African continent. https://investors.biontech.de/news-releases/news-release-details/biontech-provides-update-plans-develop-sustainable-solutions/ (accessed 1 October 2022).

73 Innes, E.A., Hamilton, C., Garcia, J.L. et al. (2019). A one health approach to vaccines against *Toxoplasma gondii*. *Food Waterborne Parasitol.* 15: e00053.

74 Dupont, C.D., Christian, D.A., and Hunter, C.A. (2012). Immune response and immunopathology during toxoplasmosis. *Semin. Immunopathol.* 34: 793–813.

75 Ljungberg, K. and Liljeström, P. (2015). Self-replicating alphavirus RNA vaccines. *Expert Rev. Vaccines* 14: 177–194.

76 Versteeg, L., Almutairi, M.M., Hotez, P.J., and Pollet, J. (2019). Enlisting the mRNA vaccine platform to combat parasitic infections. *Vaccines* 7: 122.

77 Maldonado, E., Morales-Pison, S., Urbina, F., and Solari, A. (2022). Vaccine design against Chagas disease focused on the use of nucleic acids. *Vaccines* 10: 587.

78 Camargo, E.P., Gazzinelli, R.T., Morel, C.M., and Precioso, A.R. (2022). Why do we still have not a vaccine against Chagas disease? *Mem. Inst. Oswaldo Cruz* 117: e200314.

79 Tarleton, R.L. (2015). CD8+ T cells in *Trypanosoma cruzi* infection. *Semin. Immunopathol.* 37: 233–238.

80 Jones, K.M., Poveda, C., Versteeg, L. et al. (2022). Preclinical advances and the immunophysiology of a new therapeutic Chagas disease vaccine. *Expert Rev. Vaccines* 0: 1–19.

81 Perera, D.J. and Ndao, M. (2021). Promising technologies in the field of helminth vaccines. *Front. Immunol.* 12: 711650.

82 Li, P., Rios Coronado, P.E., Longstaff, X.R.R. et al. (2018). Nanomedicine approaches against parasitic worm infections. *Adv. Healthc. Mater.* 7: 1701494.

83 Chavda, V.P., Pandya, A., Pulakkat, S. et al. (2021). Lymphatic filariasis vaccine development: neglected for how long? *Expert Rev. Vaccines* 20: 1471–1482.

84 Molehin, A.J., McManus, D.P., and You, H. (2022). Vaccines for human schistosomiasis: recent progress, new developments and future prospects. *Int. J. Mol. Sci.* 23: 2255.

12

Current State of mRNA Vaccine Development Against *Mycobacterium tuberculosis*

Ilke Aernout[1], Rein Verbeke[1], Stefaan C. De Smedt[1], Francis Impens[2,3,4], and Ine Lentacker[1]

[1]Ghent University, Ghent Research Group on Nanomedicines, Department Pharmaceutics, Ottergemsesteenweg 460, 9000 Ghent, Belgium
[2]VIB-UGent Center for Medical Biotechnology, VIB, Department of Biomolecular Medicine, Technologiepark-Zwijnaarde 75, 9000 Ghent, Belgium
[3]Ghent University, Department of Biomolecular Medicine, Corneel Heymanslaan 10, 9000 Ghent, Belgium
[4]Ghent University VIB Proteomics Core, VIB, Department of Biomolecular Medicine, Technologiepark-Zwijnaarde 75, 9000 Ghent, Belgium

12.1 Introduction

Mycobacterium tuberculosis (Mtb), causing tuberculosis (TB), is currently the second leading cause of death caused by a single infectious organism after SARS-CoV-2. According to the last World Health Organization (WHO) report, in 2022 10.6 million fell ill and 1.3 million died from TB [1]. Individuals carrying Mtb may be categorized as either actively infected or latently infected. In instances where TB is active, commonly referred to as primary TB, the disease tends to manifest shortly after the initial infection, predominantly impacting children. In cases of latent infection, the individual initially manages to contain Mtb, but the bacterium persists in a host-controlled manner over an extended period, often spanning many years [2, 3].

The latter condition is typically asymptomatic and 5–10% of individuals with latent infections may later progress to develop active disease [4]. With the emergence of multidrug and extensively drug-resistant strains, new tools to control this epidemic are urgently required to meet the goal of the WHO and United Nation's member states to end the global TB epidemic by 2030 [1]. While renewed efforts to discover novel antimicrobial drugs are important, vaccines are increasingly recognized as highly effective tools to mitigate antibiotic resistance as they can prevent bacterial infections thereby reducing antibiotic prescription and minimizing selective drug pressure. Therefore, the development and implementation of new TB vaccines has also been identified as a top priority by the WHO [5, 6].

Currently, the only approved Mtb vaccine is prepared from *Mycobacterium bovis* attenuated bacillus Calmette–Guérin (BCG). Although BCG demonstrates effectiveness in preventing disease in children, its efficacy in adults remains problematic. Consequently, BCG does not significantly reduce the transmission of Mtb [7]. This

Trends in mRNA Vaccine Research, First Edition. Edited by Gabor Tamas Szabo and Norbert Pardi.

deficiency in efficacy is particularly existing in countries with the highest infection rates. It has been suggested that genetic variations induced in the BCG vaccine and insufficient maintenance of the vaccine's ideal temperature during transport could have contributed to this problem [8]. However, the major explanation that has been put forward is the blocking hypothesis stating that a pre-existing immune response to antigens shared by non-TB mycobacteria and BCG can prevent multiplication of the latter, thereby limiting the induction of a protective immune response [9]. Another complicating factor to the BCG vaccine is the comorbidity with human immunodeficiency virus (HIV), as the areas with the highest rates of TB often coincide with high HIV infection rates. Based on the results of a surveillance study in a highly endemic region, it was concluded that there is an increased risk of disseminated BCG disease in HIV-infected infants and, therefore, the Global Advisory Committee on Vaccine Safety (GACVS) concluded that BCG vaccination should be contraindicated in HIV-infected children [10–12].

Thus, a more efficient TB vaccine that yields protective immunity in all age groups and allows safe vaccination even in immunocompromised people is urgently warranted and considered essential to eliminate the spread of TB [7, 13]. The recent coronavirus disease 2019 (COVID-19) pandemic has proven that mRNA-based vaccines are safe, well tolerated, and very effective in providing protective immunity against viral infections. More recently, these advancements have generated interest in leveraging this technology for the development of more effective TB vaccines. In addition to highlighting the advantages of mRNA-based vaccines in a TB context, this chapter provides an overview of the present status of mRNA vaccines against Mtb in both preclinical and clinical development.

12.2 Immune Responses Responsible for Protective Immunity Against *Mycobacterium tuberculosis*

Numerous years of research have been dedicated to gain a deeper understanding of the pathology of Mtb infections, with the aim of identifying immune correlates of protection. In fact, to this day not all aspects of the infection process are fully comprehended [1, 7]. This might be explained by the heterogeneous and complex character of the disease. Within this section, we summarize the most important findings that provide insight into the immunological aspects that are critical for the design of new TB vaccines.

Upon initial interaction with bacteria, facilitated by aerosol droplets through the airway, immune cells such as alveolar macrophages and epithelial cells create a first line of defense and recognize the pathogen-associated molecular patterns (PAMPs) of Mtb via their pattern recognition receptors (PPRs) [3, 14]. An example of such a PAMP is lipoarabinomannan (LAM), a mycobacterial cell wall component recognized by Toll-like receptor (TLR)2 [15]. These interactions are responsible for the activation of a cascade of signaling pathways that eventually result in the secretion of antimicrobial peptides, proinflammatory cytokines, and chemokines. Chemokines coordinate the attraction of immune cells such as neutrophils and monocytes from the bloodstream while complement molecules and antimicrobial peptides bind to the mycobacteria itself, thereby facilitating further immune recognition and elimination by phagocytosis, degranulation, or complement fixation. Phagocytosis takes place by various cell types, including professional antigen-presenting cells (APCs) such as macrophages and dendritic cells (DCs) and, importantly, how these cells will react might lead to either latent or active TB disease [16]. Usually after phagosome formation around the bacteria, endosomes and subsequently late endosomes are formed that finally fuse with lysosomes. The fused phagolysosomes can kill the mycobacteria through acidification, enzymatic hydrolysis, and generation of reactive oxygen species (ROS) and reactive nitrogen intermediates (RNIs), as well as by the action of antimicrobial proteins, such as cathelicidin with a known activity against Mtb [17–19].

Despite this antibacterial response, for many years it has been recognized that Mtb possesses the ability to evade host immune responses on multiple levels through various complex mechanisms. One well-documented example is that Mtb blocks phagolysosomal fusion early in infection, in which a phagosomal environment is established that fosters the survival of bacilli, enabling their further dissemination [3, 20]. Once engulfed by DCs, bacterial proteins undergo degradation, giving rise to peptide fragments that are subsequently loaded into major histocompatibility complex class II (MHC class II) molecules. These peptide–MHC II complexes are then transported to the cell surface, where they can be recognized by the T-cell receptor of $CD4^+$ T cells [3]. Simultaneously, costimulatory signals are upregulated further supporting T-cell activation as a consequence of innate immune signaling pathways. Consequently, activated $CD4^+$ T cells will proliferate into Th1, Th2, or Th17 cells depending on the cytokine milieu. The helper cells have a crucial role in B cell activation through the interaction of CD40L to the CD40 receptor on the B-cell surface. This induces immunoglobulin (Ig) isotype class switching from IgM to higher affinity IgG antibodies and generates memory B cells. Those humoral immune responses are critical in the targeted lysis of Mtb through complement-mediated killing and antibody-mediated phagocytosis [2, 17, 18]. Also, at the level of DC presentation, Mtb has developed specific mechanisms to interfere with DC maturation and antigen presentation (reviewed in [21]), leading to a delay or impairment of adaptive immune responses, indicating that DCs play an important role in the host defense against TB [3].

Activation of $CD4^+$ T cells was conventionally considered the primary immune correlate for protection in TB vaccine development. This was also supported by the fact that HIV patients, characterized by lower $CD4^+$ T-cell counts, exhibit increased susceptibility to developing active TB and reactivating latent TB [22]. Nevertheless, the failure of several TB vaccines in clinical trials, despite being selected based on this immune correlate, underscores that this parameter alone is often insufficient for ensuring disease protection [7, 23]. In contrast to $CD4^+$ T cells, the role of $CD8^+$ T cells, which contribute to direct killing of Mtb-infected macrophages, was long overlooked within the context of TB. Preclinical studies have shown that depleting $CD8^+$ T cells results in a higher susceptibility to TB infection [23]. $CD8^+$ T-cell activation occurs through DC presentation of peptides displayed on MHC class I molecules.

Peptides derived from phagolysosomal degradation, i.e. from extracellular bacteria, are more inclined to bind to MHC class II molecules, consequently triggering the activation of $CD4^+$ T cells. In contrast, MHC class I peptides primarily arise from cytosolic proteins retrieved from endogenously misfolded proteins and intracellular bacterial pathogens. These cytosolic proteins undergo initial degradation by the proteasome and the resulting peptides are subsequently translocated through the transporter associated with antigen processing (TAP) complex into the endoplasmic reticulum (ER), where further processing and coupling to MHC class I molecules occurs [21, 22]. Besides this classical presentation pathway, APCs also have the ability to present peptides from the phagolysosomal compartment on MHC class I molecules through the process of antigen cross-presentation [24]. With the central role of macrophages as Mtb-infected APCs, this further rationale has an important role for $CD8^+$ T cells in protective immunity against Mtb [25]. Antigen-specific $CD8^+$ T cells are able to recognize MHC I–peptide complexes on the cell surface and subsequently release granzymes and perforins that kill the infected cell. $CD8^+$ T cells require IL-2 secreted by Th1 $CD4^+$ T cells to become activated in the initial phase of defense against most intracellular bacteria. Both $CD8^+$ and $CD4^+$ as well as Th17 $CD4^+$ T cells are responsible for the induction of nitric oxide (NO) oxidase and NO production through interferon gamma (IFN-γ) and tumor necrosis factor alpha (TNF-α) production, which initiates mycobacterial cell death within the phagosome [26]. This process is crucial during the initial phase of bacterial infection and thus mostly in active TB, while antibodies that elicit a limited role in this phase of infection mainly act during later stages, such as during reactivation from latent infection by inhibiting receptor-mediated uptake of bacteria [17, 18, 27].

Given the intricate and diverse nature of the Mtb infection process, along with its evolved escape mechanisms, the current understanding is that a comprehensive approach will be required, rather than concentrating solely on a single immune correlate. Thus, while exact immune correlates for protection against TB have not been well defined, it is likely that a TB vaccine should induce both innate and broad adaptive immune responses [23].

12.3 Suitability and Advantages of an mRNA Vaccine Platform Against *Mycobacterium tuberculosis*

The COVID-19 pandemic has illustrated that mRNA vaccines consisting of lipid nanoparticle (LNP)-encapsulated nucleoside-modified mRNA generate a safe and effective antiviral immunity [28]. The success of this approach lies in the stimulation of both neutralizing antibodies and potent effector responses, including cytotoxic $CD8^+$ T cells and Th1 cell-biased $CD4^+$ T cells targeted against the viral spike antigen [29]. By making use of mRNA encoding the stabilized version of the transmembrane anchored spike protein of SARS-CoV-2, the protein is directed to the secretory pathway to be anchored onto the plasma membrane where it can be recognized by B cells. In addition, peptides derived from its intracellular proteolytic processing can result in both MHC II and I presentation of $CD4^+$ T and $CD8^+$ T-cell epitopes, respectively [30–32]. Besides a strong adaptive immune response, researchers found that the SARS-CoV-2 mRNA vaccines might also induce reprogramming of innate cells resulting in trained innate immunity [33]. This epigenetic and metabolic reprogramming of myeloid cells was also shown to play an essential role in the protective effect of the BCG vaccine and confers protection against a wide range of other pathogens and even cancer [34, 35]. These innate responses might also act synergistically with adaptive immunity and could be advantageous in the context of vaccination against TB. However, there remain important questions to be addressed on the durability of the effects of mRNA vaccines on myeloid cells and the biological consequences in the context of Mtb or other diseases [36, 37].

Before the COVID-19 crisis, mRNA vaccine development was mainly focused on therapeutic cancer vaccination by encoding tumor-associated or tumor-specific epitopes or antigens with the aim of inducing tumor-specific cellular immune responses. Indeed, upon mRNA or DNA transfection, the cell's internal translation machinery will lead to the cytosolic presence of the mRNA-encoded antigen. As a result, proteasomal degradation will direct the antigens preferably toward MHC-I complexation, which will mainly result in the activation of antigen-specific cytotoxic T cells. Through generation of such cytotoxic $CD8^+$ T cells, tumor cells expressing the antigen can be selectively killed [38, 39]. Also, in the context of vaccination against TB, the generation of cytotoxic T-cell responses can be especially interesting as effective killing of bacterial-infected cells could limit bacterial replication and contain the spread of Mtb [17]. In this context also, viral-vectored DNA vaccines have been developed. In comparison to mRNA vaccines, these vaccines are more likely to induce immunogenicity against the viral vector itself, which could lead to inactivation of the vaccine upon multiple administrations [40–43]. This could explain why the Modified Vaccinia Ankara/Ag85A vaccine failed to show clinical benefit [44].

A third advantage of mRNA vaccines is that they can easily be adapted to encode multiple epitopes or antigens, which allows vaccination against multiple targets from the same or different species. This exceptional versatility not only facilitates rapid development and manufacturing [28, 45, 46] but could also broaden the immune responses by encoding various antigens that are present during different stages of the disease [27, 47]. Interestingly, the use of antigen discovery approaches such as immunopeptidomics in vaccine development allows rational selection of immunodominant proteins via identification of MHC-I and MHC-II presented epitopes and could further improve the efficiency of mRNA vaccines [48, 49].

Crucially, based on their widespread use during the COVID-19 pandemic, mRNA vaccines were found to be generally well tolerated and safe. This safety profile is paramount when considering vaccination for vulnerable populations, such as the elderly and immunocompromised individuals, who are more susceptible to antimicrobial resistance (AMR) and stand to gain the most from the advancement of antibacterial vaccines [34, 35, 37, 40, 41].

Additionally, from an economic standpoint, mRNA-based vaccines hold an advantage as they have the potential to become more cost effective compared to other vaccine platforms [44]. This could be particularly interesting for TB, considering that low- and middle-income countries (LMICs) are the primary focus for vaccination efforts [1]. While progress has been made, further efforts are needed to improve the stability of current mRNA vaccines as well as to enable local production in LMICs [50, 51]. This is particularly crucial considering the current necessity for deep-freeze storage and transport of mRNA vaccines [28].

12.4 mRNA TB Vaccines in (Pre-)clinical Development

Despite their high potential, only a limited number of studies have evaluated mRNA vaccines in the context of TB (summary in Table 12.1). Already in 2004, the first RNA vaccine was evaluated in preclinical studies. In this study, naked mRNA encoding MPT83 was administered intramuscularly through direct injection. The absence of a suitable carrier resulted only in short-lasting effects, although the modest protective effect was observed in preclinical challenge experiments [52]. Also, Lorenzi et al. evaluated a naked mRNA vaccine against Mtb, encoding the HSP65 antigen from *Mycobacterium leprae*. After intranasal administration, they were able to illustrate mRNA uptake in local APCs. In a follow-up study where mice were challenged with Mtb, the mRNA vaccine showed protection although not to a similar level to subcutaneously injected BCG [53]. After these early studies, mRNA vaccines were for many years not within the focus of TB vaccine development [57].

After the COVID-19 pandemic, there seems to be a renewed interest in the development of mRNA vaccines against TB. For example, Al Tbeishat et al. made use of innovative immunoinformatic tools to design an RNA vaccine against Mtb. Interestingly, the authors also choose to include mRNA encoding Mtb resuscitation-promoting factor (RpfE), which can also serve as an adjuvant through the activation of TLR4. This adjuvant was found to decrease bacterial growth upon infection with Mtb in mice [54]. Mishra et al. evaluated a self-adjuvanted mRNA vaccine encoding a well-known mtb Antigen 85B epitope, resulting in a clear reduction of bacterial load upon challenge with Mtb [55]. In Larsen et al., the clinical candidate, protein subunit ID91 vaccine, a fusion protein consisting of four Mtb antigens esxV, RpfD, PPE60, and Ag85B, was compared with a self-amplifying RNA (saRNA) format encoding the same antigens encapsulated through a nanostructure lipid carrier. Both vaccines elicited significant cellular immune responses and achieved a reduction in bacterial burden upon challenge in mice. Interestingly, by combining both platforms during a prime-boost vaccination the highest protective effect was obtained, which was characterized by a unique profile of adaptive immune responses [23, 57]. This indicates that there could be a potential for combining various vaccine platforms and/or thus boosting BCG-vaccinated people.

For the clinical development of mRNA vaccines against TB, BioNTech is currently testing two candidates, BNT164a1 and BNT614b1, both encoding multiple MTB-derived antigens covering various stages of the infection. Interestingly, they aim to compare both modified (BNT614b1) and unmodified (BNT164a1) mRNA to determine the innate immune effects of these two mRNA vaccine platforms

Table 12.1 State of the art mRNA vaccines against Mtb.

Formulation	Antigen	(Pre-) clinical phase	Publication date	Reference
Naked mRNA	MPT 83	Preclinical	2004	Xue et al. [52]
Naked mRNA intranasal administration	Hsp65	Preclinical	2010	Lorenzi et al. [53]
LNP	Histone acetyltransferase, Rv2966c, EIS, esxL, cob, esxA, Rv3263, spoU, and erm epitopes	*In silico* prediction	2022	Al Tbeishat [54]
Adjuvant RpfE				
Nanostructured lipid carrier	ID91 fusion protein (esxV, RpfD, PPE60, and Ag85B)	Preclinical	2023	Larsen et al. [23]
SelmRp25-C5, a synthetic mRNA vaccine	Antigen-85B epitope	Preclinical	2023	Mishra et al. [55]
Multivalent mRNA vaccine LNP	Unknown (multivalent)	Phase Ia/Ib	2023	BioNTech SE [56]

in TB context [56]. Specialized teams at BioNTech's headquarters in Mainz were responsible for the antigen discovery process supporting the selection of these candidates [58].

Two clinical trials are currently active. The first, a Phase Ia study in Germany (NCT05537038), assesses the vaccine in individuals who are both BCG naïve and interferon-gamma release assay (IGRA) negative, indicating those who have never been exposed to Mtb. Simultaneously, the vaccine is being evaluated in BCG-vaccinated subjects in a Phase Ib study in Africa, where both IGRA− and IGRA+ subjects are compared (NCT05547464). Also, Moderna announced that they would work on the development of an Mtb mRNA vaccine encoding newly identified antigens in partnership with the International acquired immunodeficiency syndrome (AIDS) Vaccine Initiative [59]. Moreover, several initiatives are undertaken by academic research groups to develop mRNA vaccines against Mtb often focused on innovative technologies such as alternative delivery strategies, novel adjuvants, or novel antigens selected through innovative antigen discovery methods [60, 61].

To conclude, the development of effective vaccines against Mtb has become more urgent with the rise of drug-resistant strains. It is clear that mRNA vaccines are in the spotlight, illustrated by the renewed interest in this vaccine technology and the many developments by both academic groups and industry. First, clinical updates that are expected in 2024 may shed light on the research directions and potential of this novel vaccine technology to combat Mtb.

Acknowledgments

Ilke Aernout is funded by a PhD fellowship for strategic basic research of the Research Foundation Flanders, Belgium (FWO-vlaanderen, 1S40923N). Rein Verbeke is a postdoctoral fellow of the Research Foundation Flanders, Belgium (FWO-Vlaanderen, 1275023N). Francis Impens and Ine Lentacker acknowledge support from Ghent University Concerted Research Action under grant BOF21/GOA/033 and from the European Union's Horizon Europe Research and Innovation Program under grant agreement No. 101080544 (Baxerna2.0).

References

1 World Health Organization. (2023). Global tuberculosis report 2023. https://iris.who.int/handle/10665/373828 (accessed 8 May 2022).

2 O'Garra, A., Redford, P.S., McNab, F.W. et al. (2013). The immune response in tuberculosis. *Annu. Rev. Immunol.* 31: 475–527.

3 Chandra, P., Grigsby, S.J., and Philips, J.A. (2022). Immune evasion and provocation by *Mycobacterium tuberculosis*. *Nat. Rev. Microbiol.* 20 (12): 750–766.

4 Kumar, P. (2021). A perspective on the success and failure of BCG. *Front. Immunol.* 12: 778028.

5 Bloom, D.E., Black, S., Salisbury, D., and Rappuoli, R. (2018). Antimicrobial resistance and the role of vaccines. *Proc. Natl. Acad. Sci. U. S. A.* 115: 12868–12871.

6 Heaton, P.M. (2020). Challenges of developing novel vaccines with particular global health importance. *Front. Immunol.* 11: 517290.

7 World Health Organization. (2021). Bacterial vaccines in clinical and preclinical development 2021. https://iris.who.int/handle/10665/359172 (accessed 8 March 2022) .

8 Fine, P.E.M. (1995). Variation in protection by BCG: implications of and for heterologous immunity. *Lancet* 346: 1339–1345.

9 Brandt, L., Cunha, J.F., Olsen, A.W. et al. (2002). Failure of the *Mycobacterium bovis* BCG vaccine: some species of environmental mycobacteria block multiplication of BCG and induction of protective immunity to tuberculosis. *Infect. Immun.* 70: 672–678.

10 WHO. (2017). GACVS meeting of 7–8 June 2017. https://www.who.int/groups/global-advisory-committee-on-vaccine-safety/topics/bcg-vaccines#cms (accessed 14 December 2023).

11 Taştan, Y. Comment on Hesseling, et al. "The risk of disseminated Bacille Calmette-Guerin (BCG) disease in HIV-infected children" [*Vaccine* 25 (2006) 14–18]. *Vaccine* 2007, 25: 4513.

12 Hesseling, A.C., Marais, B.J., Gie, R.P. et al. (2007). The risk of disseminated Bacille Calmette-Guerin (BCG) disease in HIV-infected children. *Vaccine* 25: 14–18.

13 Hesseling, A.C., Rabic, II., Marais, B.J. et al. (2006). Bacille Calmette-Guérin vaccine—induced disease in HIV-infected and HIV-uninfected children. *Clin. Infect. Dis.* 42: 548–558.

14 Van Crevel, R., Kleinnijenhuis, J., Oosting, M. et al. (2011). Innate immune recognition of *Mycobacterium tuberculosis*. *Clin. Dev. Immunol.* 2011: 405310.

15 Kumar, S., Ingle, H., Prasad, D.V.R., and Kumar, H. (2013). Recognition of bacterial infection by innate immune sensors. *Crit. Rev. Microbiol.* 39: 229–246.

16 Frieden, T.R., Sterling, T.R., Munsiff, S.S. et al. (2003). Tuberculosis. *Lancet* 362: 887–899.

17 Osterloh, A. (2022). Vaccination against bacterial infections: challenges, progress, and new approaches with a focus on intracellular bacteria. *Vaccines (Basel)* 10: 571.

18 Thakur, A., Mikkelsen, H., and Jungersen, G. (2019). Intracellular pathogens: host immunity and microbial persistence strategies. *J. Immunol. Res.* 2019: 1356540.

19 Castañeda-Delgado, J., Hernández-Pando, R., Serrano, C.J. et al. (2010). Kinetics and cellular sources of cathelicidin during the course of experimental latent tuberculous infection and progressive pulmonary tuberculosis. *Clin. Exp. Immunol.* 161 (3): 542–550.

20 Petit, T.J.P. and Lebreton, A. (2022). Adaptations of intracellular bacteria to vacuolar or cytosolic niches. *Trends Microbiol.* 30: 736–748.

21 Ankley, L., Thomas, S., and Olive, J.A. (2020). Fighting persistence: how chronic infections with *Mycobacterium tuberculosis* evade T cell-mediated clearance and new strategies to defeat them. *Infect. Immun.* 88: e00916–e00919. https://doi.org/10.1128/iai.00916-19.

22 Bruchfeld, J., Correia-Neves, M., and Kallenius, G. (2015). Tuberculosis and HIV coinfection. *Cold Spring Harb. Perspect. Med.* 5: a017871.

23 Larsen, S.E., Erasmus, J.H., Reese, V.A. et al. (2023). An RNA-based vaccine platform for use against *Mycobacterium tuberculosis*. *Vaccines (Basel)* 11: 130.

24 Joffre, O.P., Segura, E., Savina, A., and Amigorena, S. (2012). Cross-presentation by dendritic cells. *Nat. Rev. Immunol.* 12: 557–569.

25 Baena, A. and Porcelli, S.A. (2009). Evasion and subversion of antigen presentation by *Mycobacterium tuberculosis*. *Tissue Antigens* 74: 189–204.

26 Jamaati, H., Mortaz, E., Pajouhi, Z. et al. (2017). Nitric oxide in the pathogenesis and treatment of tuberculosis. *Front. Microbiol.* 8: 2008.

27 Mayer, R.L. and Impens, F. (2021). Immunopeptidomics for next-generation bacterial vaccine development. *Trends Microbiol.* 29: 1034–1045.

28 Kumar, A., Blum, J., Thanh Le, T. et al. (2022). The mRNA vaccine development landscape for infectious diseases. *Nat. Rev. Drug Discov.* 21: 333–334.

29 Jeyanathan, M., Afkhami, S., Smaill, F. et al. (2020). Immunological considerations for COVID-19 vaccine strategies. *Nat. Rev. Immunol.* 20: 615–632.

30 Grifoni, A., Weiskopf, D., Ramirez, S.I. et al. (2020). Targets of T cell responses to SARS-CoV-2 coronavirus in humans with COVID-19 disease and unexposed individuals. *Cell* 181: 1489–1501.e15.

31 Heinz, F.X. and Stiasny, K. (2021). Distinguishing features of current COVID-19 vaccines: knowns and unknowns of antigen presentation and modes of action. *NPJ Vaccines* 6: 104.

32 Verbeke, R., Lentacker, I., De Smedt, S.C., and Dewitte, H. (2021). The dawn of mRNA vaccines: the COVID-19 case. *J. Control. Release* 333: 511–520.

33 Föhse, F.K., Geckin, B., Overheul, G.J. et al. (2021). The BNT162b2 mRNA vaccine against SARS-CoV-2 reprograms both adaptive and innate immune responses. *SSRN Electron. J.* 255: 1–24.

34 O'Neill, L.A.J. and Netea, M.G. (2020). BCG-induced trained immunity: can it offer protection against COVID-19? *Nat. Rev. Immunol.* 20: 335–337.

35 Netea, M.G., Domínguez-Andrés, J., Barreiro, L.B. et al. (2020). Defining trained immunity and its role in health and disease. *Nat. Rev. Immunol.* 20: 375–388.

36 Stevens, N.E., Ryan, F.J., Messina, N.L. et al. (2023). No evidence of durable trained immunity after two doses of adenovirus-vectored or mRNA COVID-19 vaccines. *J. Clin. Invest.* 133: e171742.

37 Yamaguchi, Y., Kato, Y., Edahiro, R. et al. (2022). Consecutive BNT162b2 mRNA vaccination induces short-term epigenetic memory in innate immune cells. *JCI Insight* 7: e163347.

38 Pardi, N., Hogan, M.J., Porter, F.W., and Weissman, D. (2018). mRNA vaccines-a new era in vaccinology. *Nat. Rev. Drug Discov.* 17: 261–279.

39 Iavarone, C., O'hagan, D.T., Yu, D. et al. (2017). Mechanism of action of mRNA-based vaccines. *Expert Rev. Vaccines* 16: 871–881.

40 Gebre, M.S., Brito, L.A., Tostanoski, L.H. et al. (2021). Novel approaches for vaccine development. *Cell* 184: 1589–1603.

41 Zhang, C., Maruggi, G., Shan, H., and Li, J. (2019). Advances in mRNA vaccines for infectious diseases. *Front. Immunol.* 10: 1–13.

42 Ulmer, J.B. and Geall, A.J. (2016). Recent innovations in mRNA vaccines. *Curr. Opin. Immunol.* 41: 18–22.

43 Yin, H., Kanasty, R.L., Eltoukhy, A.A. et al. (2014). Non-viral vectors for gene-based therapy. *Nat. Rev. Genet.* 15: 541–555.

44 Tameris, M.D., Hatherill, M., Landry, B.S. et al. (2013). Safety and efficacy of MVA85A, a new tuberculosis vaccine, in infants previously vaccinated with BCG: a randomised, placebo-controlled phase 2b trial. *Lancet* 381: 1021–1028.

45 Nitika, W.J. and Hui, A.M. (2021). The development of mRNA vaccines for infectious diseases: recent updates. *Infect. Drug Resist.* 14: 5271–5285.

46 Cobelens, F., Suri, R.K., Helinski, M. et al. (2022). Accelerating research and development of new vaccines against tuberculosis: a global roadmap. *Lancet Infect. Dis.* 22: e108–e120.

47 Freyn, A.W., Ramos da Silva, J., Rosado, V.C. et al. (2020). A multi-targeting, nucleoside-modified mRNA influenza virus vaccine provides broad protection in mice. *Mol. Ther.* 28: 1569–1584.

48 Bettencourt, P., Müller, J., Nicastri, A. et al. (2020). Identification of antigens presented by MHC for vaccines against tuberculosis. *NPJ Vaccines* 5: 2.

49 Mayer, R.L., Verbeke, R., Asselman, C. et al. (2022). Immunopeptidomics-based design of mRNA vaccine formulations against *Listeria monocytogenes*. *Nat. Commun.* 13: 6075.

50 Meulewaeter, S., Nuytten, G., Cheng, M.H.Y. et al. (2023). Continuous freeze-drying of messenger RNA lipid nanoparticles enables storage at higher temperatures. *J. Control. Release* 357: 149–160.

51 Muramatsu, H., Lam, K., Bajusz, C. et al. (2022). Lyophilization provides long-term stability for a lipid nanoparticle-formulated, nucleoside-modified mRNA vaccine. *Mol. Ther.* 30: 1941–1951.

52 Xue, T., Stavropoulos, E., Yang, M. et al. (2004). RNA encoding the MPT83 antigen induces protective immune responses against *Mycobacterium tuberculosis* infection. *Infect. Immun.* 72: 6324–6329.

53 Lorenzi, J.C.C., Trombone, A.P.F., Rocha, C.D. et al. (2010). Intranasal vaccination with messenger RNA as a new approach in gene therapy: use against tuberculosis. *BMC Biotechnol.* 10: 1–11.

54 Al Tbeishat, H. (2022). Novel in silico mRNA vaccine design exploiting proteins of *M. tuberculosis* that modulates host immune responses by inducing epigenetic modifications. *Sci. Rep.* 12: 1–19.

55 Mishra, A., Singh, V., Court, K.P. et al. (2023). A novel self-adjuvanted mRNA vaccine expressing the Antigen-85B-p25 epitope of *Mycobacterium tuberculosis* protects mice against tuberculosis. *J. Immunol.* 210: 141.03.

56 Crowell, C., Vogel, A., and van der Most, R.2023). *BioNTech Workshop – Development of mRNA-based Medicines, ISV Congress*, Lausanne.

57 Larsen, S.E., Baldwin, S.L., and Coler, R.N. (2023). Tuberculosis vaccines update: is an RNA-based vaccine feasible for tuberculosis? *Int. J. Infect. Dis.* 130 (Suppl 1): S47–S51.

58 BioNTech. (2021). BioNTech provides update on plans to develop sustainable solutions to address infectious diseases on the African continent. p. 2. https://investors.biontech.de/news-releases/news-release-details/biontech-provides-update-plans-develop-sustainable-solutions (accessed 4 August 2022).

59 Youngdahl, K. (2022). IAVI and Moderna partner to tackle broad global health priorities using mRNA for vaccines and antibodies. https://www.iavi.org/news-resources/press-releases/2022/iavi-and-moderna-partner-to-tackle-broad-global-health-priorities-using-mrna-for-vaccines-and-antibodies (accessed 16 October 2023).

60 Certest Biotec. (2023). Development of an mRNA vaccine against tuberculosis. https://www.certest.es/news/development-of-an-mrna-vaccine-against-tuberculosis/ (accessed 21 December 2023).

61 Baxerna. (2023). Baxerna: next-generation bacterial mRNA vaccines. https://www.baxerna.eu/ (accessed 21 December 2023)

13

Cancer Vaccines Based on mRNA: Hype or Hope?

Wout de Mey, Dorien Autaers, Giada Bertazzon, Arthur Esprit, Marta Marco Aragon, Lorenzo Franceschini, and Karine Breckpot

Vrije Universiteit Brussel (VUB), Transaltional Oncology Research Center (TORC), Laboratory for Molecular and Cellular Therapy (LMCT), Laarbeeklaan 103, 1090 Brussels, Belgium

13.1 Tumors: Setting the Scene for Cancer Immunotherapy

Human cancer cells result from genetic and epigenetic alterations that induce hallmarks such as sustaining proliferative signaling, evading growth suppressors, resisting cell death, enabling replicative immortality, inducing angiogenesis, and activating invasion and metastasis [1]. Genetic alterations further give rise to neoantigens, a class of tumor-specific antigens (TSAs) [2, 3]. Epigenetic alterations give rise to tumor-associated antigens (TAAs, e.g. melanoma-associated antigens [MAGEs]), a class of antigens also expressed to a certain extent by healthy cells [4–7].

The immune system can recognize both tumor antigen types to identify and destroy cancer cells [8]. To that end, tumor antigen-derived peptides generated by proteasomal degradation need to be presented in human leukocyte antigen (HLA) class I molecules on the cancer cell surface. As such, activated tumor antigen-specific $CD8^+$ cytotoxic T lymphocytes (CTLs) can bind cancer cells with their T-cell receptor (TCR), enabling the destruction of cancer cells [9]. The activation of CTLs relies on antigen-presenting cells (APCs), such as dendritic cells (DCs), which can acquire antigens at the tumor microenvironment (TME) and can cross-present them to CTLs [10, 11]. Further, DCs can present tumor antigen-derived peptides in the context of HLA class II to $CD4^+$ T cells that, when activated into T helper 1 (T_H1) cells, can support CTL activation [12]. Though tumor antigen-specific T_H1 cells and CTLs, activated by DCs, are considered the main players in eliminating cancer cells, many other immune cell types can assist in this process, among other classically activated macrophages, natural killer (NK) cells, innate-like T cells, including type I NKT cells and Vγ9δV2 T cells, and B cells [13–15]. The concerted action of these immune cells, if effective, results in cancer cell rejection. However, under the pressure of the immune system, cancer cells

Trends in mRNA Vaccine Research, First Edition. Edited by Gabor Tamas Szabo and Norbert Pardi.

can develop resistance mechanisms, for instance, evasion of immune recognition, disruption of T-cell signaling, or induction of tolerance. This allows them to escape immune destruction, which results in the formation of tumors. A tumor is a malignant tissue consisting of cancer cells interwoven with stroma and stromal cells that promote cancer progression, among others by inhibition of T_H1 cells and CTLs [16]. Among the immune cells that promote tumor progression are alternatively activated macrophages, monocytic and granulocytic myeloid-derived suppressors cells (MDSCs), tolerogenic DCs (tolDCs), regulatory T (T_{REG}) cells, and regulatory B (B_{REG}) cells [13, 17]. Type II NKT cells and several subsets of $\gamma\delta$ T cells can exert tumor-promoting activity as well [14, 18]. These tumor-promoting immune cells outnumber T_H1 cells and CTLs in most if not all of tumors (Figure 13.1).

Several approaches have been studied to tip the balance in favor of cancer-rejecting instead of cancer-promoting immune cells in the TME (Figure 13.2). This endeavor is the field of cancer immunotherapy, which has moved from a field with anecdotal success to a highly regarded field in which monoclonal antibodies (mAbs) that block inhibitory immune checkpoint (ICP) axis have revolutionized the treatment of advanced cancer [19, 20]. Though ICP therapy has been proven effective, it is clear that there are limitations, with a sizable cohort of patients failing to benefit from this cancer immunotherapy [21]. Response to ICP-blocking mAbs is correlated to a tumor immune contexture characterized by classically activated macrophages, activated memory $CD4^+$ T cells, T follicular helper (T_{FH}) cells, $CD8^+$ T cells, and a

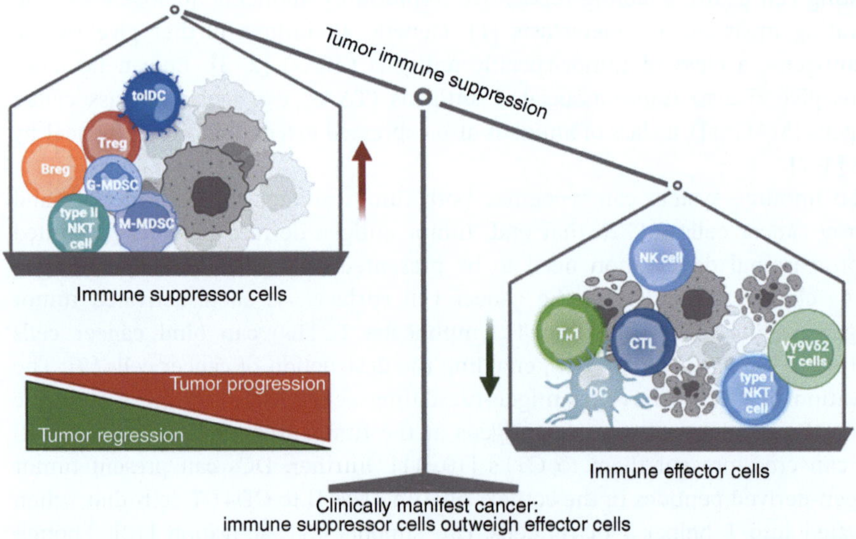

Figure 13.1 Immune suppressor versus immune effector cells in the TME of established tumors. Immune suppressor cells, such as tolDCs, alternatively activated macrophages, G- and M-MDSCs, type II NKT cells, B_{REG} and T_{REG} cells, outweigh immune effector cells, such as cross-presenting DCs, NK cells, type 1 NKT cells, Vγ9δV2 T cells, T_H1 cells, and CTLs, in clinically manifest tumors. As a result, tumors progress. Abbreviations: B_{REG}, regulatory B cell; DC, dendritic cell; G, granulocytic; NK, natural killer; M, monocytic; MDSC, myeloid-derived suppressor cell; tolDC, tolerogenic DC; T_{REG}, regulatory T cell.

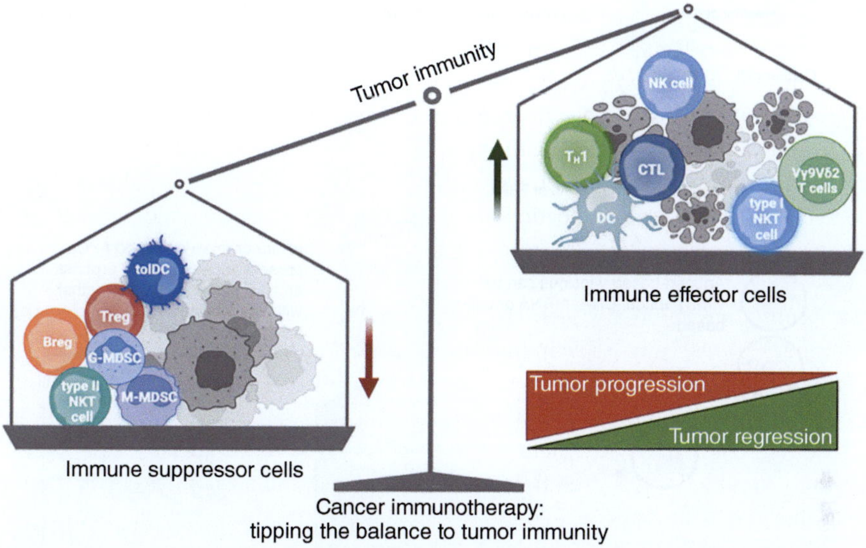

Figure 13.2 Immune suppressor versus immune effector cells in the TME: tipping the balance. Immunotherapy aims to tip the balance toward immune effector cells, such as cross-presenting DCs, NK cells, type 1 NKT cells, Vγ9δV2 T cells, T_H1 cells, and CTLs, to facilitate tumor regression. Abbreviations: B_{REG}, regulatory B cell; DC, dendritic cell; G, granulocytic; NK, natural killer; M, monocytic; MDSC, myeloid-derived suppressor cell; tolDC, tolerogenic DC; T_{REG}, regulatory T cell.

typical interferon (IFN)-γ signature [22]. This observation has rekindled the interest in cancer vaccines [23, 24]. Cancer vaccines have a long-standing history characterized by periods of scientific discoveries and technological advances that raised enthusiasm. However, they were often followed by periods of skepticism when the cancer vaccines under development did not generate the expected results. Nonetheless, immune activation has been reported across various vaccine formulations, and, even in some cases, significant clinical responses have been observed in early-phase clinical trials, highlighting the promise of cancer vaccination [25].

13.2 Cancer Vaccination

The aim of a cancer vaccine, either being preventive (e.g. human papillomavirus [HPV] vaccines [26]) or therapeutic, is to activate the adaptive immune system against tumor antigens (Figure 13.3) [27]. In that way, tumor cells that express and present these tumor antigens, whether newly arising or established, could be recognized and killed. Cancer vaccination is particularly interesting in tumors characterized as "cold" or "immune desert," i.e. tumors that for various reasons did not naturally provoke a strong response by the immune system [24]. Examples hereof are glioblastomas, ovarian, prostate, pancreatic, and microsatellite stable (MSS) colorectal cancer (CRC) [28].

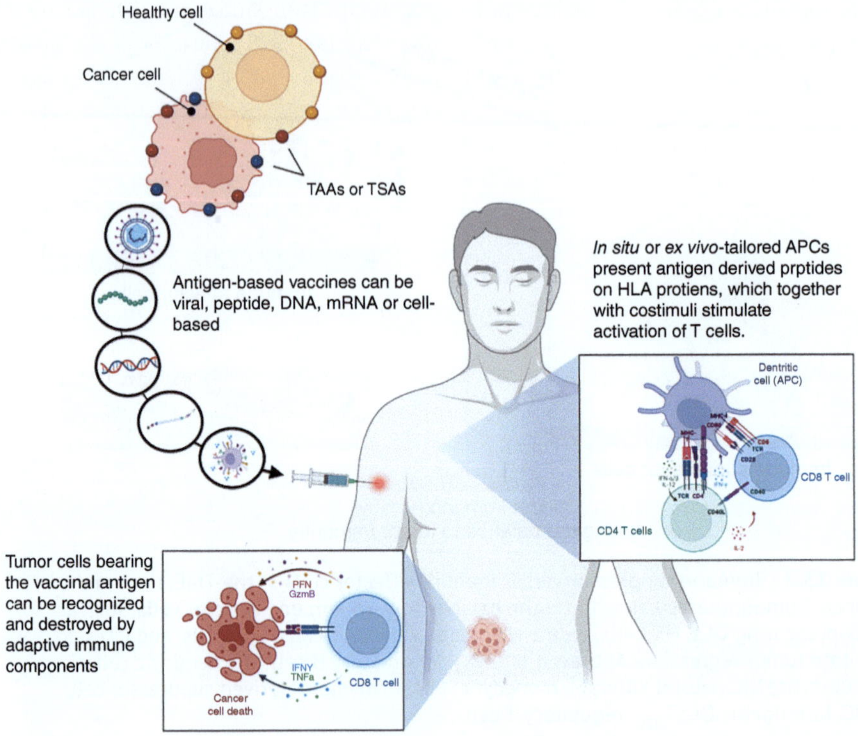

Figure 13.3 Cancer vaccination. Cancer vaccines based on viral vectors, nucleic acids (mRNA or DNA), peptides, or APCs stimulate adaptive immunity against TAAs, which are scarce in healthy cells yet highly expressed on cancer cells, or TSAs, which are unique to cancer cells. Therefore, the cancer vaccine contains TAAs/TSAs and adjuvants. APCs, tailored *in situ* or *ex vivo*, among which DCs, activate adaptive immunity, including CD4$^+$ T$_H$1 cells and CD8$^+$ CTLs that can cooperate in rejecting cancer cells, potentially instigating a self-propagating process, leading to a broad T-cell response and an immunological memory. Abbreviations: APC, antigen-presenting cell; CTL, cytotoxic T lymphocyte; Ig, immunoglobulin; TAA, tumor-associated antigen; T$_H$1, T helper 1; TSA, tumor-specific antigen.

The success of cancer vaccination critically depends on professional APCs, specifically DCs, that need to be tailored to present considerable levels [29] of highly immunogenic [30] tumor antigen-derived peptides to CD4$^+$ and CD8$^+$ T cells, while providing costimulatory ligands (e.g. CD70 [31] and CD83 [32]) and cytokines (e.g. interleukin [IL]-12p70 and IFN-α/β [33]) to stimulate a T$_H$1 and CTL-mediated antitumor response. Though DCs are the main players in vaccination, it is known that other APCs such as macrophages can induce antitumor responses [34] and can act in concert with DCs to increase vaccine efficacy [35].

Engineering DCs can be accomplished by delivering tumor antigens and adjuvants to endogenous DCs [36] or DCs *in vitro* cultured [37]. Reverting endogenous DCs into APCs that can elicit strong antitumor immunity, also referred to as *in situ* vaccination, can be achieved in various ways. Up to this moment, it is well established that most of the successful cancer cell death-inducing therapies evoke immunogenic cell death and as such provide tumor antigens and damage-associated molecular patterns (DAMPs) that act as adjuvants for DCs. These DCs can subsequently activate tumor-specific T-cell responses [38]. More traditional *in situ* vaccines based on peptides, mRNA, DNA, or viral vectors, rely on careful selection and preparation of tumor antigens and adjuvants (e.g. pathogen-associated molecular patterns [PAMPs]) for injection into patients [39]. Though this brings along several challenges, including the selection of the best-suited antigen, adjuvant, and vaccine delivery platform, nevertheless, it has the main advantage that the vaccination condition is more controlled. In this regard, any uncertainty about the activity of the tailored DCs is taken away by generating DC vaccines *ex vivo*. Manufacturing *ex vivo* DC vaccines is undoubtedly more cumbersome due to its patient-specific nature, yet allows controlling every step of the process, i.e. DC yield, viability, phenotype, and functionality, before and after delivery of tumor antigens and adjuvants, thereby lowering the risk of failing to induce T-cell responses. Table 13.1 provides an overview of the advantages and disadvantages of *in vivo* versus *ex vivo* tailoring of DCs.

It has been shown that antitumor immune responses, elicited upon vaccination, can lead to the accumulation of immunostimulants that can amplify and broaden the T-cell response [40, 41]. Various cancer vaccines have exhibited the ability to unleash tumor-specific T cells, eradicate tumors, and establish an immunological memory in several mouse cancer models. Still, the results of most clinical trials

Table 13.1 Advantages and disadvantages of *in vivo* versus *ex vivo* targeting of DCs.

	In Vivo	*Ex Vivo*
Advantages	1. Off-the-shelf → Warehouse of tumor (neo)antigen vaccines 2. Lower manufacturing cost 3. Lower batch-to-batch variations 4. Delivery of antigens and adjuvants to natural APCs → Targeting allows to reach multiple or specific APCs (cDCs, pDCs, macrophages)	1. Highly controlled antigen delivery 2. Highly controlled activation (adjuvant delivery) → Analysis of the DC yield, viability, phenotype, antigen presentation, and the T-cell-activating capacity can be performed before vaccination
Disadvantages	1. Delivery of antigens and adjuvants to natural APCs → Only a few receptors, utilized for DC targeting, are truly DC specific → The adjuvant should be carefully considered to ensure full activation of different APCs	1. Patient specific → Autologous cellular vaccine 2. Requires leukapheresis → Not feasible for every patient 3. Limited to DC subsets that can be isolated in sufficient numbers or cultured *in vitro* 4. Considerable manufacturing cost 5. Higher batch-to-batch variability

Abbreviations: APC, antigen-presenting cell; cDC, conventional DC; DC, dendritic cell; pDC, plasmacytoid DC.

have been unfulfilling, failing to show convincing objective clinical responses [25, 37]. To date, the United States Food and Drug Administration (FDA) approved only one cell-based vaccine for the treatment of hormone-refractory prostate cancer, Sipuleucel-T (Provenge®) [42]. No other therapeutic cancer vaccines have been approved since 2010, even though some vaccines tested in small-scale phase I/II clinical trials have shown promising results. An example hereof is the TriMixDC-MEL vaccine: an autologous DC vaccine used to vaccinate melanoma patients. This vaccine consists of monocyte-derived DCs (moDCs) that have been electroporated with mRNA-encoding TAAs (MAGE-A3, MAGE-C2, tyrosinase, or gp100), engineered to allow presentation of TAA-derived peptides in HLA-I and HLA-II, and mRNA-encoding two DC-activating proteins, CD40 ligand (CD40L) and a constitutively active (ca) variant of toll-like receptor (TLR) 4 (caTLR4), supplemented with mRNA encoding the T-cell-costimulatory protein CD70. This mRNA mix, referred to as TriMix, endows the DCs with strong T-cell-activating capacity [43], while circumventing the inhibitory activity of T_{REG} cells [44]. Several clinical trials have been performed using TriMixDC-MEL in patients with grade III/IV melanoma to study their efficacy as a monotherapy [45, 46] or in combination with ICP therapy (Ipilimumab, an anti-CTLA-4 mAb) [47]. These studies showed a considerably improved life expectancy of melanoma patients with few and mild adverse events (AEs) of the vaccination procedure. Immunomonitoring data have further demonstrated that the level of activated tumor-specific T cells after vaccination correlates with clinical objective responses [48]. This TriMixDC-MEL with IFN-α2b has also been used to treat melanoma patients following complete resection of their metastasis, showing that this adjuvant therapy is tolerable and results in encouraging long-term overall survival (OS) rates [49]. Studies in mice further showed that delivery of TAAs and TriMix mRNA to DCs within lymph nodes [50] or TriMix mRNA to DCs within tumors [51] has high potential as a cancer vaccine. These strategies are currently under clinical evaluation. This work performed by researchers at the Vrije Universiteit Brussel and many other preclinical and clinical studies, testing numerous cancer vaccine formulations, provided valuable knowledge, resulting in a number of guidelines for effective cancer vaccine development, worth mentioning (i) prioritize multiple and highly immunogenic TSAs; (ii) use a potent adjuvant to activate APCs, in particular for DCs; (iii) select an efficacious, flexible, safe, and preferably low-cost vaccine vector; (iv) choose the best route of delivery; and (v) incorporate strategies to subdue tumor-mediated immunosuppression.

13.3 Vaccine Development Rules: A Brief Overview of Lessons Learned

13.3.1 Use Multiple and Highly Immunogenic Tumor-Specific Antigens

Cancer vaccination could be considered self-defeating, when it is performed with only one tumor antigen, as the activated T cells will put selection pressure on the cancer cells to escape by downregulating the tumor antigen, particularly if the tumor antigen is not crucial for survival of the cancer cells [52–54]. Hence, it is important to include multiple antigens in a cancer vaccine to reduce the chance of immune escape. The finding that higher objective clinical responses were observed in 1711 patients vaccinated with an irradiated whole-tumor vaccine relative to 1733 patients vaccinated with molecularly defined tumor antigens might be partly explained by a difference in the number of tumor antigens [55]. However, other factors such as higher immunogenicity of the tumor antigens (including TSAs) in the irradiated whole-tumor vaccines versus the molecularly defined tumor antigen vaccines should not be ignored. Early vaccines, with defined tumor antigens, were mainly based on TAAs that stimulate a low-avidity T-cell repertoire, which is suboptimal for *in vivo* tumor control [56–58]. Studies on TCR avidity have shown a strong correlation with the capacity of $CD8^+$ T cells to lyse target cells. However, a plateau in T-cell functionality is reached above a certain TCR avidity threshold [57, 58]. In contrast, vaccines that contain TSAs, neoantigens, that are not subject to thymic tolerance, stimulate a high avidity T-cell repertoire [59, 60]. Notably, it is expected that different TCRs can interact with a given neoepitope [2, 61]. Further, mutated peptides may be recognized by cross-reactive memory T cells that were primed against an unrelated antigen, e.g. from pathogens [54]. Therefore, current vaccine research focuses on TSAs rather than TAAs. The latter has been facilitated due to continuously improving technologies, including DNA/RNA sequencing and computational analysis (reviewed in [62, 63]), allowing identification and prioritization of neoantigens. These can be classified based on molecular characteristics in single-nucleotide variants (SNVs), insertions or deletions of nucleotides (INDELs), fusion genes and splice variants, or on potential functional impact in guarding, restrained, and ignored neoantigens (Table 13.2) [2]. The functional classification was introduced to provide a framework, linking neoantigen biology to proficiency to induce antitumor responses with clinical benefit [58].

13.3.2 Use a Potent Adjuvant

The role of an adjuvant in vaccines is to regulate the type and magnitude of the immune response to the selected antigens by acting on APCs, preferably DCs. In cancer vaccines, the adjuvant should stimulate the maturation of DCs to activate a T_H1-supported CTL response that is dominated by an IFN-γ signature. A lot of work has been invested in designing safe, effective adjuvants for cancer immunotherapy, resulting in several adjuvants acting on various pathways within APCs to activate them. Many vaccine modalities are on the market. Therefore, research has also focused on optimizing the formulation and administration of adjuvants and tumor antigens, as this might strengthen the immune activation and antitumor effects. Despite considerable efforts, few adjuvants have been approved by the FDA for cancer therapy applications, though there is convincing evidence that most adjuvants enhance antitumor immunity [64].

Clinical-grade incomplete Freund's adjuvant (IFA) has been widely used in clinical research in the context of whole tumor cell (protein) vaccines [65]. Montanide

Table 13.2 Classification of neoantigens [58, 64, 65].

Molecular	**Functional**
1. SNV: high frequency → Exchange of single nucleotides within the genome → Shared mutations exist (e.g. KRAS^{G12D}in CRC) → SNV burden is predictive of the clinical efficacy of ICP therapy	1. Guarding: low frequency (<2% of all mutations) → Neoantigens driving early CTL expansion or cross-recognized by pathogen-specific memory T cells → Prognostically significant executors of antitumor immunity in the immunotherapy naive host
2. INDEL: 16–20% of all mutations → Single insertions or deletions of nucleotides that lead to a frameshift mutation or to a stop codon (prone to nonsense-mediated decay of RNA) → INDELs correlate with clinical efficacy of ICP therapy	2. Restrained: low frequency (<2% of all mutations) → Inactive in the immunotherapy naive host due to immunosuppression in the TME → Neoantigens that induce PD-1$^+$ memory T cells under ICP therapy in the immunotherapy-naive host
3. Fusion genes: very low frequency (rare) → Intra- and inter-chromosomal rearrangements that join two unrelated genes to form a fusion gene → Value in immunotherapy is uncertain though T-cell responses to fusion antigens occur upon ICP therapy	3. Ignored: 15–25% of all mutations → Neoantigens that are not naturally recognized → Neoantigens that do not impact tumor growth under ICP therapy → Memory T cells can be induced by vaccination
4. Splice variants: high frequency → Abnormal regulation of alternative splicing produces different protein isoforms that can be immunogenic → The role of splicing-derived neoantigens in enabling ICP therapy needs further investigation	

Abbreviations: CRC, colorectal cancer; CTL, cytotoxic T lymphocyte; ICP, immune checkpoint; INDEL, insertion/deletion; KRAS, Kirsten rat sarcoma viral oncogene homolog; PD-1, programmed death-1; SNV, single-nucleotide variant; TME, tumor microenvironment.

ISA-51, a water-in-oil emulsion, has been studied to improve synthetic long peptide (SLP)-based vaccination. This emulsion forms a depot at the injection site, trapping SLPs for controlled release, while inducing inflammation. A clinical trial showed induction of T-cell responses in patients vaccinated with SLPs of the HPV oncoproteins E6 and E7 [66]. Vaccine adjuvants that act on pattern recognition receptors (PRRs), including TLRs and stimulator of IFN genes (STING), have gained increasing attention as these may reverse CD8$^+$ T-cell tolerance, making them particularly attractive for cancer vaccination [67, 68]. Agonists of various TLRs have been evaluated in clinical trials as adjuvants for cancer vaccines based on proteins, DNA, and mRNA. Examples hereof are TLR3 agonist, based on polyinosinic–polycytidylic acid (polyI:C) [69, 70], the TLR4 agonist monophosphoryl lipid A (MPLA) [71, 72], the TLR7 agonist imiquimod (R-837) [73], the TLR7/8 agonist resiquimod [74], and the TLR9 agonist CpG oligodeoxynucleotide (CpG ODN) [75, 76]. Among these, only MPLA and imiquimod have been approved by the FDA in cancer therapy [77]. Agonists of STING, synthetic cyclic dinucleotides (CDNs), delivered at low doses using various formulations to avoid their enzymatic degradation and to increase their delivery to APCs, also showed vaccine adjuvant properties in various preclinical mouse cancer studies [78]. Despite encouraging preclinical data, the results from clinical trials with STING agonists remain elusive, likely as they are most often studied as a monotherapy or combined with ICP therapy rather than a vaccine adjuvant [79]. Agonists of the costimulatory receptor CD40 are also attractive as vaccine adjuvants. CD40, capable of triggering DCs, leads to early endosomal location of antigens, mediating cross-presentation, and stimulates expression of IL-12 as well as CD70, enabling activation of long-lived memory $CD8^+$ T cells [80]. Various preclinical studies have shown that combining signaling via CD40 and TLRs in a vaccination strategy creates considerable synergy [31, 81–84], and a vaccine that incorporates CD40 and TLR4 signaling together with CD70 expression has translated into clinical efficacy [45]. Notably, the efficacy of this vaccine has been linked to the production of IL-12p70 [45], an immunostimulatory cytokine. Similar to IL-12p70, other cytokines have been studied as vaccine adjuvants, such as ILs (IL-2 and IL-15), IFNs (IFN-α/β and IFN-γ), and granulocyte-macrophage colony-stimulating factor (GM-CSF) [80, 85]. It is noteworthy that cytokines can act on different cell types and as a result can elicit different kinds of responses, which call for caution when using cytokines in the context of cancer therapy. For example, GM-CSF, widely studied in view of whole tumor cell cancer vaccination, has been shown to stimulate DC activation and accumulation [86]. In contrast, other studies suggested that GM-CSF can promote tumor progression by inducing MDSCs [87]. A cytokine demonstrated to act in concert with CD40 and TLR4 agonists is IFN-γ [88]. These adjuvants increase the capacity of DCs to express CCR7 and as a result migrate to chemokines expressed in secondary lymphoid organs (SLOs), to produce IL-12 and activate T_H1 cells [88]. Moreover, activating DCs via CD40, TLR4, and IFN-γ lowered their capacity to produce IL-10 and phosphorylate signal transducer and activator of transcription 3 (STAT3), two well-known negative factors in T-cell stimulation [88–90]. Various adjuvants with interesting immunostimulating effects on APCs and T cells have been identified to date. To ensure their optimal use, it is tremendously important to rationally combine adjuvants and to optimize their delivery regime (formulation, dose, and route), which should be defined on a case-by-case basis for a given vaccine modality, e.g. SLPs versus mRNA.

13.3.3 Use an Efficacious, Flexible, Safe, and Preferably Low-Cost Vaccine Vector

Since the dawn of medical science, many historical events show that vaccines, as defined by modern medicine, have been exploited for cancer treatment.

The Egyptian physician Imhotep induced infection to treat tumors as early as 2600 BCE, a strategy that was adopted in the eighteenth and nineteenth centuries and that became more standardized by the practice of the New York surgeon William Coley, who published antitumor responses to treatment with "Coley's Toxin," a concoction of bacteria [91]. This bacterial immunization relied on APCs that already acquired the tumor cells' antigens, while cancer vaccines based on tumor cells and tumor lysates, first developed in the 1980s for treatment of CRC patients, delivered an unbiased pool of tumor antigens [92]. The identification of MAGE-1, the first human TAA [93], followed by continued efforts to discover new TAAs and their immunogenic epitopes [94, 95], opened new avenues for cancer vaccination. Clinical trials with peptide-based vaccines soon followed, inducing immunity against TAAs such as mucin-1 (MUC-1) [96], MAGE-A3 [97], and human epidermal growth factor receptor 2 (HER2; also known as ERBB2 and NEU) [98]. Meanwhile, DCs gained increasing attention as nature's adjuvant, and protocols to generate and mature DCs *in vitro* became more established [99–102]. As a result, vectors to deliver TAAs to DCs were intensively studied, including vectors based on viruses, bacteria, proteins, and nucleic acids (i.e. DNA and mRNA) [103, 104], leading to hundreds of clinical trials using DC-based vaccines in different cancer types [105]. In 2010, the DC-based vaccine, Sipuleucel-T (Provenge®), was used to treat prostate cancer, proving the viability of cancer vaccines and leading to its approval by the FDA [42]. Most of the different vectors that have been used to load TAAs to DCs *in vitro* were also developed into *in situ* vaccines [106–109], which all have their advantages and disadvantages, as depicted in Figure 13.4.

To date, cancer vaccines are focusing on using TSAs, demanding a flexible vaccine vector that requires minimal time for *in silico* design, *in vitro* manufacturing, and *in vivo* administration [62]. The outbreak of severe acute respiratory syndrome coronavirus 2 (SARS-CoV2), which required rapid development of vaccines capable of controlling this pandemic, has shown that mRNA is a flexible, efficacious, time, and cost-effective vaccine platform. Manufacturing of mRNA is a cell-free and swift process that avoids the need to grow pathogenic organisms (e.g. viral or bacterial vectors) on a large scale. As a consequence, the safety profile of mRNA as a pharmaceutical ingredient is ideal with little risk of biological contaminants. The flexible nature of the mRNA vaccine platform negates the need for a dedicated product-specific production facility. Nevertheless, once the production process is established for one vaccine, only the *in silico* design, that is the mRNA molecule sequence, needs to be changed if another vaccine (peptide) needs to be targeted or produced. Consequently, the manufacturing process can be streamlined, including its encapsulation in nanoparticles (NPs), allowing time and cost-effective mRNA vaccine development [110]. These features make mRNA vaccines particularly helpful in a personalized TSA-based vaccine scenario, where time is crucial.

13.3.4 Choose the Best Route of Delivery

In addition to the features of the cancer vaccine, i.e. the selected tumor antigen(s), adjuvant, and vaccine platform, the route of administration can have an important

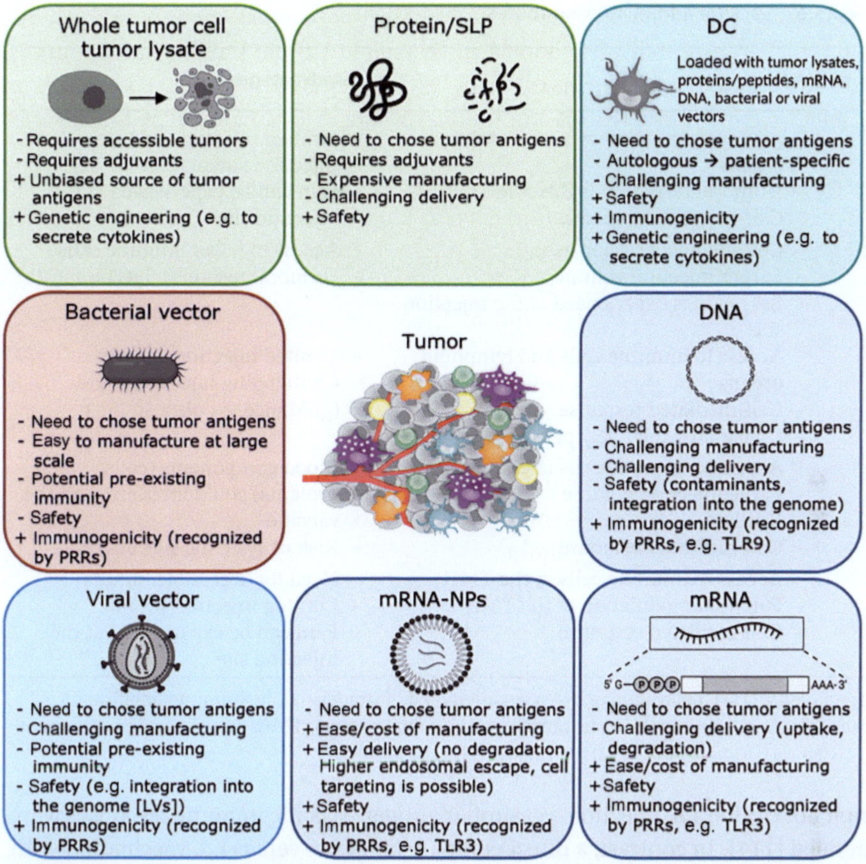

Figure 13.4 Cancer vaccination platforms. A plethora of cancer vaccines have been developed. They loosely group into vaccines based on whole tumor cells or tumor lysates, proteins or peptides, DCs, DNA, mRNA, viral vectors, and bacterial vectors. Abbreviations: DC, dendritic cell; NP, nanoparticle; PRR, pattern recognition receptor; SLP, synthetic long peptide; TLR, toll-like receptor.

impact on the safety profile, ability to induce long-lasting immunity, and linked herewith the therapeutic outcome. Routes of delivery that have been frequently exploited in cancer vaccination are the intradermal (i.d.), subcutaneous (s.c.), intranodal (i.n.) or intralymphatic, intravenous (i.v.), and intratumoral (i.t.) route of delivery (Table 13.3) [111]. Though APCs and lymphoid organs are the common targets in vaccination, the optimal route of vaccine delivery is dependent on the context (tumor type and stage) and the vaccine formulation. Therefore, the optimal route of vaccine delivery should be considered on a case-by-case basis.

DC or molecular vaccination via the i.d. delivery route has been shown to result in low levels of antigen-presenting DCs in draining lymph nodes [112–114]. However, several clinical trials in diverse cancer types and with different vaccine types have shown T-cell activation and clinical benefits [114–121]. Comparison of i.d. versus i.n. injection of a DC vaccine showed that more DCs reached the T-cell areas in

Table 13.3 Vaccine administration routes.

Route	Advantages	Disadvantages
i.d.	– Access to immune cells and lymphoid organs – Humoral response: IgG2a > IgG1 – Cell-mediated response	– Limited injection volume – Injection site reaction (DTH) – Pain can be experienced at the injection site
s.c.	– Cell-mediated response – Larger injection volume – Less pain is experienced at the injection site	– Access to fewer immune cells – Humoral response: IgG1 > IgG2a
i.n.	– Access to immune cells and lymphoid organs – Cell-mediated response – Considered relatively painless	– Limited injection volume – Challenging injection route (guidance via ultra-sound)
i.v.	– Access to immune cells in circulation – Large injection volume – Painless – Cell-mediated response	– Blood components (cells, proteins) could interfere with the vaccine – Risk of systemic side effects
i.t.	– Access to immune cells in the TME – Potential modulation of the TME – Cell-mediated response	– Need for accessible tumors – Limited injection volume – Pain can be experienced at the injection site

Abbreviations: DTH, delayed-type hypersensitivity; i.d., intradermal; Ig, immunoglobulin; i.n., intranodal; i.t., intratumoral; i.v., intravenous; s.c., subcutaneous; TME, tumor microenvironment.

lymph nodes after i.n. injection, yet similar antigen-specific immune responses were generated [114]. In contrast, a direct comparison of i.n. versus i.d. vaccination with unprotected mRNA in mice has proven that the former delivery route is superior, likely as the access to APCs is facilitated [122]. This difference in DC versus mRNA vaccines illustrates the earlier claim that the optimal delivery route is vaccine dependent. The maximum volume that can be injected i.d. or i.n. is limited compared to the volumes that can be injected subcutaneously. Also, this skin layer contains fewer immune cells than the dermis [123], explaining the need for considerably higher antigen quantities for s.c. vaccination when compared to i.d. or i.n. vaccination [124–126]. Moreover, it has been shown in mice with ovalbumin-loaded particles that s.c. vaccination is less proficient in stimulating IFN-γ and IgG2a responses compared to i.d. or intralymphatic vaccination [127]. These differences have been reproduced using a model vaccine of modified vaccinia virus Ankara in nonhuman primates (NHPs) [128]. Despite the observation of a less favorable T_H2 cell-oriented immune response, following s.c. vaccination, stimulation of $CD8^+$ T-cell responses has been achieved using s.c. delivery of SLP and DC cancer vaccines [129–132]. In mice, it was shown that i.d. and s.c. vaccination with DCs was superior to i.v. vaccination, though i.v. delivery of DCs could facilitate their migration to SLOs [133, 134]. In contrast, i.v. delivery of a peptide vaccine stimulated higher CTL responses compared to s.c. delivery, resulting in more pronounced antitumor effects [135]. Also, mRNA-NP vaccines have been delivered i.v., modifying splenic DCs and eliciting strong T-cell responses [136–139], which were more pronounced compared to the T-cell responses elicited after s.c. or i.m. injection of the mRNA-NP vaccine [137]. A newer route of vaccine delivery is the i.t. route. This route of delivery, though limited to accessible tumors and limited in injection volume, has been shown to achieve significantly higher antitumor results than s.c. injection of the same NP vaccine [140]. Using an mRNA vaccine, it has been shown that tumor-associated DCs are key to stimulate T cells, yet only a limited number of these DCs find their way to draining lymph nodes to stimulate T cells *de novo* [51]. Moreover, i.t. delivery of vaccines can modulate the TME, acting on myeloid cells and tumor-infiltrating lymphocytes (TILs) [51, 140].

The route of vaccine administration has also been shown to affect the balance between tumor-specific circulating memory T cells versus tissue-resident memory T (T_{RM}), which should not be underestimated as both are necessary to induce meaningful antitumor immunity [141–143]. It has been shown in early-stage nonsmall-cell lung carcinoma, pulmonary squamous cell carcinoma, and high-grade serous epithelial ovarian cancer that infiltration of these tumors by T_{RM} cells positively correlates with OS [142, 144, 145]. Evidence that vaccines, depending on the route of delivery, can divert T cells from tumors or promote infiltration of T_{RM} cells in tumors has been shown in various studies [146–149]. Moreover, it has been shown that the capacity of T cells to migrate to specific tissues is defined at the site of antigen capture by cross-presenting APCs [150]. These studies provide a rationale for combining multiple routes of vaccine delivery to generate T cells that might migrate to multiple tissue sites, inducing robust immune responses in patients with metastatic tumors, the target population in most vaccine studies [151]. This idea is supported by the observation that combined i.d. and i.v. delivery of the TriMixDC-MEL vaccine resulted in objective responses in 27% of the treated stage III/IV melanoma patients. In contrast, the same vaccine failed to induce any objective responses after i.d. delivery, despite evidence of activated T cells (in DTH and blood) following both vaccination regimes [46, 152, 153]. Thus, for a given cancer type (location, e.g. gut versus skin) and stage (local versus metastatic), and a given vaccine modality, a comparison of diverse delivery routes will help to define the most suitable injection method and, therefore, promote the development of an efficacious cancer vaccine.

13.3.5 Incorporate Strategies to Subdue Tumor-Mediated Immunosuppression

A plethora of preclinical and clinical studies with therapeutic cancer vaccines based on various antigens and vaccine formulations have evidenced that inducing strong antitumor immunity is feasible.

However, only a handful of studies have shown that cancer vaccination can result in the long-term survival of patients [46, 49, 154]. One study in particular reported that the 12-year survival of patients with nonresectable metastatic melanoma vaccinated i.d. with a moDC vaccine was 19% [154], which is comparable to the survival rates documented for melanoma patients treated with mAbs that block CTLA-4

[155, 156]. The fact remains that the majority of cancer patients enrolled in clinical cancer vaccination trials have not benefited from this immunotherapy, despite eliciting tumor-specific T-cell responses upon vaccination with a wide variety of antigens, adjuvants, and vaccine platforms. It is now well established that the response to cancer vaccination is likely suppressed in patients with advanced-stage disease, the target population in most vaccine clinical trials [105].

As mentioned in Section 13.1, the TME of established tumors is typically characterized by the presence of several suppressive immune cell types, including alternatively activated macrophages, monocytic and granulocytic MDSCs, tolDCs, T_{REG} cells, B_{REG} cells [13, 17], type II NKT cells, and tumor-promoting $\gamma\delta$ T-cell subsets [14, 18]. Moreover, coinhibitory pathways that reduce the activation state of T cells are abundant in the TME and are being exploited by immunosuppressive immune cells as well as cancer cells to paralyze cancer-rejecting T cells [157–159]. This knowledge has driven researchers to look into strategies to overcome immunosuppression and develop specific reagents that reduce immunosuppressive actions at the TME [160, 161]. Such reagents have been used in combination with cancer vaccination to improve clinical outcomes (e.g. angiogenesis inhibiting agents to promote T-cell homing to tumors, chemotherapies to deplete immunosuppressive immune cells, and radiotherapy to increase antigen presentation on cancer cells) [162]. Notably, pharmaceutical companies have heavily invested in developing ICP therapy targeting coinhibitory pathways that curtail the T-cell function. In particular, mAbs that block PD-1 and its ligand PD-L1 have shown unprecedented success with acceptable toxicity in cancer types like melanoma, Hodgkin lymphoma, squamous cell carcinoma, and Merkel carcinoma (50–80% response). However, some cancer types are nonresponsive (e.g. pancreatic cancer, glioma, and MSS-CRC) to PD-1/PD-L1 blockade, while the response in most cancers is between 15% and 30% [163]. As response to ICP therapy has been correlated to the presence of tumor-specific T cells (mostly in tumors with a high mutational burden), interest in cancer vaccines has been renewed as a strategy to increase T-cell numbers. To date, several clinical trials address the synergy between cancer vaccines and ICP therapy (targeting CTLA-4 or PD-1/PD-L1), providing encouraging results, i.e. improved therapy outcomes without raising toxicity compared to ICP monotherapy [162, 164]. Moreover, two studies in advanced melanoma patients, one combining the TriMixDC-MEL vaccine with anti-CTLA-4 mAbs (Ipilimumab) and one combining an mRNA vaccine with anti-PD-1 mAbs (pembrolizumab), suggested that the level of T-cell activation positively correlated with the clinical response [48, 165]. Hence, combining cancer vaccination with ICP therapy is a promising avenue. To optimize the treatment regimen, it would be of interest to dynamically evaluate the expression of ICPs after vaccination, e.g. via noninvasive imaging [166, 167], as this would allow to define which ICP is dominantly expressed and which timing would be optimal to start ICP therapy. Both are key to rationally design a combination therapy, as it has been shown that anti-CTLA-4 therapy better synergizes with cancer vaccination when provided during boost vaccination rather than during prime vaccination [83], while blocking PD-1/PD-L1 interactions during T-cell priming has been shown to be beneficial [168].

13.4 mRNA: From Discovery to Application in Vaccinology

As outlined in Section 13.3.3, mRNA has turned out to be a successful technology for immunotherapy. The pandemic caused by SARS-CoV2 resulted in a breakthrough for mRNA vaccines, rewarding the efforts of many scientists who pioneered research into mRNA and its use for vaccination [169]. However, the history of mRNA is a tangled one as covered in various reports that do not see eye to eye when it comes to the question: "who discovered mRNA?" [170, 171]. As shown in Figure 13.5, mRNA was first found in 1869, when Friedrich Miescher isolated a phosphate-rich substance from the nuclei of human blood cells termed Nuclein. A few years later, Miescher isolated Nuclein from salmon sperm. This Nuclein was shown to contain uracil, therefore RNA, by modern scientists who reproduced this experiment [172]. Though several researchers made progress from this discovery, Richard Altman changed the name Nuclein to nucleic acid, and Albrecht Kossel described the building units of the nucleotides (cytosine [C], guanine [G], adenine, and uracil [U]). Further, Phoebes Levene together with Walter Jacobs differentiated the nucleic acid DNA from RNA [170, 173], and almost after 100 years, Sydney Brenner discovered the true nature of mRNA, the nucleic acid that transfers information from DNA in the nucleus to initiate protein synthesis in the cytoplasm of the cell (Figure 13.6a) [174].

The timeline then shifts from the history of mRNA discovery to the history of using mRNA for vaccination (Figure 13.5). Credit should be given to Melton and colleagues, who used bacteriophage SP6 RNA polymerase to produce biologically active mRNA *in vitro* [175]. This mRNA was injected into frog eggs, resulting in its translation into the encoded protein [176]. However, the use of *in vitro* transcribed

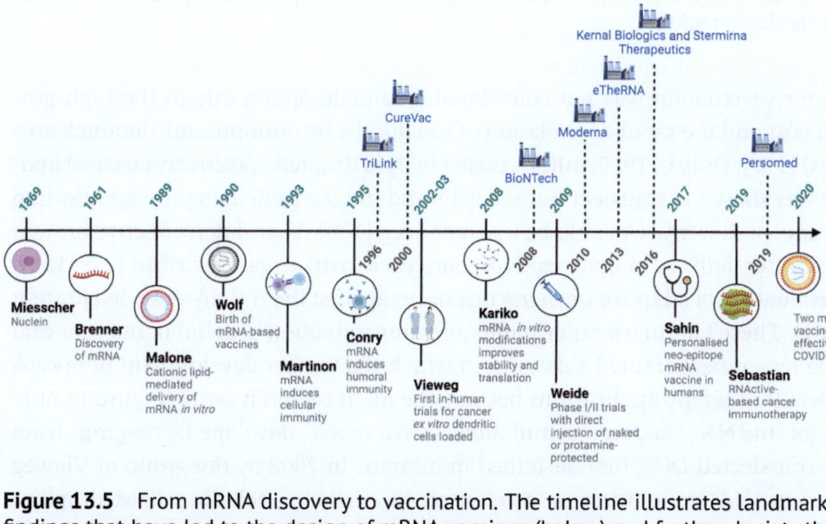

Figure 13.5 From mRNA discovery to vaccination. The timeline illustrates landmark findings that have led to the design of mRNA vaccines (below) and further depicts the foundation of companies focusing on mRNA therapies (above).

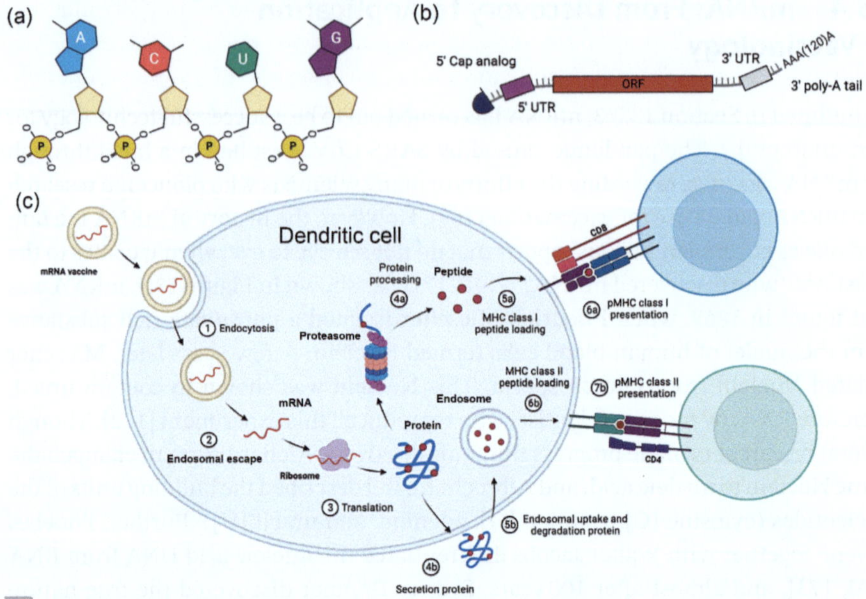

Figure 13.6 From the building blocks of mRNA to lab-made mRNA for antigen delivery. (a) mRNA nucleotide single chain. Each nucleotide is constituted by a ribose carbon sugar, an intercalating phosphate group, and a nitrogenous base. The phosphate group is attached to the 5′ carbon of the ribose and the following nitrogenous base to the 3′ carbon. The RNA chain is made out of four different nitrogenous bases, indicated as guanine (G), cytosine (C), adenine (A), and uracil (U). The alternation and combination of these four nitrogenous bases in the polymer serves as a code to communicate to the ribosomes in the cell, giving precise instructions for the synthesis of proteins. (b) *In vitro* manufactured mRNA representation showing the ORF sequence flanked by a 5′ and 3′ UTR. A 5′-cap analog and the 3′ poly(A) tail. (c) mRNA delivery to DCs resulting in protein expression, procession, and presentation. Abbreviations: MHC, major histocompatibility complex; ORF, open reading frame; U, uracil; UTR, untranslated region.

mRNA for vaccination was not considered a suitable option due to the high production cost and the rapid degradation of the mRNA by omnipresent ribonucleases (RNases) [177]. Only in 1989, mRNA mixed in lipid droplets (positively charged liposomes) was shown to transfect human cells and induce protein expression, leading to the concept that mRNA could be a potent drug [178]. Years later, effective protein synthesis after delivery of lipid–mRNA complexes to mice was described [179] leading to evaluation of adaptive immune responses against the mRNA-encoded protein [180, 181]. These landmark experiments showing induction of cellular and humoral immune responses heralded a new era in which the further development of mRNA for molecular therapy applications became the main research focus (Figure 13.6b).

Various mRNA vaccine formulations have been developed, ranging from mRNA-transfected DCs, first described in humans in 2002 by the group of Vieweg [182], to mRNA in solution or condensed in carriers, including lipid droplets, polymers, and peptides (Figure 13.6c) [183]. Several clinical trials have shown promising results of *in vivo* delivery of mRNA for the stimulation of immune reactivity in cancer patients [117, 120, 136, 184–186]. These studies (and the preclinical work preceding them) have shown that *in vivo* mRNA vaccines mimic infection with RNA viruses, resulting in stimulation of several PRRs and production of an antiviral innate response characterized by IFN-α/β release [187]. The release of IFN-α/β can have a double effect on the activity of the RNA vaccine. On one hand, it harbors the potential to activate the immune system, which can facilitate T-cell activation [137, 138]. However, on the other hand, it can also shut down the translational machinery, reducing expression of the mRNA-encoded antigenic protein, affecting its bioavailability, and therefore compromising the mRNA vaccine efficiency [50, 188]. Moreover, the potent proinflammatory features of IFN-α/β are linked to dose-limiting toxicity. Karikó et al. introduced nucleotide analogs such as pseudouridine (Ψ) in 2008 to generate chemically modified, immunosilent mRNA, allowing increased protein production *in vivo* [189]. Since then, other strategies have been employed to ensure little self-adjuvant activity and high protein expression (e.g. mRNA purification, increased capping efficiency, and codon optimization) [62]. Despite vast improvements in mRNA vaccines, cancer vaccines using mRNA have not reached governmental approval. Nevertheless, several companies have been focusing on the development of different platforms for utilizing mRNA for vaccination purposes, showing the continued hope that mRNA-based cancer vaccines will have an impact on the standard of care for cancer patients (Figure 13.5) [62].

13.5 mRNA Manufacturing and Design

In vitro manufacturing of mRNA is still based on the protocol introduced by Melton et al. [175]. Key reagents in this enzymatic reaction are the DNA template, typically a plasmid DNA template (PDT), a T7 bacteriophage RNA polymerase, and modified nucleotides, including the cap analog. *In silico* sequence design and consequently PDT cloning are the first steps for the mRNA *in vitro* transcription process. Nonetheless, it is very important for a good manufacturing process of an RNA vaccine that the DNA template used should not be contaminated with traces of bacterial genomic DNA and other forms of plasmid DNA (pDNA), including supercoiled, relaxed circle, and linear genomic DNA [190]. Therefore, preparation of pure pDNA, as required for a vaccine, is highly demanding. Efforts to generate mRNA using pDNA-free protocols have been reported. However, to date, synthetic RNA production protocols are limited only to short oligonucleotides [191, 192].

When preparing mRNA, all residual DNA (bacterial and pDNA) is removed after the linearized PDT has been transcribed to mRNA [62]. Moreover, compared to pDNA, mRNA offers safety advantages, as it only contains limited elements that are required to express only the encoded protein. Generally, mRNA does not integrate into the genome, though integration via L1 retroelements is theoretically possible [193]. Still, mRNA is generally considered a highly safe vaccine platform, as mRNA is a transient carrier of information that metabolically decays within a few days [194–196].

To produce biologically active mRNA *in vitro* (Figure 13.6b), the PDT contains a promotor sequence (RNA polymerase binding site), an open reading frame (ORF flanked by 5′ and 3′ untranslated regions [UTRs]), and a unique restriction site for template linearization, ensuring transcription termination [190]. The 3′-end poly(A) tail can be included in the PDT. However, this can also be achieved by enzymatic reaction performed after the *in vitro* mRNA transcription reaction [62, 197]. The actual mRNA synthesis process begins with linearization of the PDT to produce multiple copies of the encoded mRNA using bacteriophage RNA polymerases (e.g. T3, T7, and SP6 RNA polymerases) and rNTPs, which can be chemically modified rNTPs (e.g. N1 methyl pseudouridine [N1mΨ]) [189, 198]. The cap, a 7-methyl-guanosine residue joined to the 5′ end via a 5′,5′ triphosphate (m7GpppG), can be added during or after *in vitro* transcription [199–202]. After iVT, the sample contains the transcribed mRNA and remaining reagents, RNA polymerase, rNTPs, PDT, and impurities, including aberrant mRNA (from abortive cycling during initiation [203], longer mRNA from not linearized PDT [204]), and double-stranded RNA (dsRNA, from the RNA-dependent RNA polymerase activity of bacteriophage polymerases) [205–207]. The PDT is enzymatically removed using DNase digestion followed by precipitation or selection of mRNA using LiCl/NaCl-EtOH or dT microbeads, respectively [208]. Further purification of the desired mRNA has been achieved using cellulose [209], high-performance liquid chromatography (HPLC) [210, 211], or enzymatic treatments (RNase III) [212]. Notably, these processes can all be performed according to good manufacturing practice (GMP), as pDNA, enzymes, and other reagents might be available from commercial providers as GMP-grade starting materials. Moreover, using the same workflow, the mRNA manufacturing process can be standardized, allowing rapid production of any protein of interest.

The process of manufacturing clinical-grade mRNA has notably improved in the last decade, impacting safety and enhanced protein expression. The introduction of chemically modified rNTPs and stringent purification steps has made a major impact, strongly reducing the activation of innate immune sensors, hence the production of IFN-α/β. As a result, the expression of the encoded protein was shown to be several-fold increased [120, 194, 198] and IFN-α/β-associated dose-limiting toxicity became less of an issue. Engineering each element in the mRNA molecule has further led to key findings that have been used to improve the stability and translatability of mRNA (Figure 13.7) [62]. Examples hereof are identification of the role of the 5′ cap and 3′ poly(A) tail in mRNA translation [213] and stability in the cytosol, where decay is predominantly mediated by exonucleases [195, 196]. Further, it has been shown that the stability and translation of the mRNA molecule may depend on the UTRs flanking the ORF [214, 215]. Improvements made to the mRNA design, leading to increased and prolonged protein expression, impact the bioavailability of the antigenic protein, generating better mRNA vaccines [190].

The capping process of mRNA molecules is an essential step, as the cap analog is a structure that shields mRNA from exonuclease activity, initiates mRNA translation by recruiting ribosomes, and reduces innate sensing of the mRNA molecule [190, 200]. Enzymatic, post-transcriptional or chemical, and cotranscriptional strategies have been developed to cap mRNA molecules. The Vaccinia

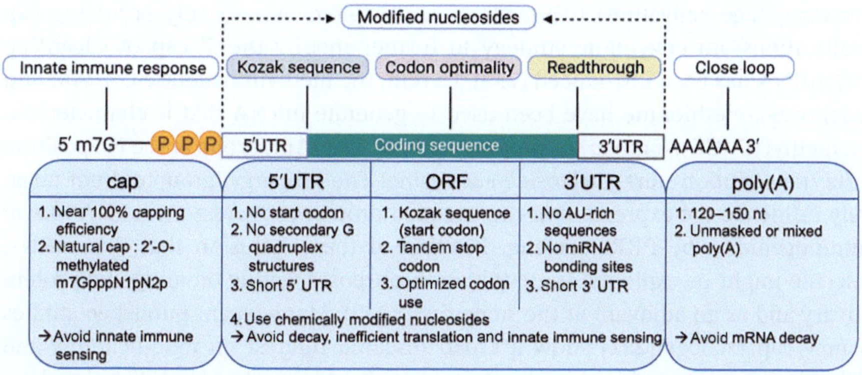

Figure 13.7 Refining the design of mRNA. The key elements in mRNA molecules are indicated, and how these have been optimized to increase stability and improve expression of the encoded protein. Abbreviations: A, adenosine; m7G, 7-methyl guanosine; miRNA, microRNA; nt, nucleotide; ORF, open reading frame.

virus capping enzyme is used for post-transcriptional capping, adding 7-methyl guanosine (m7G) to the first 5′ nucleoside through a 5′,5′-triphosphate bridge to obtain m7GpppN1pN2p [216, 217]. This enzyme is highly active with a near 100% capping efficiency [218]. Further 2′-O-methylation of the first (m7GpppN1mpN2p) or first two (m7GpppN1mpN2mp) nucleosides to mimic eukaryotic mRNA more closely is performed to prevent recognition of the exogenous mRNA by innate immune sensors [219, 220]. An alternative strategy to the enzymatic capping is chemical capping, in which the cap analog is added during the *in vitro* transcription (cotranscriptionally), resulting in more convenient production for a large-scale mRNA vaccine. This cotranscriptional capping has the downside that the m7G cap analog can be reversely incorporated into the mRNA molecule, generating Gpppm7GpNpN instead of m7GpppN1pN2p. As a result, one out of three mRNA molecules has a free phosphate at the 5′ position that can activate PRRs [221, 222]. Antireverse cap analogs (ARCAs) that are O-methylated at the C3 position ensure the addition of a nucleotide solely at the nonmethylated guanosine during cotranscriptional capping [200, 223, 224] and have been further improved (triphosphate linkage) to inhibit decapping and to increase the affinity for the eukaryotic translation initiation factor 4E (eIF4E) [202, 225]. However, issues such as the artificial O-methylation of the cap, low capping efficiency (±70%, leaving 30% uncapped immunogenic mRNA molecules), and generation of a m7GpppN1pN2p cap that is more immunogenic than the 2′-O-methylated m7GpppN1pN2p cap do not support the use of ARCAs. The mRNA could be further improved by enzymatic 2′-O-methylation of the m7GpppN1pN2p cap and purified removing the immunogenic 5′-triphosphate molecules [226]. CleanCap™ (TriLink) uses an initiating capped trimer to reproducibly generate 90–99% mRNA molecules with a natural 5′ cap that is 2′-O-methylated at the first nucleoside (m7GpppN1mpN2p) [222, 227, 228]. Unexpectedly, side-by-side evaluation of mRNA produced with ARCAs, ARCAs, and methyltransferases for 2′-O-methylation, or CleanCap has not revealed differences in protein expression or immunogenicity (measured by macrophage activation) [229]. Moreover, inspired by naturally occurring cap modifications, an enzymatic strategy to further modify the 5′ cap of CleanCap (CC) mRNA has been introduced [230]. Herein, the methyltransferase CAPAM and S-adenosyl-L-methionine have been used to generate mRNA that is characterized by a methyl (5′-CC-N6mAm) or propargyl (5′-CC-N6pAm) group at the N6 position of the transcription start nucleoside adenosine. The propargyl group did not negatively influence the expression of the encoded protein or increase the RNA innate immunogenicity, by PRRs sensing. Leading to the conclusion that this mRNA molecule might be exploited for vaccination purposes, acting on antigenic protein delivery and as an adjuvant at the same time [230]. Many recent published studies on new cap analogs [231] show a broad research interest on modifications and further improvement of the cap structure of *in vitro* transcribed mRNA molecules.

The 5′ UTR has been shown to impact the stability and translatability of the mRNA molecule [232, 233]. Several 5′ UTRs have been compared leading to some selection criteria that can be followed when selecting the 5′-UTR sequence [222, 232, 234]. Start codons such as the canonical AUG and noncanonical CUG should be avoided in the 5′ UTR, as it has been shown to interfere with the translation of the ORF and to trigger mRNA decay. Stable secondary structures, generated by G quadruplex or other hybridization sequences, have been shown to prevent ribosome recruitment, codon recognition, and promote mRNA decay [232]. Therefore, sequences leading to such secondary structures should be identified and optimized. Short 5′ UTRs are more conducive to mRNA translation [234]. It has been shown that a short stretch of consecutive adenosines within the 5′ UTR allows mRNA translation in a cap-independent fashion [232]. This work showed that the translational output can be increased by different sequence combinations, computed by bioinformatic tools that help predict the optimal 5′ UTR sequence [235]. To date, the 5′ UTR of the β globin gene of Xenopus [176, 236], tobacco etch virus [237], and human heat shock protein 70 [238] have been shown to improve mRNA translation. Of these, the β globin UTR is widely used to design *in vitro* transcribed mRNA for vaccination [100, 239–241].

Enhanced ORF translation has been shown by altering the start and stop codon sequences and via codon optimization tools [234]. The fidelity with which the ribosomes recognize the start codon AUG is influenced by the codon content and initiation factors. The start codon should be part of the Kozak sequence, reported as gccRccAUGG. Herein, the start codon is flanked by highly conserved nucleotides [242]. Moreover, noncanonical start codons (e.g. CUG, GUG, UUG, and ACG), present in many mammalian genes, have been shown to introduce shorter ORFs upstream of the main ORF, leading to polycistronic transcripts [234, 243]. These codons should be modified without changing the protein sequence. This is possible due to codon degeneracy: a single amino acid can be coded by multiple codon combinations. Codon optimization using the codon degeneracy principle has been frequently used to improve the stability and translatability of mRNA by increasing the GC content [244–246] and introducing sequence features that interfere with protein expression (secondary RNA structures) [247]. The *in silico* sequence design is widely exploited in the codon optimization process of mRNA-encoding antigenic proteins [248–250] and is facilitated by the availability of many bioinformatic algorithms that assess the codon adaptation index, GC richness, and RNA secondary structure [251]. As described in the context of the mRNA production process, chemically modified nucleosides have been used in mRNA vaccines to silence immune responses mediated by PRR and increase protein expression levels [189, 252–254]. Thess et al. showed that codon-optimized mRNA produced with nonmodified nucleosides allowed higher protein expression than noncodon-optimized mRNA produced with chemically modified nucleosides, underlining the role that codon optimization can play in improving mRNA expression efficiency [255]. Moreover, it has been shown that chemically modified nucleosides could affect the decoding speed and fidelity when present in particular codon combinations, resulting in miscoding [256]. These results warrant the research effort into the use of chemically modified nucleosides in mRNA transcripts, and on how the cellular machinery processes them [257]. Ribosomal termination and further abortion of the mRNA translation process requires a specific coding sequence indicated as stop codons such as UAA, UAG, or UGA [258]. Moreover, sequences down and upstream of the stop codon have been shown to influence the termination of the translation process [259, 260]. Readthrough or extended translation into the 3′ UTR and poly(A) tail initiates mRNA decay [261]. In the design of *in vitro* transcribed mRNA, stop codon readthrough has been prevented by the incorporation of a second in-frame stop codon, downstream of the primary stop codon [262]. It is important to mention that engineered fusion proteins have been encoded by mRNA transcripts in which sorting signals for the MHC-II pathway have been fused to the antigen. Examples hereof are the MHC-II sorting signal of the invariant chain (Ii), the lysosomal-associated membrane protein (LAMP), and DC-LAMP [249, 263–266]. As a result, presentation of antigenic peptides is achieved in both classes MHC-II and MHC-I, aimed to recruit both $CD4^+$ and $CD8^+$ T cells in the triggered immune response.

The 3′ UTR, similar to the 5′ UTR, is involved in various regulatory functions, impacting the mRNA stability and translatability, including several cis-acting destabilizing sequences [267] and microRNA (miRNA) binding sites [268]. In this regard, short 3′ UTRs that escape miRNA-mediated destruction are preferable in the design of mRNA. To date, the 3′ UTR of the β globin gene of Xenopus is commonly used [176, 263, 269, 270], though other 3′ UTR sequences, such as the bovine growth hormone and hepatitis B virus, have been investigated [271]. As for 5′ UTR optimization, high-throughput approaches, e.g. library screening in cells, have been used to analyze and optimize the 3′ UTR [272, 273].

Multiple consecutive adenosines at the 3′ end of the mRNA transcript, known as the poly(A) tail, have been proven to be an essential element to protect the mRNA molecule from RNA exonuclease activity and therefore prolonging mRNA lifetime, increasing the RNA stability, enhancing the translation efficiency, and reducing the immunogenicity [222]. Naturally, the poly(A) tail in mammalian cells consists of 250 consecutive adenosines. However, it has been described that the optimal length of the poly(A) tail in human moDCs should be in the range of 120 up to 150 nucleotides [274]. Notably, proteins that bind the poly(A) sequence can interact with the 5′ cap via translational initiation factors (e.g. eIF4E), which also depends on the poly(A) length. This results in forming a closed-loop structure that helps mRNA translation. This structure further hampers deadenylation from exonuclease activity, and therefore mRNA degradation [275, 276]. It has been reported that a mixed poly(A) tail, containing one or more non-A residues intermittently (e.g. G) could further hamper mRNA degradation [277]. Moreover, the poly(A) length has been linked to the immunostimulatory activity of *in vitro* transcribed mRNA, suggesting that enzymatic 3′-polyadenylation with a minimum of 150 added adenines to the RNA molecule reduces immunostimulation [278, 279].

Every component in the mRNA backbone can be modified, impacting mRNA stability, translatability, and immunogenicity. Combining different modifications in the mRNA molecule design has been exploited to improve mRNA vaccine performance, and continuous efforts are made in this direction to ensure that mRNA achieves a reputation as a powerful and versatile vaccine platform.

13.6 mRNA Delivery and Formulation

The cytosol is the cellular playground in which mRNA is active. Therefore, mRNA-encoding antigenic proteins for vaccination should be delivered to the cytosol of APCs, preferably DCs [280]. Delivery of mRNA to DCs has been achieved using various strategies for both transfection of DCs in culture (*ex vivo*) and endogenous DCs (*in vivo*) [152, 183, 281, 282]. The simplest form of mRNA delivery relies on the capacity of DCs to acquire mRNA in solution [50, 194, 283–285]. More sophisticated strategies to enhance the uptake of mRNA include its encapsulation in carriers, such as lipid- or polymer-based NPs [137, 138, 286, 287], cell-penetrating peptides [288], or the use of strategies to permeabilize the cell membrane to allow passive influx of the mRNA, e.g. electroporation [289–291] or sonoporation [292] (Figure 13.8).

Several studies have investigated the mechanisms and kinetics of cellular entry of mRNA, dissolved in buffers such as phosphate-buffered saline (PBS) and Ringer lactate (RL). It has been shown *in vitro* that various primary cells, including smooth muscle cells and DCs, can acquire mRNA in solution. This process depends on the temperature and the mRNA dose, reaching a point of saturation [285]. *In vitro* it has been further shown that mRNA primarily enters cells via caveolae, implying a role for scavenger receptors [293]. At the same time, macropinocytosis only plays a minor role in the mRNA uptake [285]. Codelivery of various maturation stimuli (e.g. lipopolysaccharide [LPS], MPLA, and poly I:C) reduced protein expression [50], which could be explained by the fact that processes such as macropinocytosis are downregulated following maturation [294]. The validity of these *in vitro* findings has mainly been confirmed *in vivo* after i.d. delivery of mRNA. It has been shown that i.d. delivery of mRNA in solution resulted in an ion (calcium) and dose-dependent transfection for various cells. This local uptake of mRNA in solution is mediated by a saturable mechanism, which is a specific process for nucleic acids and depends on moving vesicles before entering the cytosol. Also here, macropinocytosis only played

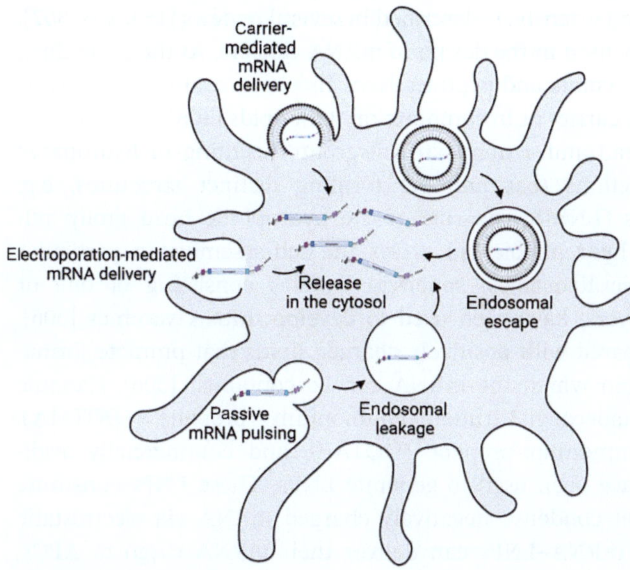

Figure 13.8 Entry of mRNA in DCs. Several methods have been applied to deliver *in vitro* transcribed mRNA to DCs. These can be broadly divided into passive pulsing with mRNA in solution, active transfection of mRNA in solution, or delivery of mRNA in carriers. Depending on the mode of delivery, mRNA passes through endosomes before being released into the cytosol where it can be translated to protein.

a minor role [194]. In contrast, i.t. [51] and i.n. [50, 283] delivery of mRNA in solution predominantly resulted in transfection of DCs, which had taken up the mRNA via micropinocytosis [283]. This finding suggests that the mechanism of acquiring mRNA in solution depends on the delivery route and likely the targeted cell type. It has been calculated that the uptake rate is <1 in 10 000 molecules when DCs take up mRNA in solution [295]. Strategies such as electroporation have been developed to increase mRNA uptake, as this permeabilizes the cell membrane and allows the mRNA to enter into the cytosol directly. This strategy is widely used to deliver mRNA to *ex vivo* generated DCs, as it is by far the most efficient method [289, 296]. Such *ex vivo* mRNA-electroporated DCs have shown some clinical success as an autologous cellular cancer vaccine [45–47, 49, 152, 297–300]. Also, electroporation has been optimized for i.d. delivery of mRNA in solution in mice [291]. However, there are no studies to support this approach's efficacy in humans [301].

Naked mRNA (mRNA in solution) is not ideal for *in vivo* applications, as it is prone to rapid degradation by omnipresent extracellular ribonucleases. Therefore, carriers have been developed to encapsulate and protect the mRNA following its delivery *in situ*. Overall, mRNA encapsulated in carriers, forming mostly NPs, follows different kinetics and intracellular routes as the naked mRNA in solution [301–303]. Endocytosis is the primary route of acquiring encapsulated mRNA, followed by endosomal escape, and release of the mRNA into the cytosol, where translation occurs. In this process, the endosomes and the endosomal membrane represent a considerable barrier [304]. The components of carriers applied in mRNA vaccines are multifold and have been extensively described in several reviews [183, 305–307]. Lipids are most frequently used in the design of mRNA carriers. At the same time, other components like polymers and peptides have also been evaluated, either as the sole component of the carrier or in combination with lipids [308].

Lipids have a polar head and a nonpolar tail group, resulting in hydrophilic and hydrophobic interactions that promote forming distinct structures, e.g. liposomes and lipid NPs (LNPs). The size of the hydrophilic head group relative to the size of the hydrophobic tail drives the self-assembly in particular structures [309]. Cationic liposomes, spherical vesicles consisting of one or multiple phospholipid layers, have been used to develop mRNA vaccines [306]. These liposomes are prepared with positively charged lipids that promote formation of an aqueous core in which the mRNA can be contained [306]. Cationic lipids like 1,2-di-*O*-octadecenyl-3-trimethylammonium propane (DOTMA), 1,2-dioleoyl-3-trimethylammonium-propane (DOTAP), and commercially available proprietary lipids have been used to generate LNPs. These LNPs constitute multilayer complexes that condense negatively charged mRNA via electrostatic interactions [183]. Such mRNA–LNPs can deliver their mRNA cargo to APCs, eliciting strong immune responses, in part owing to their intrinsic adjuvant properties [136, 137]. Moreover, mRNA–LNPs that increase delivery to APCs via the inclusion of tri-mannose have been described [138]. In the clinic, i.v. delivery of TAA mRNA–LNPs consisting of the cationic lipid DOTMA combined with the fusogenic helper phospholipid 1,2-dioleoyl-*sn*-glycero-3-phosphoethanolamine (DOPE) has been studied in melanoma patients [136]. However, the main issue when using positively charged LNPs for mRNA delivery is their toxicity [310]. In contrast, LNPs produced with ionizable lipids have a neutral charge under physiological pH, while this charge becomes positive and promotes membrane fusion at endosomal pH [311]. Therefore, it is not surprising that the LNPs approved by the FDA for delivery of mRNA for SARS-CoV2 vaccine contain ionizable lipids in addition to three other components; cholesterol, a helper lipid, and polyethylene glycol (PEG)-lipid [309]. Each of these elements has a specific function within the mRNA–LNP. The cationic or ionizable lipids mediate self-assembly, facilitate membrane fusion, and promote endosomal escape. Cholesterol functions as a stabilizing agent and also together with neutral helper phospholipids support the bilayer structure of the LNPs. The PEG, anchored to the lipids, has several functions, including preventing aggregation through steric hindrance and increasing the half-life time of the mRNA–LNP, thereby prolonging circulation time [282, 309, 312]. Despite the renowned LNP formulations used by BioNTech, Moderna, and Curevac in their SARS-CoV2 mRNA vaccine [312], efforts continue to design mRNA–LNPs with improved traits for delivery of mRNA for cancer vaccination. These many efforts are justified for various reasons. In cancer, it has been suggested that circulating and tissue-resident T cells are required to elicit meaningful immune responses [141–143]. It has been shown that s.c. [313] and i.m. [311] delivery of mRNA–LNPs, targeting local APCs, results in only moderate antigen-specific $CD8^+$ T-cell levels in the circulation. In contrast, i.v. delivery of cationic mRNA–LNPs has demonstrated mRNA delivery to splenic DCs with strong T-cell responses and antitumor immunity [136–138].

However, cationic mRNA–LNPs might be less proficient in mRNA delivery and less favorable in terms of toxicity than mRNA–LNPs produced with ionizable lipids. Moreover, many LNP formulations end up transfecting liver cells instead of APCs upon i.v. delivery [314, 315], requiring novel formulations that effectively reach APCs. Finally, it is well known that the lipid structure alters how LNPs interact with cells [316, 317], ensuring that the quest for an mRNA–LNP formulation for i.v. delivery and mRNA transfection into APCs is not idle. Libraries of dozens to thousands of chemically distinct lipid delivery systems exist [318, 319] and allow the design of experiments and Bayesian-based analysis to identify the optimal mRNA–LNP for i.v. cancer vaccination. This strategy has been applied by Bevers et al. [139], showing the selection of an ionizable mRNA–LNP that induced a high level of tumor-specific $CD8^+$ T cells within a single round of screening. Tweaking of the LNP composition further enhanced the uptake of mRNA by multiple splenic immune cell populations, including type I IFN-producing phagocytes and B cells that both stimulated the T-cell response. A similar biodistribution was observed in NHPs without histopathological changes in the liver and spleen, implying a lack of toxicity.

The first polymer tested for mRNA delivery was diethyl aminoethyl dextran [178]. Since then, other cationic polymers have been evaluated as carriers for mRNA, including polyethyleneimine (PEI), poly-β-amino ester (PBAE), poly-lactic-*co*-glycolic acid (PLGA), and dendrimers [320–325]. But polymer-based carriers were shown to have a high polydispersity, high molecular weight, and unfavorable toxicity profile, instigating research into modifications to remedy these drawbacks [183, 282]. For instance, PEI that forms complexes with anionic mRNA via electrostatic interactions with its cationic amine has been grafted with PEG, resulting in nontoxic NPs that mediate mRNA delivery to immune cells in the lungs [320]. *In vivo* mRNA vaccination has also been achieved with cyclodextrin-PEI conjugates, showing induction of IgG2a antibodies against ovalbumin following i.d. and i.m. delivery [321]. Dendrimers (poly-amidoamine) together with PLGA and PEG have been formulated into mRNA-NPs that delivered ovalbumin mRNA and a TLR7/8 agonist, resulting in tumor control [322]. Also, PBAEs containing cationic amines and biodegradable ester bonds formulated with PEG and/or lipids have been used to deliver mRNA to cells *in vitro* and *in vivo* [323–325]. Variants of PBAEs have been used to generate charge-altering releasable transports (CARTs) that undergo dynamic changes (esters to amides) via which the cationic backbone is transformed into small neutral molecules, releasing mRNA [325]. Notably, the small neutral molecules remaining after the degradation of CARTs are likely less toxic than cationic materials (e.g. cationic lipids or polymers) [310]. Codelivery of mRNA and the TLR9 agonist CpG via CARTs or mRNA via CARTs combined with coinjected adjuvants (e.g. anti-CD40 mAb) in an established mouse cancer model has been shown to transfect and activate APCs, stimulating curative immune responses [326].

Protamine, a small nucleotide-binding peptide rich in amino acid arginine, can be used to complex mRNA, stabilizing the mRNA and enhancing its delivery to the cytosol [302]. However, the electrostatic interaction between protamine and mRNA is strong and hinders the release of mRNA for translation. Moreover, the protamine–mRNA complex acts as an agonist of TLR7/8, an adjuvant able to stimulate T_H1-supported immunity [327]. This finding led to a formulation referred to as RNActive® for cancer vaccination, consisting of protamine-condensed mRNA and noncomplexed mRNA-encoding antigenic proteins, showing safety, tolerability, and immunogenicity in preclinical and clinical studies [120, 121, 328, 329]. Another arginine-rich peptide with cell-penetrating capacity RALA has been used to condense mRNA into complexes, facilitating transfection of *ex vivo* DCs and stimulating CTL responses after i.d. injection of these DCs [288]. From the same family, the peptides KALA (lysine rich) [330] and GALA (glutamic acid rich) [330] have been used to enhance mRNA delivery to DCs, albeit combined with other delivery platforms, i.e. lipids and/or polymers. Likewise, the cationic peptide DP7, modified with cholesterol (DP7-C), has been used in combination with the lipid DOTAP, showing transfer of mRNA to DCs *in vitro* and delay of lung tumor growth following s.c. vaccination with this mRNA-DOTAP/DP7-C complex [331].

To date, there are several strategies to use mRNA as a cancer vaccination platform ranging from mRNA-transfected *ex vivo* DCs to platforms that allow efficient and safe *in vivo* delivery of mRNA. Considering the multitude of carriers that can be used for mRNA delivery to APCs, a key question remains how do these compare to each other in terms of efficacy and safety. In this regard, a recent study has compared mRNA–LNPs to *ex vivo* mRNA-transfected DCs to stimulate antigen-specific T cells, confirming that the route of delivery is a major determinant for the biodistribution of the vaccine and as a result its T-cell-activating capacity [332]. This study further showed that mRNA–LNPs transfected stromal cells within lymph nodes, which are considered tolerogenic APCs [333], warranting in-depth mechanistic analysis of mRNA-NP vaccines that are under development.

13.7 Controlling the Innate Immune Sensing of mRNA

Several PRRs, located in the endosomes and cytosol, can bind *in vitro* transcribed mRNA and some of the by-products present in unpurified mRNA (Figure 13.9) [187, 222, 334]. In the endosomes, ssRNA is bound by TLR7/8, resulting in activation of the myeloid differentiation marker 88 (MyD88) [335–337]. Also, TLR3 can be activated upon release of *in vitro* transcribed mRNA in the endosomes, mainly when secondary dsRNA structures are formed or when dsRNA fragments (contaminants) are not removed during the mRNA manufacturing process [336]. This TLR3 engagement leads to activation of toll-IL1 receptor (TIR) domain-containing adapter-inducing IFN-β (TRIF). Activation of the adaptor molecules MyD88 and TRIF results in a signaling cascade that converges in the upregulation of transcription factors like interferon regulatory factors (IRFs) and nuclear factor-κB (NF-κB). While IRFs enable transcription of genes encoding type I IFNs, NF-κB enables the transcription of genes encoding proinflammatory cytokines (e.g. IL-6 and tumor necrosis factor-α [TNF-α]) [101]. Distinct RNA species can also be sensed by various PRRs located in the cytosol, including retinoic acid-inducible gene-I

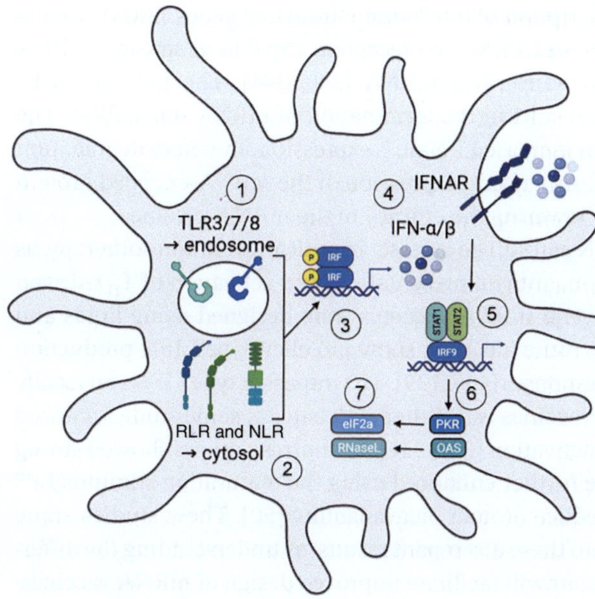

Figure 13.9 Innate immune sensing of mRNA. (1) Endosomal TLR3/7/8 and (2) cytosolic RLRs and NLRs bind several RNA species, e.g. ssRNA containing canonical nucleotides and dsRNA. (3) This starts a signaling cascade that ends in upregulation of transcription factors such as IRFs. (4) IRFs drive IFN-α/β production and as such activation of its receptor: IFNAR. (5) In turn, IFNAR activation results in a signaling cascade ending in transcription of ISGs. (6) Among these are genes coding for PKR and OAS that can bind dsRNA and improperly designed mRNA. (7) PKR deters translation of mRNA by eIF2a, while OAS mediates degradation of mRNA by RNase L. Abbreviations: eIF2a, elongation initiation factor 2a; IFN, interferon; IFNAR, IFN-α receptor; IRF, IFN regulatory factor; NLR, NOD-like receptor; NOD, nucleotide oligomerization domain; OAS, oligoadenylate synthetase; PKR, protein kinase R; RIG-I, retinoic acid-inducible gene-I; RLR, RIG-I-like receptor; RNase L, ribonuclease L; TLR, toll-like receptor.

(RIG-I)-like receptors (RLRs) [219, 338, 339], oligoadenylate synthetase (OAS) receptors [340, 341], and RNA-dependent protein kinase (PKR) [342–344]. In the cytosol, nucleotide oligomerization domain (NOD)-like receptors (NLRs) might be involved in sensing ssRNA [345, 346], although further studies are required to confirm this. It has been shown that mRNA without a cap (free 5′ triphosphate) or with a cap that has not been 2-O′-methylated stimulates RIG-I [219, 343, 347–349]. In addition, 2-O′-unmethylated capped mRNA can be detected by the RLR, melanoma differentiation-associated protein 5 (MDA5) [338]. Both RLRs are further activated by dsRNA, their natural ligands, and potential impurities in mRNA preparations [301]. Activation of both RLRs leads to conformational changes and a signaling cascade that starts with the interaction with the mitochondrial antiviral signaling (MAVS) protein and ends with upregulation of IRFs and NF-κB, again resulting in type I IFN and proinflammatory cytokine production [187]. Notably, type I IFNs activate the Janus kinase-signal transducer activator of transcription (JAK-STAT) pathway following engagement of its receptor. The activation of the JAK-STAT pathway will lead to the transcription of interferon-stimulated genes (ISGs), among which the genes coding OAS and PKR, two receptors capable of sensing dsRNA and poorly designed *in vitro* transcribed mRNA [340, 344]. The latter is to be avoided as activation of PKR results in the termination of mRNA translation. The activation of OAS will result in increased RNase L expression, therefore degradation of exogenous RNA [340, 350]. As a result, expression of the mRNA-encoded protein could be reduced, potentially lowering the efficacy of the mRNA vaccine.

The production of type I IFN can still be an asset in anticancer immunotherapy, as it can stimulate DC maturation, antigen presentation, and activation of T_H1-driven adaptive immunity [222]. Several mRNA vaccines were designed using lipids and administered utilizing the i.v. route has been shown to elicit type I IFN production and to promote $CD8^+$ T-cell responses [136, 139]. The impact of type I IFNs on locally delivered lipid-based mRNA vaccines is a matter of debate, as some studies showed an inhibitory effect on T-cell activation [351, 352]. In contrast, others showed strong T-cell activation that could be further enhanced using the maturation stimulus LPS [313], previously shown to reduce protein bioavailability [50]. These studies argue for more in-depth research into these discrepant results, as understanding the differences and how these came about will facilitate improved design of mRNA vaccines. In this regard, a comparison could be made with vaccines based on ssRNA viruses for which studies indicate that differences in transfected cell types are at the basis of the observed differences in T-cell activation [353].

Even if the type I IFN response could be exploited to our advantage, one should not ignore that type I IFNs are not harmless, as these can mediate unwanted toxicity, induce pathological damage, and inflammatory or autoimmune syndromes [354, 355]. Therefore, it is warranted that the mRNA vaccine is designed to induce minimal type I IFN production by transfected cells.

Several strategies can be adopted to reduce the immunogenicity of mRNA. These involve refinements of the mRNA molecule and its encoding PDT, manufacturing process, and delivery method [187]. The modifications to the mRNA molecule and its PDT that reduce the immunogenicity of *in vitro* transcribed mRNA will be briefly described covering the mRNA molecule from cap to tail. Note, to our knowledge the sequence of UTRs has not been described to directly influence the immune-activating potential of *in vitro* transcribed mRNA [222, 346]; therefore, UTRs are not covered in this section. A natural cap that is 2′-O-methylated at the first or first two nucleosides has been shown to prevent recognition of the mRNA by RIG-I [219, 220]. Such cap structure can be added post-transcriptionally using the enzymes guanylyl transferase and 2′-*O*-methyltransferases [216, 217]. Also, the CleanCap technology can be used to obtain m7GpppN1mpN2p during the transcription [222, 227, 228]. These processes show almost 100% efficiency [218, 224]. Further, treatment with phosphatases could remove any remaining uncapped mRNA, preventing innate recognition of free 5′ di- and triphosphates by RIG-I and PKR [343, 348, 349]. The coding sequence or ORF can be optimized to avoid highly stable secondary structures, hairpin loops [241], and uridine-rich regions [222]. This can be achieved by optimizing the codon use, for instance, increasing the GC content to eliminate as many uridines as possible [279]. Concerning the uridine content, it is important to link the use of chemically modified nucleosides and the modulation of the poly(A) tail. Chemically modified nucleosides, 5-methylcytidine (m5C), N6-methyladenosine (m6A), 5-methyluridine (m5U), 2-thiouridine (s2U), or pseudouridine (Ψ), have been used by Karikó et al. [336] to reduce and even abolish activation of TLR3, TLR7, and TLR8 following mRNA transfection in DCs. Replacing uridine with Ψ has further reduced detection by PKR [343, 344] and OAS [341]. A further reduction in immunogenicity of the mRNA has been achieved by using N1mΨ [252]. In addition, increasing the length of the poly(A) tail has been used to reduce the relative uridine content or shield uridines in the mRNA sequence, lowering the mRNA's capacity to elicit proinflammatory cytokine production by APCs [279].

Short ssRNA and dsRNA are generated during the *in vitro* transcription of mRNA and can activate PPRs. Therefore, strategies to avoid these impurities in the final mRNA product have been developed, including minimizing their occurrence during the *in vitro* transcription or removing them afterwards [208–212]. Minimizing the generation of dsRNA impurities has been achieved by lowering the concentration of Mg^{2+} or increasing the temperature during *in vitro* transcription [274]. The generation of dsRNA fragments can also be avoided by synthesizing the mRNA using a solid phase method [356]. Herein, short RNA fragments (~70 nucleotides) are produced and ligated into the full-length mRNA. Removing impurities after traditional *in vitro* transcription of mRNA has been achieved using various methods, including the use of dT microbeads [208], cellulose [209] or HPLC [210, 211] purification, or RNase III enzymatic treatment [212].

The formulation and delivery of mRNA, and as a result the mode of cell entry, endosomal versus direct cytoplasmic entry, determines the type of PRRs encountered by the mRNA. There is ample evidence showing that mRNA delivered by carriers such as protamine, DOTAP, and PEI exhibit immunogenicity [302, 327, 335, 357], likely as these enable interaction with endosomal and cytosolic PRRs. As explained in the Section 13.8, this feature has sometimes been exploited to the advantage of cancer vaccination. In contrast, physical methods, such as electroporation [289–291] or sonoporation [292], permeabilize the cell membrane and allow the mRNA to reach the cytosol directly. These techniques have mainly been applied to deliver mRNA to DCs cultured *in vitro*. In these studies, it has been shown that electroporation using mRNA in solution does not activate DCs [289–291], while sonoporation using mRNA in carriers (attached to microbubbles) does lead to moderate activation of DCs [292]. The latter suggests that some encapsulated mRNA is still acquired via the endosomal route. Nonetheless, additional adjuvants to fully mature the mRNA-transfected DCs were required to reach therapeutic efficacy of such DC vaccines [50, 292]. Based hereon, it is fair to claim that physical and carrier-free methods of mRNA delivery abolish the immunogenicity of mRNA. However, whether such techniques will be efficacious for mRNA delivery *in vivo* is underexplored [291, 301] and the efforts of most researchers are focused on the design of carriers that elicit minimal type I IFN production.

13.8 Adjuvants for mRNA-Based Vaccines

As mentioned in Section 13.3.2, adjuvants aim to improve the T-cell-priming capacity of DCs. In the context of mRNA, these need to be well thought out to ensure high expression levels of the antigen mRNA. As a result, a branch of mRNA vaccine research is devoted to studying adjuvants suited for mRNA vaccination (Figure 13.10).

The compatibility between mRNA vaccines and agonists of TLR3, 4, 7, and 8 has been shown. The TLR3 agonist polyI:C, which also signals via RIG-I and MDA5 [358], has been used to mature moDCs electroporated with mRNA encoding the HPV E7/HLA-A2 epitope, showing DC maturation and strong T-cell activation [359]. The TLR3 agonist polyI:C_{12}U, which does not engage MDA5 [358], has been coelectroporated with TAA (MelanA) mRNA into immature moDCs, avoiding maturation by exogenous maturation stimuli and toxicity as observed with polyI:C [360]. This study showed maturation of the moDCs and strong capacity to stimulate TAA-specific CTLs *in vitro* [360]. Further, the T-cell-activating capacity of these moDCs could significantly be increased by coelectroporating them with polyI:C_{12}U, TAA mRNA and small-interfering RNA (siRNA) to increase the activity of NF-κB and remove IL-10 [89]. Recently, Uchida et al. [361] incorporated a dsRNA portion into the design of the mRNA molecule by hybridizing part of the poly(A) tail with antisense RNA, resulting in mRNA:pU. This mRNA:pU simultaneously allowed

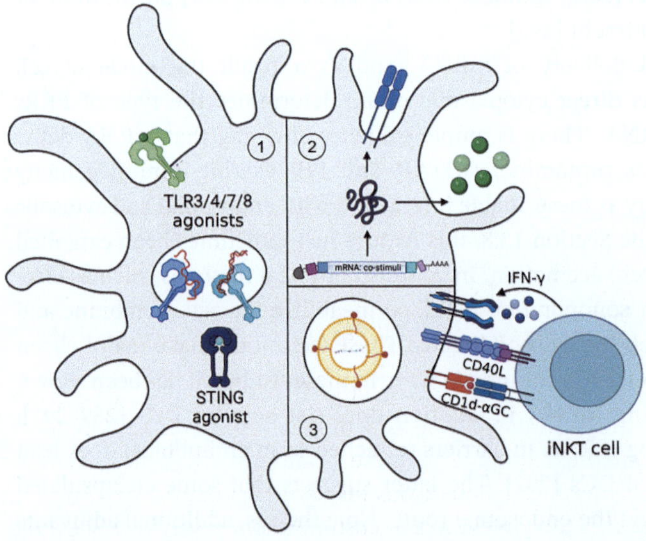

Figure 13.10 mRNA compatible adjuvants. Adjuvants compatible with mRNA for *ex vivo* DC or *in vivo* mRNA vaccination can be categorized into three classes: (1) agonists of PRRs such as TLRs and STING, (2) mRNA-encoding costimulatory proteins (e.g. CD70) and cytokines (e.g. IL-15), and (3) adjuvants acting on DC licensing immune cells such as αGC. Abbreviations: αGC, α-galactosyl ceramide; CD40L, CD40 ligand; IFN, interferon; iNKT, invariant natural killer T cells; PRR, pattern recognition receptor; TLR, toll-like receptor; STING, stimulator of interferon genes.

efficient translation and immune stimulation via TLR3 and RIG-I. It was shown *in vivo* that i.n. delivery of ovalbumin mRNA:pU in solution significantly enhanced the ovalbumin-specific cellular and humoral immune response compared to conventional mRNA. Another *in vivo* study showed that MPLA, a TLR4 agonist, could be efficiently incorporated into LNPs encapsulating immunosilent mRNA [287]. Codelivery of MPLA and mRNA did not hamper the expression of the mRNA-encoded protein and allowed strong activation of T cells. In contrast, codelivery of LPS, a related TLR4 agonist, and mRNA in solution was not a suitable combination [50], showing that adjuvants could affect mRNA vaccines in a distinct way depending on the delivery platform. Activation of TLR7/8 has also been exploited to improve the outcome of mRNA-NP vaccines. An NP, consisting of a lipid-PEG shell loaded with ovalbumin mRNA and C16-R848 (palmitic acid-modified R848, a TLR7/8 agonist), improved the transfection efficiency (>95%) and MHC-I presentation of ovalbumin by APCs. Following *in vivo* vaccination, more ovalbumin-specific $CD8^+$ T cells were retrieved in tumors when mice were treated with the C16-R848 adjuvant mRNA-NP relative to the mRNA-NP without adjuvant. As a result, this mRNA cancer vaccine showed good therapeutic responses in various mouse cancer models [322]. Also, RNA condensed by protamine and referred to as RNActive® has been shown to be a potent TLR7/8 adjuvant that induces strong cell-mediated antitumor immunity when codelivered with mRNA in solution [302].

It has recently been shown by Miao et al. that certain LNPs have the intrinsic ability to activate STING and as such have adjuvant activity [362, 363]. These LNPs were identified during experiments designed to optimize mRNA delivery materials. From over 1000 lipid formulations; the STING-activating lipids were identified that contain unsaturated lipid tail groups, cyclic amine head groups, and dihydroimidazole linkers [362]. Vaccines manufactured with these cyclic lipids boosted the maturation of APCs, triggered T-cell responses, and showed strong antitumor efficacy in several mouse cancer models [362, 363]. Also, Tse et al. [364] used STING activation to enhance the outcome of an mRNA–LNP vaccine. In this case, mRNA encoding a mutated, active variant of STING ($STING^{V155M}$) was included in the mRNA–LNP in addition to antigen mRNA. This mRNA–LNP vaccine was shown to result in strong $CD8^+$ T-cell stimulation and have tumor controlling capacity following i.m. delivery of the mRNA–LNP to mice.

Activation of PRRs induces maturation of APCs characterized by the expression of costimulatory surface proteins and the production of proinflammatory cytokines. Knowledge on the relevance of these costimuli in the activation of adaptive T-cell-mediated immune responses has instigated research into the use of mRNA-encoding proinflammatory cytokines or costimulatory proteins to boost the antitumor potential of mostly mRNA-transfected DC vaccines. Various cytokines have been encoded in mRNA and combined with TAA mRNA for engineering *ex vivo* DCs, including GM-CSF, IL-12, and IL-15 [365–367]. Preclinical studies showed improved antitumor efficacy of the transfected DCs in both *in vivo* mouse models [365] and *in vitro* human models [366, 367] of cancer vaccination. In a more direct approach, Van der Jeught et al. [368] delivered mRNA-encoding Fβ2, an engineered cytokine based on interferon-β (IFN-β) fused to a transforming growth factor-β (TGF-β) antagonist to tumor-residing DCs. This Fβ2 mRNA increased the cytolytic capacity of $CD8^+$ T cells and delayed tumor progression in several mouse cancer models, likely by stimulating T-cell activation by DCs and by modulating the TME. Likewise, i.t. delivery of mRNA-encoding IL-23, IL-36γ, and T-cell-costimulatory OX40L has been shown to overcome the suppressive TME and produce effective systemic antitumor immunity [369]. Also, mRNA-encoding costimulatory ligands have been codelivered with antigen mRNA to *ex vivo* DCs in several preclinical studies. Among the costimulatory proteins that were delivered in that way are OX40 ligand (OX40L), 4-1BB ligand (4-1BBL), glucocorticoid-induced tumor necrosis factor receptor ligand (GITRL), CD40L, ca CD40, inducible T-cell-costimulatory ligand (ICOSL), CD70, and CD83 [32, 370–375]. These different preclinical studies showed that increased costimulation enhanced T-cell priming. However, Rocapuldencel-T, an autologous DC vaccine modified with TAA and CD40L mRNA, largely failed in a phase III clinical trial, as there was little improvement of the OS of patients with metastatic renal cell carcinoma (mRCC) that also received sunitinib [376, 377].

Combination of mRNA-encoding costimulatory proteins, in particular, CD70, CD40L, and caTLR4, referred to as TriMix mRNA, has also been explored to enhance the T-cell-activating capacity of *ex vivo* DCs [43, 50] and DCs located in lymph nodes [50] or tumors [51]. A preclinical study performed in a human cancer vaccination model has shown the key role of the three components of TriMix mRNA in the priming of $CD8^+$ T cells by TriMixDC-MEL [31]. Also, preclinical studies in mouse cancer models evidenced that this TriMix mRNA can be an interesting adjuvant when applying mRNA vaccines *in vivo* [50, 51]. As discussed in the Section 13.9, the use of TriMixDC in clinical trials has delivered on its promise.

Combination of antigen mRNA with suitable adjuvants is still actively researched though adjuvants should be used with caution. For example, the adjuvant α-galactosyl ceramide (αGC) has been incorporated into mRNA–LNPs to recruit iNKT cells through expression of CD40L and IFN-γ license DCs [378]. This vaccine considerably improves priming of T-cell responses but upon boost anergy was observed within the iNKT cell population. Such findings warrant a full understanding of the mode-of-action of adjuvants (and their formulation) before translating their use to the clinic.

13.9 Clinical Application

A multitude of clinical trials using mRNA in cancer vaccines have been registered on ClinicalTrials.gov [301]. These vaccines are used alone or in combination with other cancer therapies in indications such as acute myeloid leukemia (AML), CRC, mRCC, melanoma, glioblastoma, and cancer of the breast, lung, prostate, pancreas, ovarian, and head and neck. With few exceptions, vaccination trials using mRNA in solution or in carriers are mostly sponsored by companies (e.g. eTheRNA Immunotherapies, BioNTech, CureVac, and Moderna). In contrast, trials using mRNA-transfected DCs are mainly investigator driven.

The ease of delivering mRNA to DCs via electroporation, together with improved protocols to generate and mature moDCs as well as to control every step of these processes, has instigated research into their use for cancer vaccination [152]. Moreover, it is well known how mRNA-transfected DCs distribute when injected i.v., i.d., or s.c. in patients with metastatic breast, lung, and colon cancer [379], providing solid anchor points for a rationally designed treatment regimen. Vaccines consisting of mRNA-electroporated moDCs have been studied for the treatment of mRCC, glioblastoma, AML, and melanoma, mostly in phase I/II clinical trials. Only the vaccine Rocapuldencel-T has been tested in a phase III clinical trial in a combination with sunitinib in mRCC [376, 377]. A large cohort of patients was enrolled yet failed to show a substantial increase in clinical objective responses, resulting in untimely termination of the trial.

Nonetheless, immune activity was documented in 70% of patients treated with Rocapuldencel-T. The magnitude of the immune response positively correlated with OS and the amount of IL-12 produced by the DCs was shown to predict OS [377]. Other mRNA- and DC-based vaccine studies, though at a smaller scale, have shown more encouraging results. Batich et al. [300] showed that the long-term progression-free survival (PFS) and OS were considerably increased in glioblastoma patients when they applied the strategy described by Mitchell et al. [298]. Herein, the vaccination site is conditioned with tetanus toxoid before i.d. injection of moDC electroporated with mRNA encoding a cytomegalovirus antigen (pp65) and matured with a cytokine cocktail. To address the limitation of small patient cohorts, three distinct clinical trials were set up in patients with newly diagnosed glioblastoma, assessing reproducibility [380]. All trials including randomized and two-arm trial phase II trials showed that one out of three patients showed exceptional long-term survival. Also, multiple trials have been performed with mRNA- and DC-based vaccines in the context of AML. In these trials, mRNA-encoding leukemia-associated antigens such as Wilms' tumor 1, human telomerase reverse transcriptase, and preferentially expressed antigen in melanoma (PRAME) have been used to endow moDCs with anti-AML T-cell-activating capacity [299, 381–384]. Maturation of the moDCs was obtained through a cocktail of cytokines [381, 383] or a cocktail of cytokines and TLR agonists [384]. In these studies, the vaccine was also administered via the i.d. route in patients with low disease burden. Clinically and molecular complete remission [299] and long-term absence of disease recurrence [383] have been reported. Follow-up studies combining mRNA-electroporated DC vaccines with salvage treatment such as chemotherapy and/or allogeneic hematopoietic stem cell transplantation [381] and hypomethylating agents [385] are ongoing. Further efforts are ongoing to improve the DC vaccine, e.g. through codelivery of mRNA-encoding IL-15 variants to include NK cells in the antitumor response [367]. Three strategies were exploited to improve DC vaccination in melanoma patients with metastatic disease. First, moDCs were electroporated with mRNA-encoding TAAs (MAGE-A3, MAGE-C2, tyrosinase, or gp100) and TriMix (CD40L, CD70, and caTLR4), resulting in the TriMixDC-MEL vaccine. This approach allows maturation of the moDCs *in situ* instead of in a culture dish. As a result, proinflammatory cytokines (e.g. IL-12) and T-cell-attracting chemokines are fully exploited during vaccination [43]. Yet, none of the melanoma patients showed objective responses despite the stimulation of T cells in about 60% of patients after i.d. vaccination, prompting subsequent treatment with IFNα2b. This combination resulted in disease control of over six months in 6 out of 17 evaluable patients [45]. Second, the vaccine was injected both via the i.d. and i.v. route to widen the distribution of the moDCs. Tumor antigen-specific $CD4^+$ and $CD8^+$ T cells were detected in peripheral blood and skin biopsies [46, 386] and both complete responses (CRs) and partial responses (PRs) were observed using only the TriMixDC-MEL vaccine, resulting in objective responses in 27% of patients [46]. Notably, a correlation between IL-12 production by the TriMixDC-MEL vaccine and vaccine efficacy was also reported [45]. Finally, i.d./i.v. TriMixDC-MEL vaccination was combined with ICP therapy, blocking CTLA-4 with the mAb ipilimumab. In this study, 39 patients were included and a disease control rate of 51% was reported [47]. Monitoring of the T-cell-activating capacity of this treatment regimen showed T-cell stimulation in 80% of patients, which was significantly higher, broader, and polyfunctional in patients with CRs or PRs [48]. As for AML, the TriMixDC-MEL vaccine has been used as adjuvant therapy in melanoma patients with no clinically evident disease after resection of their metastasis [49]. It was reported that the median OS was not reached after a follow-up of over six years, advocating the use of cancer vaccination in minimal disease settings. Another strategy to improve cancer vaccination would be shifting from using TAAs to using TSAs. To our knowledge, clinical trials with moDCs that have been loaded *ex vivo* with neoantigen mRNA have not yet been performed. However, the Flemish-based consortium "Persomed" has set up a roadmap to develop such a vaccine for the treatment of patients with CRC [62].

Various clinical trials that rely on the delivery of *in vitro* transcribed mRNA-encoding TAAs or TSAs to APCs *in situ* have been described. These are highly variable in setup, differing in the formulation of the mRNA (in solution or in complex with protamine, polymers, or lipids with variations in the composition of carriers) as well as in the delivery of the mRNA (routes of delivery are i.m., i.d., s.c., i.n., i.v., and i.t.). As a result, the APCs that are involved in the ensuing immune response are different as well. This is important to keep in mind as these are determinants of the vaccine efficacy [222]. Therefore, we will discuss the current state-of-the-art according to treatment regimen rather than cancer type. Note, mRNA cancer vaccines have been mostly used to treat metastatic tumors, including mRCC, CRC, melanoma, and cancer of the lung, prostate, pancreas, ovarian, and head and neck. Weide et al. [186] described the first phase I/II clinical trial in which metastatic melanoma patients were vaccinated via the i.d. route with noncomplexed mRNA that was *in vitro* transcribed yet based on the transcriptome of tumors. This mRNA vaccination was combined with the adjuvant GM-CSF (delivered s.c.) in 15 patients, showing that this therapy was safe and tolerable, inducing humoral responses in some patients [186]. Noncomplexed mRNA-encoding TAAs (survivin, MUC-1, HER2, carcinoembryonic antigen, telomerase, and MAGE-A1) have also been administered following a similar regimen to treat 30 patients with mRCC. This study confirmed that vaccination with noncomplexed mRNA is well tolerated and further showed induction of T-cell responses for several of the TAAs used for vaccination [117]. Short-term clinical responses included one PR and stable disease (SD) in 50% of the patients, while long-term follow-up showed that the median OS exceeded the predicted OS [117, 387]. Further activities with mRNA in solution build on the TriMix technology, which has been licensed to eTheRNA Immunotherapies. A phase I trial in melanoma patients has been conducted mimicking the adjuvant setting that was previously shown to be successful with the TriMixDC-MEL vaccine [49]. Herein, 20 melanoma patients with clinically undetectable disease after resection of tumors have received i.n. injection of mRNA-encoding TriMix and the TAAs: tyrosinase, gp100, MAGE-A3, MAGE-C2, and PRAME (ECI-006). This therapy was well tolerated, and vaccine-induced immune responses were detected in patients treated with 600 and 1800 μg of the mRNA mixture [388]. Weide et al. [184] used protamine to complex mRNA-encoding MelanA, tyrosinase, gp100, MAGE-A1, MAGE-A3, and survivin and as such improve mRNA delivery in melanoma patients. To that end, protamine in RL was added to mRNA in a 1:2 mass ratio. The resulting stable protamine–mRNA complex does not allow translation of the mRNA. Hence, noncomplexed TAA mRNA was mixed with the complex in a 1:1 mass ratio in RL. The vaccination regimen involved i.d. delivery of mRNA combined with s.c. delivery of GM-CSF. It was shown in 21 metastatic melanoma patients that the treatment was tolerable (AEs were grade 1 or 2). Moreover, the magnitude of TAA-specific T cells was increased compared to baseline in two of the four evaluated patients. More importantly, one out of seven patients with measurable disease showed a CR. To date, mRNA condensed in protamine is known as the RNActive® technology of CureVac. Different mRNA vaccines based on this technology have been and are still being evaluated in several clinical trials, treating patients with prostate cancer [121, 302, 389] or lung cancer [390]. An example hereof is the phase I/II trial in which patients with hormone-refractory prostate cancer are treated with an i.d. injection of self-adjuvanted (RNActive®) mRNA-encoding four distinct prostate-specific antigens (CV9103).

Only grade 1 to 2 AEs occurred, confirming the tolerability of this therapy even at doses of 1280 μg. Most patients receiving this high dose developed TAA-specific immune responses and showed a favorable median OS [121]. RNActive®-based vaccination (CV9202) has moreover been evaluated in combination with local radiation to enhance immune responses in patients with advanced-stage lung cancer treated with chemotherapy or tyrosine kinase inhibitors [328, 329]. The CV9202 vaccine encodes six different antigens, including MAGE-C1, MAGE-C2, New York esophageal squamous cell carcinoma 1 (NY-ESO-1), trophoblast glycoprotein (5T4), survivin, and MUC-1. Some grade 3 AEs were reported of which some related to the radiation therapy. However, in general the therapy regimen was tolerable. The majority of patients showed increased humoral and T-cell responses, resulting in 1 out of 26 patients with a PR and 12 out of 26 patients with SD [329]. To date, the CV9202 vaccine is being tested in combination with ICP therapy, blocking the negative feedback provided via CTLA-4 as well as PD-1 [391]. Another type of TAA mRNA vaccines that has been evaluated in the clinical setting under impulse of BioNTech is based on formulation in LNPs, which are administered via the i.v. route. The vaccine BNT111, consisting of a mix of mRNA-encoding

NY-ESO-1, tyrosinase, MAGE-A3, and transmembrane phosphatase with tensin homology, has been evaluated for treatment of patients with advanced melanoma in a phase I/II trial, known as Lipo-MERIT [136, 165]. Increased plasma levels of proinflammatory cytokines, including IFN-α, were observed a few hours following each vaccination but normalized within 24 h. This cytokine profile parallels the transient and self-limiting AE profile, which was mild to moderate. Stimulation of TAA-specific CTLs was demonstrated. Three out of 25 patients treated with BNT111 had PR and 7 out of 25 patients had SD. This vaccine was further combined with cemiplimab, a mAb that blocks PD-1 signals, showing the safety of this combination as well as PRs in 6 out of 17 patients [165]. Similar mRNA vaccines have been developed for the treatment of prostate cancer (BNT112: five prostate cancer-specific antigens), HPV16$^+$ head and neck cancer (BNT113: HPV16-E6 and E7 antigens), and ovarian cancer (BNT115: three ovarian-associated antigens) [392]. Given the knowledge that TSAs or neoantigens are prime vaccine antigens, BioNTech has also evaluated mRNA vaccines based on neoantigens. The first vaccine BNT121 was delivered via the i.n. route in 13 patients with metastatic melanoma and consisted of mRNA-encoding 10 neoepitopes [185]. Lack of severe AEs, detection of immunological responses, and evidence of clinical efficacy encouraged further research into neoantigen-based mRNA vaccines. The following vaccine, BNT122 consisting of up to 20 neoepitopes, was injected via the i.v. route and used as a monotherapy or in combination with atezolizumab, a mAb that binds PD-L1. This therapy has been shown to have an acceptable safety profile in melanoma patients with transient AEs and is further under evaluation for the treatment of patients with cancer of the breast, colon, pancreas, ovarian, and lung [62, 392, 393]. Also, Moderna has launched vaccines based on mutated antigens: mRNA-5671 and mRNA-4157. The vaccine designated mRNA-5671 encodes the four most common Kirsten rat sarcoma viral oncogene homolog (KRAS) mutations (G12D, G12V, G13D, and G12C). The phase I clinical trial studying mRNA-5671 as a monotherapy or combined with pembrolizumab in patients with solid tumors has been completed. The vaccine mRNA-4157 encodes up to 34 neoepitopes in one single mRNA molecule and is under investigation in ongoing phase I/II clinical trials as a monotherapy or combined with pembrolizumab in patients with solid tumors. At this time, little results are available, except for early communications on the safety of these vaccines [394].

The data arising from the clinical vaccination studies employing mRNA, whether delivered as a DC vaccine, in solution or in carriers, all point toward the safety and tolerability of mRNA-based vaccine approaches.

Any reactogenicity has so far been transient and self-limiting, likely resulting from cytokine release at the moment of vaccine delivery [45, 136, 165]. Vaccination trials eliciting immune responses against TAAs have shown encouraging immune activation and correlations with clinical outcomes [48, 165], raising high hope for trials in which multiple neoantigens are encoded in mRNA vaccines. Complete datasets are still lacking for most of these neoantigen targeting trials. However, early data [185] and the finding that mRNA vaccines can be combined with ICP therapy as well as other cancer therapies [47, 165, 328, 329, 381, 385] warrant optimism and demand that mRNA vaccines are introduced early in the standard-of-care of cancer patients.

13.10 Conclusion

Since its first description as an intermediate between DNA and proteins, significant investments have been made in research on exploiting mRNA in medicine. Progress in this field of research was at first slow. However, a turning point was reached in the last decade, allowing to respond quickly to the SARS-CoV2 pandemic by mass manufacturing mRNA vaccines and using them clinically on a global scale. The vast amount of positive data from this global treatment provides the incentive to further invest in cancer vaccines that exploit mRNA to deliver an antitumor message to our immune system.

However, several points merit attention to fully capitalize on the potential of cancer vaccines based on mRNA. These points are related to the rules for obtaining a well-functioning cancer vaccine. We established in this chapter that mRNA is a favorable vaccination platform. Because of its nature, mRNA facilitates multiple and rapid refinements with almost limitless combinations, allowing the pursuit of optimization in a cost- and time-efficient way. Refining the production workflow of mRNA is one of the challenges ahead, particularly as TSAs, neoantigens, are favored for vaccination and demand a workflow that is flexible, fast, and exploitable in both testing of and immunization with immunogens [62]. Without a doubt, mRNA has that potential. Native and *in silico* designed proteins (e.g. fusion proteins and multimeric proteins) that would be difficult to produce in a bioreactor can be encoded in mRNA for production in the patient's own cells such as APCs, either *ex vivo* or *in situ*. Efforts are made to develop PDT-free manufacturing protocols prone to automation [191, 192]. These genuinely synthetic mRNA production protocols, avoiding bacteria for pDNA production, could speed up the process and lower the cost of mRNA production considerably. Another challenge lies within the introduction of mRNA to patients. Many carriers are under development for direct delivery of mRNA to APCs in the patient's body. The vast number of preclinical studies on this matter has shown that mRNA delivered *in situ* is recognized as foreign, eliciting type I IFN responses. These can reach toxic levels, limiting mRNA vaccine dosing. Therefore, mRNA needs to be rendered immunosilent via the introduction of chemically modified nucleotides. Alternatively, DCs generated in the lab have been modified with mRNA *ex vivo*, exhibiting little activation of PRRs. Whether immunosilent mRNA is delivered to a patient's APCs or whether mRNA-transfected DCs are reinjected to that patient, one issue has to be kept in mind: without an adjuvant the immune response to the antigenic protein will likely not reach its full potential. As outlined in this chapter, several adjuvants are compatible with mRNA cancer vaccines. However, the adjuvant composed of TriMix mRNA is likely the most advanced in terms of clinical testing [388]. We learned from clinical trials that IL-12 is a cytokine linked to vaccine efficacy and clinical outcome [45, 377]. Therefore, efforts to ensure long-lasting production of high amounts of IL-12 could be further pursued. Key in this pursuit will be finding the optimal balance between immune and inflammatory activation to establish an acceptable risk–benefit profile of the vaccine. This will likely be codetermined by the route of vaccine delivery and as a result the vaccine biodistribution. Considering the spatiotemporal biodistribution of vaccines and trying to grasp the interactions with immune cells could allow for a more rational development of vaccines. This requires nonempirical testing in animal models such as NHPs that are more closely related to humans than mice. However, testing in NHPs is restricted by ethical considerations. In this regard, noninvasive imaging of vaccine biodistribution in NHP could be a helpful strategy [395].

The parameters of a given vaccine, including adjuvant, delivery vehicle, and route of administration, profoundly impact the type of immune response generated and subsequent vaccine efficacy [222, 396]. With each vaccination approach having its advantages and disadvantages based on the treatment setting, understanding, and reverse engineering the spatiotemporal kinetics of successful vaccines could allow for the rational development of vaccines that share similar trafficking characteristics. In other words, knowing the "why" and "how" of a successful vaccine can aid in improving the efficacy of other less efficacious vaccines.

Decades of slow progress have proved that cancer vaccines can elicit systemic tumor regression, durable remission, and improvement in OS [397]. We believe that the mRNA technology will take the forefront in cancer vaccination and cause acceleration, building upon the success during the SARS-CoV-2 pandemic. Overall, with significant advances in mRNA biology, delivery, and manufacturing, the biotechnology and vaccine industries are poised for further investment in developing novel products.

References

1 Hanahan, D. and Weinberg, R.A. (2011). Hallmarks of cancer: the next generation. *Cell* 144 (5): 646–674.

2 Lang, F., Schrörs, B., Löwer, M. et al. (2022). Identification of neoantigens for individualized therapeutic cancer vaccines. *Nat. Rev. Drug Discov.* 21 (4): 261–282.

3 Zhang, Z., Lu, M., Qin, Y. et al. (2021). Neoantigen: a new breakthrough in tumor immunotherapy. *Front. Immunol.* 12: 672356.

4 Schumacher, T.N., Scheper, W., and Kvistborg, P. (2019). Cancer neoantigens. *Annu. Rev. Immunol.* 37: 173–200.

5 De Plaen, E., Lurquin, C., Van Pel, A. et al. (1988). Immunogenic (tum-) variants of mouse tumor P815: cloning of the gene of tum- antigen P91A and identification of the tum- mutation. *Proc. Natl. Acad. Sci. U. S. A.* 85 (7): 2274–2278.

6 De Smet, C., De Backer, O., Faraoni, I. et al. (1996). The activation of human gene MAGE-1 in tumor cells is correlated with genome-wide demethylation. *Proc. Natl. Acad. Sci. U. S. A.* 93 (14): 7149–7153.

7 Coulie, P.G., Van den Eynde, B.J., van der Bruggen, P., and Boon, T. (2014). Tumour antigens recognized by T lymphocytes: at the core of cancer immunotherapy. *Nat. Rev. Cancer* 14 (2): 135–146.

8 Heemskerk, B., Kvistborg, P., and Schumacher, T.N. (2013). The cancer antigenome. *EMBO J.* 32 (2): 194–203.

9 Vose, B.M. and Moore, M. (1985). Human tumor-infiltrating lymphocytes: a marker of host response. *Semin. Hematol.* 22 (1): 27–40.

10 Noubade, R., Majri-Morrison, S., and Tarbell, K.V. (2019). Beyond cDC1: emerging roles of DC crosstalk in cancer immunity. *Front. Immunol.* 10: 1014.

11 Hildner, K., Edelson, B.T., Purtha, W.E. et al. (2008). Batf3 deficiency reveals a critical role for CD8alpha+ dendritic cells in cytotoxic T cell immunity. *Science* 322 (5904): 1097–1100.

12 Bonehill, A., Heirman, C., and Thielemans, K. (2005). Genetic approaches for the induction of a CD4+ T cell response in cancer immunotherapy. *J. Gene Med.* 7 (6): 686–695.

13 Awad, R.M., De Vlaeminck, Y., Maebe, J. et al. (2018). Turn back the TIMe: targeting tumor infiltrating myeloid cells to revert cancer progression. *Front. Immunol.* 9: 1977.

14 Nair, S. and Dhodapkar, M.V. (2017). Natural killer T cells in cancer immunotherapy. *Front. Immunol.* 8: 1178.

15 Silva-Santos, B., Serre, K., and Norell, H. (2015). γδ T cells in cancer. *Nat. Rev. Immunol.* 15 (11): 683–691.

16 O'Donnell, J.S., Teng, M.W.L., and Smyth, M.J. (2019). Cancer immunoediting and resistance to T cell-based immunotherapy. *Nat. Rev. Clin. Oncol.* 16 (3): 151–167.

17 Michaud, D., Steward, C.R., Mirlekar, B., and Pylayeva-Gupta, Y. (2021). Regulatory B cells in cancer. *Immunol. Rev.* 299 (1): 74–92.

18 Chabab, G., Barjon, C., Bonnefoy, N., and Lafont, V. (2020). Pro-tumor γδ T cells in human cancer: polarization, mechanisms of action, and implications for therapy. *Front. Immunol.* 11: 2186.

19 Finck, A., Gill, S.I., and June, C.H. (2020). Cancer immunotherapy comes of age and looks for maturity. *Nat. Commun.* 11 (1): 3325.

20 Couzin-Frankel, J. (2013). Breakthrough of the year 2013. Cancer immunotherapy. *Science* 342 (6165): 1432–1433.

21 Jenkins, R.W., Barbie, D.A., and Flaherty, K.T. (2018). Mechanisms of resistance to immune checkpoint inhibitors. *Br. J. Cancer* 118 (1): 9–16.

22 Liu, R., Yang, F., Yin, J.Y. et al. (2021). Influence of tumor immune infiltration on immune checkpoint inhibitor therapeutic efficacy: a computational retrospective study. *Front. Immunol.* 12: 685370.

23 Kim, J.M. and Chen, D.S. (2016). Immune escape to PD-L1/PD-1 blockade: seven steps to success (or failure). *Ann. Oncol.* 27 (8): 1492–1504.

24 Galon, J. and Bruni, D. (2019). Approaches to treat immune hot, altered and cold tumours with combination immunotherapies. *Nat. Rev. Drug Discov.* 18 (3): 197–218.

25 Antonarelli, G., Corti, C., Tarantino, P. et al. (2021). Therapeutic cancer vaccines revamping: technology advancements and pitfalls. *Ann. Oncol.* 32 (12): 1537–1551.

26 Markowitz, L.E. and Schiller, J.T. (2021). Human papillomavirus vaccines. *J. Infect. Dis.* 224 (12 Suppl 2): S367–S378.

27 Melief, C.J., van Hall, T., Arens, R. et al. (2015). Therapeutic cancer vaccines. *J. Clin. Invest.* 125 (9): 3401–3412.

28 Bonaventura, P., Shekarian, T., Alcazer, V. et al. (2019). Cold tumors: a therapeutic challenge for immunotherapy. *Front. Immunol.* 10: 168.

29 Alexander-Miller, M.A., Derby, M.A., Sarin, A. et al. (1998). Supraoptimal peptide-major histocompatibility complex causes a decrease in bc1-2 levels and allows tumor necrosis factor alpha receptor II-mediated apoptosis of cytotoxic T lymphocytes. *J. Exp. Med.* 188 (8): 1391–1399.

30 Ma, H. and Kapp, J.A. (2000). Antigenic epitopes regulate the phenotype of CD8+ CTL primed by exogenous antigens. *J. Immunol.* 164 (11): 5698–5703.

31 Bonehill, A., Tuyaerts, S., Van Nuffel, A.M. et al. (2008). Enhancing the T-cell stimulatory capacity of human dendritic cells by co-electroporation with CD40L, CD70 and constitutively active TLR4 encoding mRNA. *Mol. Ther.* 16 (6): 1170–1180.

32 Aerts-Toegaert, C., Heirman, C., Tuyaerts, S. et al. (2007). CD83 expression on dendritic cells and T cells: correlation with effective immune responses. *Eur. J. Immunol.* 37 (3): 686–695.

33 Tüting, T., Gambotto, A., Robbins, P.D. et al. (1999). Co-delivery of T helper 1-biasing cytokine genes enhances the efficacy of gene gun immunization of mice: studies with the model tumor antigen beta-galactosidase and the BALB/c Meth A p53 tumor-specific antigen. *Gene Ther.* 6 (4): 629–636.

34 Muraoka, D., Harada, N., Hayashi, T. et al. (2014). Nanogel-based immunologically stealth vaccine targets macrophages in the medulla of lymph node and induces potent antitumor immunity. *ACS Nano* 8 (9): 9209–9218.

35 Goyvaerts, C., Kurt, D.G., Van Lint, S. et al. (2014). Immunogenicity of targeted lentivectors. *Oncotarget* 5 (3): 704–715.

36 Goyvaerts, C. and Breckpot, K. (2015). Pros and cons of antigen-presenting cell targeted tumor vaccines. *J. Immunol. Res.* 2015: 785634.

37 Anguille, S., Smits, E.L., Lion, E. et al. (2014). Clinical use of dendritic cells for cancer therapy. *Lancet Oncol.* 15 (7): e257–e267.

38 Garg, A.D., Galluzzi, L., Apetoh, L. et al. (2015). Molecular and translational classifications of DAMPs in immunogenic cell death. *Front. Immunol.* 6: 588.

39 Jou, J., Harrington, K.J., Zocca, M.B. et al. (2021). The changing landscape of therapeutic cancer vaccines - novel platforms and neoantigen identification. *Clin. Cancer Res.* 27 (3): 689–703.

40 Chen, D.S. and Mellman, I. (2013). Oncology meets immunology: the cancer-immunity cycle. *Immunity* 39 (1): 1–10.

41 Brossart, P. (2020). The role of antigen spreading in the efficacy of immunotherapies. *Clin. Cancer Res.* 26 (17): 4442–4447.

42 Kantoff, P.W., Higano, C.S., Shore, N.D. et al. (2010). Sipuleucel-T immunotherapy for castration-resistant prostate cancer. *N. Engl. J. Med.* 363 (5): 411–422.

43 Bonehill, A., Van Nuffel, A.M., Corthals, J. et al. (2009). Single-step antigen loading and activation of dendritic cells by mRNA electroporation for the purpose of therapeutic vaccination in melanoma patients. *Clin. Cancer Res.* 15 (10): 3366–3375.

44 Pen, J.J., De Keersmaecker, B., Maenhout, S.K. et al. (2013). Modulation of regulatory T cell function by monocyte-derived dendritic cells matured through electroporation with mRNA encoding CD40 ligand, constitutively active TLR4, and CD70. *J. Immunol.* 191 (4): 1976–1983.

45 Wilgenhof, S., Van Nuffel, A.M., Corthals, J. et al. (2011). Therapeutic vaccination with an autologous mRNA electroporated dendritic cell vaccine in patients with advanced melanoma. *J. Immunother.* 34 (5): 448–456.

46 Wilgenhof, S., Van Nuffel, A.M.T., Benteyn, D. et al. (2013). A phase IB study on intravenous synthetic mRNA electroporated dendritic cell immunotherapy in pretreated advanced melanoma patients. *Ann. Oncol.* 24 (10): 2686–2693.

47 Wilgenhof, S., Corthals, J., Heirman, C. et al. (2016). Phase II study of autologous monocyte-derived mRNA electroporated dendritic cells (TriMixDC-MEL) plus ipilimumab in patients with pretreated advanced melanoma. *J. Clin. Oncol.* 34 (12): 1330–1338.

48 De Keersmaecker, B., Claerhout, S., Carrasco, J. et al. (2020). TriMix and tumor antigen mRNA electroporated dendritic cell vaccination plus ipilimumab: link between T-cell activation and clinical responses in advanced melanoma. *J. Immunother. Cancer* 8 (1): e000329.

49 Wilgenhof, S., Corthals, J., Van Nuffel, A.M. et al. (2015). Long-term clinical outcome of melanoma patients treated with messenger RNA-electroporated dendritic cell therapy following complete resection of metastases. *Cancer Immunol. Immunother.* 64 (3): 381–388.

50 Van Lint, S., Goyvaerts, C., Maenhout, S. et al. (2012). Preclinical evaluation of TriMix and antigen mRNA-based antitumor therapy. *Cancer Res.* 72 (7): 1661–1671.

51 Van Lint, S., Renmans, D., Broos, K. et al. (2016). Intratumoral delivery of TriMix mRNA results in T-cell activation by cross-presenting dendritic cells. *Cancer Immunol. Res.* 4 (2): 146–156.

52 Dullaers, M., Van Meirvenne, S., Heirman, C. et al. (2006). Induction of effective therapeutic antitumor immunity by direct in vivo administration of lentiviral vectors. *Gene Ther.* 13 (7): 630–640.

53 Jhunjhunwala, S., Hammer, C., and Delamarre, L. (2021). Antigen presentation in cancer: insights into tumour immunogenicity and immune evasion. *Nat. Rev. Cancer* 21 (5): 298–312.

54 Leng, Q., Tarbe, M., Long, Q., and Wang, F. (2020). Pre-existing heterologous T-cell immunity and neoantigen immunogenicity. *Clin. Transl. Immunol.* 9 (3): e01111.

55 Neller, M.A., López, J.A., and Schmidt, C.W. (2008). Antigens for cancer immunotherapy. *Semin. Immunol.* 20 (5): 286–295.

56 Dutoit, V., Rubio-Godoy, V., Dietrich, P.Y. et al. (2001). Heterogeneous T-cell response to MAGE-A10(254-262): high avidity-specific cytolytic T lymphocytes show superior antitumor activity. *Cancer Res.* 61 (15): 5850–5856.

57 Schmid, D.A., Irving, M.B., Posevitz, V. et al. (2010). Evidence for a TCR affinity threshold delimiting maximal CD8 T cell function. *J. Immunol.* 184 (9): 4936–4946.

58 Zhong, S., Malecek, K., Johnson, L.A. et al. (2013). T-cell receptor affinity and avidity defines antitumor response and autoimmunity in T-cell immunotherapy. *Proc. Natl. Acad. Sci. U. S. A.* 110 (17): 6973–6978.

59 Carreno, B.M., Magrini, V., Becker-Hapak, M. et al. (2015). Cancer immunotherapy. A dendritic cell vaccine increases the breadth and diversity of melanoma neoantigen-specific T cells. *Science* 348 (6236): 803–808.

60 Hilf, N., Kuttruff-Coqui, S., Frenzel, K. et al. (2019). Actively personalized vaccination trial for newly diagnosed glioblastoma. *Nature* 565 (7738): 240–245.

61 Nelson, R.W., Beisang, D., Tubo, N.J. et al. (2015). T cell receptor cross-reactivity between similar foreign and self peptides influences naive cell population size and autoimmunity. *Immunity* 42 (1): 95–107.

62 Esprit, A., de Mey, W., Bahadur Shahi, R. et al. (2020). Neo-antigen mRNA vaccines. *Vaccines (Basel)* 8 (4): 776.

63 Schaap-Johansen, A.L., Vujović, M., Borch, A. et al. (2021). T cell epitope prediction and its application to immunotherapy. *Front. Immunol.* 12: 712488.

64 Hu, H.G. and Li, Y.M. (2020). Emerging adjuvants for cancer immunotherapy. *Front. Chem.* 8: 601.

65 Chiang, C.L., Kandalaft, L.E., and Coukos, G. (2011). Adjuvants for enhancing the immunogenicity of whole tumor cell vaccines. *Int. Rev. Immunol.* 30 (2–3): 150–182.

66 Kenter, G.G., Welters, M.J., Valentijn, A.R. et al. (2009). Vaccination against HPV-16 oncoproteins for vulvar intraepithelial neoplasia. *N. Engl. J. Med.* 361 (19): 1838–1847.

67 Yang, Y., Huang, C.T., Huang, X., and Pardoll, D.M. (2004). Persistent Toll-like receptor signals are required for reversal of regulatory T cell-mediated CD8 tolerance. *Nat. Immunol.* 5 (5): 508–515.

68 Foote, J.B., Kok, M., Leatherman, J.M. et al. (2017). A STING agonist given with OX40 receptor and PD-L1 modulators primes immunity and reduces tumor growth in tolerized mice. *Cancer Immunol. Res.* 5 (6): 468–479.

69 Ammi, R., De Waele, J., Willemen, Y. et al. (2015). Poly(I:C) as cancer vaccine adjuvant: knocking on the door of medical breakthroughs. *Pharmacol. Ther.* 146: 120–131.

70 Ogino, H., Taylor, J.W., Nejo, T. et al. (2022). Randomized trial of neoadjuvant vaccination with tumor-cell lysate induces T cell response in low-grade gliomas. *J. Clin. Invest.* 132 (3): e151239.

71 Vosika, G.J., Barr, C., and Gilbertson, D. (1984). Phase-I study of intravenous modified lipid A. *Cancer Immunol. Immunother.* 18 (2): 107–112.

72 Shetab Boushehri, M.A. and Lamprecht, A. (2018). TLR4-based immunotherapeutics in cancer: a review of the achievements and shortcomings. *Mol. Pharm.* 15 (11): 4777–4800.

73 Chi, H., Li, C., Zhao, F.S. et al. (2017). Anti-tumor activity of Toll-like receptor 7 agonists. *Front. Pharmacol.* 8: 304.

74 Sabado, R.L., Pavlick, A., Gnjatic, S. et al. (2015). Resiquimod as an immunologic adjuvant for NY-ESO-1 protein vaccination in patients with high-risk melanoma. *Cancer Immunol. Res.* 3 (3): 278–287.

75 Anwar, M.A., Shah, M., Kim, J., and Choi, S. (2019). Recent clinical trends in Toll-like receptor targeting therapeutics. *Med. Res. Rev.* 39 (3): 1053–1090.

76 Zhang, Z., Kuo, J.C., Yao, S. et al. (2021). CpG oligodeoxynucleotides for anticancer monotherapy from preclinical stages to clinical trials. *Pharmaceutics* 14 (1): 73.

77 Wang, Y., Zhang, S., Li, H. et al. (2020). Small-molecule modulators of Toll-like receptors. *Acc. Chem. Res.* 53 (5): 1046–1055.

78 Su, T., Zhang, Y., Valerie, K. et al. (2019). STING activation in cancer immunotherapy. *Theranostics* 9 (25): 7759–7771.

79 Amouzegar, A., Chelvanambi, M., Filderman, J.N. et al. (2021). STING agonists as cancer therapeutics. *Cancers (Basel)* 13 (11): 2695.

80 Paston, S.J., Brentville, V.A., Symonds, P., and Durrant, L.G. (2021). Cancer vaccines, adjuvants, and delivery systems. *Front. Immunol.* 12: 627932.

81 Ahonen, C.L., Gibson, S.J., Smith, R.M. et al. (1999). Dendritic cell maturation and subsequent enhanced T-cell stimulation induced with the novel synthetic immune response modifier R-848. *Cell. Immunol.* 197 (1): 62–72.

82 Bullock, T.N. and Yagita, H. (2005). Induction of CD70 on dendritic cells through CD40 or TLR stimulation contributes to the development of CD8+ T cell responses in the absence of CD4+ T cells. *J. Immunol.* 174 (2): 710–717.

83 Cho, H.I., Jung, S.H., Sohn, H.J. et al. (2015). An optimized peptide vaccine strategy capable of inducing multivalent CD8. *Oncoimmunology* 4 (11): e1043504.

84 Stevens, A.D. and Bullock, T.N.J. (2021). Therapeutic vaccination targeting CD40 and TLR3 controls melanoma growth through existing intratumoral CD8 T cells without new T cell infiltration. *Cancer Immunol. Immunother.* 70 (8): 2139–2150.

85 Conlon, K.C., Miljkovic, M.D., and Waldmann, T.A. (2019). Cytokines in the treatment of cancer. *J. Interf. Cytokine Res.* 39 (1): 6–21.

86 Zarei, S., Schwenter, F., Luy, P. et al. (2009). Role of GM-CSF signaling in cell-based tumor immunization. *Blood* 113 (26): 6658–6668.

87 Dufait, I., Schwarze, J.K., Liechtenstein, T. et al. (2015). Ex vivo generation of myeloid-derived suppressor cells that model the tumor immunosuppressive environment in colorectal cancer. *Oncotarget* 6 (14): 12369–12382.

88 Frasca, L., Nasso, M., Spensieri, F. et al. (2008). IFN-gamma arms human dendritic cells to perform multiple effector functions. *J. Immunol.* 180 (3): 1471–1481.

89 Breckpot, K., Aerts-Toegaert, C., Heirman, C. et al. (2009). Attenuated expression of A20 markedly increases the efficacy of double-stranded RNA-activated dendritic cells as an anti-cancer vaccine. *J. Immunol.* 182 (2): 860–870.

90 Cheng, F., Wang, H.W., Cuenca, A. et al. (2003). A critical role for Stat3 signaling in immune tolerance. *Immunity* 19 (3): 425–436.

91 Nauts, H.C., Fowler, G.A., and Bogatko, F.H. (1953). A review of the influence of bacterial infection and of bacterial products (Coley's toxins) on malignant tumors in man; a critical analysis of 30 inoperable cases treated by Coley's mixed toxins, in which diagnosis was confirmed by microscopic examination selected for special study. *Acta Med. Scand. Suppl.* 276: 1–103.

92 Hoover, H.C., Surdyke, M.G., Dangel, R.B. et al. (1985). Prospectively randomized trial of adjuvant active-specific immunotherapy for human colorectal cancer. *Cancer* 55 (6): 1236–1243.

93 van der Bruggen, P., Traversari, C., Chomez, P. et al. (1991). A gene encoding an antigen recognized by cytolytic T lymphocytes on a human melanoma. *Science* 254 (5038): 1643–1647.

94 Finn, O.J. (2017). Human tumor antigens yesterday, today, and tomorrow. *Cancer Immunol. Res.* 5 (5): 347–354.

95 Breckpot, K., Heirman, C., De Greef, C. et al. (2004). Identification of new antigenic peptide presented by HLA-Cw7 and encoded by several MAGE genes using dendritic cells transduced with lentiviruses. *J. Immunol.* 172 (4): 2232–2237.

96 Goydos, J.S., Elder, E., Whiteside, T.L. et al. (1996). A phase I trial of a synthetic mucin peptide vaccine. Induction of specific immune reactivity in patients with adenocarcinoma. *J. Surg. Res.* 63 (1): 298–304.

97 Marchand, M., van Baren, N., Weynants, P. et al. (1999). Tumor regressions observed in patients with metastatic melanoma treated with an antigenic peptide encoded by gene MAGE-3 and presented by HLA-A1. *Int. J. Cancer* 80 (2): 219–230.

98 Disis, M.L., Grabstein, K.H., Sleath, P.R., and Cheever, M.A. (1999). Generation of immunity to the HER-2/neu oncogenic protein in patients with breast and ovarian cancer using a peptide-based vaccine. *Clin. Cancer Res.* 5 (6): 1289–1297.

99 Tuyaerts, S., Aerts, J.L., Corthals, J. et al. (2007). Current approaches in dendritic cell generation and future implications for cancer immunotherapy. *Cancer Immunol. Immunother.* 56 (10): 1513–1537.

100 Tuyaerts, S., Noppe, S.M., Corthals, J. et al. (2002). Generation of large numbers of dendritic cells in a closed system using Cell Factories. *J. Immunol. Methods* 264 (1-2): 135–151.

101 Breckpot, K. and Escors, D. (2009). Dendritic cells for active anti-cancer immunotherapy: targeting activation pathways through genetic modification. *Endocr. Metab. Immune Disord. Drug Targets* 9 (4): 328–343.

102 Breckpot, K., Corthals, J., Bonehill, A. et al. (2005). Dendritic cells differentiated in the presence of IFN-beta and IL-3 are potent inducers of an antigen-specific CD8(+) T cell response. *J. Leukoc. Biol.* 78 (4): 898–908.

103 Hernández-Luna, M.A., Luria-Pérez, R., and Huerta-Yépez, S. (2013). Therapeutic intervention alternatives in cancer, using attenuated live bacterial vectors: Salmonella enterica as a carrier of heterologous molecules. *Rev. Investig. Clin.* 65 (1): 65–73.

104 Breckpot, K., Heirman, C., Neyns, B., and Thielemans, K. (2004). Exploiting dendritic cells for cancer immunotherapy: genetic modification of dendritic cells. *J. Gene Med.* 6 (11): 1175–1188.

105 Finn, O.J. (2018). The dawn of vaccines for cancer prevention. *Nat. Rev. Immunol.* 18 (3): 183–194.

106 Yu, M. and Finn, O.J. (2006). DNA vaccines for cancer too. *Cancer Immunol. Immunother.* 55 (2): 119–130.

107 Toussaint, B., Chauchet, X., Wang, Y. et al. (2013). Live-attenuated bacteria as a cancer vaccine vector. *Expert Rev. Vaccines* 12 (10): 1139–1154.

108 Goyvaerts, C. and Breckpot, K. (2018). The journey of *in vivo* virus engineered dendritic cells from bench to bedside: a bumpy road. *Front. Immunol.* 9: 2052.

109 De Mey, W., Esprit, A., Thielemans, K. et al. (2022). RNA in cancer immunotherapy: unlocking the potential of the immune system. *Clin. Cancer Res.* 28 (18): 3929–3939.

110 Rosa, S.S., Prazeres, D.M.F., Azevedo, A.M., and Marques, M.P.C. (2021). mRNA vaccines manufacturing: challenges and bottlenecks. *Vaccine* 39 (16): 2190–2200.

111 Maeng, H.M. and Berzofsky, J.A. (2019). Strategies for developing and optimizing cancer vaccines. *F1000Res.* 8: https://doi.org/10.12688/f1000research.18693.1.

112 Liu, H., Moynihan, K.D., Zheng, Y. et al. (2014). Structure-based programming of lymph-node targeting in molecular vaccines. *Nature* 507 (7493): 519–522.

113 Fifis, T., Gamvrellis, A., Crimeen-Irwin, B. et al. (2004). Size-dependent immunogenicity: therapeutic and protective properties of nano-vaccines against tumors. *J. Immunol.* 173 (5): 3148–3154.

114 Verdijk, P., Aarntzen, E.H., Lesterhuis, W.J. et al. (2009). Limited amounts of dendritic cells migrate into the T-cell area of lymph nodes but have high immune activating potential in melanoma patients. *Clin. Cancer Res.* 15 (7): 2531–2540.

115 Karbach, J., Neumann, A., Atmaca, A. et al. (2011). Efficient in vivo priming by vaccination with recombinant NY-ESO-1 protein and CpG in antigen naive prostate cancer patients. *Clin. Cancer Res.* 17 (4): 861–870.

116 Stebbing, J., Dalgleish, A., Gifford-Moore, A. et al. (2012). An intra-patient placebo-controlled phase I trial to evaluate the safety and tolerability of intradermal IMM-101 in melanoma. *Ann. Oncol.* 23 (5): 1314–1319.

117 Rittig, S.M., Haentschel, M., Weimer, K.J. et al. (2011). Intradermal vaccinations with RNA coding for TAA generate CD8+ and CD4+ immune responses and induce clinical benefit in vaccinated patients. *Mol. Ther.* 19 (5): 990–999.

118 Sampson, J.H., Heimberger, A.B., Archer, G.E. et al. (2010). Immunologic escape after prolonged progression-free survival with epidermal growth factor receptor variant III peptide vaccination in patients with newly diagnosed glioblastoma. *J. Clin. Oncol.* 28 (31): 4722–4729.

119 Lesterhuis, W.J., de Vries, I.J., Schreibelt, G. et al. (2011). Route of administration modulates the induction of dendritic cell vaccine-induced antigen-specific T cells in advanced melanoma patients. *Clin. Cancer Res.* 17 (17): 5725–5735.

120 Sebastian, M., Schröder, A., Scheel, B. et al. (2019). A phase I/IIa study of the mRNA-based cancer immunotherapy CV9201 in patients with stage IIIB/IV non-small cell lung cancer. *Cancer Immunol. Immunother.* 68 (5): 799–812.

121 Kübler, H., Scheel, B., Gnad-Vogt, U. et al. (2015). Self-adjuvanted mRNA vaccination in advanced prostate cancer patients: a first-in-man phase I/IIa study. *J. Immunother. Cancer.* 3: 26.

122 Kreiter, S., Selmi, A., Diken, M. et al. (2010). Intranodal vaccination with naked antigen-encoding RNA elicits potent prophylactic and therapeutic antitumoral immunity. *Cancer Res.* 70 (22): 9031–9040.

123 Ibrahim, M.M. (2010). Subcutaneous and visceral adipose tissue: structural and functional differences. *Obes. Rev.* 11 (1): 11–18.

124 de Vos van Steenwijk, P.J., van Poelgeest, M.I., Ramwadhdoebe, T.H. et al. (2014). The long-term immune response after HPV16 peptide vaccination in women with low-grade pre-malignant disorders of the uterine cervix: a placebo-controlled phase II study. *Cancer Immunol. Immunother.* 63 (2): 147–160.

125 Maloy, K.J., Erdmann, I., Basch, V. et al. (2001). Intralymphatic immunization enhances DNA vaccination. *Proc. Natl. Acad. Sci. U. S. A.* 98 (6): 3299–3303.

126 Johansen, P., Häffner, A.C., Koch, F. et al. (2005). Direct intralymphatic injection of peptide vaccines enhances immunogenicity. *Eur. J. Immunol.* 35 (2): 568–574.

127 Mohanan, D., Slütter, B., Henriksen-Lacey, M. et al. (2010). Administration routes affect the quality of immune responses: a cross-sectional evaluation of particulate antigen-delivery systems. *J. Control. Release* 147 (3): 342–349.

128 Rosenbaum, P., Tchitchek, N., Joly, C. et al. (2021). Vaccine inoculation route modulates early immunity and consequently antigen-specific immune response. *Front. Immunol.* 12: 645210.

129 Ott, P.A., Hu, Z., Keskin, D.B. et al. (2017). An immunogenic personal neoantigen vaccine for patients with melanoma. *Nature* 547 (7662): 217–221.

130 Welters, M.J., Kenter, G.G., de Vos van Steenwijk, P.J. et al. (2010). Success or failure of vaccination for HPV16-positive vulvar lesions correlates with kinetics and phenotype of induced T-cell responses. *Proc. Natl. Acad. Sci. U. S. A.* 107 (26): 11895–11899.

131 Baek, S., Kim, C.S., Kim, S.B. et al. (2011). Combination therapy of renal cell carcinoma or breast cancer patients with dendritic cell vaccine and IL-2: results from a phase I/II trial. *J. Transl. Med.* 9: 178.

132 Oshita, C., Takikawa, M., Kume, A. et al. (2012). Dendritic cell-based vaccination in metastatic melanoma patients: phase II clinical trial. *Oncol. Rep.* 28 (4): 1131–1138.

133 Okada, N., Tsujino, M., Hagiwara, Y. et al. (2001). Administration route-dependent vaccine efficiency of murine dendritic cells pulsed with antigens. *Br. J. Cancer* 84 (11): 1564–1570.

134 Eggert, A.A., Schreurs, M.W., Boerman, O.C. et al. (1999). Biodistribution and vaccine efficiency of murine dendritic cells are dependent on the route of administration. *Cancer Res.* 59 (14): 3340–3345.

135 Sultan, H., Kumai, T., Nagato, T. et al. (2019). The route of administration dictates the immunogenicity of peptide-based cancer vaccines in mice. *Cancer Immunol. Immunother.* 68 (3): 455–466.

136 Kranz, L.M., Diken, M., Haas, H. et al. (2016). Systemic RNA delivery to dendritic cells exploits antiviral defence for cancer immunotherapy. *Nature* 534 (7607): 396–401.

137 Broos, K., Van der Jeught, K., Puttemans, J. et al. (2016). Particle-mediated intravenous delivery of antigen mRNA results in strong antigen-specific T-cell responses despite the induction of type I interferon. *Mol. Ther. Nucleic Acids* 5 (6): e326.

138 Van der Jeught, K., De Koker, S., Bialkowski, L. et al. (2018). Dendritic cell targeting mRNA lipopolyplexes combine strong antitumor T-cell immunity with improved inflammatory safety. *ACS Nano* 12 (10): 9815–9829.

139 Bevers, S., Kooijmans, S.A.A., Van de Velde, E. et al. (2022). mRNA-LNP vaccines tuned for systemic immunization induce strong antitumor immunity by engaging splenic immune cells. *Mol. Ther.* 30 (9): 3078–3094.

140 Jiang, X., Wang, J., Zheng, X. et al. (2022). Intratumoral administration of STING-activating nanovaccine enhances T cell immunotherapy. *J. Immunother. Cancer* 10 (5): e003960.

141 Enamorado, M., Iborra, S., Priego, E. et al. (2017). Enhanced anti-tumour immunity requires the interplay between resident and circulating memory CD8. *Nat. Commun.* 8: 16073.

142 Djenidi, F., Adam, J., Goubar, A. et al. (2015). CD8+CD103+ tumor-infiltrating lymphocytes are tumor-specific tissue-resident memory T cells and a prognostic factor for survival in lung cancer patients. *J. Immunol.* 194 (7): 3475–3486.

143 Ganesan, A.P., Clarke, J., Wood, O. et al. (2017). Tissue-resident memory features are linked to the magnitude of cytotoxic T cell responses in human lung cancer. *Nat. Immunol.* 18 (8): 940–950.

144 Koh, J., Kim, S., Kim, M.Y. et al. (2017). Prognostic implications of intratumoral CD103+ tumor-infiltrating lymphocytes in pulmonary squamous cell carcinoma. *Oncotarget* 8 (8): 13762–13769.

145 Webb, J.R., Milne, K., Watson, P. et al. (2014). Tumor-infiltrating lymphocytes expressing the tissue resident memory marker CD103 are associated with increased survival in high-grade serous ovarian cancer. *Clin. Cancer Res.* 20 (2): 434–444.

146 Fong, L., Carroll, P., Weinberg, V. et al. (2014). Activated lymphocyte recruitment into the tumor microenvironment following preoperative sipuleucel-T for localized prostate cancer. *J. Natl. Cancer Inst.* 106 (11): dju268.

147 Hailemichael, Y., Dai, Z., Jaffarzad, N. et al. (2013). Persistent antigen at vaccination sites induces tumor-specific CD8$^+$ T cell sequestration, dysfunction and deletion. *Nat. Med.* 19 (4): 465–472.

148 Sun, Y.Y., Peng, S., Han, L. et al. (2016). Local HPV recombinant vaccinia boost following priming with an HPV DNA vaccine enhances local HPV-specific CD8+ T-cell-mediated tumor control in the genital tract. *Clin. Cancer Res.* 22 (3): 657–669.

149 Nizard, M., Roussel, H., Diniz, M.O. et al. (2017). Induction of resident memory T cells enhances the efficacy of cancer vaccine. *Nat. Commun.* 8: 15221.

150 Calzascia, T., Masson, F., Di Berardino-Besson, W. et al. (2005). Homing phenotypes of tumor-specific CD8 T cells are predetermined at the tumor site by crosspresenting APCs. *Immunity* 22 (2): 175–184.

151 Mullins, D.W., Sheasley, S.L., Ream, R.M. et al. (2003). Route of immunization with peptide-pulsed dendritic cells controls the distribution of memory and effector T cells in lymphoid tissues and determines the pattern of regional tumor control. *J. Exp. Med.* 198 (7): 1023–1034.

152 Benteyn, D., Heirman, C., Bonehill, A. et al. (2015). mRNA-based dendritic cell vaccines. *Expert Rev. Vaccines* 14 (2): 161–176.

153 Benteyn, D., Van Nuffel, A.M., Wilgenhof, S. et al. (2013). Characterization of CD8+ T-cell responses in the peripheral blood and skin injection sites of melanoma patients treated with mRNA electroporated autologous dendritic cells (TriMixDC-MEL). *Biomed. Res. Int.* 2013: 976383.

154 Gross, S., Erdmann, M., Haendle, I. et al. (2017). Twelve-year survival and immune correlates in dendritic cell-vaccinated melanoma patients. *JCI Insight* 2 (8): e91438.

155 Hodi, F.S., O'Day, S.J., McDermott, D.F. et al. (2010). Improved survival with ipilimumab in patients with metastatic melanoma. *N. Engl. J. Med.* 363 (8): 711–723.

156 Schadendorf, D., Hodi, F.S., Robert, C. et al. (2015). Pooled analysis of long-term survival data from phase II and phase III trials of ipilimumab in unresectable or metastatic melanoma. *J. Clin. Oncol.* 33 (17): 1889–1894.

157 Lecocq, Q., Keyaerts, M., Devoogdt, N., and Breckpot, K. (2020). The next-generation immune checkpoint LAG-3 and its therapeutic potential in oncology: third time's a charm. *Int. J. Mol. Sci.* 22 (1): 75.

158 Broos, K., Lecocq, Q., Raes, G. et al. (2018). Noninvasive imaging of the PD-1:PD-L1 immune checkpoint: embracing nuclear medicine for the benefit of personalized immunotherapy. *Theranostics* 8 (13): 3559–3570.

159 Qin, S., Xu, L., Yi, M. et al. (2019). Novel immune checkpoint targets: moving beyond PD-1 and CTLA-4. *Mol. Cancer* 18 (1): 155.

160 Van der Jeught, K., Bialkowski, L., Daszkiewicz, L. et al. (2015). Targeting the tumor microenvironment to enhance antitumor immune responses. *Oncotarget* 6 (3): 1359–1381.

161 Bejarano, L., Jordão, M.J.C., and Joyce, J.A. (2021). Therapeutic targeting of the tumor microenvironment. *Cancer Discov.* 11 (4): 933–959.

162 Cuzzubbo, S., Mangsbo, S., Nagarajan, D. et al. (2020). Cancer vaccines: adjuvant potency, importance of age, lifestyle, and treatments. *Front. Immunol.* 11: 615240.

163 Esfahani, K., Roudaia, L., Buhlaiga, N. et al. (2020). A review of cancer immunotherapy: from the past, to the present, to the future. *Curr. Oncol.* 27 (Suppl 2): S87–S97.

164 Collins, J.M., Redman, J.M., and Gulley, J.L. (2018). Combining vaccines and immune checkpoint inhibitors to prime, expand, and facilitate effective tumor immunotherapy. *Expert Rev. Vaccines* 17 (8): 697–705.

165 Sahin, U., Oehm, P., Derhovanessian, E. et al. (2020). An RNA vaccine drives immunity in checkpoint-inhibitor-treated melanoma. *Nature* 585 (7823): 107–112.

166 Broos, K., Lecocq, Q., Xavier, C. et al. (2019). Evaluating a single domain antibody targeting human PD-L1 as a nuclear imaging and therapeutic agent. *Cancers (Basel)* 11 (6): 872.

167 Lecocq, Q., Awad, R.M., De Vlaeminck, Y. et al. (2021). Single-domain antibody nuclear imaging allows noninvasive quantification of LAG-3 expression by tumor-infiltrating leukocytes and predicts response of immune checkpoint blockade. *J. Nucl. Med.* 62 (11): 1638–1644.

168 Broos, K., Lecocq, Q., Keersmaecker, B. et al. (2019). Single domain antibody-mediated blockade of programmed death-ligand 1 on dendritic cells enhances CD8 T-cell activation and cytokine production. *Vaccines (Basel)* 7 (3): 85.

169 Dolgin, E. (2021). The tangled history of mRNA vaccines. *Nature* 597 (7876): 318–324.

170 Minchin, S. and Lodge, J. (2019). Understanding biochemistry: structure and function of nucleic acids. *Essays Biochem.* 63 (4): 433–456.

171 Cobb, M. (2015). Who discovered messenger RNA? *Curr. Biol.* 25 (13): R526–R532.

172 Thess, A., Hoerr, I., Panah, B.Y. et al. (2021). Historic nucleic acids isolated by Friedrich Miescher contain RNA besides DNA. *Biol. Chem.* 402 (10): 1179–1185.

173 Veigl, S.J., Harman, O., and Lamm, E. (2020). Friedrich Miescher's discovery in the historiography of genetics: from contamination to confusion, from nuclein to DNA. *J. Hist. Biol.* 53 (3): 451–484.

174 Brenner, S., Jacob, F., and Meselson, M. (1961). An unstable intermediate carrying information from genes to ribosomes for protein synthesis. *Nature* 190: 576–581.

175 Melton, D.A., Krieg, P.A., Rebagliati, M.R. et al. (1984). Efficient in vitro synthesis of biologically active RNA and RNA hybridization probes from plasmids containing a bacteriophage SP6 promoter. *Nucleic Acids Res.* 12 (18): 7035–7056.

176 Krieg, P.A. and Melton, D.A. (1984). Functional messenger RNAs are produced by SP6 in vitro transcription of cloned cDNAs. *Nucleic Acids Res.* 12 (18): 7057–7070.

177 Houseley, J. and Tollervey, D. (2009). The many pathways of RNA degradation. *Cell* 136 (4): 763–776.

178 Malone, R.W., Felgner, P.L., and Verma, I.M. (1989). Cationic liposome-mediated RNA transfection. *Proc. Natl. Acad. Sci. U. S. A.* 86 (16): 6077–6081.

179 Wolff, J.A., Malone, R.W., Williams, P. et al. (1990). Direct gene transfer into mouse muscle in vivo. *Science* 247 (4949 Pt 1): 1465–1468.

180 Martinon, F., Krishnan, S., Lenzen, G. et al. (1993). Induction of virus-specific cytotoxic T lymphocytes in vivo by liposome-entrapped mRNA. *Eur. J. Immunol.* 23 (7): 1719–1722.

181 Conry, R.M., LoBuglio, A.F., Wright, M. et al. (1995). Characterization of a messenger RNA polynucleotide vaccine vector. *Cancer Res.* 55 (7): 1397–1400.

182 Heiser, A., Coleman, D., Dannull, J. et al. (2002). Autologous dendritic cells transfected with prostate-specific antigen RNA stimulate CTL responses against metastatic prostate tumors. *J. Clin. Invest.* 109 (3): 409–417.

183 Zeng, C., Zhang, C., Walker, P.G., and Dong, Y. (2022). Formulation and delivery technologies for mRNA vaccines. *Curr. Top. Microbiol. Immunol.* 440: 71–110.

184 Weide, B., Pascolo, S., Scheel, B. et al. (2009). Direct injection of protamine-protected mRNA: results of a phase 1/2 vaccination trial in metastatic melanoma patients. *J. Immunother.* 32 (5): 498–507.

185 Sahin, U., Derhovanessian, E., Miller, M. et al. (2017). Personalized RNA mutanome vaccines mobilize poly-specific therapeutic immunity against cancer. *Nature* 547 (7662): 222–226.

186 Weide, B., Carralot, J.P., Reese, A. et al. (2008). Results of the first phase I/II clinical vaccination trial with direct injection of mRNA. *J. Immunother.* 31 (2): 180–188.

187 Devoldere, J., Dewitte, H., De Smedt, S.C., and Remaut, K. (2016). Evading innate immunity in nonviral mRNA delivery: don't shoot the messenger. *Drug Discov. Today* 21 (1): 11–25.

188 Kuhn, A.N., Diken, M., Kreiter, S. et al. (2011). Determinants of intracellular RNA pharmacokinetics: implications for RNA-based immunotherapeutics. *RNA Biol.* 8 (1): 35–43.

189 Karikó, K., Muramatsu, H., Welsh, F.A. et al. (2008). Incorporation of pseudouridine into mRNA yields superior nonimmunogenic vector with increased translational capacity and biological stability. *Mol. Ther.* 16 (11): 1833–1840.

190 Schlake, T., Thess, A., Fotin-Mleczek, M., and Kallen, K.J. (2012). Developing mRNA-vaccine technologies. *RNA Biol.* 9 (11): 1319–1330.

191 Holstein, J.M. and Rentmeister, A. (2016). Current covalent modification methods for detecting RNA in fixed and living cells. *Methods* 98: 18–25.

192 de Mey, W., De Schrijver, P., Autaers, D. et al. (2022). A synthetic DNA template for fast manufacturing of versatile single epitope mRNA. *Mol. Ther. Nucleic Acids* 29: 943–954.

193 Domazet-Lošo, T. (2022). mRNA vaccines: why is the biology of retroposition ignored? *Genes (Basel)* 13 (5): 719.

194 Probst, J., Weide, B., Scheel, B. et al. (2007). Spontaneous cellular uptake of exogenous messenger RNA in vivo is nucleic acid-specific, saturable and ion dependent. *Gene Ther.* 14 (15): 1175–1180.

195 Parker, R. and Song, H. (2004). The enzymes and control of eukaryotic mRNA turnover. *Nat. Struct. Mol. Biol.* 11 (2): 121–127.

196 Yamashita, A., Chang, T.C., Yamashita, Y. et al. (2005). Concerted action of poly(A) nucleases and decapping enzyme in mammalian mRNA turnover. *Nat. Struct. Mol. Biol.* 12 (12): 1054–1063.

197 Munroe, D. and Jacobson, A. (1990). mRNA poly(A) tail, a 3′ enhancer of translational initiation. *Mol. Cell. Biol.* 10 (7): 3441–3455.

198 Andries, O., De Filette, M., De Smedt, S.C. et al. (2013). Innate immune response and programmed cell death following carrier-mediated delivery of unmodified mRNA to respiratory cells. *J. Control. Release* 167 (2): 157–166.

199 Martin, S.A. and Moss, B. (1975). Modification of RNA by mRNA guanylyltransferase and mRNA (guanine-7-)methyltransferase from vaccinia virions. *J. Biol. Chem.* 250 (24): 9330–9335.

200 Stepinski, J., Waddell, C., Stolarski, R. et al. (2001). Synthesis and properties of mRNAs containing the novel "anti-reverse" cap analogs 7-methyl(3′-O-methyl)GpppG and 7-methyl (3′-deoxy)GpppG. *RNA* 7 (10): 1486–1495.

201 Grudzien-Nogalska, E., Stepinski, J., Jemielity, J. et al. (2007). Synthesis of anti-reverse cap analogs (ARCAs) and their applications in mRNA translation and stability. *Methods Enzymol.* 431: 203–227.

202 Grudzien-Nogalska, E., Jemielity, J., Kowalska, J. et al. (2007). Phosphorothioate cap analogs stabilize mRNA and increase translational efficiency in mammalian cells. *RNA* 13 (10): 1745–1755.

203 Gong, P. and Martin, C.T. (2006). Mechanism of instability in abortive cycling by T7 RNA polymerase. *J. Biol. Chem.* 281 (33): 23533–23544.

204 Schenborn, E.T. and Mierendorf, R.C. (1985). A novel transcription property of SP6 and T7 RNA polymerases: dependence on template structure. *Nucleic Acids Res.* 13 (17): 6223–6236.

205 Arnaud-Barbe, N., Cheynet-Sauvion, V., Oriol, G. et al. (1998). Transcription of RNA templates by T7 RNA polymerase. *Nucleic Acids Res.* 26 (15): 3550–3554.

206 Krupp, G. (1989). Unusual promoter-independent transcription reactions with bacteriophage RNA polymerases. *Nucleic Acids Res.* 17 (8): 3023–3036.

207 Cazenave, C. and Uhlenbeck, O.C. (1994). RNA template-directed RNA synthesis by T7 RNA polymerase. *Proc. Natl. Acad. Sci. U. S. A.* 91 (15): 6972–6976.

208 Geall, A.J., Mandl, C.W., and Ulmer, J.B. (2013). RNA: the new revolution in nucleic acid vaccines. *Semin. Immunol.* 25 (2): 152–159.

209 Baiersdörfer, M., Boros, G., Muramatsu, H. et al. (2019). A facile method for the removal of dsRNA contaminant from in vitro-transcribed mRNA. *Mol. Ther. Nucleic Acids* 15: 26–35.

210 Karikó, K., Muramatsu, H., Ludwig, J., and Weissman, D. (2011). Generating the optimal mRNA for therapy: HPLC purification eliminates immune activation and improves translation of nucleoside-modified, protein-encoding mRNA. *Nucleic Acids Res.* 39 (21): e142.

211 Weissman, D., Pardi, N., Muramatsu, H., and Karikó, K. (2013). HPLC purification of in vitro transcribed long RNA. *Methods Mol. Biol.* 969: 43–54.

212 Foster, J.B., Choudhari, N., Perazzelli, J. et al. (2019). Purification of mRNA encoding chimeric antigen receptor is critical for generation of a robust T-cell response. *Hum. Gene Ther.* 30 (2): 168–178.

213 Gallie, D.R. (1991). The cap and poly(A) tail function synergistically to regulate mRNA translational efficiency. *Genes Dev.* 5 (11): 2108–2116.

214 Wilkie, G.S., Dickson, K.S., and Gray, N.K. (2003). Regulation of mRNA translation by 5′- and 3′-UTR-binding factors. *Trends Biochem. Sci.* 28 (4): 182–188.

215 Kozak, M. (1989). Circumstances and mechanisms of inhibition of translation by secondary structure in eucaryotic mRNAs. *Mol. Cell. Biol.* 9 (11): 5134–5142.

216 Ensinger, M.J., Martin, S.A., Paoletti, E., and Moss, B. (1975). Modification of the 5'-terminus of mRNA by soluble guanylyl and methyl transferases from vaccinia virus. *Proc. Natl. Acad. Sci. U. S. A.* 72 (7): 2525–2529.

217 Muttach, F., Muthmann, N., and Rentmeister, A. (2017). Synthetic mRNA capping. *Beilstein J. Org. Chem.* 13: 2819–2832.

218 Fuchs, A.L., Neu, A., and Sprangers, R. (2016). A general method for rapid and cost-efficient large-scale production of 5' capped RNA. *RNA* 22 (9): 1454–1466.

219 Devarkar, S.C., Wang, C., Miller, M.T. et al. (2016). Structural basis for m7G recognition and 2′-O-methyl discrimination in capped RNAs by the innate immune receptor RIG-I. *Proc. Natl. Acad. Sci. U. S. A.* 113 (3): 596–601.

220 Ramanathan, A., Robb, G.B., and Chan, S.H. (2016). mRNA capping: biological functions and applications. *Nucleic Acids Res.* 44 (16): 7511–7526.

221 Schuberth-Wagner, C., Ludwig, J., Bruder, A.K. et al. (2015). A conserved histidine in the RNA sensor RIG-I controls immune tolerance to N1-2'O-methylated self RNA. *Immunity* 43 (1): 41–51.

222 Miao, L., Zhang, Y., and Huang, L. (2021). mRNA vaccine for cancer immunotherapy. *Mol. Cancer* 20 (1): 41.

223 Zohra, F.T., Chowdhury, E.H., Tada, S. et al. (2007). Effective delivery with enhanced translational activity synergistically accelerates mRNA-based transfection. *Biochem. Biophys. Res. Commun.* 358 (1): 373–378.

224 Grudzien, E., Kalek, M., Jemielity, J. et al. (2006). Differential inhibition of mRNA degradation pathways by novel cap analogs. *J. Biol. Chem.* 281 (4): 1857–1867.

225 Rydzik, A.M., Kulis, M., Lukaszewicz, M. et al. (2012). Synthesis and properties of mRNA cap analogs containing imidodiphosphate moiety–fairly mimicking natural cap structure, yet resistant to enzymatic hydrolysis. *Bioorg. Med. Chem.* 20 (5): 1699–1710.

226 Hadas, Y., Sultana, N., Youssef, E. et al. (2019). Optimizing modified mRNA. *Mol. Ther. Methods Clin. Dev.* 14: 300–305.

227 Henderson, J.M., Ujita, A., Hill, E. et al. (2021). Cap 1 messenger RNA synthesis with co-transcriptional CleanCap. *Curr. Protoc.* 1 (2): e39.

228 Pardi, N., Hogan, M.J., and Weissman, D. (2020). Recent advances in mRNA vaccine technology. *Curr. Opin. Immunol.* 65: 14–20.

229 Moradian, H., Roch, T., Anthofer, L. et al. (2022). Chemical modification of uridine modulates mRNA-mediated proinflammatory and antiviral response in primary human macrophages. *Mol. Ther. Nucleic Acids* 27: 854–869.

230 van Dülmen, M., Muthmann, N., and Rentmeister, A. (2021). Chemo-enzymatic modification of the 5′ cap maintains translation and increases immunogenic properties of mRNA. *Angew. Chem. Int. Ed. Eng.* 60 (24): 13280–13286.

231 Bollu, A., Peters, A., and Rentmeister, A. (2022). Chemo-enzymatic modification of the 5' cap to study mRNAs. *Acc. Chem. Res.* 55 (9): 1249–1261.

232 Cao, J., Novoa, E.M., Zhang, Z. et al. (2021). High-throughput 5' UTR engineering for enhanced protein production in non-viral gene therapies. *Nat. Commun.* 12 (1): 4138.

233 Leppek, K., Das, R., and Barna, M. (2018). Functional 5' UTR mRNA structures in eukaryotic translation regulation and how to find them. *Nat. Rev. Mol. Cell Biol.* 19 (3): 158–174.

234 Jia, L. and Qian, S.B. (2021). Therapeutic mRNA engineering from head to tail. *Acc. Chem. Res.* 54 (23): 4272–4282.

235 Sample, P.J., Wang, B., Reid, D.W. et al. (2019). Human 5' UTR design and variant effect prediction from a massively parallel translation assay. *Nat. Biotechnol.* 37 (7): 803–809.

236 Wang, Z., Day, N., Trifillis, P., and Kiledjian, M. (1999). An mRNA stability complex functions with poly(A)-binding protein to stabilize mRNA in vitro. *Mol. Cell. Biol.* 19 (7): 4552–4560.

237 Gallie, D.R., Tanguay, R.L., and Leathers, V. (1995). The tobacco etch viral 5' leader and poly(A) tail are functionally synergistic regulators of translation. *Gene* 165 (2): 233–238.

238 Vivinus, S., Baulande, S., van Zanten, M. et al. (2001). An element within the 5' untranslated region of human Hsp70 mRNA which acts as a general enhancer of mRNA translation. *Eur. J. Biochem.* 268 (7): 1908–1917.

239 Carralot, J.P., Probst, J., Hoerr, I. et al. (2004). Polarization of immunity induced by direct injection of naked sequence-stabilized mRNA vaccines. *Cell. Mol. Life Sci.* 61 (18): 2418–2424.

240 Kreiter, S., Selmi, A., Diken, M. et al. (2008). Increased antigen presentation efficiency by coupling antigens to MHC class I trafficking signals. *J. Immunol.* 180 (1): 309–318.

241 Linares-Fernández, S., Moreno, J., Lambert, E. et al. (2021). Combining an optimized mRNA template with a double purification process allows strong expression of. *Mol. Ther. Nucleic Acids* 26: 945–956.

242 Kozak, M. (1986). Point mutations define a sequence flanking the AUG initiator codon that modulates translation by eukaryotic ribosomes. *Cell* 44 (2): 283–292.

243 Mehdi, H., Ono, E., and Gupta, K.C. (1990). Initiation of translation at CUG, GUG, and ACG codons in mammalian cells. *Gene* 91 (2): 173–178.

244 Kudla, G., Lipinski, L., Caffin, F. et al. (2006). High guanine and cytosine content increases mRNA levels in mammalian cells. *PLoS Biol.* 4 (6): e180.

245 Mordstein, C., Savisaar, R., Young, R.S. et al. (2020). Codon usage and splicing jointly influence mRNA localization. *Cell Syst.* 10 (4): 351–362.e8.

246 Hia, F., Yang, S.F., Shichino, Y. et al. (2019). Codon bias confers stability to human mRNAs. *EMBO Rep.* 20 (11): e48220.

247 Mauger, D.M., Cabral, B.J., Presnyak, V. et al. (2019). mRNA structure regulates protein expression through changes in functional half-life. *Proc. Natl. Acad. Sci. U. S. A.* 116 (48): 24075–24083.

248 Frelin, L., Ahlén, G., Alheim, M. et al. (2004). Codon optimization and mRNA amplification effectively enhances the immunogenicity of the hepatitis C virus nonstructural 3/4A gene. *Gene Ther.* 11 (6): 522–533.

249 De Keersmaecker, B., Heirman, C., Allard, S. et al. (2010). Lumenal part of the DC-LAMP protein is not required for induction of antigen-specific T cell responses by means of antigen-DC-LAMP messenger RNA-electroporated dendritic cells. *Hum. Gene Ther.* 21 (4): 479–485.

250 Van Gulck, E.R., Ponsaerts, P., Heyndrickx, L. et al. (2006). Efficient stimulation of HIV-1-specific T cells using dendritic cells electroporated with mRNA encoding autologous HIV-1 Gag and Env proteins. *Blood* 107 (5): 1818–1827.

251 Gould, N., Hendy, O., and Papamichail, D. (2014). Computational tools and algorithms for designing customized synthetic genes. *Front. Bioeng. Biotechnol.* 2: 41.

252 Andries, O., Mc Cafferty, S., De Smedt, S.C. et al. (2015). N(1)-methylpseudouridine-incorporated mRNA outperforms pseudouridine-incorporated mRNA by providing enhanced protein expression and reduced immunogenicity in mammalian cell lines and mice. *J. Control. Release* 217: 337–344.

253 Kormann, M.S., Hasenpusch, G., Aneja, M.K. et al. (2011). Expression of therapeutic proteins after delivery of chemically modified mRNA in mice. *Nat. Biotechnol.* 29 (2): 154–157.

254 Durbin, A.F., Wang, C., Marcotrigiano, J., and Gehrke, L. (2016). RNAs containing modified nucleotides fail to trigger RIG-I conformational changes for innate immune signaling. *mBio* 7 (5): e00833-16.

255 Thess, A., Grund, S., Mui, B.L. et al. (2015). Sequence-engineered mRNA without chemical nucleoside modifications enables an effective protein therapy in large animals. *Mol. Ther.* 23 (9): 1456–1464.

256 Hoernes, T.P., Heimdörfer, D., Köstner, D. et al. (2019). Eukaryotic translation elongation is modulated by single natural nucleotide derivatives in the coding sequences of mRNAs. *Genes (Basel)* 10 (2): 84.

257 Roy, B. (2021). Effects of mRNA modifications on translation: an overview. *Methods Mol. Biol.* 2298: 327–356.

258 Wangen, J.R. and Green, R. (2020). Stop codon context influences genome-wide stimulation of termination codon readthrough by aminoglycosides. *Elife* 9: e52611.

259 Beznosková, P., Gunišová, S., and Valášek, L.S. (2016). Rules of UGA-N decoding by near-cognate tRNAs and analysis of readthrough on short uORFs in yeast. *RNA* 22 (3): 456–466.

260 Floquet, C., Hatin, I., Rousset, J.P., and Bidou, L. (2012). Statistical analysis of readthrough levels for nonsense mutations in mammalian cells reveals a major determinant of response to gentamicin. *PLoS Genet.* 8 (3): e1002608.

261 van Hoof, A., Frischmeyer, P.A., Dietz, H.C., and Parker, R. (2002). Exosome-mediated recognition and degradation of mRNAs lacking a termination codon. *Science* 295 (5563): 2262–2264.

262 Adachi, M. and Cavalcanti, A.R. (2009). Tandem stop codons in ciliates that reassign stop codons. *J. Mol. Evol.* 68 (4): 424–431.

263 Benteyn, D., Anguille, S., Van Lint, S. et al. (2013). Design of an optimized Wilms' tumor 1 (WT1) mRNA construct for enhanced WT1 expression and improved immunogenicity in vitro and in vivo. *Mol. Ther. Nucleic Acids* 2: e134.

264 Bonehill, A., Heirman, C., Tuyaerts, S. et al. (2003 Sep). Efficient presentation of known HLA class II-restricted MAGE-A3 epitopes by dendritic cells electroporated with messenger RNA encoding an invariant chain with genetic exchange of class II-associated invariant chain peptide. *Cancer Res.* 63 (17): 5587–5594.

265 Bonehill, A., Heirman, C., Tuyaerts, S. et al. (2004). Messenger RNA-electroporated dendritic cells presenting MAGE-A3 simultaneously in HLA class I and class II molecules. *J. Immunol.* 172 (11): 6649–6657.

266 Dullaers, M., Breckpot, K., Van Meirvenne, S. et al. (2004). Side-by-side comparison of lentivirally transduced and mRNA-electroporated dendritic cells: implications for cancer immunotherapy protocols. *Mol. Ther.* 10 (4): 768–779.

267 Barreau, C., Paillard, L., and Osborne, H.B. (2005). AU-rich elements and associated factors: are there unifying principles? *Nucleic Acids Res.* 33 (22): 7138–7150.

268 Fang, Z. and Rajewsky, N. (2011). The impact of miRNA target sites in coding sequences and in 3'UTRs. *PLoS One* 6 (3): e18067.

269 Ross, J. and Sullivan, T.D. (1985). Half-lives of beta and gamma globin messenger RNAs and of protein synthetic capacity in cultured human reticulocytes. *Blood* 66 (5): 1149–1154.

270 Karikó, K., Kuo, A., and Barnathan, E. (1999). Overexpression of urokinase receptor in mammalian cells following administration of the in vitro transcribed encoding mRNA. *Gene Ther.* 6 (6): 1092–1100.

271 Zinckgraf, J.W. and Silbart, L.K. (2003). Modulating gene expression using DNA vaccines with different 3'-UTRs influences antibody titer, seroconversion and cytokine profiles. *Vaccine* 21 (15): 1640–1649.

272 Zhao, W., Pollack, J.L., Blagev, D.P. et al. (2014). Massively parallel functional annotation of 3' untranslated regions. *Nat. Biotechnol.* 32 (4): 387–391.

273 Orlandini von Niessen, A.G., Poleganov, M.A., Rechner, C. et al. (2019). Improving mRNA-based therapeutic gene delivery by expression-augmenting 3' UTRs identified by cellular library screening. *Mol. Ther.* 27 (4): 824–836.

274 Linares-Fernández, S., Lacroix, C., Exposito, J.Y., and Verrier, B. (2020). Tailoring mRNA vaccine to balance innate/adaptive immune response. *Trends Mol. Med.* 26 (3): 311–323.

275 Eckmann, C.R., Rammelt, C., and Wahle, E. (2011). Control of poly(A) tail length. *Wiley Interdiscip. Rev. RNA* 2 (3): 348–361.

276 Lima, S.A., Chipman, L.B., Nicholson, A.L. et al. (2017). Short poly(A) tails are a conserved feature of highly expressed genes. *Nat. Struct. Mol. Biol.* 24 (12): 1057–1063.

277 Lim, J., Kim, D., Lee, Y.S. et al. (2018). Mixed tailing by TENT4A and TENT4B shields mRNA from rapid deadenylation. *Science* 361 (6403): 701–704.

278 Koski, G.K., Karikó, K., Xu, S. et al. (2004). Cutting edge: innate immune system discriminates between RNA containing bacterial versus eukaryotic structural features that prime for high-level IL-12 secretion by dendritic cells. *J. Immunol.* 172 (7): 3989–3993.

279 Weissman, D. and Karikó, K. (2015). mRNA: fulfilling the promise of gene therapy. *Mol. Ther.* 23 (9): 1416–1417.

280 Balan, S., Saxena, M., and Bhardwaj, N. (2019). Dendritic cell subsets and locations. *Int. Rev. Cell Mol. Biol.* 348: 1–68.

281 Van Lint, S., Renmans, D., Broos, K. et al. (2015). The ReNAissanCe of mRNA-based cancer therapy. *Expert Rev. Vaccines* 14 (2): 235–251.

282 Kowalski, P.S., Rudra, A., Miao, L., and Anderson, D.G. (2019). Delivering the messenger: advances in technologies for therapeutic mRNA delivery. *Mol. Ther.* 27 (4): 710–728.

283 Diken, M., Kreiter, S., Selmi, A. et al. (2011). Selective uptake of naked vaccine RNA by dendritic cells is driven by macropinocytosis and abrogated upon DC maturation. *Gene Ther.* 18 (7): 702–708.

284 Selmi, A., Vascotto, F., Kautz-Neu, K. et al. (2016). Uptake of synthetic naked RNA by skin-resident dendritic cells via macropinocytosis allows antigen expression and induction of T-cell responses in mice. *Cancer Immunol. Immunother.* 65 (9): 1075–1083.

285 Lorenz, C., Fotin-Mleczek, M., Roth, G. et al. (2011). Protein expression from exogenous mRNA: uptake by receptor-mediated endocytosis and trafficking via the lysosomal pathway. *RNA Biol.* 8 (4): 627–636.

286 Boczkowski, D., Nair, S.K., Snyder, D., and Gilboa, E. (1996). Dendritic cells pulsed with RNA are potent antigen-presenting cells in vitro and in vivo. *J. Exp. Med.* 184 (2): 465–472.

287 Verbeke, R., Lentacker, I., Wayteck, L. et al. (2017). Co-delivery of nucleoside-modified mRNA and TLR agonists for cancer immunotherapy: restoring the immunogenicity of immunosilent mRNA. *J. Control. Release* 266: 287–300.

288 Udhayakumar, V.K., De Beuckelaer, A., McCaffrey, J. et al. (2017). Arginine-rich peptide-based mRNA nanocomplexes efficiently instigate cytotoxic T cell immunity dependent on the amphipathic organization of the peptide. *Adv. Healthc. Mater.* 6 (13): https://doi.org/10.1002/adhm.201601412.

289 Van Tendeloo, V.F., Ponsaerts, P., Lardon, F. et al. (2001). Highly efficient gene delivery by mRNA electroporation in human hematopoietic cells: superiority to lipofection and passive pulsing of mRNA and to electroporation of plasmid cDNA for tumor antigen loading of dendritic cells. *Blood* 98 (1): 49–56.

290 Michiels, A., Tuyaerts, S., Bonehill, A. et al. (2005). Electroporation of immature and mature dendritic cells: implications for dendritic cell-based vaccines. *Gene Ther.* 12 (9): 772–782.

291 Knudsen, M.L., Ljungberg, K., Liljeström, P., and Johansson, D.X. (2014). Intradermal electroporation of RNA. *Methods Mol. Biol.* 1121: 147–154.

292 Dewitte, H., Van Lint, S., De Smedt, S. et al. (2012). mRNA sonoporation as a novel tool in dendritic cell-based cancer immunotherapy. *Hum. Gene Ther.* 23 (10): A92–A93.

293 Pearson, A.M., Rich, A., and Krieger, M. (1993). Polynucleotide binding to macrophage scavenger receptors depends on the formation of base-quartet-stabilized four-stranded helices. *J. Biol. Chem.* 268 (5): 3546–3554.

294 Canton, J. (2018). Macropinocytosis: new insights into its underappreciated role in innate immune cell surveillance. *Front. Immunol.* 9: 2286.

295 Sahin, U., Karikó, K., and Türeci, Ö. (2014). mRNA-based therapeutics–developing a new class of drugs. *Nat. Rev. Drug Discov.* 13 (10): 759–780.

296 Van Meirvenne, S., Straetman, L., Heirman, C. et al. (2002). Efficient genetic modification of murine dendritic cells by electroporation with mRNA. *Cancer Gene Ther.* 9 (9): 787–797.

297 Van Lint, S., Wilgenhof, S., Heirman, C. et al. (2014). Optimized dendritic cell-based immunotherapy for melanoma: the TriMix-formula. *Cancer Immunol. Immunother.* 63 (9): 959–967.

298 Mitchell, D.A., Batich, K.A., Gunn, M.D. et al. (2015). Tetanus toxoid and CCL3 improve dendritic cell vaccines in mice and glioblastoma patients. *Nature* 519 (7543): 366–369.

299 Van Tendeloo, V.F., Van de Velde, A., Van Driessche, A. et al. (2010). Induction of complete and molecular remissions in acute myeloid leukemia by Wilms' tumor 1 antigen-targeted dendritic cell vaccination. *Proc. Natl. Acad. Sci. U. S. A.* 107 (31): 13824–13829.

300 Batich, K.A., Reap, E.A., Archer, G.E. et al. (2017). Long-term survival in glioblastoma with cytomegalovirus pp65-targeted vaccination. *Clin. Cancer Res.* 23 (8): 1898–1909.

301 Kowalzik, F., Schreiner, D., Jensen, C. et al. (2021). mRNA-based vaccines. *Vaccines (Basel)* 9 (4): 390.

302 Fotin-Mleczek, M., Duchardt, K.M., Lorenz, C. et al. (2011). Messenger RNA-based vaccines with dual activity induce balanced TLR-7 dependent adaptive immune responses and provide antitumor activity. *J. Immunother.* 34 (1): 1–15.

303 Van Lint, S., Thielemans, K., and Breckpot, K. (2011). mRNA: delivering an antitumor message? *Immunotherapy* 3 (5): 605–607.

304 Dewitte, H., Verbeke, R., Breckpot, K. et al. (2014). Nanoparticle design to induce tumor immunity and challenge the suppressive tumor microenvironment. *Nano Today* 9 (6): 743–758.

305 Verbeke, R., Lentacker, I., De Smedt, S.C., and Dewitte, H. (2019). Three decades of mRNA development. *Nano Today* 28: 100766.

306 Liu, T., Liang, Y., and Huang, L. (2021). Development and delivery systems of mRNA vaccines. *Front. Bioeng. Biotechnol.* 9: 718753.

307 Karmacharya, P., Patil, B.R., and Kim, J.O. (2022). Recent advancements in lipid-mRNA nanoparticles as a treatment option for cancer immunotherapy. *J. Pharm. Investig.* 52 (4): 415–426.

308 Pardi, N., Hogan, M.J., Porter, F.W., and Weissman, D. (2018). mRNA vaccines - a new era in vaccinology. *Nat. Rev. Drug Discov.* 17 (4): 261–279.

309 Paunovska, K., Loughrey, D., and Dahlman, J.E. (2022). Drug delivery systems for RNA therapeutics. *Nat. Rev. Genet.* 23 (5): 265–280.

310 Lv, H., Zhang, S., Wang, B. et al. (2006). Toxicity of cationic lipids and cationic polymers in gene delivery. *J. Control. Release* 114 (1): 100–109.

311 Reichmuth, A.M., Oberli, M.A., Jaklenec, A. et al. (2016). mRNA vaccine delivery using lipid nanoparticles. *Ther. Deliv.* 7 (5): 319–334.

312 Schoenmaker, L., Witzigmann, D., Kulkarni, J.A. et al. (2021). mRNA-lipid nanoparticle COVID-19 vaccines: structure and stability. *Int. J. Pharm.* 601: 120586.

313 Oberli, M.A., Reichmuth, A.M., Dorkin, J.R. et al. (2017). Lipid nanoparticle assisted mRNA delivery for potent cancer immunotherapy. *Nano Lett.* 17 (3): 1326–1335.

314 Pardi, N., Tuyishime, S., Muramatsu, H. et al. (2015). Expression kinetics of nucleoside-modified mRNA delivered in lipid nanoparticles to mice by various routes. *J. Control. Release* 217: 345–351.

315 Ramaswamy, S., Tonnu, N., Tachikawa, K. et al. (2017). Systemic delivery of factor IX messenger RNA for protein replacement therapy. *Proc. Natl. Acad. Sci. U. S. A.* 114 (10): E1941–E1950.

316 Semple, S.C., Akinc, A., Chen, J. et al. (2010). Rational design of cationic lipids for siRNA delivery. *Nat. Biotechnol.* 28 (2): 172–176.

317 Sago, C.D., Lokugamage, M.P., Paunovska, K. et al. (2018). High-throughput in vivo screen of functional mRNA delivery identifies nanoparticles for endothelial cell gene editing. *Proc. Natl. Acad. Sci. U. S. A.* 115 (42): E9944–E9952.

318 Altınoglu, S., Wang, M., and Xu, Q. (2015). Combinatorial library strategies for synthesis of cationic lipid-like nanoparticles and their potential medical applications. *Nanomedicine (Lond)* 10 (4): 643–657.

319 Zhang, Y., Sun, C., Wang, C. et al. (2021). Lipids and lipid derivatives for RNA delivery. *Chem. Rev.* 121 (20): 12181–12277.

320 Ke, X., Shelton, L., Hu, Y. et al. (2020). Surface-functionalized PEGylated nanoparticles deliver messenger RNA to pulmonary immune cells. *ACS Appl. Mater. Interfaces* 12 (32): 35835–35844.

321 Tan, L., Zheng, T., Li, M. et al. (2020). Optimization of an mRNA vaccine assisted with cyclodextrin-polyethyleneimine conjugates. *Drug Deliv. Transl. Res.* 10 (3): 678–689.

322 Islam, M.A., Rice, J., Reesor, E. et al. (2021). Adjuvant-pulsed mRNA vaccine nanoparticle for immunoprophylactic and therapeutic tumor suppression in mice. *Biomaterials* 266: 120431.

323 Su, X., Fricke, J., Kavanagh, D.G., and Irvine, D.J. (2011). In vitro and in vivo mRNA delivery using lipid-enveloped pH-responsive polymer nanoparticles. *Mol. Pharm.* 8 (3): 774–787.

324 Kaczmarek, J.C., Patel, A.K., Kauffman, K.J. et al. (2016). Polymer-lipid nanoparticles for systemic delivery of mRNA to the lungs. *Angew. Chem. Int. Ed. Eng.* 55 (44): 13808–13812.

325 Patel, A.K., Kaczmarek, J.C., Bose, S. et al. (2019). Inhaled nanoformulated mRNA polyplexes for protein production in lung epithelium. *Adv. Mater.* 31 (8): e1805116.

326 Haabeth, O.A.W., Blake, T.R., McKinlay, C.J. et al. (2018). mRNA vaccination with charge-altering releasable transporters elicits human T cell responses and cures established tumors in mice. *Proc. Natl. Acad. Sci. U. S. A.* 115 (39): E9153–E9161.

327 Scheel, B., Teufel, R., Probst, J. et al. (2005). Toll-like receptor-dependent activation of several human blood cell types by protamine-condensed mRNA. *Eur. J. Immunol.* 35 (5): 1557–1566.

328 Sebastian, M., Papachristofilou, A., Weiss, C. et al. (2014). Phase Ib study evaluating a self-adjuvanted mRNA cancer vaccine (RNActive®) combined with local radiation as consolidation and maintenance treatment for patients with stage IV non-small cell lung cancer. *BMC Cancer* 14: 748.

329 Papachristofilou, A., Hipp, M.M., Klinkhardt, U. et al. (2019). Phase Ib evaluation of a self-adjuvanted protamine formulated mRNA-based active cancer immunotherapy, BI1361849 (CV9202), combined with local radiation treatment in patients with stage IV non-small cell lung cancer. *J. Immunother. Cancer* 7 (1): 38.

330 Tateshita, N., Miura, N., Tanaka, H. et al. (2019). Development of a lipoplex-type mRNA carrier composed of an ionizable lipid with a vitamin E scaffold and the KALA peptide for use as an ex vivo dendritic cell-based cancer vaccine. *J. Control. Release* 310: 36–46.

331 Zhang, R., Tang, L., Tian, Y. et al. (2020). DP7-C-modified liposomes enhance immune responses and the antitumor effect of a neoantigen-based mRNA vaccine. *J. Control. Release* 328: 210–221.

332 Firdessa-Fite, R. and Creusot, R.J. (2020). Nanoparticles versus dendritic cells as vehicles to deliver mRNA encoding multiple epitopes for immunotherapy. *Mol. Ther. Methods Clin. Dev.* 16: 50–62.

333 Ciré, S., Da Rocha, S., Ferrand, M. et al. (2016). In vivo gene delivery to lymph node stromal cells leads to transgene-specific CD8+ T cell anergy in mice. *Mol. Ther.* 24 (11): 1965–1973.

334 Schlee, M. and Hartmann, G. (2016). Discriminating self from non-self in nucleic acid sensing. *Nat. Rev. Immunol.* 16 (9): 566–580.

335 Heil, F., Hemmi, H., Hochrein, H. et al. (2004). Species-specific recognition of single-stranded RNA via toll-like receptor 7 and 8. *Science* 303 (5663): 1526–1529.

336 Karikó, K., Buckstein, M., Ni, H., and Weissman, D. (2005). Suppression of RNA recognition by Toll-like receptors: the impact of nucleoside modification and the evolutionary origin of RNA. *Immunity* 23 (2): 165–175.

337 Diebold, S.S., Massacrier, C., Akira, S. et al. (2006). Nucleic acid agonists for Toll-like receptor 7 are defined by the presence of uridine ribonucleotides. *Eur. J. Immunol.* 36 (12): 3256–3267.

338 Züst, R., Cervantes-Barragan, L., Habjan, M. et al. (2011). Ribose 2'-O-methylation provides a molecular signature for the distinction of self and non-self mRNA dependent on the RNA sensor Mda5. *Nat. Immunol.* 12 (2): 137–143.

339 Li, C., Lee, A., Grigoryan, L. et al. (2022). Mechanisms of innate and adaptive immunity to the Pfizer-BioNTech BNT162b2 vaccine. *Nat. Immunol.* 23 (4): 543–555.

340 Torrence, P.F., Johnston, M.I., Epstein, D.A. et al. (1981). Activation of human and mouse 2-5A synthetases and mouse protein P1 kinase by nucleic acids. Structure-activity relationships and correlations with inhibition of protein synthesis and interferon induction. *FEBS Lett.* 130 (2): 291–296.

341 Anderson, B.R., Muramatsu, H., Jha, B.K. et al. (2011). Nucleoside modifications in RNA limit activation of 2'-5'-oligoadenylate synthetase and increase resistance to cleavage by RNase L. *Nucleic Acids Res.* 39 (21): 9329–9338.

342 Bevilacqua, P.C., George, C.X., Samuel, C.E., and Cech, T.R. (1998). Binding of the protein kinase PKR to RNAs with secondary structure defects: role of the tandem A-G mismatch and noncontiguous helixes. *Biochemistry* 37 (18): 6303–6316.

343 Nallagatla, S.R. and Bevilacqua, P.C. (2008). Nucleoside modifications modulate activation of the protein kinase PKR in an RNA structure-specific manner. *RNA* 14 (6): 1201–1213.

344 Anderson, B.R., Muramatsu, H., Nallagatla, S.R. et al. (2010). Incorporation of pseudouridine into mRNA enhances translation by diminishing PKR activation. *Nucleic Acids Res.* 38 (17): 5884–5892.

345 Sabbah, A., Chang, T.H., Harnack, R. et al. (2009). Activation of innate immune antiviral responses by Nod2. *Nat. Immunol.* 10 (10): 1073–1080.

346 Minnaert, A.K., Vanluchene, H., Verbeke, R. et al. (2021). Strategies for controlling the innate immune activity of conventional and self-amplifying mRNA therapeutics: getting the message across. *Adv. Drug Deliv. Rev.* 176: 113900.

347 Hornung, V., Ellegast, J., Kim, S. et al. (2006). 5'-Triphosphate RNA is the ligand for RIG-I. *Science* 314 (5801): 994–997.

348 Nallagatla, S.R., Hwang, J., Toroney, R. et al. (2007). 5'-triphosphate-dependent activation of PKR by RNAs with short stem-loops. *Science* 318 (5855): 1455–1458.

349 Pardi, N., Muramatsu, H., Weissman, D., and Karikó, K. (2013). In vitro transcription of long RNA containing modified nucleosides. *Methods Mol. Biol.* 969: 29–42.

350 Pulit-Penaloza, J.A., Scherbik, S.V., and Brinton, M.A. (2012). Activation of Oas1a gene expression by type I IFN requires both STAT1 and STAT2 while only STAT2 is required for Oas1b activation. *Virology* 425 (2): 71–81.

351 De Beuckelaer, A., Pollard, C., Van Lint, S. et al. (2016). Type I interferons interfere with the capacity of mRNA lipoplex vaccines to elicit cytolytic T cell responses. *Mol. Ther.* 24 (11): 2012–2020.

352 Pollard, C., Rejman, J., De Haes, W. et al. (2013). Type I IFN counteracts the induction of antigen-specific immune responses by lipid-based delivery of mRNA vaccines. *Mol. Ther.* 21 (1): 251–259.

353 Goyvaerts, C., De Vlaeminck, Y., Escors, D. et al. (2017). Antigen-presenting cell-targeted lentiviral vectors do not support the development of productive T-cell effector responses: implications for in vivo targeted vaccine delivery. *Gene Ther.* 24 (6): 370–375.

354 Trinchieri, G. (2010). Type I interferon: friend or foe? *J. Exp. Med.* 207 (10): 2053–2063.

355 Pascual, V., Chaussabel, D., and Banchereau, J. (2010). A genomic approach to human autoimmune diseases. *Annu. Rev. Immunol.* 28: 535–571.

356 Shivalingam, A., Taemaitree, L., El-Sagheer, A.H., and Brown, T. (2020). Squaramides and ureas: a flexible approach to polymerase-compatible nucleic acid assembly. *Angew. Chem. Int. Ed. Eng.* 59 (28): 11416–11422.

357 Diebold, S.S., Kaisho, T., Hemmi, H. et al. (2004). Innate antiviral responses by means of TLR7-mediated recognition of single-stranded RNA. *Science* 303 (5663): 1529–1531.

358 Yang, J.X., Tseng, J.C., Yu, G.Y. et al. (2022). Recent advances in the development of Toll-like receptor agonist-based vaccine adjuvants for infectious diseases. *Pharmaceutics* 14 (2): 423.

359 Ponsaerts, P., Van den Bosch, G., Cools, N. et al. (2002). Messenger RNA electroporation of human monocytes, followed by rapid in vitro differentiation, leads to highly stimulatory antigen-loaded mature dendritic cells. *J. Immunol.* 169 (4): 1669–1675.

360 Michiels, A., Breckpot, K., Corthals, J. et al. (2006). Induction of antigen-specific CD8+ cytotoxic T cells by dendritic cells co-electroporated with a dsRNA analogue and tumor antigen mRNA. *Gene Ther.* 13 (13): 1027–1036.

361 Uchida, S., Yoshinaga, N., Yanagihara, K. et al. (2018). Designing immunostimulatory double stranded messenger RNA with maintained translational activity through hybridization with poly A sequences for effective vaccination. *Biomaterials* 150: 162–170.

362 Miao, L., Li, L., Huang, Y. et al. (2019). Delivery of mRNA vaccines with heterocyclic lipids increases anti-tumor efficacy by STING-mediated immune cell activation. *Nat. Biotechnol.* 37 (10): 1174–1185.

363 Miao, L., Lin, J., Huang, Y. et al. (2020). Synergistic lipid compositions for albumin receptor mediated delivery of mRNA to the liver. *Nat. Commun.* 11 (1): 2424.

364 Tse, S.W., McKinney, K., Walker, W. et al. (2021). mRNA-encoded, constitutively active STING. *Mol. Ther.* 29 (7): 2227–2238.

365 Naka, T., Iwahashi, M., Nakamura, M. et al. (2008). Tumor vaccine therapy against recrudescent tumor using dendritic cells simultaneously transfected with tumor RNA and granulocyte macrophage colony-stimulating factor RNA. *Cancer Sci.* 99 (2): 407–413.

366 Bontkes, H.J., Kramer, D., Ruizendaal, J.J. et al. (2007 Feb). Dendritic cells transfected with interleukin-12 and tumor-associated antigen messenger RNA induce high avidity cytotoxic T cells. *Gene Ther.* 14 (4): 366–375.

367 Van den Bergh, J., Willemen, Y., Lion, E. et al. (2015). Transpresentation of interleukin-15 by IL-15/IL-15Rα mRNA-engineered human dendritic cells boosts antitumoral natural killer cell activity. *Oncotarget* 6 (42): 44123–44133.

368 Van der Jeught, K., Joe, P.T., Bialkowski, L. et al. (2014). Intratumoral administration of mRNA encoding a fusokine consisting of IFN-β and the ectodomain of the TGF-β receptor II potentiates antitumor immunity. *Oncotarget* 5 (20): 10100–10113.

369 Hewitt, S.L., Bai, A., Bailey, D. et al. (2019). Durable anticancer immunity from intratumoral administration of IL-23, IL-36γ, and OX40L mRNAs. *Sci. Transl. Med.* 11 (477).

370 Tuyaerts, S., Van Meirvenne, S., Bonehill, A. et al. (2007). Expression of human GITRL on myeloid dendritic cells enhances their immunostimulatory function but does not abrogate the suppressive effect of CD4+CD25+ regulatory T cells. *J. Leukoc. Biol.* 82 (1): 93–105.

371 Dannull, J., Nair, S., Su, Z. et al. (2005). Enhancing the immunostimulatory function of dendritic cells by transfection with mRNA encoding OX40 ligand. *Blood* 105 (8): 3206–3213.

372 Grünebach, F., Kayser, K., Weck, M.M. et al. (2005). Cotransfection of dendritic cells with RNA coding for HER-2/neu and 4-1BBL increases the induction of tumor antigen specific cytotoxic T lymphocytes. *Cancer Gene Ther.* 12 (9): 749–756.

373 Tcherepanova, I.Y., Adams, M.D., Feng, X. et al. (2008). Ectopic expression of a truncated CD40L protein from synthetic post-transcriptionally capped RNA in dendritic cells induces high levels of IL-12 secretion. *BMC Mol. Biol.* 9: 90.

374 Daneshmandi, S., Pourfathollah, A.A., and Forouzandeh-Moghaddam, M. (2018). Enhanced CD40 and ICOSL expression on dendritic cells surface improve anti-tumor immune responses; effectiveness of mRNA/chitosan nanoparticles. *Immunopharmacol. Immunotoxicol.* 40 (5): 375–386.

375 Levin, N., Pato, A., Cafri, G. et al. (2017). Spontaneous activation of antigen-presenting cells by genes encoding truncated homo-oligomerizing derivatives of CD40. *J. Immunother.* 40 (2): 39–50.

376 Amin, A., Dudek, A.Z., Logan, T.F. et al. (2015). Survival with AGS-003, an autologous dendritic cell-based immunotherapy, in combination with sunitinib in unfavorable risk patients with advanced renal cell carcinoma (RCC): phase 2 study results. *J. Immunother. Cancer* 3: 14.

377 Figlin, R.A., Tannir, N.M., Uzzo, R.G. et al. (2020). Results of the ADAPT phase 3 study of rocapuldencel-T in combination with sunitinib as first-line therapy in patients with metastatic renal cell carcinoma. *Clin. Cancer Res.* 26 (10): 2327–2336.

378 Verbeke, R., Lentacker, I., Breckpot, K. et al. (2019). Broadening the message: a nanovaccine co-loaded with messenger RNA and α-GalCer induces antitumor immunity through conventional and natural killer T cells. *ACS Nano* 13 (2): 1655–1669.

379 Morse, M.A., Coleman, R.E., Akabani, G. et al. (1999). Migration of human dendritic cells after injection in patients with metastatic malignancies. *Cancer Res.* 59 (1): 56–58.

380 Batich, K.A., Mitchell, D.A., Healy, P. et al. (2020). Once, twice, three times a finding: reproducibility of dendritic cell vaccine trials targeting cytomegalovirus in glioblastoma. *Clin. Cancer Res.* 26 (20): 5297–5303.

381 Van Driessche, A., Van de Velde, A.L., Nijs, G. et al. (2009). Clinical-grade manufacturing of autologous mature mRNA-electroporated dendritic cells and safety testing in acute myeloid leukemia patients in a phase I dose-escalation clinical trial. *Cytotherapy* 11 (5): 653–668.

382 Anguille, S., Van de Velde, A.L., Smits, E.L. et al. (2017). Dendritic cell vaccination as postremission treatment to prevent or delay relapse in acute myeloid leukemia. *Blood* 130 (15): 1713–1721.

383 Khoury, H.J., Collins, R.H., Blum, W. et al. (2017). Immune responses and long-term disease recurrence status after telomerase-based dendritic cell immunotherapy in patients with acute myeloid leukemia. *Cancer* 123 (16): 3061–3072.

384 Subklewe, M., Geiger, C., Lichtenegger, F.S. et al. (2014). New generation dendritic cell vaccine for immunotherapy of acute myeloid leukemia. *Cancer Immunol. Immunother.* 63 (10): 1093–1103.

385 Van Acker, H.H., Versteven, M., Lichtenegger, F.S. et al. (2019). Dendritic cell-based immunotherapy of acute myeloid leukemia. *J. Clin. Med.* 8 (5): 579.

386 Van Nuffel, A.M., Benteyn, D., Wilgenhof, S. et al. (2012). Intravenous and intradermal TriMix-dendritic cell therapy results in a broad T-cell response and durable tumor response in a chemorefractory stage IV-M1c melanoma patient. *Cancer Immunol. Immunother.* 61 (7): 1033–1043.

387 Rittig, S.M., Haentschel, M., Weimer, K.J. et al. (2016). Long-term survival correlates with immunological responses in renal cell carcinoma patients treated with mRNA-based immunotherapy. *Oncoimmunology* 5 (5): e1108511.

388 Fernandez, A.M.A., Baurain, J.-F., Vulsteke, C. et al. (2019). A phase I study (E011-MEL) of a TriMix-based mRNA immunotherapy (ECI-006) in resected melanoma patients: analysis of safety and immunogenicity. *J. Clin. Oncol.* 37 (15_suppl): 2641.

389 Rausch, S., Schwentner, C., Stenzl, A., and Bedke, J. (2014). mRNA vaccine CV9103 and CV9104 for the treatment of prostate cancer. *Hum. Vaccin. Immunother.* 10 (11): 3146–3152.

390 Hong, H.S., Koch, S.D., Scheel, B. et al. (2016). Distinct transcriptional changes in non-small cell lung cancer patients associated with multi-antigenic RNActive® CV9201 immunotherapy. *Oncoimmunology* 5 (12): e1249560.

391 Sabari, J., Ramirez, K.A., Schwarzenberger, P. et al. (2019). Abstract B209: phase 1/2 study of mRNA vaccine therapy + durvalumab (durva) ± tremelimumab (treme) in patients with metastatic non-small cell lung cancer (NSCLC). *Cancer Immunol. Res.* 7 (2_Supplement): B209.

392 Barbier, A.J., Jiang, A.Y., Zhang, P. et al. (2022). The clinical progress of mRNA vaccines and immunotherapies. *Nat. Biotechnol.* 40 (6): 840–854.

393 BioNTech. (2021). Next generation immunotherapy. https://investors.biontech.de/static-files/057be080-d0bd-4b58-8ad5-6acb6f7e421b (accessed 1 August 2022).

394 Bauman, J., Burris, H., Clarke, J. et al. (2020). 798 safety, tolerability, and immunogenicity of mRNA-4157 in combination with pembrolizumab in subjects with unresectable solid tumors (KEYNOTE-603): an update. *J. ImmunoTher. Cancer* 8 (Suppl 3): A477.

395 Lindsay, K.E., Bhosle, S.M., Zurla, C. et al. (2019). Visualization of early events in mRNA vaccine delivery in non-human primates via PET-CT and near-infrared imaging. *Nat. Biomed. Eng.* 3 (5): 371–380.

396 Saxena, M., van der Burg, S.H., Melief, C.J.M., and Bhardwaj, N. (2021). Therapeutic cancer vaccines. *Nat. Rev. Cancer* 21 (6): 360–378.

397 Lin, M.J., Svensson-Arvelund, J., Lubitz, G.S. et al. (2022). Cancer vaccines: the next immunotherapy frontier. *Nat. Cancer* 3 (8): 911–926.

Index